MOSBY'S®
MASSAGE THERAPY EXAM REVIEW

MOSBY'S®
MASSAGE THERAPY EXAM REVIEW

EDITION 5

Sandy Fritz
MS, NCTMB
Founder, Owner, Director,
and Head Instructor
Health Enrichment Center
School of Therapeutic
Massage and Bodywork
Lapeer, Michigan

Luke Fritz
BA, LMT
Instructor
Health Enrichment Center
School of Therapeutic
Massage and Bodywork
Lapeer, Michigan

ELSEVIER

Elsevier
3251 Riverport Lane
St. Louis, Missouri 63043

MOSBY'S® MASSAGE THERAPY EXAM REVIEW, FIFTH EDITION

ISBN: 978-0-323-88150-0

Notice

Practitioners and researchers must always rely on their own experience and knowledge in evaluating and using any information, methods, compounds or experiments described herein. Because of rapid advances in the medical sciences, in particular, independent verification of diagnoses and drug dosages should be made. To the fullest extent of the law, no responsibility is assumed by Elsevier, authors, editors or contributors for any injury and/or damage to persons or property as a matter of products liability, negligence or otherwise, or from any use or operation of any methods, products, instructions, or ideas contained in the material herein.

Previous editions copyrighted 2002, 2006, 2010, and 2015.

Content Strategist: Melissa Rawe
Senior Content Development Specialist: Shilpa Kumar
Publishing Services Manager: Deepthi Unni
Project Manager: Nayagi Anandan
Design Direction: Amy Buxton

Printed in India

Last digit is the print number: 9 8 7 6 5 4 3 2 1

Working together to grow libraries in developing countries

www.elsevier.com • www.bookaid.org

To those beginning their massage therapy practice journey

This 5th edition of *Mosby's Massage Therapy Exam Review* reflects an increased level of knowledge required for the professional practice of therapeutic massage as measured in various licensing and certification processes. The text is much more than a collection of facts and various practice questions. It is a complete review system to help you organize your study process and integrate your various learning endeavors, such as formal education, continuing education, and self-education. This book is a platform for you to become your own best teacher and is based on solid learning theory. Learning is more than memorization—it is comprehension and utilization. To truly learn something, you need repeated exposure to the content. Your brain, however, will not effectively focus on data that it has previously processed unless the same information is presented multiple times in different ways. This review guide does just that.

The body of knowledge for therapeutic massage is vast. Learning it requires repetition, but memorization does not support comprehension. Memorization is important, especially for learning terminology, but it is only one aspect of the process. The words need to be understood in context to support comprehension. The learning system developed for this revision of *Mosby's Massage Therapy Exam Review* begins with facts and evolves to comprehension through creative repetition.

Remember that no therapeutic massage review guide on the market has the exact questions that will appear on the exams. You may answer all questions correctly on the practice tests offered in review guides, but this will not guarantee that you will pass the real exams. On the other hand, true comprehension allows you to use your knowledge and reasoning skills to solve each problem presented by exam questions. Excellence, future success, and leadership in the therapeutic massage profession rely on thorough comprehension of massage therapy knowledge and service. This review guide presents a learning process to guide you down the path of therapeutic massage service by preparing you to successfully pass the exams that will allow you to provide massage therapy safely and effectively.

BACKGROUND

When the first edition of this text was published years ago, massage was on the verge of professional recognition. Now massage therapists are held to professional standards measured by licensing in most states. Licensing is not an option. You have to pass licensing exams. The main licensing exam for massage therapy is provided by the Federation of State Massage Boards and called the MBLEx. To prove excellence, you seek board certification through exams. Certification is voluntary and provided by the National Certification Board for Therapeutic Massage and Bodywork. Regardless, you need to know how to pass a multiple-choice exam. The current exams contain questions that require comprehension. Exams in the past contained more definition-type questions, and you could simply memorize definitions and pass the test. Not anymore. You have to really think and problem-solve to pass exams today. Today you need a review system that results in an understanding of massage therapy professional practice. This is the goal of the fifth edition of this unique review system.

WHO WILL BENEFIT FROM THIS BOOK?

Anyone who will be taking a licensing or certification exam will benefit from this text and support materials. It can be used as a core text in a review course and the end of formal education or by an individual studying to take an exam.

CONCEPTUAL APPROACH

A review guide is not the same as a textbook. A textbook takes you from knowing nothing to knowing something. A review guide assumes you know the material and are seeking support for comprehension and practice for taking exams. *Mosby's Massage Therapy Exam Review* is developed using information on how people learn. Repetition is key, but it needs to be done in a novel way so your brain continues to be intrigued by it. The challenge was to develop a review process that creatively and uniquely presented the facts and concepts required to successfully pass massage therapy licensing and certification exams that kept your brain involved. The result is this five-step review system based on novel but repetitive exposure to the information you need.

There are five parts of the review process. In Chapter 1, you will learn about the licensing and certification process. In Chapter 2, you will learn how to study for multiple-choice exams.

PART 1: How to Study for Credentialing Exams
Chapter 1: Overview of the Licensing Process
Chapter 2: How to Study for Exams

Part 2 provides an illustrated and activity-based, factual review based on terminology. There are many figures, which support the saying "one picture is worth a million words." This content is expanded on the Evolve website that supports this textbook.

PART 2: Reviewing for Factual Recall
Chapter 3: Review of Massage Application
Chapter 4: Anatomy and Physiology

Part 3 provides a narrative that uses the terminology from Part 2 and weaves a language-based presentation of the combined sciences and theory and practice of massage. This aspect of the review system is essential and missing in most review guides. Test questions are word-based. You need to be able to decode the concepts presented in the words. This part of the review process moves you from memorization to understanding. Your brain can only stay focused on the written page for about 15 minutes. To support comprehension, there is a "Take Five" feature in Part 3 that breaks up the narratives into chunks to support your brain's need for variety. There is also a list of defined key terms found in the narratives to support comprehension. There are various animations to support the narrative content on the accompanying EVOLVE website that accompanies this textbook for another unique review process.

PART 3: Reviewing for Comprehension
Chapter 5: Massage Theory and Application
Chapter 6: Functional Anatomy and Physiology

Part 4 presents the content again, but this time it is in the form of a concise word review and practice questions. Content areas are related clusters of information, such as ethics or the skeletal systems. All questions in each section are specific to each content area. Two categories of practice questions are presented. The factual recall category reinforces the terminology recall, and the concept identification lets you master the relationship of information.

PART 4: Review Questions by Content Area
Chapter 7: Therapeutic Massage
Chapter 8: Anatomy, Physiology, and Pathology

Finally, Part 5 consists of Practice Exams. Question types and content are interspersed as they are in the actual licensing or certification exam. There is a feature on the Evolve website that randomizes hundreds of test questions, providing an ongoing supply of different exams for you can study.

The appendixes are an added benefit.

Appendix A: Indications and Contraindications to Massage: Many of the questions on exams are about safe practice. Therefore, this content is especially important.

Appendix B: Glossary: A comprehensive list of massage therapy terms.

Appendix C: Answer Keys to the labeling exercises and practice questions, including rationales. The book is fully indexed as well.

As you can see, a well-organized review system is provided, and the comprehensive and sequential presentation leads you all the way through your review and exam preparation.

NEW TO THIS EDITION

- Expanded information on the Federation of State Massage Boards MBLEx exam
- Evolve website that takes the review guide into another dimension
- Reorganized presentation supporting a five-step review system
- Expanded full-color art
- Comprehensive narratives on the theory and practice of massage and relevant anatomy and physiology
- Comprehensive content outline used for exam development

LEARNING AIDS

- Art and labeling exercises
- Step-by-step review guidelines
- Review tips
- Quick content review
- Rationales for test question answers
- More than 2000 practice questions

NOTE TO THE STUDENT

Your future depends on your ability to pass the exam. I am an educator, and my students have to pass the exams as well. This review guide gives you the support you need to succeed. If you follow the recommendations and progress through all five parts of the review process, your chances for passing will dramatically increase. Study smart!

ACKNOWLEDGMENTS

Writing a book is a team effort. Many thanks to my team:

Luke Fritz (my son) for being my co-author
Laura Cochran (my daughter) for proofreading
The Elsevier groups:
Melissa Rawe, Content Strategist
Shilpa Kumar, Senior Content Development Specialist
Nayagi Anandan, Project Manager
Joshua Caparas, Marketing Manager
Amy Buxton, Designer

All the sales representatives who work hard to sell this book

CONTENTS

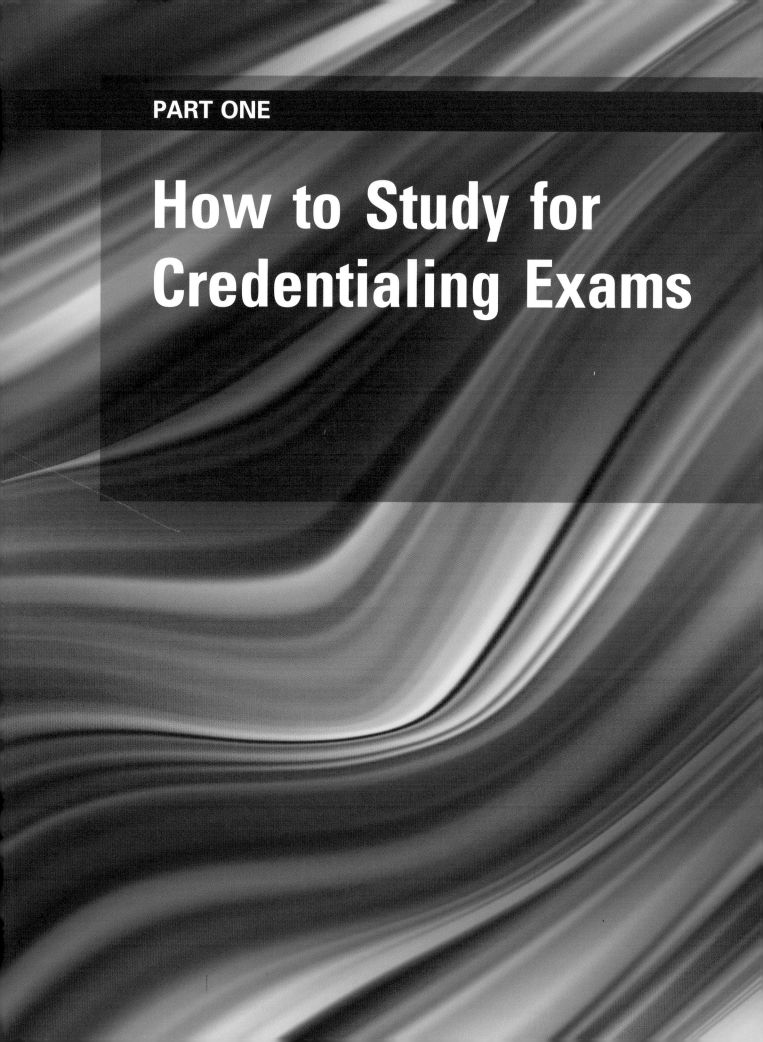

PART ONE

How to Study for Credentialing Exams

CHAPTER 1

Overview of the Licensing Process

Licensure is a governmental regulation. You must be licensed to practice massage legally if your state requires it. Governmental licensing is often confused with professional credentialing (certification) because the meanings of the terms are frequently interchanged. Licensing is mandatory, whereas certification involves self-regulation of a profession and is voluntary. The massage profession is experiencing changes in terminology and types of credentialing, and it is common for people to be confused. You must be licensed first. Then you may want to become board certified by meeting the eligibility requirements of the National Certification Board for Therapeutic Massage and Bodywork.

This review guide covers three types of examinations:
1. *School-based exams* are developed and administered by the school that is issuing the certificate or diploma. These exams are administered by course instructors. Examples include exams for individual classes such as business ethics and anatomy, as well as midterm and final exams.
2. *Licensing exams* are required by law for practice and are developed to protect the public.
3. *Board Certification exams* are administered by professional organizations such as the National Certification Board for Therapeutic Massage and Bodywork. This exam is developed to assess knowledge and skills beyond entry level. Licensure is required to be eligible for the Board Certification Exam. Occasionally Board Certification is used in a state or local regulation.

LICENSURE

Obtaining a license in order to practice a profession is mandatory by law in many areas of the United States. Licensure is the process by which the government (federal, state, province, or local governmental agency) grants an individual permission to practice an occupation or profession that is subject to regulation under the government's authority. Licensing is used to protect the public from harm. Entry-level education is required for licensure and is considered the most basic, fundamental level of professional practice needed to safely work. Each state indicates the amount and content of entry-level education for massage therapy in the licensing legislation. Most states use the Massage & Bodywork Licensing Examination (MBLEx) through the Federation of State Massage Therapy Boards (FSMTB).

The Federation of State Massage Therapy Boards

FSMTB is an organization of states that currently have massage licensing and aids those states that are seeking to license massage therapy. The mission of the FSMTB is to support its member boards in their work to ensure that the practice of massage therapy is provided to the public in a safe and effective manner.

The FSMTB has developed a model licensing exam called the MBLEx (Massage & Bodywork Licensing Exam) for states. Note that the exam is called "MASSAGE & BODYWORK." What does this mean? Are massage and bodywork the same or different? This remains an area of confusion. The intent of the MBLEx is to be inclusive enough in the exam content so that the exam can be used to evaluate entry-level practice readiness for all the name variations. For example, Swedish/classical massage is only one form of massage. There are many other systems and most often multiple systems are combined in what is considered therapeutic massage. The term *bodywork* can embrace forms of manual therapy similar to massage but uniquely named. Neuromuscular therapy is an example, and there are many more, which adds to confusion when attempting to credential with licensing. The term *western massage therapy* is broader in scope. There are also cultural forms of massage/bodywork, some of which fall under the term *Eastern bodywork*. The methods are often, but not exclusively, derived from Traditional Chinese Medicine, Ayurvedic Medicine, Shiatsu, etc. The MBLEx exam has been developed to ensure the provision of a valid and reliable licensing examination by which entry-level competence can be determined. The terms *massage practitioner*, *bodywork*, and *bodywork practitioner* are all used in the exam.

The distribution of topics tested is as follows:
- Anatomy and Physiology (11%)
- Kinesiology (12%)
- Pathology, Contraindications, Areas of Caution, Special Population (14%)
- Benefits and Physiological Effects of Techniques that Manipulate Soft Tissue (15%)
- Client Assessment, Reassessment, Treatment Planning (17%)
- Ethics, Boundaries, Laws and Regulations (16%)
- Guidelines for Professional Practice (15%)

Contact information is as follows:

Federation of State Massage Therapy Boards.

7300 College Boulevard, Suite 650, Overland Park, KS 66210.

913.681.0380 | info@fsmtb.org.

Massage & Bodywork Licensing Examination (MBLEx)

866.962.3926 | mblex@fsmtb.org

Website: https://www.fsmtb.org/

National Certification Board for Therapeutic Massage and Bodywork

Board Certification is voluntary and a goal after licensing. The Board Certification exam contains 140 questions. You will have 140 minutes to complete the exam. Content found on this exam embraces application of technique and is assessment based—simulating real-life scenarios you will most likely encounter as a certified massage therapist.

The Board Certification Exam is Built Around the Below Main Categories

- Assessment (25%)
- Applied Science, including Anatomy, Physiology, Kinesiology, Pathology/Injury, and Pharmacology (25%)
- Massage Modalities, Techniques, and Manual Forces (20%)
- Professional Communication (15%)
- Professionalism and Ethics (10%)
- Laws and Business Practices (5%)

https://www.ncbtmb.org/

WHICH EXAM WILL I TAKE?

Almost always the MBLEx exam is used for licensing. A couple of states still use a state developed exam. It is the responsibility of those who are seeking to take an exam for licensing to contact their governmental regulatory body or local jurisdiction to identify which exam is administered for licensing. This review guide is developed to help you prepare to take any massage therapy exam intended for licensure.

WHAT INFORMATION IS COVERED ON THE LICENSING EXAMS?

Information presented in most educational curricula and information required to function as a massage professional can be divided into four areas. These categories form the basis of most licensing and certifying examinations. The four categories are as follows: Human anatomy, physiology, and kinesiology; Clinical pathology and indications and contraindications for massage application; Massage therapy and bodywork theory and application; and Professional ethics, business practices, and wellness practices.

1. *Human anatomy, physiology, and kinesiology—about 25% of the exam content.* General education in human anatomy, physiology, and kinesiology prepares the student to understand the benefits of massage and lays the foundation for the following category.
2. *Clinical pathology and indications and contraindications for massage application—about 25% of exam content.* The focus is to provide sufficient information to support safe and beneficial professional practice.

Human anatomy, physiology, kinesiology, clinical pathology, and indications and contraindications for massage application make up half of the content on most exams. Usually, these two categories are studied most effectively in an integrated format. For example, discussion of the anatomy of the nervous system leads to an understanding of the functions of the nervous system. Subsequently, an understanding of how massage affects the nervous system leads to identification of indications for massage, pathologic conditions of the nervous system, and contraindications for massage, including cautions for use of massage when pathologic conditions are present.

Many find the sciences a difficult area of study. The terminology can seem overwhelming—almost like learning another language. If we can agree that the various methods and theoretic bases of the many different bodywork modalities provide diversity, then the sciences provide commonality. The human body remains consistent in structure and function; therefore, it makes sense that an understanding of the sciences is essential and relevant to massage.

3. *Massage therapy and bodywork theory and application—about 30% of exam content.* This area covers methods used to obtain a database about the client and proper method usage. Competency in this area indicates that the massage professional is able to apply methods appropriately in a safe and beneficial way. A commonality exists in most bodywork approaches. In addition to therapeutic massage, general knowledge about complementary bodywork modalities, such as hydrotherapy, Asian theory, and applications such as acupressure, trigger points, and connective tissue massage, often is measured.
4. *Professional ethics, business practices, and wellness practices—about 20% of exam content.* The professional standards, ethics, and business practices area of the exam relates to the professional abilities needed to conduct oneself in a manner that reflects decision-making to support ethical standards and sound business practices.

This review guide is based on information obtained by consolidating multiple curriculum guidelines and exam content outlines. The review material and questions for study and practice should prepare the reader to address these areas on massage licensing and certification exams. The Federation of State Massage Boards and National Certification Board for Therapeutic Massage and Bodywork websites provide specifics on the exam content outline (Box 1.1).

REALITY CHECK

✓ It is important to not become overwhelmed as you review the content outline. Although it is comprehensive, it is not insurmountable. You should have received this information while completing your schooling and reading your textbooks. Importantly you must be your own best teacher. The general scope of entry-level massage therapy education as defined by the Entry Level Analysis Project (elapmassage.org) is 625 contact hours. It is difficult for the following content to be covered during actual class time. It is necessary to follow a self-teaching plan using textbooks typically published by academic publishers that are current and have been peer reviewed. Commonly revision cycles for academic textbooks are 5–6 years. It is prudent to identify and use textbooks other than the ones used during formal entry-level education. The content outline is provided for informational purposes and to help you understand the big picture of content that questions are written about on exams. The actual study portion is presented later in the book. As you read the content outline, if you find an area that is unfamiliar to you, mark it, so you can look it up in your textbooks. *Remember, this review book is not intended to replace textbooks. You need your books to help you study.*

BOX 1.1   Exam Content Outline

The content outline that follows is compiled from multiple sources including, but not limited to, the following: The Entry Level Analysis Project (ELAP) The Core: Entry-Level Analysis Project Report (Final Report) and The Core: Entry-Level Massage Education Blueprint (the Blueprint)
- National Certification Board for Therapeutic Massage and

Bodywork Job Task Analysis and Content Outline for board certification
- Federation of State Massage Therapy Boards (FSMTB) and the Massage & Bodywork Licensing Examination (MBLEx)
- Commission on Massage Therapy Training and Accreditation (COMTA)
- The Massage Therapy Body of Knowledge document (MTBOK)

COMPREHENSIVE LICENSING EXAMINATION CONTENT OUTLINE

The Sciences: Human Anatomy, Physiology, and Kinesiology

- Define anatomy and physiology.
- Define the structural organization of the body.
- Define life processes.
- List the most important functions of each body system.
- Define homeostasis; describe its generalized process and relationship to health and disease.
- Define directional terms, anatomic planes, and body cavities.
- Review the benefits and physiologic effects of massage techniques by which soft tissue is manipulated.

Anatomy and Physiology
This area of content explores the structure and function of the human body and their relationship to applications of massage therapy and bodywork.

The Chemical Level

- Define atoms, molecules, and elements.
- Identify different types of chemical bonds.
- Explain basic chemical reactions and the concept of pH.
- List organic and inorganic compounds.
- Explain the action of enzymes.
- Explain the structure of DNA and RNA.

The Cellular Level

- List the components of a generalized cell.
- Describe the function of each component.
- Describe the movement of substances into and out of cells.
- Describe the phases of cell division.

The Tissue Level

- Define the four tissue types.
- List and describe the general features of the two types of epithelial tissues and their locations.
- List and describe the general features of connective tissues and their locations.
- List and describe the types of membranes.
- Describe tissue repair.
- Discuss system structure and function.

Circulatory/Cardiovascular

- Describe the relationship of blood to interstitial fluid and lymph.
- Describe the general functions of blood.
- Describe the components of blood.
- Describe the formation of blood cells.

- Describe the functions of erythrocytes, leukocytes, and thrombocytes.
- Describe the flow of blood through the heart and the systemic and pulmonary circulation.
- Describe the structure of the heart and pericardium.
- Describe coronary circulation.
- Describe the cardiac conduction system and the regulation of heart rate.
- Describe the cardiac cycle and electrocardiogram.
- Describe normal heart sounds during a cardiac cycle.
- Explain the benefits for the heart of regular exercise.
- Describe the structure and function of arteries, veins, and capillaries.
- Describe the concepts of blood distribution and capillary exchange.
- Explain blood pressure regulation.
- Define shock.
- Describe pulmonary and systemic circulation.
- Describe the location and direction of flow of all major blood vessels.
- Describe hepatic portal circulation.

Digestive System

- List the structures of the digestive system.
- List the accessory structures of the digestive system.
- Describe the six basic processes of the digestive system.
- Describe the peritoneum and its associated structures.
- Describe the structure and function of the accessory glands of digestion.

Endocrine System

- List major groups of hormones.
- Briefly describe the mechanisms of hormonal actions.
- Describe the location, histology, and major functions of the endocrine glands, as well as their hormones and target tissues.
- Describe how the body responds to stress.

Integumentary System

- List and describe the layers of the skin.
- Describe the accessory structures of the skin.
- List and describe the functions of the skin.
- Explain how epidermal and deep wounds heal.
- Describe the effects of aging on the integumentary system.

Immune System

- List the components of the immune system.
- Describe the mechanisms of nonspecific resistance to disease.
- Describe the mechanisms of specific resistance to disease.
- Describe the relationship of the immune system to other body systems.

Lymphatic System

- Describe the function and formation of lymph.
- Identify and describe lymphatic vessels.
- Name the major lymphatic vessels and describe the direction of lymph flow.
- Describe the structure and function of bone marrow, the thymus gland, lymph nodes, spleen, and lymphatic nodules.

Muscular System

- List the types and functions of muscle tissue and fascia.
- Describe skeletal, cardiac, and smooth muscle.
- Describe the anatomy of skeletal muscle fibers.
- List and describe the different types of muscle actions.
- List and explain the structure of a neuromuscular junction and a motor unit.
- Describe the sliding filament theory.
- Describe aerobic and anaerobic activity and its relationship to muscle physiology.
- Explain the types of skeletal muscle fibers.

Kinesiology and Biomechanics

- Define, compare, and locate the three types of levers.
- Describe skeletal muscle as a functional unit or organ (skeletal muscle fibers, connective tissue, nervous and vascular tissue).
- Describe and palpate the proximal (origin) and distal (insertion) attachments, their actions, and innervations associated with the following muscle groups:
  1. Muscles of mastication
  2. Muscles of the neck
  3. Muscles of the vertebral column
  4. Muscles of the abdominal wall and breathing
  5. Muscles of the pectoral girdle
  6. Muscles that move the humerus
  7. Muscles that move the forearm, wrist, hand, and fingers
  8. Muscles of the pelvic girdle
  9. Muscles that move the femur
  10. Muscles that move the leg, ankle, foot, and toes
- Identify the general location of the following muscle groups:
  1. Muscles of facial expression
  2. Extrinsic eye muscles
  3. Anterior neck muscles, including hyoids
  4. Pelvic floor muscles

Nervous System

- Describe the function of neuroglia.
- Describe the structure and function of a generalized neuron.
- Describe the difference between gray matter and white matter.
- Describe and identify the main parts of the brain and its protective coverings.

- Identify and describe the structure and functions of the brainstem, cerebellum, diencephalon, and cerebrum.
- List the 12 cranial nerves and describe their functions.
- Discuss the general components of somatic sensory and motor pathways.
- Describe the organization of the sensory and motor cortex.
- Describe the phase of action potential and signal transmission at synapses.
- List the connective tissue coverings and branches of the spinal nerve.
- Describe the major branches of the cervical, brachial, lumbar, and sacral plexuses.
- Identify the assessment importance of dermatomes.
- Describe the damage and repair processes of peripheral neurons.
- Describe the classes and functions of neurotransmitters.
- Describe the spinal cord and its protective coverings.
- Identify sensory and motor tracts in the spinal cord.
- Describe a reflex arc.
- Describe four types of somatic reflexes—the stretch reflex, the Golgi tendon reflex, the withdrawal reflex, and the crossed extensor reflex.
- Classify sensory receptors according to location and type of stimulus.
- Identify and describe somatic sensations.
- Describe the processes of learning and memory, wakefulness and sleep.
- Compare and contrast the somatic nervous system with the autonomic nervous system (ANS).
- Describe the anatomic components of the sympathetic and parasympathetic divisions.
- Describe the enteric division of the ANS.
- Identify the neurotransmitters and receptors of the ANS.
- Describe, compare, and contrast the responses of most organs of the body to sympathetic and parasympathetic activity.

Reproductive System

- Describe the anatomy of the structures and functions of the male reproductive system.
- Describe the anatomy of the structures of the female reproductive system.
- Describe the normal function of pregnancy, including trimesters and labor and delivery.
- List the common sexually transmitted diseases.

Respiratory System

- Describe the functions and structures of the respiratory system.
- Describe external and internal respiration.
- Describe how respiratory rates are controlled.

Skeletal System (Bones and Joints)

- Discuss the functions of bone.
- Identify the parts of a long bone.

- Describe compact and spongy bone.
- Describe types of fractures and explain the process of fracture repair.
- Describe the effects of exercise and aging on bone tissue (mass).
- Classify bones into one of six categories.
- Define bone surface markings.
- Differentiate bones of the axial skeleton from bones of the appendicular skeleton.
- Identify, describe, locate, and palpate the bones of the skull (differentiate cranial from facial bones).
- Identify, describe, and locate the sutures, paranasal sinuses, bones of the orbit, and nasal septum.
- Identify, locate, and palpate the bones of the vertebral column, and discuss normal and abnormal curvatures of the spine.
- Identify and locate the bones of the thorax.
- List, identify, and locate the bony landmarks of the axial skeleton.
- Identify and describe the bones of the appendicular skeleton.
- List, identify, and locate the bony landmarks of the appendicular skeleton.
- List the bones that make up the shoulder and pelvic girdles.
- Differentiate bones of the appendicular skeleton from bones of the axial skeleton.
- Define the types of bone surface markings/bony landmarks.
- Classify joints into structural and functional categories.
- Define and demonstrate joint movements in the frontal, sagittal, and transverse (horizontal) planes.
- Describe the structure of a typical diarthrotic/synovial joint and list the six types.
- List and define movements of the diarthrotic/synovial joints.
- List and describe the structures of the shoulder, hip, elbow, knee, wrist, and ankle, and explain the typical range of motion of each.
- List and explain the factors that affect range of motion of joints.
- Differentiate between a sprain and a strain.

Special Senses

- Describe the sense of smell.
- Describe the sense of taste.
- Describe the anatomy of the eye and its accessory structures.
- Describe the physiology of vision.
- Describe the anatomy of the ear.
- Describe the physiology of hearing.
- Describe the physiology of vestibular function/equilibrium.

Urinary System

- List, identify, and describe the structures of the urinary system.

- List, identify, and describe the functions of the urinary system.

CLINICAL PATHOLOGY, INDICATIONS, AND CONTRAINDICATIONS FOR MASSAGE APPLICATION

- Define and explain the concept of standard precautions.
- Identify current recommendations from the Centers for Disease Control and Prevention (CDC).
- Describe appropriate personal hygiene for practicing massage.
- Identify potential sources for transmission of pathogenic organisms.
- Explain the prevention of transmission of pathogens in a therapeutic environment.
- Identify the physiologic and psychological effects of stress.
- Identify various stress reduction techniques and explain their benefits.
- Demonstrate knowledge of the physiologic and emotional effects of touch, massage, and bodywork techniques.
- Identify and define "endangerment area," and list vulnerable structures in each "endangerment area."
- Define and list indications and contraindications for the application of manual massage and bodywork procedures.
- Identify anatomic, physiologic, and structural conditions in which the localized or general application of massage procedures would be indicated or contraindicated.
- Identify signs and symptoms that determine indication or contraindication for a specific massage procedure.
- Identify physical and psychological conditions in which specific massage procedures are contraindicated or must be altered.
- Identify physical conditions that would require a referral and evaluation by another healthcare provider before massage procedures are applied.
- Describe physical changes that require emergency measures.
- Identify specific indications, contraindications, and precautions, and describe the signs and symptoms of common conditions/diseases.
- Identify and describe the signs and symptoms of a contagious disease.
- Identify the signs and symptoms of local and systemic contraindicated conditions/diseases in various populations.
- Identify common pathologies, and determine indications, contraindications, and cautions.
- Describe massage application adaptations based on areas of caution, special populations, and pathologic conditions.

PHARMACOLOGY

- Identify and explain the following classes of medications, and describe procedural contraindications that apply when a client is taking a particular class of medication:

- Analgesics, including opioids and nonopioids
- Antibacterials, including antibiotics
- Anticonvulsants
- Anticoagulants
- Antidepressants
- Antifungals
- Antiinflammatory agents, including corticosteroids and nonsteroidal antiinflammatory drugs (NSAIDs)
- Antineoplastics
- Antiparasitics
- Antipsychotics
- Antivirals
- Anxiolytic (antianxiety) agents
- Blood glucose regulators, including insulin and other diabetes medications
- Cardiovascular agents, including beta-blockers and ACE inhibitors
- Central nervous system agents, including amphetamines
- Gastrointestinal agents, including H2 blockers and proton pump inhibitors
- Hormonal agents
- Immunological agents, including vaccines
- Respiratory tract agents, including antihistamines and bronchodilators
- Sedatives and hypnotics
- Skeletal muscle relaxants
- Therapeutic nutrients, minerals, and electrolytes
- Describe synergistic and antagonistic interactions of massage with medication.

PHYSIOLOGIC EFFECTS OF TECHNIQUES BY WHICH SOFT TISSUE IS MANIPULATED

- Compare and contrast similarities and differences between common massage/bodywork styles (i.e., Swedish/classical massage, chair massage, deep tissue, lymphatic drainage, medical/clinical massage, myofascial/connective tissue massage, neuromuscular therapy, trigger point therapy, orthopedic massage), special populations (infants, pregnant women, geriatric clients, athletes), joint movement and stretching, and cultural-based massage systems (Amma, ayurveda, shiatsu, Thai, Tui Na).
- Use healthcare and massage and bodywork terminology in communicating assessment findings and therapeutic results.
- Identify the physiologic effects of soft tissue manipulation.
- Identify the psychological aspects and benefits of touch.
- List and describe the benefits of soft tissue manipulation for specific client populations.
- List, explain, and define three major categories of physiologic effects: mechanical, chemical, and neurological.
- Identify specific physiologic effects of massage on the following systems: integumentary, skeletal, muscular, nervous, cardiovascular, lymphatic, digestive, respiratory, and urinary.

- Describe how to vary each of the following in primary massage procedures:
  1. Location of application
  2. Level of pressure
  3. Speed
  4. Direction
  5. Drag
  6. Duration
  7. Mechanical stresses (tension, compression, shear, torsion, bend) and their results
- Perform and describe massage application using the following:
  1. Hands
  2. Fists
  3. Fingers
  4. Forearms
  5. Elbows
  6. Feet
- Identify and compare the following primary massage procedures:
  1. Gliding/effleurage
  2. Kneading/pétrissage—superficial kneading, skin rolling
  3. Compression (ischemic compression)—pressure touch
  4. Friction/cross-fiber friction
  5. Percussion/tapotement
  6. Oscillation—vibration, rocking, shaking
  7. Joint movement——active, active assisted, active resisted, passive
  8. Stretching/elongation—passive and active lengthening of muscle and connective tissue to achieve normal resting length
- Explain the physiologic effects and therapeutic applications for each of the primary massage procedures and variations.
- Describe how to vary the choice and application of techniques as appropriate to the client's needs, including those of special populations.
- Identify and practice appropriate methods of sanitation and personal hygiene in the performance of massage.
- Explain how to use standard precautions at all times.
- Describe the importance and function of draping.
- Describe various draping materials and styles of draping.
- Describe how to sanitize and launder draping materials.
- Describe and demonstrate four positions for massage application, including draping, appropriate bolstering, and use of supports.
- Describe the use and care of a massage table, mat, and chair.
- Describe the use of appropriate equipment and supplies [such as adjustable massage tables, bolsters, pillows, gloves, linens, and lubricants (oil, lotion, gel)].

Ergonomics/Body Mechanics

- Demonstrate efficient application of massage methods in an ergonomically and biomechanically effective manner.

- Identify strategies that can be used to prevent self-injury and enhance the efficacy of techniques through the use of proper body mechanics, centering, focusing, and breathing.
- Identify and practice the biomechanical skills necessary for the safe and effective performance of massage.
- Identify and discuss how the lifestyle habits that influence physical fitness can affect performance and stress management for the massage therapist.

Adjunct Methods

Application of Adjunct Methods
Adjunct approaches are methods that are not massage but combine well with massage such as aromatherapy, craniosacral, thermotherapy, hot stone, scraping, suction, percussion, hydrotherapy, polarity, Reiki, reflexology, therapeutic touch, structural integration, and others.

- Describe the basis of and safe practice for adjunct approaches.
- Identify various hot and cold hydrotherapy techniques (such as cold or hot packs [Hydrocollator therapy packs], immersion baths, paraffin, and ice massage).
- Identify the physiologic principles and mechanisms involved in the effects of hydrotherapy.
- Identify and explain the physiologic effects of heat and cold application on the human body.
- Identify and explain the physiologic effects of hot and cold water application on the human body.
- Demonstrate the appropriate use of heat and cold for specific therapeutic applications.
- Define, identify, and explain contraindications for the application of hydrotherapy.
- Define, demonstrate, and contrast hot and cold applications.
- Describe the safe application of hot and cold stones or other thermo applications.

Essential Oils
- List contraindications for essential oil use during massage.
- Describe the mode of action of essential oils.
- List common essential oils used during massage application that generally are considered safe.
- Describe the importance of a carrier oil for the proper dilution of essential oils.

Tools: Scraping, Suction, Percussion
- List contraindications for tool use during massage.
- Describe the mode of action of scraping, suction, and percussion tools.
- Maintain sanitation of tools.
- Use tools safely.

CLIENT ASSESSMENT, REASSESSMENT, AND TREATMENT PLANNING ASSESSMENT

- Demonstrate knowledge of the wellness model and describe its relationship to massage therapy and bodywork practice.
- Identify the scope of practice of massage therapy and bodywork in relation to the components of a wellness model.
- Identify and demonstrate an appropriate assessment of anatomic structures through the use of palpatory skills.
- Perform assessment and data collection to determine contraindications and formulate a client-centered treatment strategy.
- Perform assessment and data collection:
  1. History taking
  2. Observation
  3. Palpation
  4. Range of motion (ROM)
  5. Functional testing
  6. Pain assessment
  7. Formulation and documentation of a treatment strategy based on assessment findings, client goals, and client response to previous applications of massage and bodywork techniques (treatment/care plan)
- Integrate methods of clinical reasoning with methods of assessment, treatment outcome measures, and quantified and qualified client goals in the formulation of an organized, safe, and effective application of massage therapy/bodywork in a treatment plan.
- Use effective clinical reasoning skills in the development and execution of the treatment/care plan based on knowledge of anatomy and physiology and on interpretation and prioritization of all assessment and client information (i.e., client history, assessment, referral letters, and other sources of information).
- Formulate and provide informed consent information to client for signature before beginning the treatment protocol.
- Modify the treatment plan and therapeutic approach used during a client session based on client response to the application of massage and bodywork techniques.
- Manage time within a client session.
- Explain the importance of the client's level of comfort and feedback to the massage therapist.
- Demonstrate an understanding of integrated and interdisciplinary care and wellness information.
- Write clear, concise, and accurate client notes based on treatment sessions.
- Discuss and explain client history, including medication, nutritional supplements and herbs, medical reports, and referrals from other professionals, family members, and friends.
- Demonstrate and create client charts (documentation) consisting of subjective data, objective data, assessment, and plan (SOAP); charting; and other forms of medical records.
- Make appropriate referrals to other professionals for interdisciplinary care, knowing when, to whom, and how to refer, and provide release and authorization forms.
- Demonstrate the ability to provide client intake and assessment that includes the following:
  1. Verbal intake
  2. Health history form
  3. Written data collection
  4. Visual assessment (general, postural)
  5. Palpation assessment
  6. Muscle assessment
  7. ROM assessment
  8. Gait assessment
- Demonstrate the ability to use clinical reasoning to do the following:
  1. Guide client treatment goal setting
  2. Rule out contraindications
  3. Adapt massage applications related to assessment data
  4. Evaluate response to previous treatment
  5. Determine appropriate massage approach
  6. Justify massage treatment approach as beneficial and not harmful
- Discuss therapeutic education (e.g., self-massage techniques).
- Discuss ergonomics.
- Educate clients and others about massage therapy, including results and benefits, goals and expectations, and the concepts of informed consent and right of refusal.

PROFESSIONALISM, ETHICS, BOUNDARIES, LEGAL ISSUES, AND BUSINESS PRACTICES

Professionalism

- Professional behavior
- Ethical behavior
- Professional boundaries
- Code of ethics violations
- The therapeutic relationship
- Dual relationships
- Sexual misconduct
- Massage/bodywork-related laws and regulations
- Scope of practice
- Professional communication
- Confidentiality
- Cultural competency
- Implicit bias
- Health Insurance Portability and Accountability Act (HIPAA)
- Americans with Disabilities Act (ADA)
- Recognizing human trafficking

Communication

- Oral/verbal
- Written
- Nonverbal

Business Practices and Policies

- Describe insurance, including the concepts of liability and reimbursement.
- Comply with the Health Insurance Portability and Accountability Act of 1996 (HIPAA) when required.
- Explain how to implement marketing strategies and create a business plan.
- Explain pertinent business laws, including local, state, federal, and discrimination laws.
- Demonstrate a working understanding of basic accounting principles, including bookkeeping, tax preparation, and financial planning.
- Define the right to refuse service.
- Use effective strategies for dealing with difficult clients.
- Identify and demonstrate appropriate professional referrals.
- Identify confidentiality principles related to massage therapy/bodywork practice, including HIPAA compliance and responsibilities and liability for maintaining client confidentiality and privileged communication.
- Identify professional/clinical conditions that might present ethical dilemmas.
- Describe professional behavior that would be considered unethical by most "reasonable" professionals.
- Identify and explain the ethical, emotional/legal implications for establishing a personal/intimate/sexual relationship with a client.
- Identify and explain the role and purpose of a code of ethics.
- Identify the role and purpose of standards of practice specific to massage therapy and bodywork.
- Develop successful and ethical therapeutic relationships with clients.
- Use effective communication in the therapist–client relationship.
- Define and demonstrate active listening, rapport, empathy, and feedback.
- Identify strategies that can be used to deal effectively with emotional and behavioral client responses to massage therapy and bodywork treatment.
- Describe the principles of conflict resolution and apply conflict resolution skills effectively in the therapist–client relationship.
- Establish and maintain safe and respectful boundaries with clients.
- Self-assess needs, behaviors, beliefs, attitudes, and knowledge relevant to the practice of massage therapy and bodywork.

- Identify how personal and cultural values, attitudes, and ethics influence professional values, attitudes, and ethics.
- Develop a strategy for a successful practice, business, or employment situation.
- Identify and describe basic business practices relevant to the practice of massage therapy/bodywork.
- Identify common business practices and structures as applied to proprietorships, partnerships, and corporations in massage therapy and bodywork practice.
- Formulate a business plan or outline an employment strategy that includes short- and long-term goals related to the student's professional goals.
- Explain the basic aspects of legal agreements, contracts, employment agreements, and professional insurance.
- Create and maintain client, financial, and tax records, and identify legal requirements for retaining records.
- Demonstrate knowledge of federal, state, and local regulations as they pertain to massage therapy and bodywork practice.
- Demonstrate knowledge of Americans with Disabilities Act (ADA) requirements and explain the implications of this law for the practice of massage therapy and bodywork.
- Apply knowledge in writing a clear and concise résumé.
- Identify strategies that can be used to develop and maintain a client base and promote client retention.
- Discuss the process that should be followed to identify the scope of practice of allied professions.
- Identify strategies for effective management of the work environment.
- Identify and design effective methods for time management, client scheduling, and maintenance of the work environment.
- Discuss the process of establishing and maintaining professional boundaries and relationships with peers, in the workplace, and with other professionals.
- Identify strategies that can be used to participate in professional activities and pursue personal professional development.
- Discuss the influences of history on the massage therapy and bodywork profession and describe the role of professional associations in the lives of massage therapists and bodyworkers today.
- Identify strategies that can be used to attain new knowledge and support continuing education.
- Discuss the importance of ongoing education and skill development for the professional.
- Describe methods of identifying advanced training programs that will enhance performance, knowledge, and skills in relation to student goals.
- Demonstrate the ability to read and evaluate research and technical information found in articles in health-related journals and identify biases and limitations in the findings or premises on which the articles are based.
- Explain the value of research to the profession.
- Locate research literature on therapeutic massage.
- Critically read and evaluate a published article in the field of massage therapy and bodywork.

- Access appropriate information resources as needed, and apply the information gathered to the practice of massage therapy and bodywork.

Professional Boundaries

- Identify the qualities and characteristics of professional boundaries.
- Discuss and demonstrate the use of draping during treatment as a professional boundary issue.
- Identify cultural differences related to boundary issues.
- Define and discuss transference and countertransference.
- Define and discuss the differences between a personal and a professional relationship.

Technology and Equipment

- Massage equipment (i.e., tables)
- Computers and other office equipment
- Software programs for business practices
- Social media
- Websites
- Smart phone tablet applications

REALITY CHECK

WOW, no wonder it takes a comprehensive education to be a massage therapist!

CHAPTER 2

How to Study for Exams

First, review terminology. This is the goal of Part 2 of this guide. Second, review how the content relates to massage. Next, consider each question in Parts 3 and 4 of this review guide as a mini lesson. It really is not that important to get the right answer to the study question, but rather the question should be used as a platform for study and for seeing how the content could be incorporated into the question. None of the review guides for massage exams includes the questions and answers for the licensing exams, so remember that this review guide is targeted toward promoting an understanding of the questioning process, not just getting the right answer.

It is important that you use your textbooks as reference material; many resources are provided in the review book as well as the Evolve site. With each question, first, make sure you know the definition of all the words in the question and of the possible answers. A glossary is provided in the review guide to help you. After you are sure you know the meaning of all the words, next ask yourself, "What is this question trying to teach me?" Once you understand the mini lesson provided by the questions, look at each answer. At the beginning of the review guide, an explanation is provided of how wrong answers are developed. It is important to understand why only one possible answer is correct and the other possible answers are wrong. Rationales as to why the correct answer is correct and the other answers are incorrect are included for you to read, but sometimes the issue purely involves vocabulary. You have to know what words mean to understand the meaning of a question.

Questions in the review guide can be easy or complex, challenging you to think. Also, attempt to write your own questions, using the patterns in the book. You will find that being able to create a really good wrong answer that appears to be right is one of the best study strategies. Finally, complete the practice exams provided in Part 5 and on the Evolve site.

How Do I Use Textbooks and Reference Materials as I Study?

When you study, you should have your textbooks, a medical dictionary, and an anatomy atlas of some sort available for reference. The study tool resources in this guide and on the accompanying website called Evolve—the comprehensive glossary, the various charts and review content, the labeling exercises, review games, animations, and more—do not replace the textbooks but enhance and guide the study process.

It is best to study for exams by using accepted textbooks and references. Most exams use standardized textbooks to reference the questions written for the exam. It may not be prudent to invest in study guides that "rewrite" textbook content because the content has not actually been referenced to the exams. The purpose of a study helper such as this book is to guide you through the review process and assist you in using problem-solving methods to identify correct answers. You can use other textbooks as resources as well by looking up relevant content in the index.

The questions in Part 4 of this review guide are presented by content area. Consistent with this format, specific content areas, such as the nervous system, assessment, ethics, and massage methods, are grouped together. Readers can determine which content they are proficient in, and in which areas they need more study.

The questions for each content area are presented in two blocks. First, factual recall questions are listed with answers and other material. Concept identification and clinical reasoning questions with answers and rationales follow. In an actual exam, the content will be mixed up.

How to Use This Review Guide

Repetition and memorization are necessary. Understanding and comprehension are even more important. This guide is based on a four-step review process that provides the necessary content repetition but presents the information in different ways to solidify comprehension.

Step 1: Review terminology, using various labeling activities and vocabulary review with illustrations. There are many activities on the Evolve website to expand this step in the review process (Part 2, Chapters 3 and 4).

Step 2: Understand the relationships regarding all information. A functional narrative is provided that links and integrates theory and practice. You should read this part numerous times to support comprehension, but do not attempt to memorize this material. It is supported with animations and demonstration clips on the accompanying Evolve website (Part 3, Chapters 5 and 6).

Step 3: Study the questions by content area. Use this part to assess proficiency in related areas such as muscles or ethics (Part 4, Chapters 7 and 8).

Step 4: Practice exams are provided in the book to help you become confident with the multiple-choice test format (Part 5). In addition, the Evolve site provides additional practice tests.

Accompanying this review guide is the Evolve website. Two testing features are available on the Evolve site to aid you in studying for massage exams. The Tutorial mode serves questions by category and provides instant feedback. The Test mode randomly serves questions and allows for review after a test has been completed.

The practice exams on the Evolve site model the tests Chapter 1 used for licensure or certificaton. A scoring matrix is provided after each one that presents the overall number of attempted and correct questions, as well as the percentage of correct answers. The matrix also provides information regarding the four categories emphasized in the review guide (human anatomy, physiology, and kinesiology; clinical pathology and indications and contraindications for massage application; massage therapy and bodywork; and professional standards, ethics, and business practice) and indicating the student's score in each category. Following the categories is a breakdown of chapters from the review guide, which again shows the number of attempted questions, the number of correct answers, and the percentage of correct answers.

Once you have reviewed the scoring matrix, you can use the Tutorial mode to emphasize areas of weakness that have been identified. For example, if you scored a low percentage in clinical pathology and indications and contraindications for massage application, you can bring up the tutorial and practice questions in that category only.

RECOMMENDATIONS FOR STUDYING FOR AN EXAM

Important Note: One of the biggest errors readers make when using study guides such as this text is concentrating on making sure they know the answers to the questions in the study guide. *Do not do this!* The questions in this study guide,

as well as any of the others available, will not appear on the various exams. Those who administer the exams routinely screen and remove questions from the exams that appear in various review guides. Memorizing the answers to questions in any of the review guides is a waste of precious study time.

This study guide has been developed to help you understand how to take an exam. The various questions represent examples of how content may appear in an exam question. Each sample question and all of the possible answers contain the terminology you will encounter. Each sample question also teaches you how to address the various question styles found on exams.

This study tool does not replace your textbooks; instead it assists you in preparing to take exams successfully and in becoming comfortable with how textbook content may appear on exams. This study guide is designed to enhance your understanding of textbook material.

Rationales for the sample/example questions in this text are structured to teach you how to find the right answer to a test question, not restate information found in the textbooks. If a rationale tells you to look up definitions for the terminology used in the questions and possible answers, then that is the best method to use for study. In concept identification questions, some sort of relationship among the terms is evident, and this can be explained in the rationale. In clinical reasoning and synthesis questions, the rationales describe the clinical reasoning process used to solve the problem posed by the question. The computer-based exams on the Evolve website do not include rationales. The computer-based tests are designed to mimic the actual exam experience.

The following suggestions should enhance your study process:

1. Relax. Anxiety interferes with the ability to integrate and recall information.
2. Have fun and be silly. Things learned with laughter are retained more easily.
3. Study in short bursts. 15–30 minutes at a time is ideal.
4. Generally, read a chapter and then study one small part at a time.
5. Know the meaning of any words displayed in key terms lists, in bold or italic print, and in the glossary, and be able to use these words correctly in a sentence.
6. Study the illustrations and diagrams, paying attention to the labeling.
7. Manipulate the information. The interactive exercises and workbook segments of *Mosby's Fundamentals of Therapeutic Massage* and *Mosby's Essential Sciences for Therapeutic Massage* are designed to integrate information from short-term to long-term memory. Other textbooks often offer similar features.
8. Seek to understand the information; do not anticipate what questions will be on the test. Paraphrase and reword the information presented in the text.
9. Use the questions in this study guide as a study strategy. Write your own exam questions. The most difficult task is developing plausible wrong answers. (Use the questions in this book as examples.)

10. Work together in study groups by sharing information, by taking turns "teaching," or by taking each other's tests from the questions you wrote.

THE TEST

Exams are generally based on a massage therapy curriculum that contains:

- 125 hours of instruction on the body's systems and anatomy, physiology, and kinesiology
- 200 hours of in-class, supervised hands-on instruction in massage and bodywork assessment, theory, and application instruction
- 40 hours of pathology
- 10 hours of business and ethics instruction (a minimum of 6 hours in ethics)
- 125 hours of instruction in an area or related field that theoretically completes your massage program of study

The MBLEx (Federation of State Massage Boards Licensing exam is developed as an entry-level licensing exam and based on survey of the massage therapy population. The survey is called a job task analysis (JTA). Questions are developed by subject matter experts based on the JTA. The MBLEx exam is computer delivered by a professional testing company at their testing sites around the country. Each time a person takes a test the computer creates it using a large test bank. Because of this process the same test is never given twice.

Subject area categories	Percentage of test	Number of questions
Kinesiology, musculoskeletal anatomy, and physiology	20%–25%	25–32
Systemic anatomy and physiology	14%–18%	21–22
Pathology, contraindications, cautionary sites, adaptive process	10%–15%	18–25
Professional standards, business practices, ethics, boundaries	15%–20%	18–25
Massage therapy theory including benefits and physiologic effects, evaluation including client assessment, reassessment and treatment planning, method types and techniques	30%–35%	30–35

THE TEST-TAKING ENVIRONMENT: WHERE, HOW, AND HOW LONG

The exams are typically provided by Pearson VUE, the world's largest network of test centers in 175 countries across the world. The computer technology is easy to use with tutorials provided. The professional testing companies that administer the tests have multiple testing sites in every US state. As a general rule, you will have approximately 2 hours to complete the multiple-choice examination on the computer. While you are studying for the exams and using the practice exams provided, practice completing one question per minute (60 seconds).

Testing companies comply with the Americans with Disabilities Act of 1990 (ADA) and will accommodate requests from qualified candidates with a diagnosed disability for accommodations if the request is reasonable and properly documented and does not fundamentally alter the examination or jeopardize exam security.

Taking the Test

Taking exams is a secure process that ensures fairness and accuracy. Typically, you are required to bring *two* forms of identification (ID) to the test site—the primary form of identification must include a photograph and a signature and must not be expired. The secondary form of identification should include a photograph. Types of identification you can bring to the test center include the following:

- Primary (photo, signature, not expired)
- Secondary (signature, not expired)
- Government-issued driver's license
- Passport
- Military ID
- State/country ID
- Alien registration card (green card or permanent resident visa)
- Other government-issued ID
- U.S. Social Security card
- School ID
- Employee or hospital ID/work badge
- Bank ATM card
- Credit card

Scoring and Passing Exams

Many people expect an examination to have a passing score of 70%–75%. This is based on experience with examinations in schools that set the passing score.

This approach is not acceptable for the licensing examination process because it is not an appropriate measure of minimum competency. For licensing examinations, all test takers must have an equal chance of passing the examination. In addition, the examination is intended to assess who has sufficient knowledge and skills in professional practice to meet the competency standard represented by the passing score.

The criterion-referenced method results in a passing score that provides every candidate the same opportunity to pass the examination. In addition, the passing score reflects the difficulty of the individual items on the examination.

The standard setting for exams requires a group process. The group comprises qualified practitioners who represent various aspects of the practice, geographic areas, and levels of expertise. To ensure that the description of the profession represents the job tasks of practitioners who are entering the profession, input from entry-level practitioners is always included. Criterion-referenced scoring provides safeguards for both the candidate and the consumer. The total scaled score that you achieve on the examination determines whether you pass or fail. Not all questions have the same score value. The more complex the question, the more the question is worth www.bscp.org.

RECOMMENDATIONS FOR TAKING AN EXAM

1. Get plenty of rest before the exam.
2. Arrive at the exam location in plenty of time to settle into the environment.
3. Ask questions about the exam process, so that you clearly understand how to take the exam.
4. Acknowledge that you are nervous, relax as much as you can, and put the exam in perspective. The worst that can happen is that you might not pass. This only means more study and another attempt. The best that can happen is that you pass.
5. Practice time management and plan on completing a question in no more than one minute (60 seconds per question).
6. Begin at the beginning of the exam and answer the questions sequentially. YOU CANNOT GO BACK. YOU MUST ANSWER THE QUESTION. Carefully follow the specific instructions presented to you by the exam provider.
7. Acknowledge that there will be questions that you simply do not know how to answer. Do not dwell on them. Answer them the best you can and go on to the next question.
8. YOU MUST ANSWER ALL 100 QUESTIONS. Guess and follow your intuition. Do not leave a space blank. A blank is wrong whereas a guess is possibly correct.
9. Do not second-guess your answers. Change an answer only if you are sure that you were wrong with your first choice. SUBMIT the exam as instructed, and breathe.
10. You will know if you have passed before you leave the test site. You will only know if you passed or failed. If the exam was failed a report on content areas — not individual questions — will be provided. Commit to taking it again.

The exam is over. There is no sense in worrying. Remember perspective and go do something fun.

TYPES OF MULTIPLE-CHOICE QUESTIONS

The three basic types of multiple-choice questions are factual recall and comprehension, application and concept identification, and clinical reasoning and synthesis. Examples of these three types of questions follow. The questions can either be data based or scenario (story) based. Multiple choice questions can have 3 or 4 potential answer choices (i.e. a,b,c or a,b,c,d.). Research indicates that the a,b,c format is considered just as valid as the a,b,c,d format. This review guide will use both.

Factual Recall and Comprehension Questions

The information necessary to answer this type of question can be found in various textbooks and reference material in the form of descriptions and definitions. These questions are considered to represent difficulty level 1 (least difficult). Memorization of data is a method that you can use to prepare to answer these types of questions. An example of this type of question follows:
1. Which bone makes up the heel of the foot?
   a. Navicular
   b. Calcaneus
   c. Hamate
   d. Xiphoid
The answer is **b.**

Application and Concept Identification Questions

This type of question requires that you understand the language posed in the question while being able to identify simple concepts and patterns. Application and concept identification questions also address concrete information that can be described by terms, definitions, rules, laws, and other forms of structure. This information can be found directly in the textbooks and reference material. The difficulty level is considered to be 2 (moderately difficult). An example of this type of question follows:
1. Which method would be most appropriate if the client desires to remain passive during the massage?
   a. Pulsed muscle energy
   b. Contract/relax/antagonist/contract
   c. Approximation
   d. Postisometric relaxation
The answer is **c.**

Clinical Reasoning and Synthesis Questions

Clinical reasoning and synthesis questions require you to analyze information and make appropriate professional decisions. These are the most difficult questions and are considered to represent difficulty level 3. Identifying the answer to this type of question requires that you use the information in a contextual manner. The case study scenario is a common approach to this question design. The answer is not found directly in any textbook or reference material; only the language and concepts are provided in the books. An example of this type of question follows:

1. A client is taking an aspirin for osteoarthritis of the left knee. What precautions are needed for massage intervention?
   a. Avoid any type of massage to the affected knee.
   b. Avoid the use of compression above and below the knee.
   c. Reduce pressure level around the knee only.
   d. Monitor pressure levels of the massage to reduce potential bruising.

The answer is **d.**

Sample Questions

On an exam, the content areas are addressed specifically within a test question, or the content is mixed to develop combination test questions. For example, a pure science (data) question may appear as follows: "The largest of the fontanels in the infant skull is _____." An example of a question that combines content follows: "During infant massage, it is important to apply only light pressure to the anterior fontanel for which of the following reasons?"

Analyzing the Question

A good multiple-choice question presents sufficient facts so that you can identify the correct answer. Analyzing the possible answers requires a comprehensive factual base provided during your education and found in the textbooks, so that you can eliminate wrong answers and identify and justify the correct answer. You need to analyze the possible answers, based on the facts presented in the question and your knowledge, to determine the *best correct answer*. When a test question is written, all four of the possible answers should be plausible so that you cannot just guess to identify the correct answer. Incorrect answers should be clearly wrong, but only if you understand the content and not so evidently wrong that you do not have to understand the content to identify a wrong answer. As you can imagine, it is very difficult for test writers to develop a good multiple-choice question.

In this review guide, each sample question found in Parts 4 and 5 embodies a chunk of essential knowledge and represents how that knowledge can be addressed in a multiple-choice exam. Each of the possible answers also identifies important information. When using these questions to study for an exam, you should identify the information from all of the possible answers—the one correct answer and the incorrect answers—in the textbooks and reference material that you are using to study. The correct answer should stand out clearly, and the reasons why incorrect answers are false should be apparent. Many of the questions are framed in mini case studies (scenario); this is a more relevant format for massage practitioners because it allows them to use the information in the context of the client population they serve.

Questions on the actual exams may not be as complex as the ones found in this text, as the intent is to prepare you for the exam. The more complex questions are used to help you develop strategies necessary to identify the correct answers when you actually take a licensing exam.

Wrong-Answer Strategies

Developing plausible wrong answers is the most difficult aspect of writing multiple-choice questions. Wrong answers need to be clearly wrong but also must seem plausible. Good wrong answers often are developed by conflicting terminology. This is one of the reasons why studying glossaries, key terms in textbooks, and labeled illustrations is important. Often, conflicting terms are used together to make an answer wrong. Here are some examples:

- Compression is a massage application that glides and kneads.

  This is a wrong answer because compression by definition does not glide or knead. Gliding and kneading may have compression qualities. This combination of words would represent wrong usage.

- Sanitation supersedes standard precautions.

  This is a wrong answer because sanitation is an aspect of standard precautions, not something separate.

- The prone positioning of the client limits the ability to bolster and drape for modesty and warmth.

  This is a wrong answer because positioning does not affect modesty and warmth.

Another strategy for developing wrong answers is to use opposite concepts. Consider these examples:

- Flexion straightens the elbow.

  This is incorrect. Flexion bends the elbow.

- Lymphatic drainage follows a proximal-to-distal massage direction.

  This is incorrect because the direction is distal to proximal, even though the strokes begin close to the torso.

- Cross-fiber friction is applied in the direction of the muscle fibers.

  This is incorrect because cross-fiber friction is applied perpendicular to the muscle fibers.

Another strategy is to combine two or more unrelated types of information in the wrong answer. Here are a few examples:

- Geriatric massage treats sport injury.

  These two concepts are not congruent with each other.

- Body mechanics describes various draping protocols.

  These two areas are not interrelated.

- The gastrocnemius attaches on the lateral condyle of the humerus.

  The gastrocnemius muscle is located in the leg and not the arm.

Use these examples to analyze the wrong answers in the sample questions and to determine why an answer is incorrect. This is an effective study strategy. When you are actually taking an exam, it should be easier to determine the incorrect answers.

A COMPREHENSIVE STUDY SYSTEM

Remember that this text is a comprehensive study system. It is based on comprehension, which is based on repetition. For repetition to work, the content must appear over and over but in different formats. This is one of the advantages of this study system. Reviewing the same material over and over does not help. Variation is needed. This is what this system does: repetition, repetition, repetition—but presented in different formats to keep your brain engaged. Parts 2, 3, 4, and 5 are expanded on the Evolve website as an additional strategy for novel repetition.

- Part 1 provides an overview of the credentialing exam process.
- Part 2 begins the actual study process and targets terminology and basic knowledge necessary to understand what a question is asking.
- Part 3 provides a narrative for you to read that uses terminology and information from Part 2 in a context of understanding the concepts of massage theory and practice and the science information that supports safe and beneficial practice.
- Part 4 begins by using test questions as a study platform. This part is organized by content area. A mini review of the content (i.e., skeletal system or massage applications) is provided. Then, fact-based and concept and critical thinking—based questions are given.

- Part 5 consists of practice exams both in the book and on the Evolve website.

As you begin the study process, it is best to follow the process as outlined; however, it is also possible to skip around. You might want to take a practice test first from Part 5 and see how you do. Or you may want to tackle the individual questions by content area in Part 4 and go back and forth between Parts 2 and 3 if you need to look up a word or understand a concept.

Remember, the questions found in this guide (or any of the others on the market) will not appear on any exam. Instead, the questions in this comprehensive review system are written to reflect the types of questions encountered on licensing exams. Each question is a mini lesson. The questions have been thought out carefully, so if you study the question and all the possible answers (correct and incorrect), you should have the factual knowledge and the critical thinking skills needed to approach an exam confidently. Just because you can answer all the questions in this study guide does not mean that you will pass an exam.

Using the review system as outlined provides sequential study through the sciences, theory, business, and ethics of the practice of therapeutic massage and related bodywork modalities. The ability to be confident in one's knowledge and problem-solving skills—not memorization of the questions and answers in this book or any other textbook or study guide—will ensure success. Success to you!

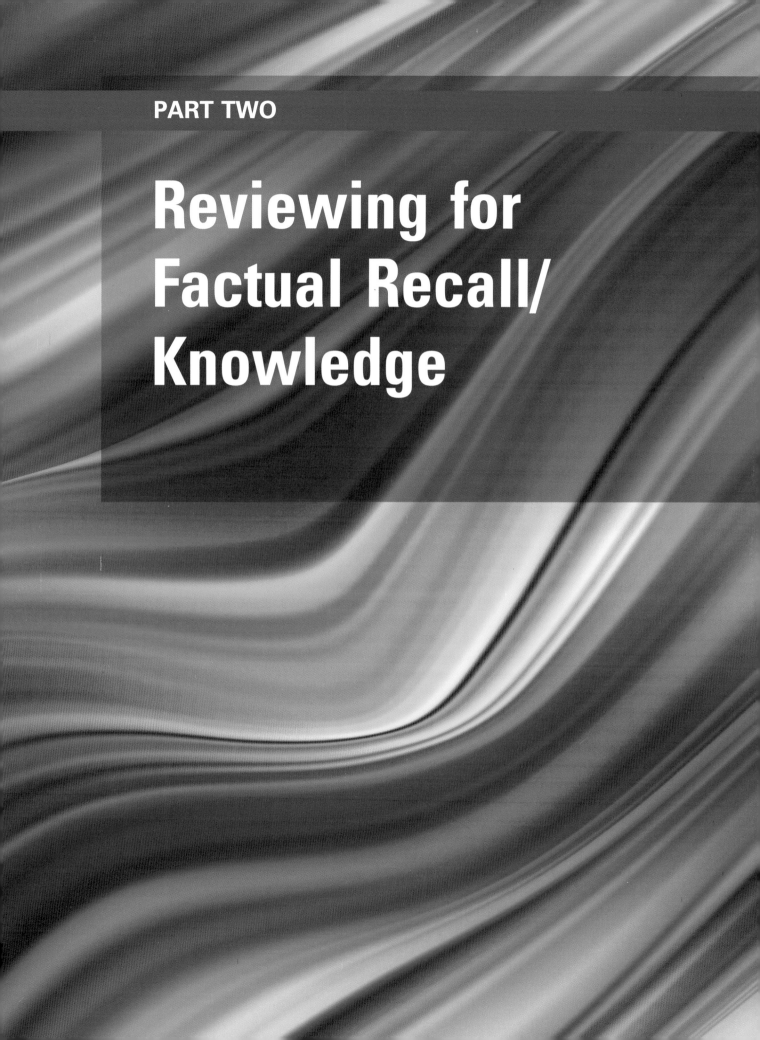

PART TWO

Reviewing for Factual Recall/ Knowledge

CHAPTER 3

Review of Massage Application

The history of massage provides an understanding of the present and guidance for the future. The timeline in Figure 3.1 presents the historical highlights. Use as an overview only, since this content is not specifically tested on MBLEx.

BODY MECHANICS

Physical ergonomics deals with the human body's responses to physical and physiologic loads. Relevant topics include handling manual materials, workstation layout, job demands, and risk factors such as repetition, vibration, force, and awkward/static posture as they relate to musculoskeletal disorders/repetitive strain injury. All work activities should permit the worker to adopt several different but equally healthy and safe postures. If muscular force needs be exerted, this should be done using the largest appropriate muscle groups available. Awkward posture is associated with an increased risk for injury, and the more a joint deviates from the neutral (natural) position, the greater the risk of injury. Every joint in the body has a neutral position at which joint spaces are even and symmetrical. The muscles around a joint in the neutral position are neither short nor long but are at their neutral physiologic resting lengths. Joint stability is provided by joint shape, joint capsule, ligaments, and normal co-contraction of the muscles around the joint. Joint stability is necessary for proper body mechanics.

Four basic concepts of body mechanics are common to all techniques used to apply mechanical force against the body tissues during massage application. These concepts are as follows:

1. Weight transfer
2. Perpendicularity
3. Stacking the joints
4. Keeping the back straight and maintaining core stability

Weight transfer allows the massage practitioner to transfer body weight by shifting the center of gravity forward to achieve a pressure that is comfortable to the client. To transfer weight, the practitioner stands, sits, or kneels with one foot forward and the other foot (or knee) back in an asymmetrical stance. In the standing position, the front leg is in a relaxed knee flexion, with the foot forward enough to be in front of the knee. The back leg is straight, and the hips and shoulders are aligned so that the back is straight. The transfer happens by taking the weight off the front leg and moving it to the heels of the hands or whichever part of the arm is being used to apply pressure. To increase pressure into the client's tissue while performing massage, put body weight into the back foot through ground reaction force. The weight of the body is distributed to the full foot of the weight-bearing leg, not just the toes.

Perpendicularity is an important concept that ensures that the pressure is sinking straight into the tissues. The line from the shoulders to the point of contact (e.g., forearm, heel of the hand) must be 90 degrees to the plane of the contact point on the client's body.

Stacking the joints one on top of another is essential to the concepts of perpendicularity and weight transfer. The practitioner's body must be a straight line from the feet through the shoulder to the forearm, or through the elbow acting as an extension of the shoulder, to the heels of the hands. The ankle, knee, hip of the back leg, and spine are stacked. The shoulder is stacked over the elbow, which in turn is stacked over the wrist. Stacking the joints in this way allows the pressure to go straight into the client's body effortlessly as the center of gravity moves forward.

A straight back and a pressure-bearing leg are other essential components of body mechanics. If the back is not straight, the practitioner often ends up pushing using upper body strength instead of the more effortless transfer of weight. The back from the iliac crest to the scull remains aligned. The trunk forward flexion occurs at the hip joint and should not move beyond 20 degrees. This is a relatively upright position supported by the table set at a higher height. The practitioner's weight should be held on the back leg and on the heel of the foot. At first, this may feel awkward; however, some of the biggest and strongest muscles in the body are those in the legs. If you carry the weight elsewhere, fatigue sets in more

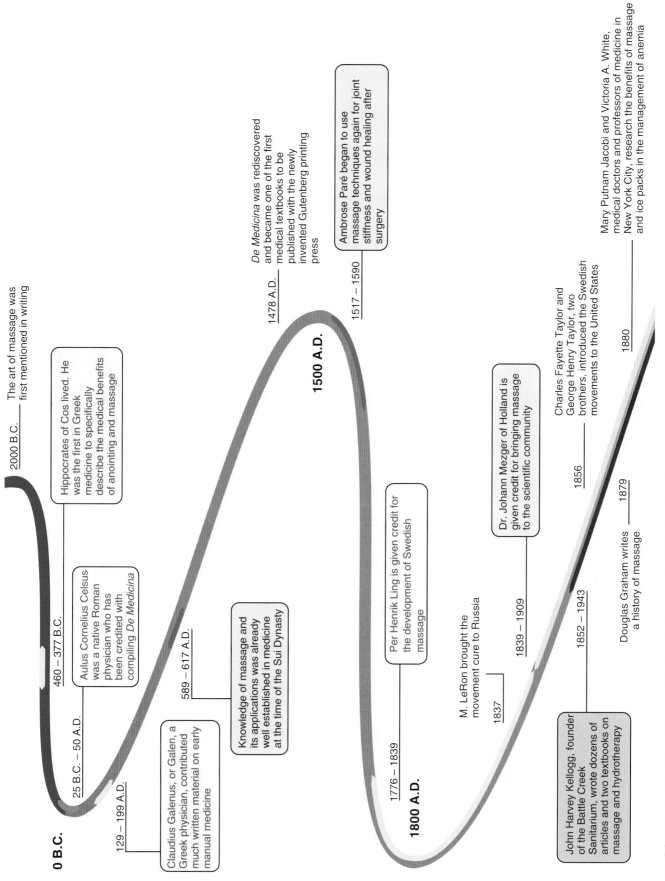

Figure 3.1 Historical timeline. (Source: Chaitow L, Delany J: *Clinical application of neuromuscular techniques: the upper body*, vol 1, ed 2, Edinburgh, 2008, Churchill Livingstone; Fritz S: *Mosby's fundamentals of therapeutic massage*, ed 5, St Louis, 2012, Mosby.)

0 B.C.

2000 B.C.   The art of massage was first mentioned in writing

460 – 377 B.C.   Hippocrates of Cos lived. He was the first in Greek medicine to specifically describe the medical benefits of anointing and massage

25 B.C. – 50 A.D.   Aulus Cornelius Celsus was a native Roman physician who has been credited with compiling *De Medicina*

129 – 199 A.D.   Claudius Galenus, or Galen, a Greek physician, contributed much written material on early manual medicine

589 – 617 A.D.   Knowledge of massage and its applications was already well established in medicine at the time of the Sui Dynasty

1500 A.D.

1478 A.D.   *De Medicina* was rediscovered and became one of the first medical textbooks to be published with the newly invented Gutenberg printing press

1517 – 1590   Ambrose Paré began to use massage techniques again for joint stiffness and wound healing after surgery

1800 A.D.

1776 – 1839   Per Henrik Ling is given credit for the development of Swedish massage

1837   M. LeRon brought the movement cure to Russia

1839 – 1909   Dr. Johann Mezger of Holland is given credit for bringing massage to the scientific community

1852 – 1943   John Harvey Kellogg, founder of the Battle Creek Sanitarium, wrote dozens of articles and two textbooks on massage and hydrotherapy

1856   Charles Fayette Taylor and George Henry Taylor, two brothers, introduced the Swedish movements to the United States

1879   Douglas Graham writes a history of massage

1880   Mary Putnam Jacobi and Victoria A. White, medical doctors and professors of medicine in New York City, research the benefits of massage and ice packs in the management of anemia

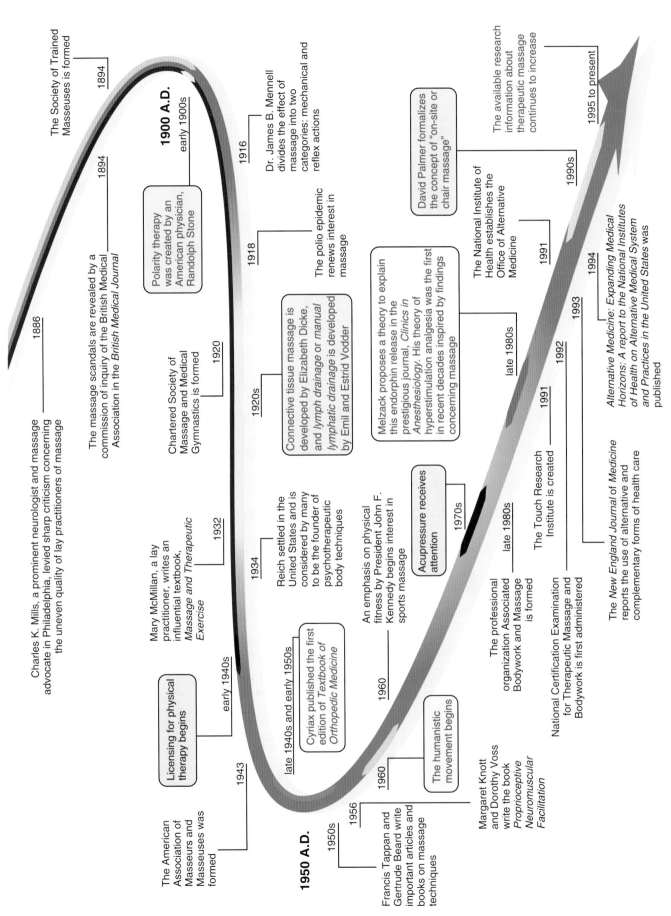

Charles K. Mills, a prominent neurologist and massage advocate in Philadelphia, levied sharp criticism concerning the uneven quality of lay practitioners of massage — 1886

The Society of Trained Masseuses is formed — 1894

The massage scandals are revealed by a commission of inquiry of the British Medical Association in the *British Medical Journal* — 1894

1900 A.D. early 1900s

Polarity therapy was created by an American physician, Randolph Stone

Dr. James B. Mennell divides the effect of massage into two categories: mechanical and reflex actions — 1916

The polio epidemic renews interest in massage — 1918

Chartered Society of Massage and Medical Gymnastics is formed — 1920

Connective tissue massage is developed by Elizabeth Dicke, and *lymph drainage* or *manual lymphatic drainage* is developed by Emil and Estrid Vodder — 1920s

Mary McMillan, a lay practitioner, writes an influential textbook, *Massage and Therapeutic Exercise* — 1932

Reich settled in the United States and is considered by many to be the founder of psychotherapeutic body techniques — 1934

The American Association of Masseurs and Masseuses was formed — early 1940s

Licensing for physical therapy begins — 1943

Cyriax published the first edition of *Textbook of Orthopedic Medicine* — late 1940s and early 1950s

An emphasis on physical fitness by President John F. Kennedy begins interest in sports massage — 1960

Acupressure receives attention — 1970s

1950 A.D. 1950s

Francis Tappan and Gertrude Beard write important articles and books on massage techniques — 1956

Margaret Knott and Dorothy Voss write the book *Proprioceptive Neuromuscular Facilitation* — 1960

The humanistic movement begins — 1960

The professional organization Associated Bodywork and Massage is formed — late 1980s

The Touch Research Institute is created — 1991

National Certification Examination for Therapeutic Massage and Bodywork is first administered — 1992

Melzack proposes a theory to explain this endorphin release in the prestigious journal, *Clinics in Anesthesiology*. His theory of hyperstimulation analgesia was the first in recent decades inspired by findings concerning massage — late 1980s

The *New England Journal of Medicine* reports the use of alternative and complementary forms of health care — 1993

David Palmer formalizes the concept of "on-site or chair massage" — 1990s

The National Institute of Health establishes the Office of Alternative Medicine — 1991

Alternative Medicine: Expanding Medical Horizons: A report to the National Institutes of Health on Alternative Medical System and Practices in the United States was published — 1994

The available research information about therapeutic massage continues to increase — 1995 to present

Figure 3.1, cont'd

quickly, and pain and injury become more likely. The core muscles and associated connective tissues of the posterior, lateral, and anterior torso are considered the core. The core includes large connective tissue structures such as the lumbar dorsal fascial and the abdominal fascia. The core muscles contract, pulling the connective tissues taut, and make a girdle-like structure to maintain upright posture. Massage therapists need core stability to maintain a straight back and stacked joints. This allows for the forward shift of the body's center of gravity to apply pressure (Figures 3.2 and 3.3).

Pressure has been defined in numerous ways: compressive force/load; force application depth; light, medium, and deep depth; and so forth. Drag is the resistance to glide. Glide moves horizontal to the tissues. If you combine pressure with drag, you create a multitude of intensities. For example, light pressure with extensive drag would significantly stretch the skin. Increase the pressure slightly and maintain significant drag, and the superficial fascia is stretched (tension load applied).

If you alter the duration (how long the technique is applied), the intensity can be modified. Generally, long duration is more intense and short duration is less intense. For specific application, short duration is 10 seconds, moderate duration 30 seconds, and long duration 60 seconds. For a whole session, short duration is 5–15 minutes, moderate duration 15–30 minutes, and long duration 45–60 minutes.

Another factor is the size of the point of contact. A large contact area is less intense than a small contact point. More pressure can be applied safely with a broad base of contact such as the forearm or full hand, rather than with a small point of contact such as the thumb. Therefore, the factors that gauge the intensity of massage applications are compressive force, drag, duration, and size of the contact point. In addition, a fast rhythmic application is more intense than a slow rhythmic application. Determining "the right pressure" is sometimes more difficult than it appears.

Beginning with compressive force, we consider that increasing force is necessary to influence various layers of soft tissue from surface to deep, as well as physiologic factors (Figure 3.4 and Table 3.1).

MASSAGE EQUIPMENT

Massage Table

The massage table must be set at a comfortable height, which depends on the body size and style of the practitioner. An individual with long arms may need a shorter table than a person with short arms. A person with a short torso, short arms, and long legs often needs a taller table.

A general rule is that the table height should begin at the hip joint level. Based on torso, arm, and leg ratios, the correct height for the table is 2–3 inches higher or lower. Torso flexion at the hip joint should be maintained at 0–20 degrees not exceeding 30 degrees. Experiment with what feels best. If one has a tendency to bend at the waist and curl the back when applying massage, the table may be too short, and raising the table will help. A higher table is needed to

efficiently use forearms so trunk flexion remains within acceptable ranges. These recommendations represent only a starting point, and each practitioner must experiment to determine the most comfortable table height.

A table that is 30 inches wide provides adequate space for the client to lie down comfortably but is not so wide that the practitioner is reaching for the client in the middle of the table.

Floor Mats

If the massage professional chooses to work on a mat on the floor, the same body mechanics principles apply. The weight-bearing balance points on the floor are then set from the knees instead of the feet.

Stools and Chairs

A low stool or chair is helpful when one is working on the face, neck, and feet. It is appropriate for the practitioner to sit while doing massage as long as the practitioner is comfortable, relaxed, and can obtain the appropriate leverage for the pressure the client needs. It is important that the stool or chair does not slip or roll while the practitioner is applying pressure.

Body Supports

The body position of the client should be adjusted as necessary. Predominately, clients should be in a comfortable, nonharmful position. Body supports are used to bolster the body during the massage and give contour to the flat working surface (Figures 3.5 and 3.6).

Draping

Draping is the process of moving sheets and towels over the client to maintain warmth, modesty, and professional boundaries. The draping materials need to be laundered in an approved sanitary fashion. Typically, the draping materials are washed in hot, soapy water with bleach (Figure 3.7).

MASSAGE/BODYWORK METHODOLOGY

The infinite variations of massage application are derived not from many different methods but from skilled use of the fundamental applications of depth, pressure, drag, direction, speed, rhythm, frequency, and duration.

All massage manipulations introduce mechanical forces into the soft tissues to stimulate various physiologic responses. It is through modification of these manipulations that various therapeutic goals are achieved.

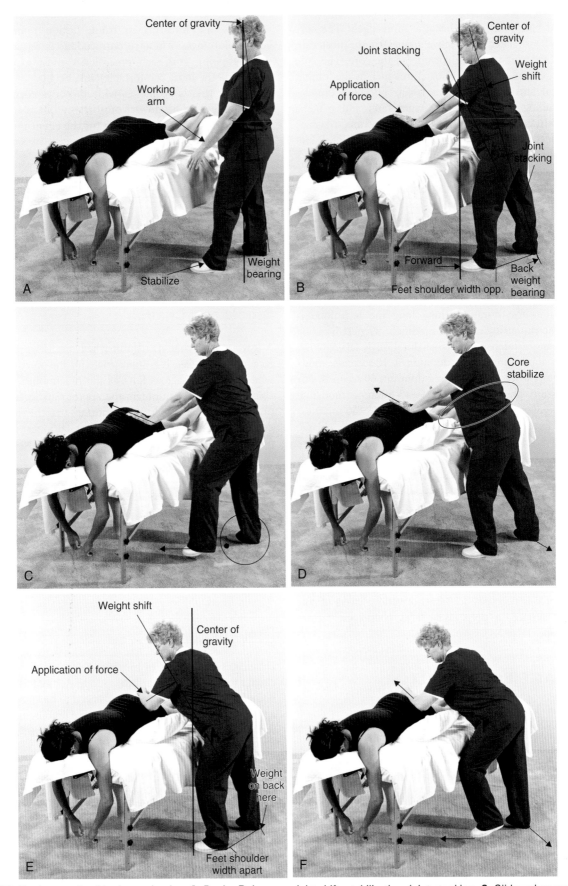

Figure 3.2 Fundamentals of body mechanics. **A**, Begin. **B**, Lean, weight shift, stabilization, joint stacking. **C**, Glide: when weight from your back foot moves forward, from the heel to the ball of your foot and your toes, it is time to reposition by taking a step. **D**, After taking the step, reestablish core stabilization and the leaning posture. **E**, Example of body mechanics. **F**, Pressure of foot into floor results in arm glide. (Source: B, Fritz S: *Mosby's fundamentals of therapeutic massage*, ed 5, St Louis, 2012, Mosby. **H**, Fritz S, Chaitow L, Hymel GM: *Clinical massage in the healthcare setting*, St Louis, 2007, Mosby.)

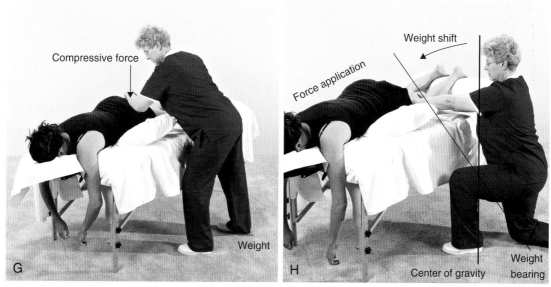

Figure 3.2, cont'd **G,** Compression down at 90 degrees. **H,** Example of application principles when kneeling.

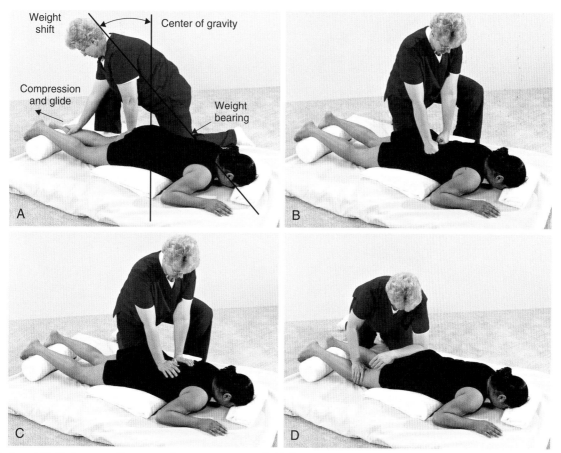

Figure 3.3 A and **B,** Mat, prone. Sequence for mat massage. **C–E,** Prone.

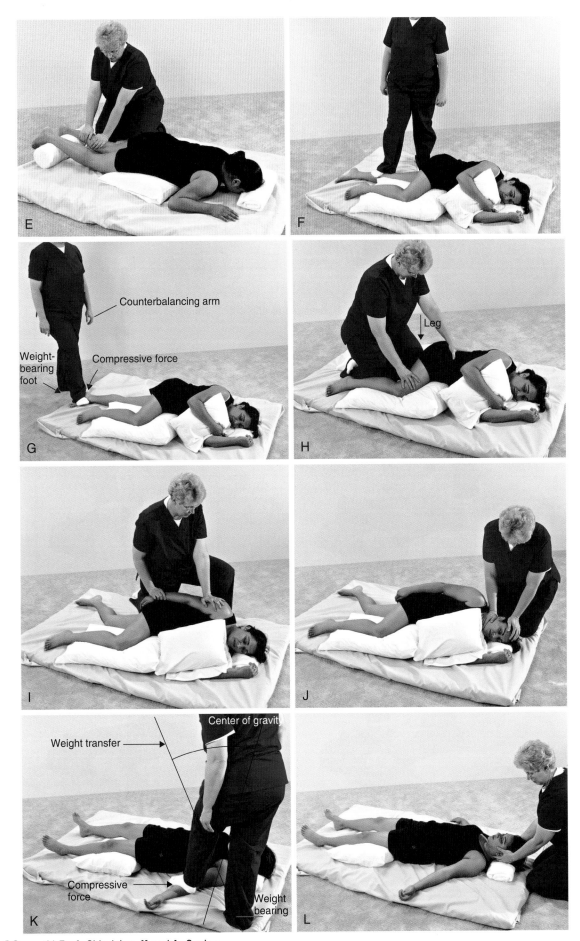

Figure 3.3, cont'd **F–J**, Side-lying. **K** and **L**, Supine.

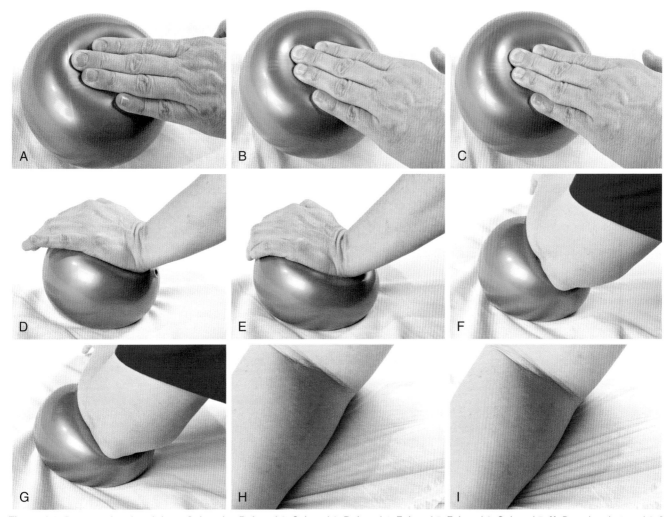

Figure 3.4 Pressure level and drag. **A**, Level 1. **B**, Level 2. **C**, Level 3. **D**, Level 4. **E**, Level 5. **F**, Level 6. **G**, Level 7. **H**, Drag levels 1 and 2. **I**, Drag level 3. (Source: Fritz S, Chaitow L, Hymel GM: *Clinical massage in the healthcare setting*, St Louis, 2007, Mosby.)

TABLE 3.1 General Guidelines for Pressure, Drag, Speed, and Duration in Massage Applications for Various Conditions

Desired Outcome	Pressure	Drag	Speed	Duration
Fragile patient (to provide comfort and to soothe)	1–2	0	Slow	Short to moderate
Palliative, wellness-based (non-fragile patient, to stimulate parasympathetic dominance)	2, 3, or 4	1	Slow	Moderate
Interstitial fluid movement lymphatic drainage, surface	2–3	2	Slow	Moderate to long
Interstitial fluid movement lymphatic drainage, deep	4–5	2	Slow	Moderate
Myofascial release (superficial fascia)	3	3	Slow	Long
General relaxation (to inhibit sympathetic arousal)	4–5	2	Slow	Moderate
Trigger point inhibition	4–6 (depending on location)	0	Moderate	Moderate
Scar tissue surface (mature scar)	2–3	2–3	Slow	Moderate
Sliding of muscle layer or layers	4–6	3	Slow	Moderate
Arterial support	4–5	0	Moderate to fast at location over artery	Short to moderate
Venous return support	3	1	Slow	Moderate
Anticoagulant use	1–2	0 to start (monitor results)	Varies	Varies
Fragile bones (osteoporosis)	1–4 (depending on muscle bulk and density)	0–3	Varies	Varies
Stimulation of sympathetic autonomic nervous system (ANS) dominance	2–5	0–1	Moderate to fast	Short to moderate

Source: Fritz S, Chaitow L, Hymel GM: *Clinical massage in the healthcare setting*, St Louis, 2007, Mosby.

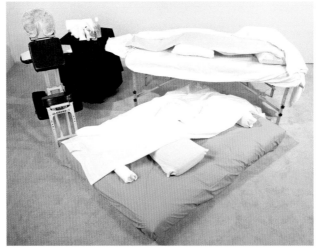

Figure 3.5 Equipment and supplies: table, chair, mat, and bolsters. (Source: Fritz S: *Mosby's fundamentals of therapeutic massage*, ed 7, St Louis, 2021, Mosby.)

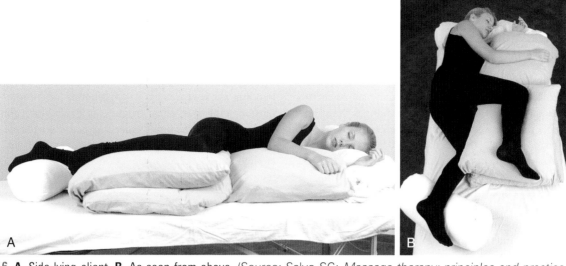

Figure 3.6 A, Side-lying client. **B**, As seen from above. (Source: Salvo SG: *Massage therapy: principles and practice*, ed 4, St Louis, 2011, Saunders.)

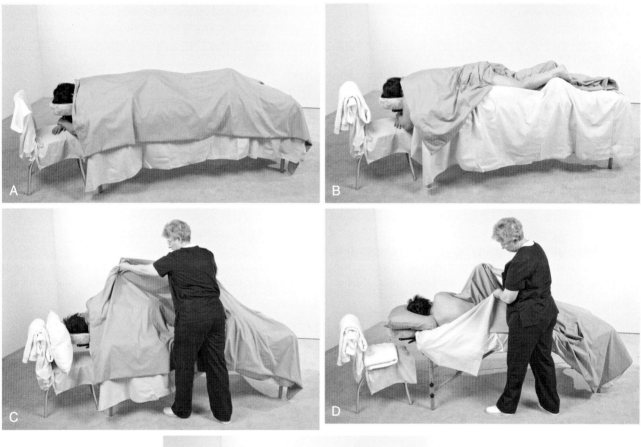

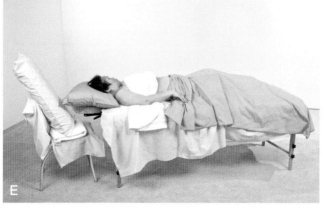

Figure 3.7 Draping examples. **A** and **B**, Prone. **C** and **D**, Side-lying. **E**, Supine. (Source: **A**, Fritz S, Chaitow L, Hymel GM: *Clinical massage in the healthcare setting*, St Louis, 2007, Mosby. **B**–**E**: Fritz S: *Mosby's fundamentals of therapeutic massage*, ed 5, St Louis, 2012, Mosby.)

Application of Mechanical Force

Mechanical force can be described as a push or a pull. A mechanical force involves contact with another object. A force exerted can cause a change in either the shape or the motion of the area. In massage, the force changes the shape of soft tissue and causes soft tissue deformation. Joint movement is a method that can influence motion. Mechanical force application that changes the shape of tissue. Motion also loads tissue creating stress to the area resulting in an adaptation-change in shape or motion. The force applied creates the stress and loads tissue which then causes the deformation or movement or both combined. Forces (pushes or pulls) may be applied in different directions such as:

• Tensile or stretching/elongation
• Compressive or squashing/crushing
• Shear or tearing/cutting
• Torsional or twisting

The five stresses that can affect the tissues of the body are "compression," "tension," "bending," "shear," and "torsion." (NOTE: The term *force* is often interchanged with stress. For example, compressive stress or compressive force.)

Compression
Compressive stress occurs when two structures are pressed together; the force is applied perpendicularly. Compression is a component of massage application used therapeutically to affect circulation, sensory and autonomic nerve stimulation, nerve chemicals, and connective tissue pliability.

Tension
Tension stress (also called tensile stress) occurs when two ends of a structure are pulled apart from one another; the force is applied more horizontally. Tension is used during massage to elongate tissues with applications that drag, glide, lengthen, and stretch.

Bending
Bending stress represents a combination of compression and tension. One side of a structure is exposed to compressive loading, while the other side is exposed to tensile loading. Bending occurs during many massage applications. Force is applied across the fiber direction of muscles, tendons, ligaments, and fascial sheaths.

Shear
Shear stress is created when the force is applied to the structure in a back-and-forth manner. Massage methods that create friction involve shear stress.

Torsion
Torsion is best understood as twisting stress. Massage methods that use kneading introduce torsion stress, which targets connective tissue changes and fluid movement (Figure 3.8).

Massage Manipulations

The methods of massage described next introduce one or a combination of these forces that load tissues creating stress to the area which then adapts and results in therapeutic benefit. This process is influenced by the quality of application, depth of pressure, drag, duration, speed, rhythm, and frequency.

Holding/Resting Position

When the massage begins, it is very important for this initial contact to be made with respect and a client-centered focus, as

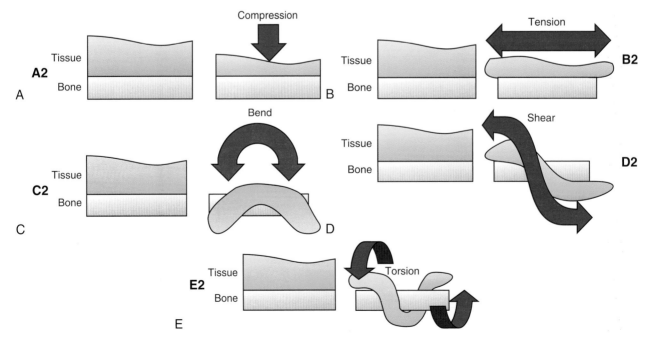

Figure 3.8 A, compression. **B**, Tension. **C**, Bending. **D**, Shear. **E**, Torsion. (Source: Fritz S, Chaitow L, Hymel GM: *Clinical massage in the healthcare setting*, St Louis, 2007, Mosby.)

well as with the intention to meet client goals. With the **holding/resting position,** we enter the client's personal boundary space. When application of the holding position has been mastered, it is easy to flow into the other methods, and gliding is often next in sequence (Figure 3.9).

Gliding

Gliding methods are historically known as "effleurage," which originates from the French verb meaning "to skim" and "to touch lightly on." The most superficial applications of this method do this, but the full spectrum is determined by pressure, drag, speed, direction, and rhythm, making this manipulation one of the most versatile. The distinguishing characteristic of gliding is that when the method is applied horizontally in relation to tissue fibers, it generates a tensile stress. Gliding also can be applied across fibers to create a bending stress. During gliding application, light pressure remains on the skin, while moderate pressure extends through

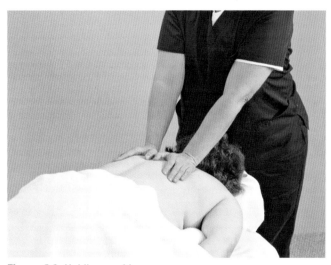

Figure 3.9 Holding position.

the subcutaneous layer of the skin to reach muscle tissue, but not so deep as to compress the tissue against underlying bony structures. Deep pressure compresses the tissue against underlying boney structures (Figure 3.10).

Kneading

During **kneading** application soft tissue is lifted, rolled, and squeezed. The main purpose of this manipulation is to lift tissue while applying bend, shear, and torsion stress. Pétrissage, the historical term for kneading, is derived from the French verb *petrir*, meaning "to knead." Just as gliding focuses horizontally on the body, kneading focuses vertically and twists (Figure 3.11).

Skin Rolling

A variation of the vertical lifting manipulation is **skin rolling.** Whereas deep kneading attempts to lift the muscular component away from the bone, skin rolling lifts only the skin and superficial fascia from the underlying muscle layer. Skin rolling is one of the very few massage methods that is safe to use directly over the spine. Because only the skin and superficial fascia are accessed and the direction of pull to the tissue is up and away from the underlying bones, the spine risks no injury, unlike when any type of downward pressure is used (Figure 3.12).

Compression

Compression moves downward into the tissue at a 90-degree angle. It can be a specific method but is also an aspect of gliding and kneading. Depth is determined by what is to be accomplished, where it is applied, and how broad or specific the contact point with the client's body (Figure 3.13).

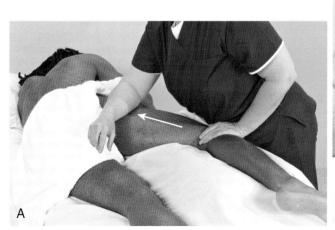

A

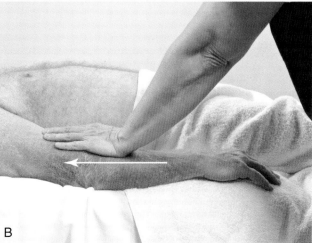

B

Figure 3.10 Gliding creates tension stress. Gliding historically has been termed effleurage. (Source: Fritz S, Chaitow L, Hymel GM: *Clinical massage in the healthcare setting*, St Louis, 2007, Mosby; Fritz S: *Mosby's fundamentals of therapeutic massage*, ed 5, St Louis, 2012, Mosby.)

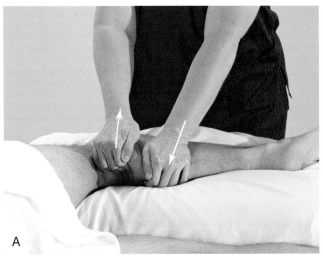

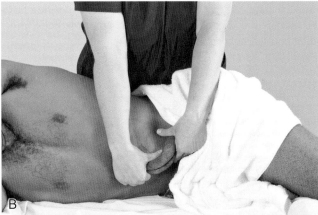

Figure 3.11 Kneading creates torsion stress. Kneading historically has been called pétrissage. (Source: Fritz S, Chaitow L, Hymel GM: *Clinical massage in the healthcare setting*, St Louis, 2007, Mosby.)

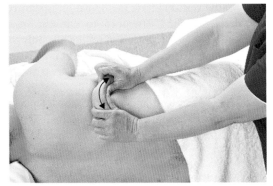

Figure 3.12 Skin rolling creates bending stress. (Source: Fritz S: *Mosby's fundamentals of therapeutic massage*, ed 5, St Louis, 2012, Mosby.)

Vibrations

The technique for producing manual **vibrations** is to set up a small amount of alternating contraction and relaxation in some of the muscles of the forearm while those of the upper arm and shoulder are kept passive (unless required for fixation purposes) (Figure 3.14).

Shaking

Shaking is a massage method that is effective in relaxing muscle groups or an entire limb. Shaking manipulations confuse the positional proprioceptors because the sensory input is too disorganized for the integrating systems of the brain to interpret; muscle relaxation is the natural response in such situations (Figures 3.15 and 3.16).

Rocking

Rocking is a soothing, rhythmic method that is used for calming. Rocking has both neurologic and chemical effects. For rocking to be most effective, the client's body must move so that the fluid in the semicircular canals of the inner ear is affected, thereby initiating parasympathetic mechanisms (Figure 3.17).

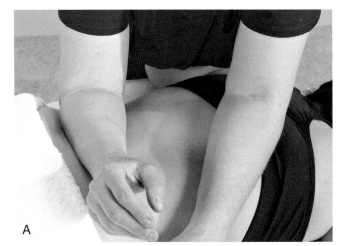

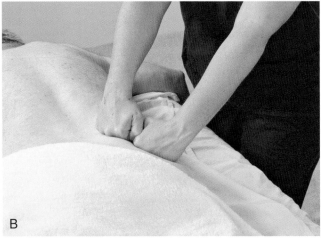

Figure 3.13 **A** and **B** compression creates compressive stress. (Source: Fritz S: *Mosby's fundamentals of therapeutic massage*, ed 5, St Louis, 2012, Mosby.)

Percussion or Tapotement

Percussion moves up and down on the tissue, creating rhythmic compression. The term "tapotement" comes from the French verb *tapoter*, which means "to rap, smack, drum, or pat." Percussion techniques require that the hands or parts of

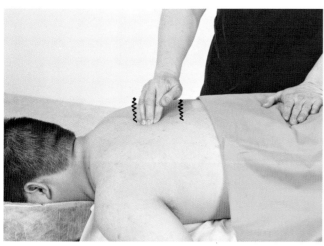

Figure 3.14 Vibration. (Source: Fritz S: *Mosby's fundamentals of therapeutic massage*, ed 5, St Louis, 2012, Mosby.)

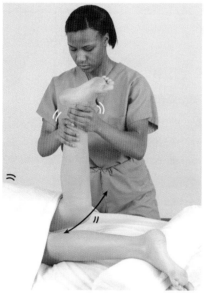

Figure 3.15 Hip joint jostling vibration with client prone. (Source: Salvo SG: *Massage therapy: principles and practice*, ed 4, St Louis, 2011, Saunders.)

the hand administer springy downward blows to the body at a fast rate.

Hacking. This method is applied with both wrists relaxed and the fingers spread, with only the little finger or the ulnar side of the hand striking the surface. The other fingers hit each other with a springy touch. Point hacking can be done by using the fingertips in the same way.

Tapping. The fingertips are used to apply targeted gentle stimulation.

Cupping. Contact is made with hands turned palm down, fingers and thumbs adducted and slightly flexed (making a cup shape). When performed on the anterior and posterior thorax, cupping is good for stimulating the respiratory system and for loosening mucus.

Slapping (splatting). The whole palm of a flattened hand makes contact with the body. This is a good method for releasing histamine to increase vasodilation and its effects on the skin.

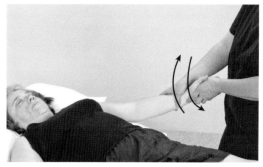

Figure 3.16 Shaking. (Source: Fritz S: *Mosby's fundamentals of therapeutic massage*, ed 5, St Louis, 2012, Mosby.)

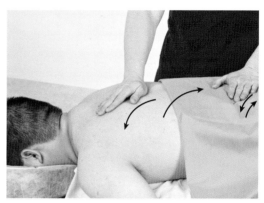

Figure 3.17 Rocking. (Source: Fritz S: *Mosby's fundamentals of therapeutic massage*, ed 7, St Louis, 2021, Mosby.)

Beating and pounding. These moves are performed by using a soft fist with knuckles down, or vertically with the ulnar side of the palm (Figure 3.18).

Friction

Friction manipulations are brisk concentrated strokes. The direction and depth can vary. One method of **friction** consists of small deep movements performed on a local area. It creates shear stress in tissue (Figure 3.19).

Joint Movement

Joint movements are methods that move each joint through various positions within the normal range of motion. These movements, which are never forced, can be active, when only the client moves; active assisted when the massage therapist helps the client move; active resisted when the massage therapist resists movement of the client; and passive when the massage therapist provides movement (Figures 3.20 and 3.21).

Muscle Energy Methods

Muscle energy methods are an intervention that uses a controlled muscle contraction to support stretching/elongation of short tissues by increasing the client's tolerance to the stretch sensation.

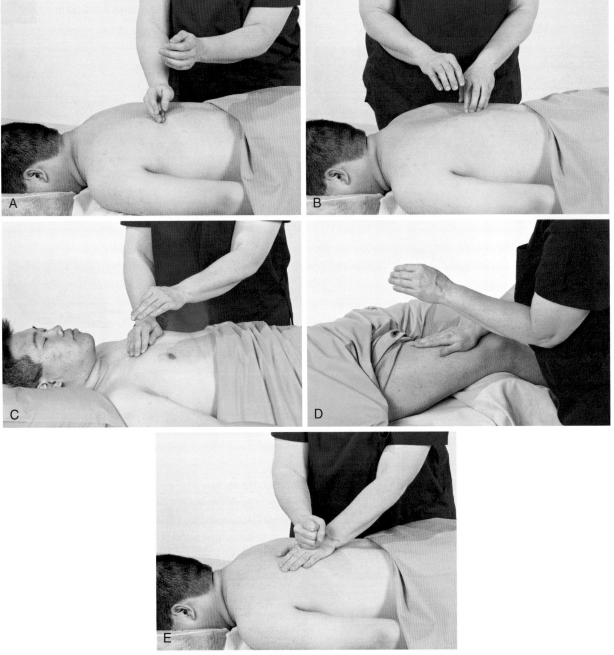

Figure 3.18 Percussion/tapotement. **A**, Hacking. **B**, Tapping. **C**, Cupping. **D**, Slapping. **E**, Beating. (Source: Fritz S: *Mosby's fundamentals of therapeutic massage*, ed 5, St Louis, 2012, Mosby.)

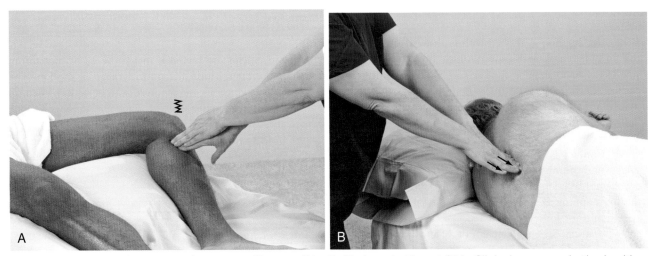

Figure 3.19 A and **B** friction creates shear stress. (Source: Fritz S, Chaitow L, Hymel GM: *Clinical massage in the healthcare setting*, St Louis, 2007, Mosby.)

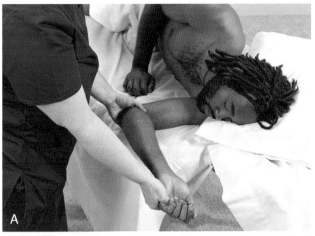

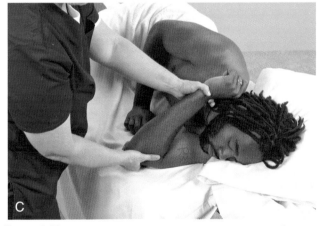

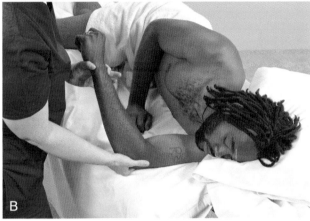

Figure 3.20 A, **B** and **C** examples of joint movement. (Source: Fritz S, Chaitow L, Hymel GM: *Clinical massage in the healthcare setting*, St Louis, 2007, Mosby.)

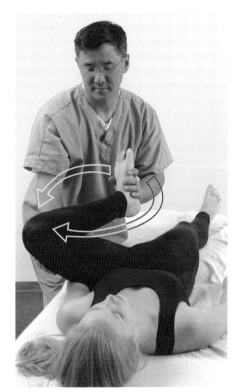

Figure 3.21 Hip circles. (Source: Salvo SG: *Massage therapy: principles and practice*, ed 4, St Louis, 2011, Saunders.)

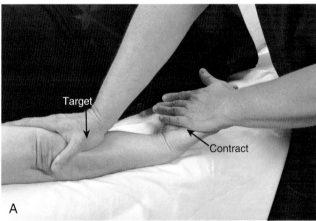

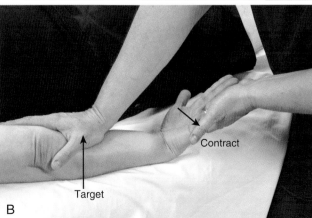

Figure 3.22 Muscle energy methods increase tolerance to stretch. **A**, Contract–relax. **B**, Antagonist contract. (Source: Fritz S, Chaitow L, Hymel GM: *Clinical massage in the healthcare setting*, St Louis, 2007, Mosby.)

Contract–Relax

This method causes isometric action in the target muscle tissue to support stretching.

Combined Methods: Contract–Relax–Antagonist–Contract

Contract–relax and antagonist–contract can be combined to enhance lengthening effects. This method can be called "contract–relax–antagonist–contract (CRAC)" (Figures 3.22 and 3.23).

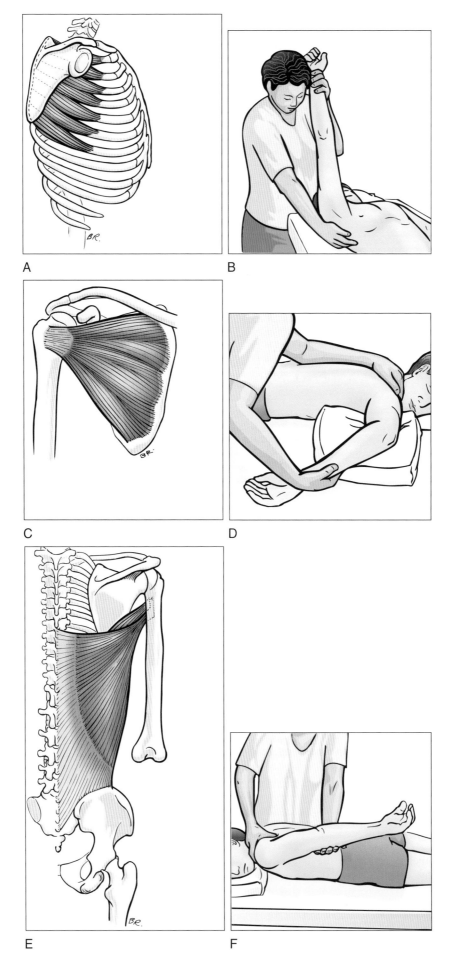

Figure 3.23 Isolation positions for muscle energy and stretching methods. **A** and **B**, Serratus anterior. **C** and **D**, Subscapularis. **E** and **F**, Latissimus dorsi. (Source: Fritz S, Chaitow L, Hymel GM: *Clinical massage in the healthcare setting*, St Louis, 2007, Mosby.)

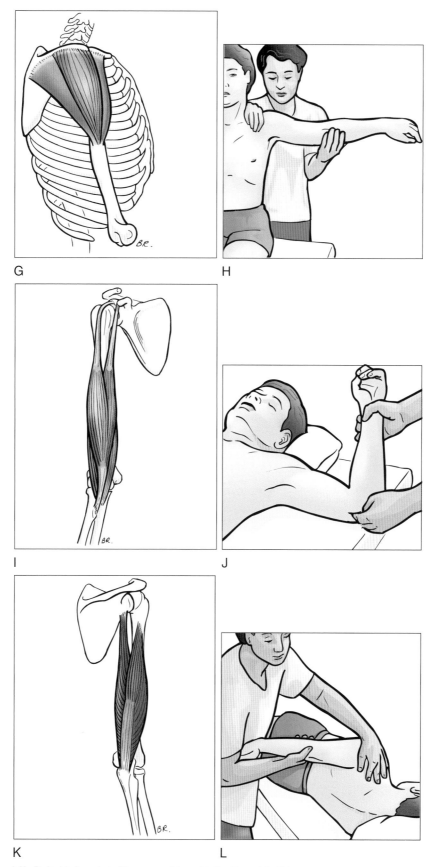

G   H

I   J

K   L

Figure 3.23, cont'd **G** and **H**, Deltoid. **I** and **J**, Biceps and brachialis. **K** and **L**, Triceps.

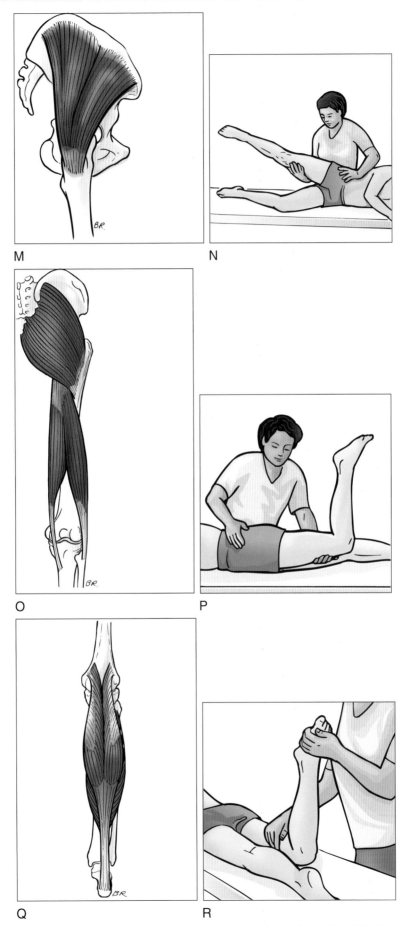

Figure 3.23, cont'd **M** and **N**, Gluteus medius. **O** and **P**, Gluteus maximus and hamstrings. **Q** and **R**, Gastrocnemius and soleus.

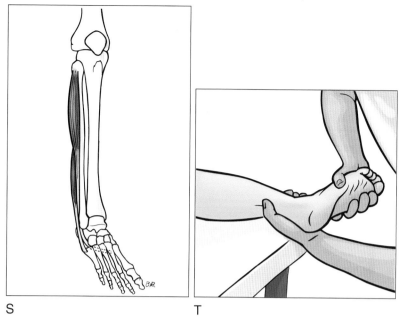

Figure 3.23, cont'd **S** and **T**, Fibularis (peroneus).

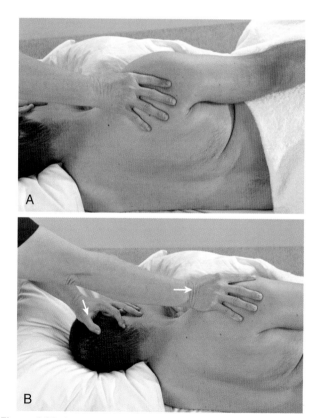

Figure 3.24 Stretching/elongation. **A**, Begin. **B**, Stretch/lengthen.

Stretching/Elongation

Stretching is a mechanical intervention method of introducing various forces to elongate areas of shortening. Muscle energy techniques prepare muscles to stretch by having the client generate a focused contraction before lengthening. The methods seem to work because the client experiences an

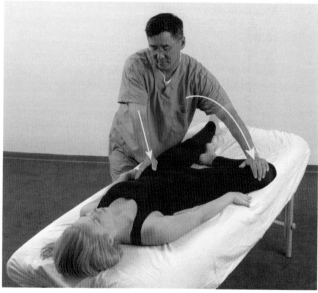

Figure 3.25 Adductor stretch. (Source: Salvo SG: *Massage therapy: principles and practice*, ed 4, St Louis, 2011, Saunders.)

increased tolerance to the stretch sensation. Longitudinal stretching pulls or pushes tissue in the direction of the fiber configuration. Cross-directional stretching pulls or pushes tissue against the fiber direction. Both accomplish the same thing, but longitudinal stretching is done in conjunction with movement at the joint. If longitudinal stretching is not advisable, such as in situations of hypermobility, cross-directional stretching is a better choice. Cross-directional stretching focuses on the tissue itself and does not depend on joint movement (Figures 3.24 and 3.25).

MASSAGE MODIFICATIONS AND ADAPTATION: ADJUNCT AND COMPLEMENTARY BODYWORK METHODS

In some instances, you may need to adapt or modify massage methods. Test questions may ask about adapting massage related to client outcomes or to support comfort. It is also common to include aspects of various bodywork models into the massage. When this is done, the applications must be safe and beneficial.

These methods include the following:

- Chair massage—modifies application to a seated position and typically over clothing (Figure 3.26).
- Mat massage—modifies application to a mat on the floor (Figures 3.27 and 3.28).
- Hydrotherapy/thermotherapy—modified temperature application using hot-cold water, stones, or rice/seed bags (Figures 3.29 and 3.30 and Boxes 3.1 and 3.2).
- Trigger point treatment—point compression/inhibitory pressure (Figures 3.31 through 3.33).
- Reflexology—a specific system of massage of the foot and hands to affect other areas of the body (Figures 3.34 and 3.35).
- Asian and Eastern methods (Figures 3.36 and 3.37 and Table 3.2).

- Connective tissue methods/myofascial release—modified introduction of mechanical forces to specific tissues (superficial fascia, deep fascia, scar tissue, etc.) resulting in pressure, pulling, movement, and stretch (Figures 3.38 and 3.39).
- Adaptive massage targeting fluid movement—interstitial fluid, lymph, and blood circulation. If massage does indeed affect the movement of fluid in the body, then somehow massage would need to mimic the natural mechanism of fluid movement. The pressure provided by massage mimics the drag and compressive forces of movement and respiration and can move various body fluids. The depth of pressure, speed and frequency, direction, rhythm, duration, and drag are adjusted to support the interstitial, lymphatic, and blood flow.
- Energy-based methods—intentional and intuitive movement of energy fields/bioenergy of the body. These methods are often based on ancient and cultural healing practices (Figures 3.40 and 3.41).
- Essential oils/aromatherapy—the use of pure concentrated oils of aromatic plants to promote health; always dilute the essential oil with a carrier oil (Table 3.3).
- Kinesiology tape—specialized tape developed by Dr. Kase is an elastic lightweight tape that is hypoallergenic and made with cotton. The thinness and elasticity of kinesiology tape is different from rigid athletic tape. Kinesiology

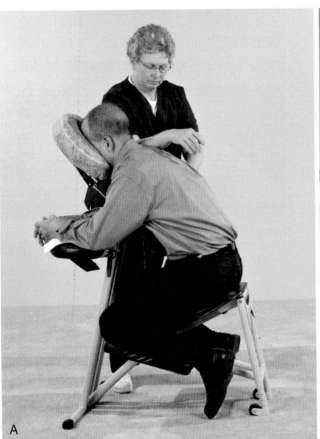
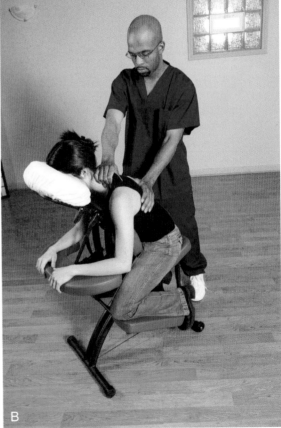

Figure 3.26 Chair massage. **A** and **B**, Two examples of massage to upper trapezius. (Source: **A**, Fritz S: *Mosby's fundamentals of therapeutic massage*, ed 5, St Louis, 2012, Mosby. **B**, Salvo SG: *Massage therapy: principles and practice*, ed 4, St Louis, 2011, Saunders.)

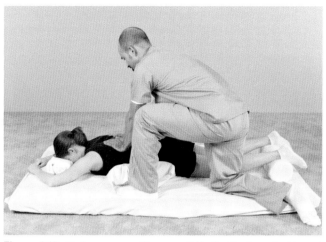

Figure 3.27 Mat massage. (Source: Fritz S, Chaitow L, Hymel GM: *Clinical massage in the healthcare setting*, St Louis, 2007, Mosby.)

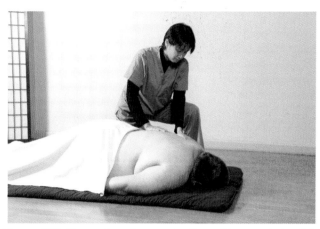

Figure 3.28 Massaging client on the floor. (Source: Salvo SG: *Massage therapy: principles and practice*, ed 4, St Louis, 2011, Saunders.)

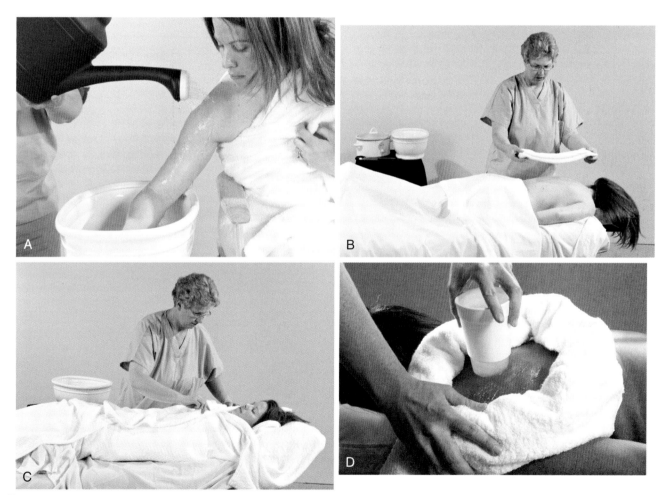

Figure 3.29 Forms of hydrotherapy. A, Bath/douche. **B,** Compress. **C,** Full sheet pack. **D,** Ice. (Source: **A–C,** Fritz S: *Mosby's fundamentals of therapeutic massage*, ed 7, St Louis, 2021, Mosby. **D,** Salvo SG: *Massage therapy: principles and practice*, ed 4, St Louis, 2011, Saunders.)

tape encourages normal movement. There are now many brands of this type of tape on the market. The tape is designed to be left in place for up to 3 days.

- Implement assisted—some sort of device that is used to augment the massage application. The device can roll and press, scrape or suction. The two main reasons for using an implement are that the device reduces the effort required to apply massage, making massage application easier for the massage therapist, and the device can apply mechanical force to the soft tissue more effectively than the massage therapist's hands, forearms, or other part of the body used to apply massage methods. A

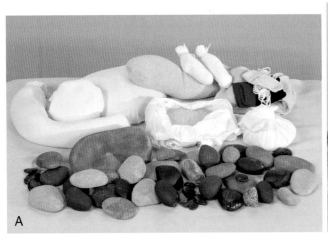 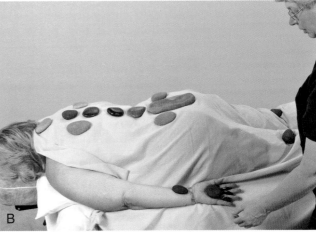

Figure 3.30 Thermotherapy. Stones or seed bags, warm and cold. **A**, Examples of stones and seed bags. **B**, Placement of stones.

BOX 3.1	Therapeutic Uses of Water		
Analgesic (relieves pain)	Hot, warm, and cold applications	Diuretic (increases urine formation)	Drinking water
		Emetic (produces vomiting)	Drinking warm water
		Expectorant (loosens mucus)	Hot and steam applications
Anesthetic (reduces sensation)	Cold application		
Antiedemic (reduces swelling)	Cold application	Immunologic enhancement (increases white cell production)	Cold application
Antipyretic (reduces fever)	Cool to cold application		
Antiseptic (kills pathogens)	Boiling water, high-pressure steam (not for use on the body)	Laxative (promotes peristalsis of the bowel)	Drinking cold water or use of an enema
		Purifier (eliminates toxins)	All forms of water
Antispasmodic (reduces muscle spasms)	Hot, warm, and cold applications	Sedative (reduces sympathetic arousal and encourages sleep)	Drinking warm water
Astringent (causes tissues to contract)	Cold application		
		Stimulant (increases sympathetic arousal)	Short hot and cold applications
Burn treatment (first-degree and mild second-degree burns only)	Cool application	Tonic (increases muscle tone)	Cold and alternating hot and cold applications
Diaphoretic (produces sweating)	Hot application		

Source: RJ Nikola: *Creatures of water: hydro & spa therapy textbook*, Salt Lake City, 2015, Europa Publishing.

BOX 3.2	Classifying Water Temperatures		
		Neutral	92–98°F	Normal skin temperature
		Warm to hot	98–104°F	Comfortable
		Very hot	104–110°F	Reddened skin
Very cold	32–56°F	Painful		
Cold	56–65°F	Uncomfortable		
Cool	65–92°F	Goosebumps		

Temperatures higher than 110°F should not be used.

Source: Fritz S: *Mosby's fundamentals of therapeutic massage*, ed 5, St Louis, 2012, Mosby.

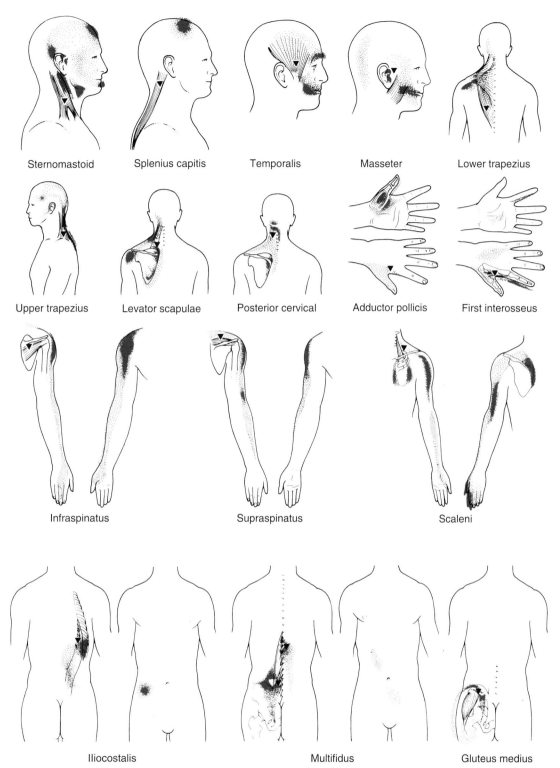

Sternomastoid   Splenius capitis   Temporalis   Masseter   Lower trapezius

Upper trapezius   Levator scapulae   Posterior cervical   Adductor pollicis   First interosseus

Infraspinatus   Supraspinatus   Scaleni

Iliocostalis   Multifidus   Gluteus medius

Figure 3.31 Common trigger points. (Source: Chaitow L: *Modern neuromuscular techniques*, ed 2, Edinburgh, 2003, Churchill Livingstone.)

suction implement, such as a silicone cup, can be helpful when lifting the superficial fascial is the outcome. However, caution is required to prevent the capillary damage by keeping the cup moving and not leaving it in one spot. The tools used to apply compression still require using the hands, so whether the tools create an advantage is questionable. The extended use of electronic percussion and vibration devices poses a risk of injury to the massage therapist. Tools that are used to scrape the skin and push and pull superficial fascia create inflammation. These implements must be used carefully.

- Health messages—teaching self-help methods and providing education to prolong the effects of massage (Figure 3.42).

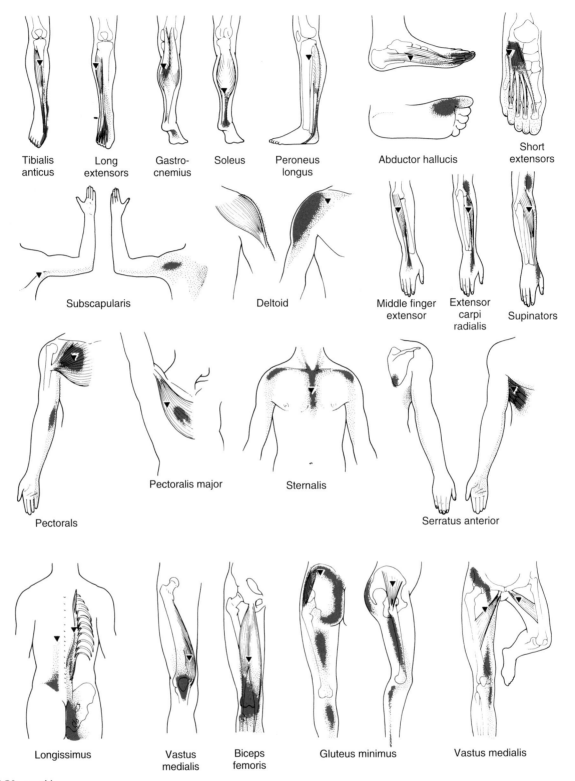

Tibialis anticus — Long extensors — Gastro-cnemius — Soleus — Peroneus longus — Abductor hallucis — Short extensors

Subscapularis — Deltoid — Middle finger extensor — Extensor carpi radialis — Supinators

Pectorals — Pectoralis major — Sternalis — Serratus anterior

Longissimus — Vastus medialis — Biceps femoris — Gluteus minimus — Vastus medialis

Figure 3.31, cont'd

Adaptations for Specific Populations

Adaptation typically takes the form of special considerations for informed consent, position, pressure levels, duration of massage, and choice of method used (Figure 3.43).

Athletes

An athlete is a person who participates in sports as an amateur or as a professional. Although fitness is necessary for everyone's wellness, the physical activity of an athlete goes beyond fitness and is performance based. Athletes require precise use of their bodies and therefore train the nervous system and muscles to perform in a specific way. Performance strain makes this population vulnerable to physical strain and mental strain, which increase the athlete's potential for injury and illness. Often the activity involves repetitive joint movement and use of one group of muscles more than others, which may result in hypertrophy, changes in strength and movement patterns, connective tissue

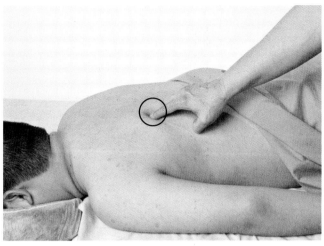

Figure 3.32 Trigger point treatment using direct inhibitory pressure. (Source: Fritz S: *Mosby's fundamentals of therapeutic massage*, ed 5, St Louis, 2012, Mosby.)

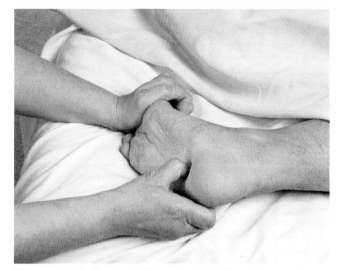

Figure 3.34 Reflexology. (Source: Fritz S: *Mosby's fundamentals of therapeutic massage*, ed 5, St Louis, 2012, Mosby.)

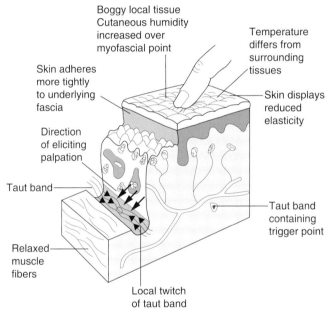

Figure 3.33 Altered physiology of tissues in the region of a myofascial trigger point.

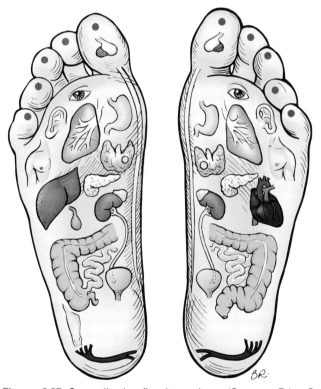

Figure 3.35 Generalized reflexology chart. (Source: Fritz S: *Mosby's fundamentals of therapeutic massage*, ed 5, St Louis, 2012, Mosby.)

formation, and compensation patterns in the rest of the body. These factors contribute to the soft tissue difficulties that often develop in athletes.

Massage Strategies

Massage can be very beneficial for athletes if the professional who is performing the massage understands the biomechanics required by the sport. If not, massage can impair optimum function in the athlete's performance. This population is complex, and in some ways massage is more difficult to manage for these individuals than for other groups. Injuries in athletes typically are of the musculoskeletal type, and illness often occurs as the result of immune suppression caused by excessive physical activity without adequate recovery.

Geriatric Populations

In general, the geriatric population consists of individuals 65 years or older. Aging is not an illness but a natural process of

being alive. As we age, our bodies do not function as efficiently as when we were 25 years old. Medical treatment can sometimes alleviate or reduce the symptoms of the natural aging process. In addition, as aging progresses, people have a greater tendency to develop age-related diseases, such as cardiovascular disease, some types of cancer, and dementia. The older body does not heal as quickly and is less able to fight off infection. Lifestyle greatly influences how well people age, and lifestyle changes can slow or even reverse some age-related changes. Exercise, diet, sleep, not smoking, moderate

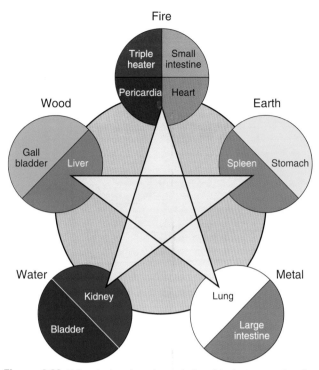

Figure 3.36 Wheel showing the relationship between the five elements and organs of the body. The center depicts the *ko*, or control cycle. Wood controls earth by covering it or holding it in place with roots. Earth controls water by damming it or containing it. Water controls fire by dousing it or extinguishing it. Fire controls metal by melting it. Metal controls wood by cutting it. The next set of lines that form a circle depicts the *sheng*, or creative cycle. Water engenders wood. Wood fuels fire. Fire creates the earth (ashes). Earth engenders metal. Metal engenders water. The two rings indicate the solid *(yin)* and hollow *(yang)* organs that are associated with the elements. (Source: Fritz S: *Mosby's fundamentals of therapeutic massage*, ed 5, St Louis, 2012, Mosby.)

use of alcohol, supportive relationships, and ongoing mental stimulation all support effective aging.

Massage Strategies

People in their advanced years can benefit greatly from massage. Although the massage methods remain consistent, older adults present specific concerns and require appropriate adjustments in the massage application. The massage therapist also needs to appreciate changes in vision, hearing, and cognitive processing speed and to use the communication skills recommended in this chapter.

To develop appropriate massage treatment plans that can address age-related symptoms, it is important to understand the natural changes that occur with aging. Muscle tissue diminishes, as does fat and connective tissue. Connective tissue in general is affected during the aging process. It becomes less pliable, is slower to reproduce, and more easily becomes fibrotic. Bones become less flexible and are prone to breaking. Joints become worn, and osteoarthritis is common. The skin is thinner, circulation is not as efficient, and fluid in the soft tissue is reduced. Medications may be prescribed to control blood pressure and other conditions, producing many side effects. The vertebral column tends to collapse a bit during aging. The spaces provided

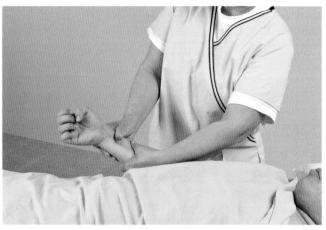

Figure 3.37 Acupressure. (Source: Fritz S: *Mosby's fundamentals of therapeutic massage*, ed 5, St Louis, 2012, Mosby.)

for the nerves are reduced, and bones and soft tissue structures can put pressure on the nerves, resulting in sciatica and thoracic outlet syndrome. The feet hurt because the intricate joint structure of the foot has broken down. Circulation to the extremities is diminished, often resulting in a burning type of pain. These conditions are not life-threatening, but they may cause a person to feel miserable.

If only temporarily, massage can ease the discomfort of these conditions. Cautionary measures for thin skin, reduced tactile sensation, pain awareness, reduced muscle mass, and circulatory changes, including increased bruising and sensitivity to heat and cold, as well as other conditions, require alteration in the massage such as using lighter pressure. With changes in the joints, the person may need additional bolstering to be comfortable. Many older adults take several medications. They also are more sensitive to the dosage level of medication and are less able to self-regulate homeostatic processes. The massage professional must be attentive to the physiologic interactions between the effects of massage and the medications. Regular massage may allow the dosages of some medications to be reduced.

Older adults may be isolated. Their spouses have passed away, and their families are busy with their own lives. We all need to be touched. If a person is not physically and emotionally stimulated, neurologic function begins to deteriorate. Interaction with a massage therapist can provide both physical/sensory and emotional/social stimulation for this population.

Older adults are sometimes depressed. This frequently occurs as a chemical depression, as well as a situational condition resulting from experiences such as loss of loved ones and friends. Massage stimulates neurochemicals that can temporarily lift mild depression. Conditions of dementia, such as Alzheimer's disease, have shown temporary improvement after massage. Wandering behavior has decreased, and an increased awareness of the current environment has been observed. If a person does not have adequate cognitive skills (e.g., dementia), he or she will be unable to give informed consent for the massage. The guardian, physician, or other healthcare professional then must give the necessary permission.

Dehydration, lack of appetite, and weight loss are problems that may be associated with advanced age. However,

TABLE 3.2 Qualities of the Five Elements

			ELEMENT		
Phase	Metal	Earth	Fire	Water	Wood
Yin	Lung	Spleen	Heart	Kidney	Liver
Yang	Large intestine	Stomach	Triple heater	Bladder Small intestine	Gallbladder
Sense	Smell	Taste	Speech	Hearing	Sight
Organ	Nose	Mouth, lips	Tongue	Ears	Eyes
Liquid	Mucus	Saliva	Sweat	Urine	Tears
Color	White	Yellow	Red	Blue/black	Green
Expression	Weeping	Singing	Laughing	Groaning	Shouting
Extreme emotion	Grief, anxiety	Worry,	reminiscence	Shock, overjoy	Fear
Anger					
Balanced emotion	Openness, receptivity	Sympathy, empathy	Joy, compassion	Resolution, trust	Assertion, motivation
Taste	Pungent, spicy	Sweet	Bitter, burned	Salty	Sour
Season	Fall	Indian summer	Summer	Winter	Spring
Related activity	Releasing	Thinking	Inspiration	Willpower and intimacy	Planning and decision-making
Times	Lung, 3–5 a.m.	Stomach, 7–9 a.m.	Heart, 11 a.m.–1 p.m.	Bladder, 3–5 p.m.	Gallbladder, 11 p.m.–1 a.m.
	Large intestine, 5–7 a.m.	Spleen, 9–11 a.m.	Small intestine, 1–3 p.m.	Kidney, 5–7 p.m. Triple heater, 9–11 p.m.	Pericardium, 7–9 p.m. Liver, 1–3 a.m.

Source: Fritz S, Chaitow L, Hymel GM: *Clinical massage in the healthcare setting*, St Louis, 2007, Mosby.

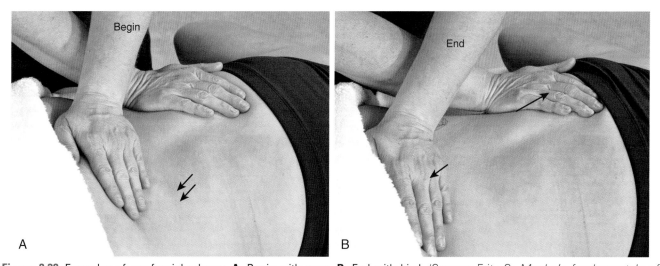

Figure 3.38 Examples of myofascial release. **A**, Begin with ease. **B**, End with bind. (Source: Fritz S: *Mosby's fundamentals of therapeutic massage*, ed 7, St Louis, 2021, Mosby.)

parasympathetic stimulation produced by massage can increase appetite and improve digestion. Massage can also improve sleep. Periods of insomnia or disrupted sleep patterns can occur as part of the aging process. Improved sleep supports restorative mechanisms and increases vitality. Any additional health concerns should be addressed, as appropriate, in the massage, with awareness that healing occurs more slowly, and adaptive mechanisms are not as effective as in younger clients. The massage application should not tire or stress the person.

Mental Health Conditions

Mental health is necessary for fitness of the body, mind, and spirit. The stresses of life strain mental health mechanisms. Mental health conditions usually consist of biologic factors, and pharmacologic treatment is an important aspect of mental healthcare that may be coupled with behavioral therapy or counseling. Psychologists and psychiatrists are the primary healthcare professionals who treat clients with mental health conditions, although nursing specialists and licensed counselors also may be involved.

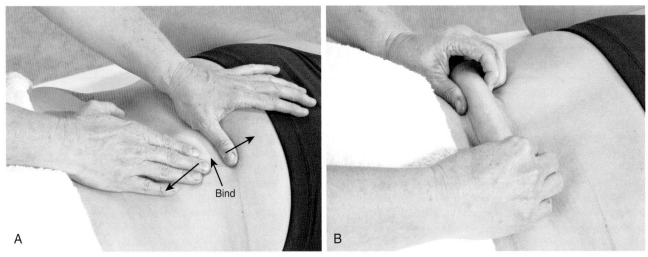

A

B

Figure 3.39 Focused tissue stretch/elongation. **A**, Bind. **B**, Lift to bind. (Source: Fritz S: *Mosby's fundamentals of therapeutic massage*, ed 7, St Louis, 2021, Mosby.)

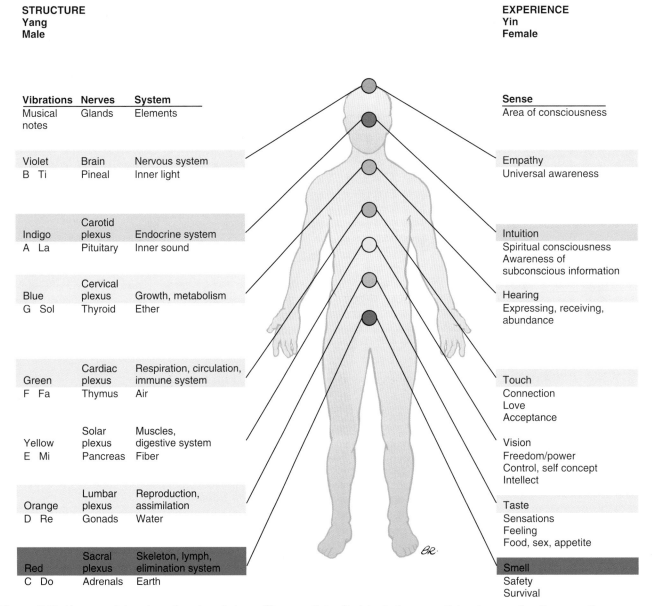

STRUCTURE
Yang
Male

EXPERIENCE
Yin
Female

Vibrations	Nerves	System
Musical notes	Glands	Elements
Violet B Ti	Brain Pineal	Nervous system Inner light
Indigo A La	Carotid plexus Pituitary	Endocrine system Inner sound
Blue G Sol	Cervical plexus Thyroid	Growth, metabolism Ether
Green F Fa	Cardiac plexus Thymus	Respiration, circulation, immune system Air
Yellow E Mi	Solar plexus Pancreas	Muscles, digestive system Fiber
Orange D Re	Lumbar plexus Gonads	Reproduction, assimilation Water
Red C Do	Sacral plexus Adrenals	Skeleton, lymph, elimination system Earth

Sense
Area of consciousness

Empathy
Universal awareness

Intuition
Spiritual consciousness
Awareness of subconscious information

Hearing
Expressing, receiving, abundance

Touch
Connection
Love
Acceptance

Vision
Freedom/power
Control, self concept
Intellect

Taste
Sensations
Feeling
Food, sex, appetite

Smell
Safety
Survival

Figure 3.40 Name and location of major chakras. (Source: Fritz S: *Mosby's essential sciences for therapeutic massage: anatomy, physiology, biomechanics, and pathology*, ed 6, St Louis, 2021, Mosby.)

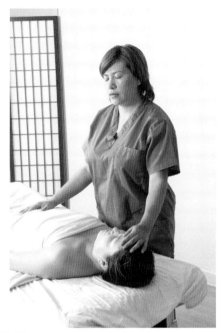

Figure 3.41 Therapist touching supine client in a quiet, focused manner. (Source: Salvo SG: *Massage therapy: principles and practice*, ed 4, St Louis, 2011, Saunders.)

Massage Strategies

Massage can be a very effective part of mental healthcare, especially for stress management. Massage affects brain chemicals by encouraging the release or utilization of serotonin, dopamine, endocannabinoids, and endorphins, which alter mood. It also affects the release of various action hormones that influence mood. Massage has a strong normalizing effect on the autonomic nervous system and can support other medical interventions for psychiatric disorders.

Pediatrics

The pediatric population starts with infancy and runs through the end of adolescence. This population is identified for special consideration because the very young are prone to illness, and adolescents experience extreme physical changes. Massage is a valuable treatment option for various conditions that develop within this population. Massage therapists are likely to find themselves teaching parents and other caregivers how to use massage to benefit a child.

The first group includes infants from birth to 3 years of age, which represents the toddler phase. A baby grows rapidly and completes the developmental process of the nervous system by at least 24 months of age. The next group, which represents the childhood phase, includes children from age 3 to the onset of puberty. Puberty can begin anywhere from 8 or 9 years of age to 15 years. Childhood typically is a stable health period allowing for physical growth and accumulated experience. Adolescence, the final phase in this part, begins with the onset of puberty and lasts until physical maturation.

Massage Strategies

All massage for infants and for minors up to 18 years of age must be done with specific parental informed consent and supervision. In the medical setting, supervision can be provided by medical personnel. The massage should follow an organized sequence, be rhythmic, and typically consist of slow gliding and gentle kneading with lubricant. It should exert sufficient pressure to stimulate the relaxation response. A light touch should be avoided because it is arousing and can trigger the tickle response. The massage should never be painful, and it is important to monitor for pain behavior such as flinching, changes in facial expression, and changes in breathing. The massage typically lasts 15–30 minutes, depending on the baby's tolerance. The lubricant should be very basic and safe for the baby's skin. Lubricants with scents or other additives should be avoided.

Medical concerns with this population include most of the potential injuries and illnesses discussed in this text. Identifying any trends based on age is difficult, but some patterns may be noted. For example, infants are prone to infection or may be dealing with birth trauma issues. Many genetic disorders are identified at this time.

Children are more apt to suffer an injury, such as falling, but concern increases with early development of stress-related diseases such as headache and stomachache. Learning disabilities usually are identified at this age. Also, some types of cancer occur more often in children, and asthma, juvenile diabetes, or rheumatoid arthritis may develop during the childhood phase.

Adolescents are most often injured in car accidents or suffer sports-type injuries. They also may have substance abuse problems, eating disorders, and early symptoms of autoimmune disease. Because of a tendency to have suppressed immune function related to lifestyle (e.g., lack of sleep, poor eating habits), adolescents are susceptible to viral infection. Type 2 diabetes is appearing in adolescents at an alarming rate. Girls may have menstrual difficulties, and adolescent sexual activity increases the potential for sexually transmitted disease.

Physical Impairments

A disability is any condition of the body or mind (impairment) that makes it more difficult for the person with the condition to do certain activities (activity limitation) and interact with the world around them (participation restrictions). Although "people with disabilities" sometimes refer to a single population, this is actually a diverse group of people with a wide range of needs. Two people with the same type of disability can be affected in very different ways. Some disabilities may be hidden or not easy to see.

Many types of disabilities can affect a person:

Vision
Movement
Thinking
Remembering
Learning
Communicating
Hearing
Mental health
Social relationships

Impairment is an absence of or significant difference in a person's body structure or function or mental functioning. For example, problems in the structure of the brain can result in difficulty with mental functions, or problems with the

TABLE 3.3 Examples of Essential Oils and Their Uses

Essential Oil	Characteristics	Uses
Balsam fir	Fresh, balsamic aroma	Used to relieve muscle aches and pains; relieve anxiety and stress-related conditions; fight colds, flu, and infections; and relieve bronchitis and coughs.
Black pepper	Warm, peppery aroma	Used to energize; increase circulation; warm and relieve muscle aches and stiffness; and fight colds, flu, and infections. Use with care; only a small amount is required (3–5 drops in 1 ounce of carrier oil).
Eucalyptus	Strong camphoraceous aroma	Used for colds, as a decongestant to relieve asthma and fever, for its bactericidal and antiviral actions, and to ease aching joints. Do not use if you or your patient has high blood pressure or epilepsy.
Geranium	Leafy, roselike scent	Used to reduce stress and tension, ease pain, balance emotions and hormones, ease premenstrual syndrome (PMS), relieve fatigue and nervous exhaustion, lift depression, and lessen fluid retention.
German chamomile	Strong, sweet, warm herbaceous aroma, blue, has many of the same properties as Roman chamomile, but its much higher azulene content gives it greater antiinflammatory activity	Used to relieve muscle pain; heal skin inflammation, acne, and wounds; also used as a sedative to ease anxiety and nervous tension and help with sleeplessness. It should not be used during early pregnancy and may cause skin reactions in some people. Before using, test a small area of skin (e.g., the medial ankle) for a reaction.
Helichrysum	Intense aroma resembling honey and tea	Used to heal bruises (internal and external), wounds, and scars; to detoxify the body, cleanse the blood, and enhance lymphatic drainage; heal colds, flu, sinusitis, and bronchitis; and relieve melancholy, migraines, stress, and tension.
Juniper berry	Fresh, pine needle aroma	Used to energize and relieve exhaustion, ease inflammation and spasms, improve mental clarity and memory, purify the body, lessen fluid retention, and disinfect. It should not be used in pregnant patients or those with kidney disease.
Lavender	Fresh, sweet scent	Used to balance emotions; relieve stress, tension, and headache; promote restful sleep; heal the skin; lower high blood pressure; help breathing; and disinfect.
Lemongrass	Powerful lemon-like aroma	Used to relieve muscle pain; ease headaches, nervous exhaustion, and other stress-related problems; and promote circulation. Use with care; only a small amount is required (3–5 drops in 1 ounce of carrier oil). Do not use during pregnancy.
Peppermint	Sweet, minty aroma	Used to boost energy, brighten mood, reduce pain, help breathing, and improve mental clarity and memory. Skin test required because it may irritate sensitive skin. Do not use during pregnancy.
Pine	Strong, coniferous, woodsy aroma	Used to ease breathing, as an immune system stimulant, to enhance energy, and to relieve muscle and joint aches.
Rosemary	Camphoraceous aroma	Used to energize, relieve muscle pains, cramps, or sprains; brighten mood and improve mental clarity and memory; ease pain; relieve headaches; and disinfect. Do not use if you or your patient is pregnant, is epileptic, or has high blood pressure.
Tea tree	Spicy, medicinal aroma; scientifically, one of the most extensively researched oils	Used as an immunostimulant, particularly against bacteria, viruses, and fungi; also used to relieve inflammation and disinfect.
Thyme	Sweet, intense, medicinal herb aroma	Used to inhibit infectious diseases, treat colds and bronchitis, relieve muscle aches and pains, aid concentration and memory, and relieve fatigue.

Source: Fritz S, Chaitow L, Hymel GM: *Clinical massage in the healthcare setting*, St Louis, 2007, Mosby.

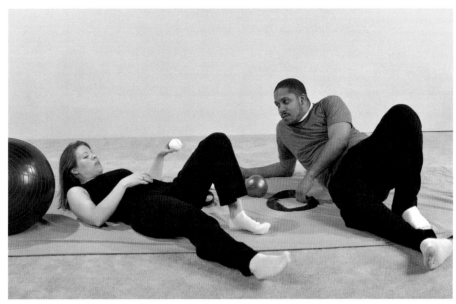

Figure 3.42 Self-help. (Source: Fritz S: *Mosby's fundamentals of therapeutic massage*, ed 5, St Louis, 2012, Mosby.)

structure of the eyes or ears can result in difficulty with the functions of vision or hearing.

The most commonly cited definitions are those provided by the World Health Organization (1980) in The International Classification of Impairments, Disabilities, and Handicaps:

Impairment—loss or abnormality of psychological, physiological, or anatomical structure or function.

Disability—any restriction or lack (resulting from an impairment) of ability to perform an activity in the manner or within the range considered normal for a human being.

Handicap—a disadvantage for a given individual that limits or prevents the fulfillment of a role that is normal.

As traditionally used, impairment refers to a problem with a structure or organ of the body; disability is a functional limitation with regard to a particular activity; and handicap refers to a disadvantage in filling a role in life relative to a peer group.

Note: The International Classification of Impairments, Disabilities, and Handicaps (ICIDH) has been succeeded by The International Classification of Functioning, Disability, and Health (ICF). The ICF is structured around three broader categories: body function/structure, activities, and information on severity/environmental factors. It is important to stay up to date regarding the labeling of persons and groups. The term "handicap" can be very offensive (ICD-ICF—International Classification of Functioning, Disability and Health [cdc.gov]).

Individuals with physical impairments can benefit from massage for all the same reasons that any other person can. These individuals often require ongoing medical treatment for rehabilitation and support services to treat illness related to the disability. They may develop compensation patterns in response to the disability. For instance, a person in a wheelchair may have increased neck and shoulder tension from moving the chair. In addition, dealing with a physical impairment can make routine daily functions more stressful. Following are some guidelines that may help

the massage therapist provide supportive services for these individuals:

- The massage therapist must never presume to know, understand, or anticipate a person's need for assistance. It is important to ask!
- A concerned massage therapist does not try to pretend that the condition does not exist, but rather responds professionally. After the individual has provided the necessary information about the condition and the accommodation required, the massage therapist should accept the impairment as part of how the person functions and should structure the treatment plan to meet the outcomes targeted for massage application.

Persons with a physical impairment often require some sort of accommodation, such as barrier-free access, restroom support, braille labeling, noninterference with service animals, etc.

Accommodating a Client With Visual Impairment

Many individuals with a visual impairment have some type of sight. Comparatively few people have no vision at all.

The conversation should begin with the massage therapist addressing the person by name, so that the person is aware that the therapist is speaking to them. It is not necessary to speak more loudly to individuals with a visual impairment; they usually can hear just fine. The therapist then should state his or her name but should not touch the individual until the person is aware of the therapist's presence in the room.

When assisting a client with a visual impairment, the therapist should never push or pull on the person. Instead, if guiding is necessary, the therapist should stand just in front and a bit to the left of the client, who can touch the massage therapist's right elbow when following.

Useful directions should be given to a person with a visual impairment. If asked where something is, the massage therapist should not point and say "over there." Instead, directions such as left, right, about 10 steps, and so on are much easier to

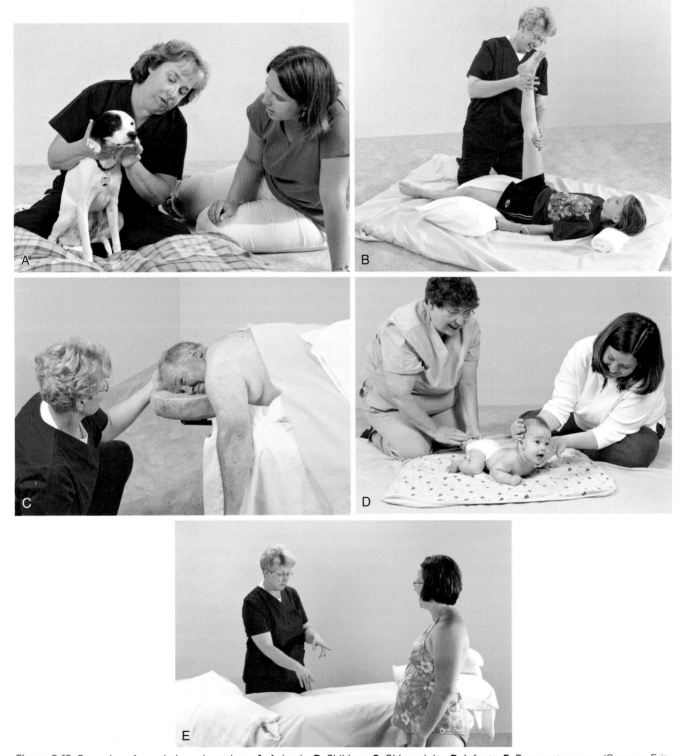

Figure 3.43 Examples of population adaptations. **A**, Animals. **B**, Children. **C**, Older adults. **D**, Infants. **E**, Pregnant person. (Source: Fritz S: *Mosby's fundamentals of therapeutic massage*, ed 5, St Louis, 2012, Mosby.)

follow. If a person with a visual impairment places anything anywhere, it should not be moved. If a door is opened, the direction of the opening (toward or away from the person) and the location of the hinges (left or right) should be explained. Allowing these clients to open the door on their own will help them to better orient to its position.

If a service dog is harnessed and working, whether it is a guide dog for someone with a visual impairment or an animal trained for any other support service, do not pet, feed, or in any other way interact with the dog. This distracts the dog and makes its important job more difficult.

Accommodating a Client With a Speech Impairment

It may be difficult to understand a person with a speech condition. The massage therapist should ask the person to repeat anything that is unclear until it is understood and then should repeat what was said so the person can clarify if necessary. The therapist should let the client know if they cannot understand what is being said. If necessary, a notepad can be used to put communication in writing. Although having an accent is not speech impairment, it can make communication difficult. Not speaking the same language also hinders communication. An interpreter may be necessary.

Accommodating a Client With Hearing Loss

Within the Deaf community, "hearing impairment" is offensive. Use of the terms "hard of hearing" or "deaf" are culturally more appropriate. To gain the attention of a person who has hearing loss, the therapist should lightly tap the person once on the shoulder or should discreetly wave a hand. If no interpreter is present, all talking should be done in a normal tone and rhythm of speech. If an individual can lip-read, it is important that the massage therapist always face the person and not cover their mouth when talking. Normal voice tone and speed should be used. If the therapist normally speaks quickly, the speed should be slowed a bit. If necessary, a notepad can be used to put communication in writing.

Hearing aids amplify sound; they do not make sound clearer. Reducing background noise helps. It may be wise to ask before using any music during the massage session. Getting too close to a hearing aid can make it squeal, so be cautious when massaging near the ears.

Accommodating a Client With a Mobility Impairment

Many types of mobility impairment occur for many reasons. It is important to remember that not all people who use a wheelchair are paralyzed. Also, many people with paralysis are able to feel sensations on certain areas of their bodies.

When speaking to a person in a wheelchair, it is best to do so from eye level. Looking up strains the individual's neck. This process obviously requires the massage therapist to sit down.

A wheelchair must never be pushed unless the person in the chair gives permission. The individual also will give directions for pushing the wheelchair over barriers.

When transferring a client from a wheelchair to the massage table, the client can give the best directions on how to proceed. The most efficient transfer is a lateral transfer to a table that is of the same height as the wheelchair. If the massage table does not have motorized height adjustment, a shift in body mechanics by the massage therapist is necessary. If necessary, massage can be provided in the chair.

Special care must be taken in giving a massage to a person with paralysis because normal feedback mechanisms may not be functioning. A person who has undergone amputation and

uses a prosthesis may or may not want the device removed during the massage; whereas one patient may readily remove the prosthesis, another may not. Ask permission before massaging the amputated area. If the client is comfortable with this, massage can be especially beneficial. Often the goal for the massage is relief of phantom pain, which requires massage at the site of the amputation.

Accommodating Size Requirements

A stool may be needed to help short clients reach the massage table, clothing hangers, or restroom fixtures. The massage professional should sit down casually to establish eye contact, so that the client does not have to look up, which strains the neck.

A very large person may not trust the massage table and may be more comfortable on a floor mat. Getting up and down from the floor may be difficult. Sometimes, seated massage is the better option. Ask the client what is preferable. If the therapist is nervous about doing the massage on the massage table, the client must be told (which is disclosure on the part of the massage therapist), because the therapist's anxiety will affect the quality of the massage.

Accommodating Clients With Physical Changes Caused by Burns, Trauma, Disease, or Congenital Conditions

Physical changes in appearance can be related to many conditions. Only those related to scar tissue formation or nerve damage might be addressed with massage therapy. Individuals who have been burned may face an assortment of challenges ranging from impaired mobility to altered appearance. As burns heal, scar tissue replaces functional epithelial tissue. All functions of the skin, including excretion, sensation, and protection, are compromised. Scar tissue tends to contract and pull, which can make the area of the healed burn feel shortened or tight and binding. Severe contractures sometimes develop, which are treated medically. Myofascial release and other connective tissue techniques can soften connective tissue. Massage of this type may reduce the effect of this shrinkage somewhat.

Massage Strategies

It is not possible to describe specific massage strategies for persons with physical impairments. Clinical reasoning is the only appropriate method for determining the best way to provide massage in a safe manner and in a comfortable environment.

Pregnancy

Pregnancy is not an illness; it is a natural event. However, it is typically managed in the healthcare environment. Early prenatal care provided by qualified healthcare professionals is needed to ensure that proper nutrition is provided for the mother and that the pregnancy is progressing normally; it also allows early identification of any potential problems. Smoking and the use of alcohol and drugs are very dangerous to the unborn child. Excessive stress also is dangerous to the developing infant.

Pregnancy is divided into three distinct segments: the first, second, and third trimesters. Massage is appropriate during all stages of pregnancy and is altered as necessary to ensure the comfort of the mother-to-be. The assumption here is that the pregnancy is planned and desired, but remember, this is not always the case. Unplanned pregnancy can be very stressful.

Massage Strategies

Unless specific circumstances or complications are involved, massage during pregnancy should be a general massage. Do not massage vigorously or extremely deeply. Do not over-stretch, and do not massage the abdomen other than with superficial stroking. Positioning in side-lying is a common adaptation. As the pregnancy progresses it may be advantageous for the client to lay more on their left side. The vena cava is the main vein that drains the entire lower half of the body. As the baby gets bigger, lying flat obstructs blood flow up toward the heart. Decreased return of blood flow to the heart will cause hypotension. Thus, lying on the back (supine) is the worst possible position in the third trimester. Lying on the right side is better, but positioning on the left side will have the least amount of weight upon the vena cava. Watch for fever, edema, varicose veins, and severe mood swings. Pregnancy is a hypercoagulable state and with an increased risk of thrombosis. After birth, postpartum depression can become a serious problem for some. Immediately refer a client with these conditions to their physician.

Hospital/Healthcare-Based Massage

Special considerations arise for massage therapists who work with clients in medical environments (e.g., hospital, rehabilitation center, extended care facility, or mental health facility). An important factor to consider is that massage therapists must be willing to work in situations where there is an increased risk of disease transmission. Even when clients do may not have a contagious disease, if they are in a hospital setting or have a chronic condition, there may still be an increased risk of infection (e.g., methicillin-resistant *Staphylococcus aureus* [MRSA]). A massage career in the healthcare/medical setting requires an increased understanding of the indications, necessary adaptations, and potential contraindications for massage methods in relationship to each client's healthcare intervention. Massage therapists need to be able to adapt to the varied environments, equipment, and rules and regulations. Massage is offered in hospitals, physical therapy practices, private physicians' practices, mental health facilities, chiropractic clinics, long-term care facilities, hospice care, and home healthcare. Each setting has policies in place to support quality care. These policies generally involve compliance with the Health Insurance Portability and Accountability Act (HIPAA), standard precautions, professional conduct, supervisor hierarchy, and incident reporting procedures. Therefore, massage therapists who want to work in healthcare settings must be skilled and knowledgeable in the following areas:

- Infection control
- Sanitation measures
- Clinical reasoning and problem-solving
- Setting qualifiable and quantifiable goals
- Medical terminology
- Pathology

- Medications
- Assessment
- Development of treatment plans
- Analysis of the effectiveness of methods used
- Charting/documentation and record-keeping
- Effective communication of information with the rest of the healthcare team
- Recognizing that the healthcare team includes experts and ultimate authorities responsible for the patient's care
- Third-party insurance reimbursement requirements
- Compliance with HIPAA

Massage therapists must also have a basic understanding of various medical tests, procedures, and treatments so that they can make safe, beneficial decisions on ways to use massage to complement the medical treatments the patient is receiving. Hospital patient conditions that may benefit from massage include the following:

- *Pain.* Through the use of massage, the subjective experience of pain is diminished, even when the use of analgesics is reduced.
- *Anxiety.* Anxiousness caused by the hospital stay and fear of procedures is reduced.
- *Nausea.* The subjective experience of nausea and the use of antiemetics are reduced.
- *Stress.* Physiologic indicators of stress are diminished.
- *Sleep.* The ability to sleep more easily and for longer periods increases with massage.

A common theme in hospital-based massage is pain management. Massage is very effective at managing acute and chronic pain and supports other pain treatments, such as medication, ultrasound, and hydrotherapy. Massage for the hospital patient is not targeted specifically to the pathologic condition or injury; rather, it is intended to provide comfort care and symptom management.

The Importance of Palliative Care

The purpose of palliative care is to reduce suffering and create comfort. Massage offers comfort and relief from aching, all of which can reduce suffering. The massage used in palliative care is based on well-being and compassion, and the focus is on reducing discomfort and providing comfort. Gentle, nonspecific massage application is used. As a reminder, gentle pressure does not necessarily mean light pressure. Gentle means slow, focused, and pleasurable. Pressure typically is not deep; however, most patients enjoy a sense of pressure that feels good.

Recommendations for a gentle, soothing, palliative massage include the following:

- Make sure the client is in a comfortable position and is physically supported/bolstered.
- Use an approved lubricant when massaging to reduce friction and add moisture to the skin.
- Target areas that have the most discomfort (i.e., have limited movement). Massage is helpful in areas related to prolonged sitting or lying. Often the neck, shoulders, low back, and calves ache as a result of immobility.
- Determine what pressure or movement is the most helpful and adjust the level and focus of pressure in response to the patient's feedback.

- If a full-body massage is not possible, provide a hand and foot massage, which can provide a sense of comfort and well-being. Gentle yet firm movements should be used.
- Encourage the person to continue to tell you what is most helpful and to let you know right away if any method causes discomfort.
- Maintain the intention of reducing suffering by focusing attention on what feels good.

Typically, the massage lasts no longer than 45 minutes; 15–30 minutes in targeted areas may be sufficient.

Adapting to the Hospital Room

One of the biggest challenges massage therapists face in the hospital or long-term care setting is providing massage when individuals are unable to lie on a massage table. Often massage is provided in the hospital bed or a standard chair. In these situations, massage therapists must pay special attention to their body mechanics. Fortunately, deep pressure requiring a lot of leverage is not usually needed. If the hospital bed can move up and down, adjust the height to a comfortable level. When possible, avoid reaching; instead, stay as close to the patient as possible. If the patient's mobility is limited, placing one knee on the bed or sitting on the bed may be helpful. However, before doing this, clear with the individual who is supervising; in some cases this is not allowed. If you sit or kneel on the bed, use a clean towel as a sanitary barrier. Place it on the bed, then sit or kneel on it. Do not get into uncomfortable positions or keep changing your position because this could disturb the patient. It is important to note that it may not be possible to access all body areas.

Working Around Medical Devices

Working with individuals in hospital beds means that you must know how to operate the bed's controls. It also is important to be able to operate the nurse call buttons. Another challenge is working around various medical devices such as monitors, intravenous (IV) lines, and so on. Be cautious when moving around in the hospital room to avoid disturbing the equipment.

Avoid all areas where something enters or exits the body, such as IV lines, catheters, drains, respiratory devices, and so forth. Avoid all surgical sites. Do not disturb or remove any bandaging. If this should occur, immediately inform the nurse so that infection control is maintained. Be cautious when working around monitoring leads, and do not dislodge them. If this should occur, immediately call the nurse. Do not attempt to replace them, because proper placement is required for accurate information. Use only the lotion provided or approved by the hospital. Do not add anything to the lotion.

The Massage Therapist's Responsibilities to the Patient and Medical Personnel

- Do not attempt to help a patient out of bed to use the restroom or for any other activity. Do not assist a patient to move into various positions. It is better to let the person move, because he or she will be protective of sensitive areas.
- Be courteous to other patients who may be sharing a hospital room. However, do not provide massage if asked unless authorized to do so.
- Leave the room when the physician, nurses, or other hospital personnel are providing care.
- Massage therapy is almost always provided as optional care in the hospital or similar medical setting.

If a patient is sleeping or does not want a massage, do not insist. Report the situation to the supervising personnel.

Long-Term Care

Although not the same as a hospital, a long-term care facility is similar, because a variety of medically based services are provided to care for people with a chronic illness or disability. In addition, long-term care helps meet personal needs. Most long-term care provides people with support services for activities such as dressing, bathing, and using the toilet. Long-term care can be provided at home, in the community, in assisted living, or in nursing homes.

Massage therapy can be integrated into long-term care services. The same adaptations used for hospital patients can be used for long-term care residents.

Terminal Illness, End-of-Life Care, and Hospice Care

No one knows when a person is going to die. However, two very powerful psychological forces influence living and dying: hope and the will to live. Attitudes about death vary. Adults usually have more fears about death than children do. They fear pain, suffering, dying alone, invasion of privacy, loneliness, and separation from family and loved ones. They worry about who will care for and support those left behind. Elderly individuals usually have fewer of these fears than younger adults. They may be more accepting that death will occur and have had more experience with death and dying. Many have lost family members and friends. Some welcome death as freedom from pain, suffering, and disability.

When nothing further can be done to prolong life, care focuses on comfort measures. Hospice is a philosophy of care, not a place. Hospice care can be provided in a hospital or long-term care setting, a specific residential hospice setting, or, most commonly, in the home.

The experts in terminal illness are the dedicated hospice nurses and staff members who treat death with dignity. It has been said that the staff members of hospices are midwives to the dying.

Massage Strategies

To work successfully with those experiencing a terminal illness, the massage practitioner must be aware of their personal feelings about death. Massage professionals who want to work with clients during this very important, challenging, and special time of life are strongly encouraged to become hospice volunteers and to take the training that hospices offer.

Massage has much to offer in comfort measures for the terminally ill. Being bedridden and immobile is painful. Massage can distract the sensory perception and provide temporary comfort measures. It provides continued human contact and can give caregivers something useful, rewarding, and positive to do for their loved one who is dying.

Massage can also become an important stress-reduction method and a means of support for family members and caregivers. Caring for someone who is terminally ill can be very stressful. The support person may need to receive massage simply to have someone take care of him or her for an hour. Teaching simple massage methods to caregivers provides them with a means of meaningful and structured interaction with their loved one, as well as a means of connecting with and supporting each other.

The massage professional should be an integral part of the team that works to make this time of passage as gentle as possible. This means that once the decision to work with someone who is terminally ill has been made, it is important to stay with the process until the client dies, if possible. The massage therapist probably will grow to care for the person and will mourn and grieve when death comes.

As always, it remains the client's choice as to what the massage therapy will entail, and they must give informed consent. The individual who is dying needs to retain as much personal empowerment as possible. It should not be discouraging if all the practitioner is asked to do during a massage session is to stroke the person's hands.

Providing Massage in the Home

It is important to move efficiently into and out of the area without disrupting the natural rhythm of the environment. It is also important to respect the client's environment. Examples include removing shoes to protect the carpet and carrying special rubber-soled shoes to wear during the massage or wiping up water splashes in the restroom after washing your hands. It is important to make sure the massage equipment and lubricants do not damage the client's floors or walls. Place a sheet on the floor under the massage table to protect the flooring.

Among other concerns, confidentiality is extremely important when providing massage and needs to be preserved. Sometimes the intimacy of the environment makes it more difficult to maintain professional boundaries and time management without seeming distant and hurried. It takes longer to enter and exit the on-site environment, not just because of the equipment setup and breakdown, but also because of the need to be respectful of the area and polite. The personal safety of the massage professional is a concern because the on-site massage environment has fewer safeguards than an office setting. Get to know those living in the home ahead of time, make sure someone always knows where you are, and check in with that person. Always carry a cell phone with you.

Oncology

The treatment of cancer, called oncology, combines disease-specific scientific knowledge, public health awareness, and psychosocial sensitivity. Cancer refers to any one of a large number of diseases characterized by the development of abnormal cells that divide uncontrollably and have the ability to infiltrate (metastasize) and destroy normal body tissue. Tumors are cell masses that are either benign or malignant and cancerous. Not all tumors are cancerous, and not all cancers form tumors. For example, leukemia is a cancer that involves blood, bone marrow, the lymphatic system, and the spleen, but it does not form a single mass or tumor. Not only do cancerous cells always invade and destroy normal tissue; they can also produce chemicals that interfere with body functions. For example, some lung cancers secrete chemicals that alter the levels of calcium in the blood, affecting nerves and muscles and causing weakness and dizziness.

Once cancer has been diagnosed, the care of the oncology patient begins with a detailed history and physical examination. Most people with cancer receive some type of therapy once a histologic diagnosis has been made. Treatment for cancer can be curative or palliative. Staging is the process of finding out how much cancer there is in the body and where it is located. Accurate staging provides a basis for both the provider and the patient to weigh individual benefits and risks associated with a treatment.

Whether treatment has a curative or a palliative intent, success depends on the patient's disease stage and acceptance of the treatment plan. If the intent of therapy is curative, both the oncology team and the patient are more apt to accept the harshness and toxicities of treatment.

Therapeutic Massage Strategies During Cancer Treatment

Massage is accepted as part of a multidisciplinary approach to cancer treatment. Massage intervention spans the time of treatment, recovery, and return to health. The benefits of massage are obvious: stress management, preoperative and postoperative pain management, management of treatment side effects, and more. There are no specific protocols for massage and cancer care. The person undergoing cancer treatment will need to be evaluated before each session, and the massage treatment must be based on the individual's status at that time.

The concern that massage increases metastasis is unfounded. However, it is prudent not to massage over any type of tissue masses. Specific, extensive, full-body lymphatic drainage may task already compromised immune function and should not be used. The areas of radiation treatment need to be avoided, because the skin is damaged by the treatment.

Cautions for Massage

- Avoid all sources of heat (hot water bottles, heating pads, and sun lamps) on the treatment field.
- Avoid exposing the treatment area to cold temperatures (ice bags or cold water treatment).
- Avoid any form of saltwater treatment.
- Avoid the use of all lotions or oils on the skin in the treatment field and use only approved lotion during massage.
- Avoid direct massage of the treatment area other than light application of an approved lotion.

Bones under areas of radiation treatment can be brittle; therefore, massage pressure levels need to be carefully monitored. Do not use any massage methods that may cause tissue damage, because chemotherapy reduces the body's ability to repair tissues.

The general protocol may be too intense during cancer treatment, but a modified palliative protocol may be appropriate.

SANITATION AND STANDARD PRECAUTIONS

- An important consideration in all licensing exams is public safety. To protect the public, it is necessary to understand how a sanitary environment can be maintained (Figures 3.44 and 3.45, Table 3.4, and Boxes 3.3 and 3.4).

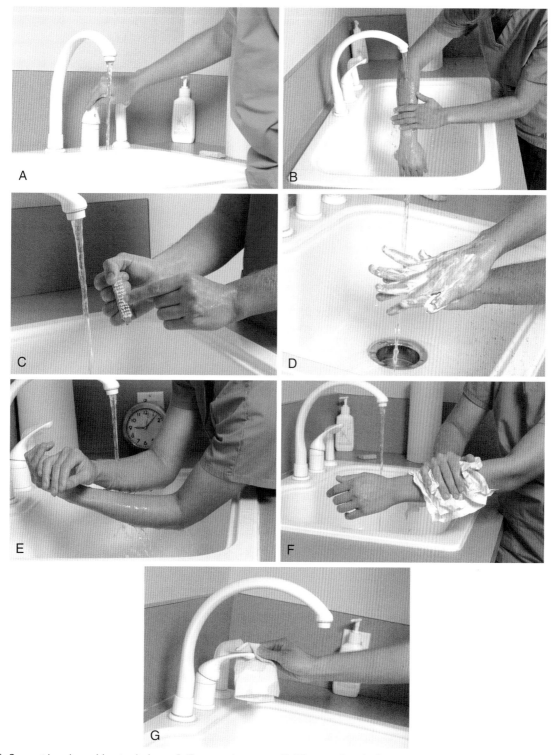

Figure 3.44 Correct hand-washing technique. **A**, Turn on the water. **B**, Wet your hands, forearms, and elbow. **C**, Clean underneath your fingernails. **D**, Soap your hands. **E**, Rinse your hands thoroughly. **F**, Dry your hands. **G**, Turn off the water. (Source: Sorrentino SA: *Mosby's textbook for nursing assistants*, ed 8, St Louis, 2012, Mosby.)

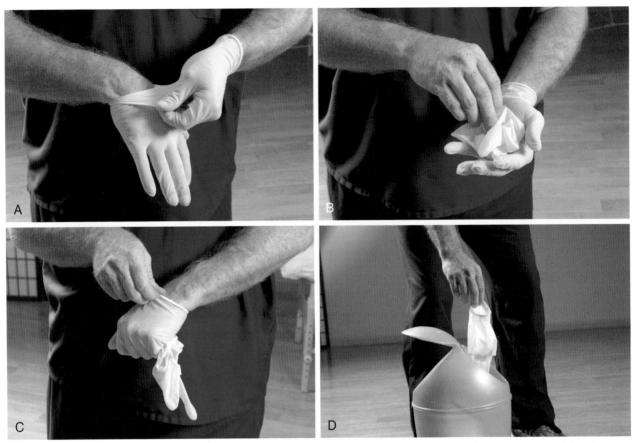

Figure 3.45 Proper removal of disposable gloves. **A,** Pulling off one glove. **B,** Putting the removed glove in the palm of the gloved hand. **C,** Removing the other glove with the first removed glove inside. **D,** Disposing of the used gloves. (Source: Salvo SG: *Massage therapy: principles and practice,* ed 4, St Louis, 2011, Saunders.)

TABLE 3.4	Common Aseptic Techniques for Preventing the Spread of Pathogens	
Sterilization	Destroys all organisms by means of heat	Pressurized steam bath, extreme temperature, irradiation
Disinfection	Destroys most pathogens (but not necessarily all microbes) on inanimate objects	Chemicals (e.g., iodine, chlorine, alcohol, soap)
Isolation	Separates potentially infectious individuals or materials from uninfected individuals	Quarantining infected clients; wearing protective apparel while giving treatments; sanitary transport, storage, and disposal of body fluids, tissues, and other materials

Source: Fritz S: *Mosby's fundamentals of therapeutic massage,* ed 7, St Louis, 2021, Mosby.

BOX 3.3	**Sanitation Practices for Massage Professionals**

The following covers sanitation requirements for practicing massage professionals. The massage professional must clean and wash the hands and forearms or feet thoroughly with soap, detergent, or antibacterial/antiviral agents before touching each client.

- Any professional known to be infected with any communicable disease or to be a carrier of such disease, or who has an infected wound or open lesion on any exposed portion of the body, is excluded from practicing massage until the communicable condition is alleviated.
- The professional must wear clean clothing. If at all possible, lockers or closets for personnel should be maintained apart from the massage room for the storage of personal clothing and effects.
- All doors and windows opening to the outside must be tight fitting and must ensure the exclusion of flies, insects, rodents, and other vermin. All floors, walks, and furniture must be kept clean, well maintained, and in good repair.
- All rooms in which massage is practiced must meet the following requirements: (1) heating must be adequate to maintain a room air temperature of 75°F; (2) ventilation must be sufficient to promote air exchange; and (3) lighting fixtures must be capable of producing a minimum of five foot-candles of light at floor level; this level of lighting should be used during cleaning.
- All sewage and liquid waste must be disposed of in a municipal sewage system or an approved septic system. All interior water distribution piping should be installed and maintained in conformity with the state plumbing code. The water supply must be adequate, deemed safe by the health department, and sanitary. Drinking fountains of an approved type or individual paper drinking cups should be provided for the convenience of employees and patrons.
- Every massage business must have a sanitary toilet facility with an adequate supply of hot and cold water under pressure, and it must be conveniently located for use by employees and patrons. Bathroom doors must be tight fitting, and the rooms must be kept clean, in good repair, and free of flies, insects, and vermin. A supply of soap in a covered dispenser and single-use sanitary towels in a dispenser must be provided at each lavatory installation, as well as a covered waste receptacle for proper disposal; a supply of toilet paper on a dispenser must be available for each toilet.
- Lavatory and toilet rooms must be equipped with fly-tight containers for garbage and refuse. These containers should be easily cleanable, well maintained, and in good repair. Any refuse must be disposed of in a sanitary manner.
- Massage lubricants, including but not limited to oil, alcohol, powders, and lotions, should be dispensed from suitable containers, to be used and stored in such a manner as to prevent contamination. The bulk lubricant must not come in contact with the massage professional. It should be poured, squeezed, or shaken into a separate container or the massage professional's hand. Any unused lubricant that comes into contact with the client or massage professional must be discarded.
- The use of unclean linen is prohibited. Only freshly laundered sheets and linens should be used for massage. All single-service materials and clean linens should be stored at least 4 inches off the floor in shelves, compartments, or cabinets used for that purpose only. All soiled linens must be placed in a covered receptacle immediately and kept there until washed in detergent and an antiviral cleaning agent (e.g., a 10% bleach solution, one part bleach to nine parts water) in a washing machine that provides a hot water temperature of at least 140°F.
- Massage tables must be covered with impervious material that is cleanable and must be kept clean and in good repair. Equipment that comes in contact with the client must be cleaned thoroughly with soap or other suitable detergent and water, followed by adequate sanitation procedures before use with each individual client (a 10% bleach solution, made daily, is recommended). All equipment must be clean, well maintained, and in good repair.
- When cleaning the massage area, observe the following rules:
  - Do not shake linen, and dust with a damp cloth to minimize the movement of dust.
  - Clean from the cleanest area to the dirtiest. This prevents soiling of a clean area.
  - Clean away from your body and uniform. If you dust, brush, or wipe toward yourself, microorganisms will be transmitted to your skin, hair, and uniform.
  - Store used linens in a closed bag or container while in the massage room or during transport.
- Floors are dirty; any object that falls on the floor should not be used on or for a client.

Modified from Oregon Board of Massage Technicians: Sanitation requirements for the state of Oregon, Oregon Administrative Rules, November 2006. Source: This text was produced from material provided by Archives Division of the Secretary of State of Oregon. The official copy of an Oregon Administration Rules is contained in the Administrative Order filed at the Archives Division, 800 Summer St., NE, Salem, Oregon 97310. Any discrepancies with the published version are satisfied in favor of the Administrative Order. The Oregon Administrative Rules and the Oregon Bulletin are copyrighted by the Oregon Secretary of State.

BOX 3.4   **Standard Precautions and Transmission-Based Precautions**

Standard precautions synthesize the major features of universal precautions (blood and body fluids), which are designed to reduce the risk of transmission of blood-borne pathogens, and body substance isolation, which is designed to reduce the risk of transmission of pathogens from moist body substances. Standard precautions apply to (1) blood; (2) all body fluids, secretions, and excretions, except sweat, regardless of whether they contain visible blood; (3) nonintact skin; and (4) mucous membranes. Standard precautions are designed to reduce the risk of transmission of microorganisms from recognized and unrecognized sources of infection in hospitals. Transmission-Based Precautions are the second tier of basic infection control and are to be used in addition to Standard Precautions for patients who may be infected or colonized with certain infectious agents for which additional precautions are needed to prevent infection transmission. Personal Protective Equipment (PPE) coupled with sanitation methods are aspects of Standard precautions. Examples of PPE include: gloves, goggles, face shields, face masks, and respiratory protection, when appropriate.

Hand Washing and Gloving

Hand washing is considered by many to be the single most important measure for reducing the risk of transmitting organisms from one person to another or from one site to another on the same patient. Washing your hands as promptly and thoroughly as possible between clients is very important. In addition to hand washing, gloves play an important role in reducing the risk of transmission of microorganisms.

Gloves are worn for two important reasons: (1) to provide a protective barrier and (2) to reduce the likelihood that microorganisms on the massage practitioner's hands will be transmitted to clients. Wearing gloves does not replace the need for hand washing because gloves may have small, inapparent defects or may be torn during use, and hands can become contaminated during the removal of gloves. Gloves must be changed and discarded after each use.

A mask provides protection against the spread of infectious large-particle droplets that are transmitted by close contact and that generally travel only short distances (up to 3 feet) from infected patients who are coughing or sneezing.

Gowns and Protective Apparel

Various types of gowns and protective apparel are worn to provide barrier protection and to reduce the opportunity for transmission of microorganisms in medical settings.

Immunocompromised Clients

Standard precautions (or the equivalent) are used for the care of all clients.

Hand Washing

1. Wash the hands after touching blood, body fluids, secretions, excretions, and contaminated items, regardless of whether gloves are worn. Wash the hands immediately after removing gloves, between client contacts, and when otherwise indicated, to avoid transfer of microorganisms to other clients or environments. It may be necessary to wash the hands between tasks and procedures on the same client to prevent cross-contamination of different body sites.
2. Use a plain (nonantimicrobial) soap for routine hand washing.
3. Use an antimicrobial agent or a waterless antiseptic agent if hand washing is not possible.

Gloves

1. Wear gloves (clean, nonsterile gloves are adequate) when touching blood, body fluids, secretions, excretions, and contaminated items. Put on clean gloves just before touching mucous membranes and nonintact skin.
2. Change gloves between tasks and procedures on the same client after contact with material that may contain a high concentration of microorganisms.
3. Remove gloves promptly after use, before touching uncontaminated items and environmental surfaces, and before going to another client, and wash hands immediately to avoid transferring microorganisms to other clients or environments.

Mask, Eye Protection, and Face Shield

Wear a mask and eye protection or a face shield to protect the mucous membranes of the eyes, nose, and mouth during procedures and client care activities that are likely to generate splashes of body fluids, secretions, and excretions.

Gown

Wear a gown (a clean, nonsterile gown is adequate) to protect skin and to prevent soiling of clothing during procedures and client care activities that are likely to generate splashes or sprays of blood, body fluids, secretions, or excretions. Select a gown that is appropriate for the activity and the amount of fluid likely to be encountered. Remove a soiled gown as promptly as possible, and wash hands to avoid transfer of microorganisms to other clients or environments.

ASSESSMENT AND TREATMENT/ CARE PLAN DEVELOPMENT

The massage therapist needs to be able to perform basic assessment procedures to determine regional and general contraindications, to plan for referrals, and to support treatment plan development (Figures 3.46 through 3.55, Table 3.5, and Boxes 3.5 and 3.6).

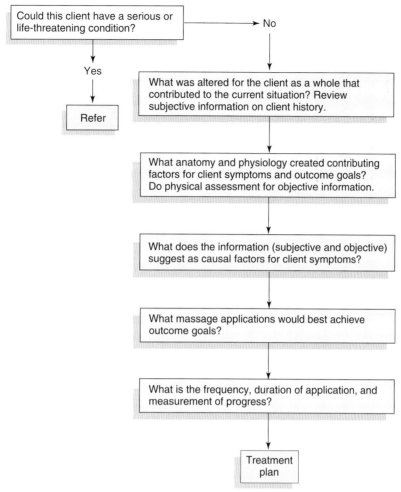

Figure 3.46 The development of a care/treatment plan.

PATHOLOGY

A major goal of licensing exams is to provide measures to ensure that those who receive a massage are safe. Many questions are related to pathology, confirming the massage professional can make responsible decisions about when to massage, when to refer, and when to alter massage application. Appendix A provides more in-depth information on pathology.

CONTRAINDICATIONS REQUIRING AVOIDANCE OF MASSAGE OR ALTERATION OF APPLICATION

Some conditions may give rise to contraindications that require the massage therapist to change the method of application or forgo the massage entirely:
- Acute illness and injury
- Acute or severe cardiac, liver, or kidney disease
- Contagious condition
- Loss of sensation
- Loss of voluntary movement

- Medication that "thins the blood" by interfering with coagulation, whether a prescription drug (e.g., warfarin [Coumadin], Plavix) or a nonprescription drug (e.g., aspirin)
- Systemic infection and acute inflammation
- Use of sensation-altering substances, whether prescribed (e.g., pain medication) or recreational (e.g., alcohol)

Specific Conditions That Present Contraindications

Acute Local Soft Tissue Inflammation

Acute inflammation can occur in any of the soft tissues, such as the skin (wounds and blisters), muscles, tendons, ligaments, bursae, synovial capsule, intervertebral disk, and periosteum. Common causes of acute inflammation are overuse, illness, injury, and surgery; common symptoms include pain and dysfunction in the affected area, heat and redness, and swelling local to the injury.

Superficial signs and symptoms usually are easy to identify. However, when inflammation occurs in deep tissues, the symptoms may not be visible, only palpable. Upon palpation,

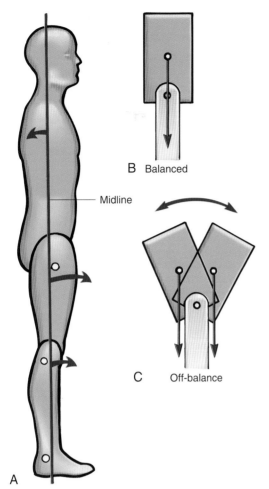

Figure 3.47 Concepts of posture assessment. (Source: Fritz S: *Mosby's fundamentals of therapeutic massage*, ed 5, St Louis, 2012, Mosby.)

Muscle Strength Grading Scale (Oxford Scale)
Medical Research Council [MRC] grading scale

Grade	Value	Muscle Strength
5	Normal	Complete range of motion (ROM) against gravity with full resistance
4	Good	• Complete ROM against gravity with some resistance: Full range of motion with decreased strength • (sometimes this category is subdivided further into $4^-/5$, 4/5, and $4^+/5$)
3	Fair	Complete ROM against gravity with no resistance; active ROM
2	Poor	Complete ROM with some assistance and gravity eliminated
1	Trace	Evidence of slight muscular contraction, no joint motion evident
0	Zero	No evidence of muscle contraction NT: Not testable

Figure 3.48 Muscle strength grading scale (Oxford scale). (Source: Whaley L, Wong D: *Nursing care of infants and children*, ed 3, St Louis, 1987, Mosby.)

areas of acute inflammation deep in the tissues feel hard and denser than surrounding tissue. Focused pressure may cause a sharp pain. These symptoms could indicate an acute problem that requires caution in massage application with a focus on lymphatic drainage.

To test for acute inflammation, apply enough pressure to the area to cause mild discomfort. Maintain this fixed pressure for up to 10 seconds. If the discomfort increases, this suggests that the tissues are in an acute state; if it decreases, it generally is safe to apply massage.

Bone and Joint Injuries

Fractures tend to cause pain and tenderness around the injury site with any movement or weight bearing. Stress fractures are difficult to diagnose. Be especially concerned if the pain persists and is accompanied by swelling and bruising in the injured area. Massage is obviously contraindicated in the acute stage of these conditions because it would cause further damage. Surgery that involves the cutting of bone (e.g., joint replacement, open heart surgery) also creates fracture-like conditions.

Myositis Ossificans

A large hematoma that occurs with a deep bruise and that goes untreated for a long time may ossify and form small pieces of bone material in the soft tissues. This is more likely to happen when a fracture is also involved because osteoblasts move into the tissues and can serve as the catalyst for calcification. Massage over the area could cause the pieces of bone to damage the surrounding soft tissues. This is a local contraindication; therefore, the area should be avoided. Although myositis ossificans is a rare condition, it should be considered a possibility if the history reveals a long recovery from a serious fracture or other major impact trauma.

Deep Vein Thrombosis

During the application of massage, a thrombus (blood clot) can form in a vein and become dislodged, or a fragment may break off and travel in the bloodstream (embolus). This is a rare occurrence, but because the results are life-threatening, extreme caution is required. The veins typically affected are those in the calf and hamstring areas. Because the veins get larger as they travel toward the heart, the clot can pass through the chambers of the heart and into the pulmonary circulation. The vessels become smaller as they divide up into the lungs, and the clot eventually blocks the vessels, occluding an area of the lung. A large clot can block the circulation to a major part of the lung (pulmonary embolism), and death can

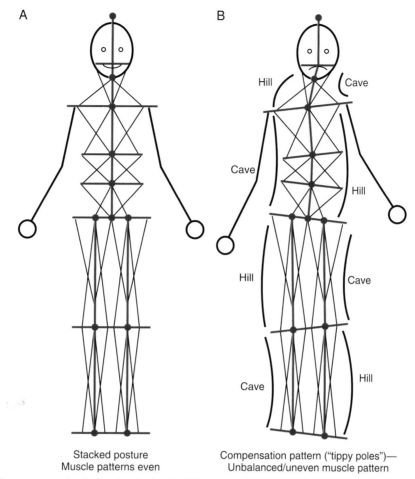

A

B

Hill   Cave

Cave

Hill

Hill   Cave

Cave   Hill

Stacked posture
Muscle patterns even

Compensation pattern ("tippy poles")—
Unbalanced/uneven muscle pattern

Figure 3.49 Postural influences on the body. Stacked pole **(A)** versus tippy pole **(B)**. Fritz S: *Mosby's fundamentals of therapeutic massage*, ed 7, St Louis, 2021, Mosby.

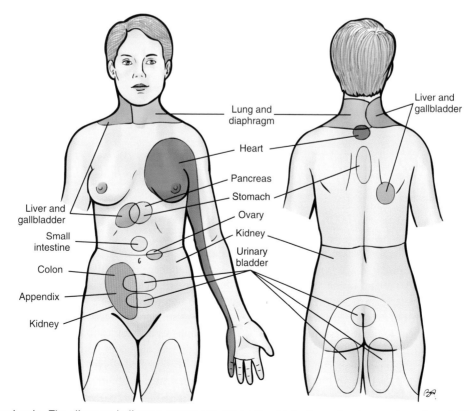

Lung and
diaphragm

Heart

Pancreas

Stomach

Ovary

Kidney

Urinary
bladder

Liver and
gallbladder

Small
intestine

Colon

Appendix

Kidney

Liver and
gallbladder

Figure 3.50 Referred pain. The diagram indicates cutaneous areas to which visceral pain may be referred. The professional who encounters pain in these areas should refer the client for diagnosis to rule out visceral dysfunction. (Source: Fritz S: *Mosby's fundamentals of therapeutic massage*, ed 5, St Louis, 2012, Mosby.)

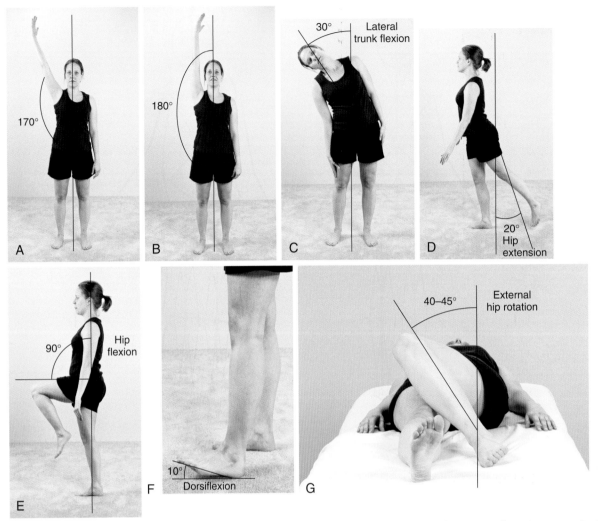

Figure 3.51 Range of motion is measured in degrees. The system presented in this book uses 0 degrees as the reference point for the standard anatomic position. Motions or positions of flexion, extension, abduction, and medial and lateral rotation are recorded as they move toward 180 degrees. **A**, 170 degrees. **B**, 180 degrees. **C**, 30 degrees, lateral trunk flexion. **D**, 20 degrees, leg extension. **E**, 90 degrees, hip flexion. **F**, 10 degrees, dorsiflexion. **G**, 40—45 degrees, internal hip rotation. (Source: Fritz S: *Mosby's fundamentals of therapeutic massage*, ed 5, St Louis, 2012, Mosby.)

result within minutes. Factors that could lead to this condition include the following:

- A long period of immobility or bed rest, which reduces circulation and can compress the veins
- Recent major surgery
- Varicose veins
- Heart disease
- Diabetes
- Use of contraceptive pills
- Impact trauma, which can cause damage inside the vein

Deep vein thrombosis (DVT) can occur in seemingly healthy people as a result of these predisposing factors. Acute pain and hard swelling, which can be confused with an acute muscle strain, may be felt when minimal pressure is applied. Some general swelling and discoloration of the distal part of the limb may be noted as a result of restricted circulation. The person may feel more pain and aching in the area when resting than would be expected with a muscle strain, and

nothing in the history would suggest an injury. These individuals must be referred to a doctor immediately; this is a medical emergency. Do not massage.

Diabetes

Diabetes can affect the peripheral circulation, especially in the feet, causing the tissues to become more brittle and fragile. It can also affect the nerves and reduce a patient's sensitivity to pressure. Deep massage techniques or methods with excessive drag can damage the brittle tissues, and with an impaired pain response, which is common in diabetes, feedback mechanisms become ineffective.

The stimulating effect of massage on the circulation sometimes seems similar to the effect of exercise on the blood sugar level of a person with diabetes. Clients with diabetes should be informed of this possibility, so they can alter their medication or diet accordingly. Although caution is required, if massage is applied correctly, it is extremely beneficial for

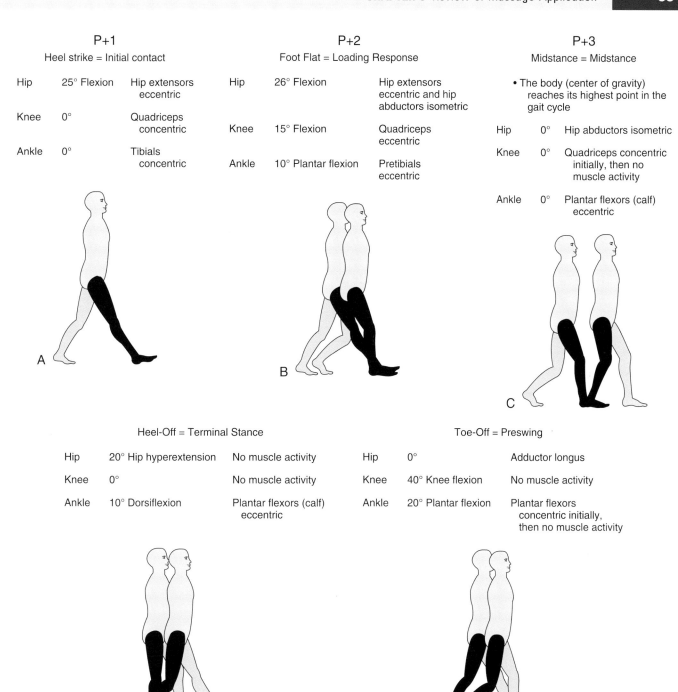

P+1

Heel strike = Initial contact

Hip	25° Flexion	Hip extensors eccentric
Knee	0°	Quadriceps concentric
Ankle	0°	Tibials concentric

P+2

Foot Flat = Loading Response

Hip	26° Flexion	Hip extensors eccentric and hip abductors isometric
Knee	15° Flexion	Quadriceps eccentric
Ankle	10° Plantar flexion	Pretibials eccentric

P+3

Midstance = Midstance

• The body (center of gravity) reaches its highest point in the gait cycle

Hip	0°	Hip abductors isometric
Knee	0°	Quadriceps concentric initially, then no muscle activity
Ankle	0°	Plantar flexors (calf) eccentric

Heel-Off = Terminal Stance

Hip	20° Hip hyperextension	No muscle activity
Knee	0°	No muscle activity
Ankle	10° Dorsiflexion	Plantar flexors (calf) eccentric

Toe-Off = Preswing

Hip	0°	Adductor longus
Knee	40° Knee flexion	No muscle activity
Ankle	20° Plantar flexion	Plantar flexors concentric initially, then no muscle activity

P+4

P+5

Figure 3.52 Gait assessment. **A–E**, Components of the stance phase. (Source: Fritz S: *Mosby's essential sciences for therapeutic massage: anatomy, physiology, biomechanics, and pathology*, ed 4, St Louis, 2012, Mosby.)

P+1

Acceleration = Initial swing

Hip	15° Hip flexion	Hip flexors concentric
Knee	60° Knee flexion	Knee flexors concentric
Ankle	10° Plantar flexion	Tibials concentric

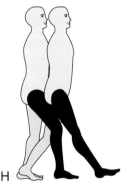

F

P+2

Midswing = Midswing

Hip	25° Hip flexion	Hip flexors concentric initially, then hamstrings eccentric
Knee	25° Knee flexion	Knee extension is created by momentum and gravity and short head of biceps femoris control rate of knee extension through eccentric control
Ankle	0°	Tibials concentric

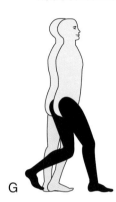

G

Deceleration = Terminal swing

Hip	25° Flexion	Hamstrings eccentric
Knee	0°	Quadriceps concentric to insure knee extension and hamstrings are active eccentrically to decelerate the leg
Ankle	0°	Tibials concentric

H

P+3

Arm swing

- The upper extremities serve an important role in counterbalancing the shifts of the center of gravity

- A reciprocal arm swing is seen in a mature gait (e.g., the left arm swings forward as the right leg swings forward and vice versa)

- As the shoulder girdle advances, the pelvis and limb trail behind. With each step, this is reversed

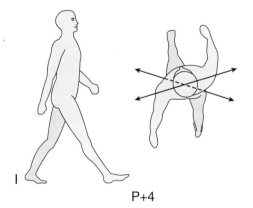

I

P+4

Figure 3.52, cont'd **F–I,** Components of the swing phase.

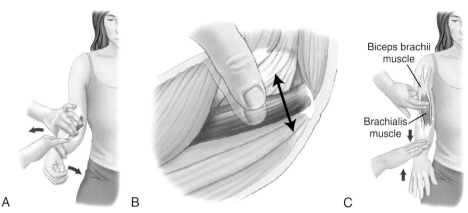

A   B   C

Figure 3.53 Five basic guidelines for palpating a muscle. **A**, Person palpating the pronator teres muscle while the client attempts to pronate the forearm at the radioulnar (RU) joints against resistance. Placement of the palpating fingers is determined by knowing the attachments of the pronator teres (palpation guideline 1). Asking the client to contract the muscle, attempting to pronate the forearm, makes the muscle become firmer and therefore more palpably discernible (palpation guideline 2). Resisting the client from performed pronation will increase the contraction of the pronator teres, making it even more discernibly palpable (palpation guideline 3). **B**, Close-up of the palpating fingers strumming perpendicular to the fiber direction of the pronator teres (palpation guideline 4). **C**, Palpation of the brachialis muscle through the biceps brachii using the neurologic reflex, reciprocal inhibition, to relax the biceps brachii (palpation guideline 5). Reciprocal inhibition is achieved in this case by having the client pronate the forearm at the RU joints, which is an action that is opposite to the action of supination of the forearm by the biceps brachii; therefore the biceps brachii relaxes, allowing the therapist to palpate the brachialis through it. Note: In **C**, the client is flexing her forearm (against gentle resistance by the therapist) to bring out the brachialis so that it can be more easily palpated. (Source: Fritz S: *Mosby's essential sciences for therapeutic massage: anatomy, physiology, biomechanics, and pathology*, ed 4, St Louis, 2012, Mosby.)

| 1+ Slight pitting, no visible distortion, disappears rapidly | 2+ Somewhat deeper pit than in 1+, no readily detectable distortion, disappears in 10-15 sec | 3+ Pit noticeably deep, may last more than a minute; the dependent extremity is swollen | 4+ Pit very deep, lasts 2-5 min; dependent extremity is grossly distorted |

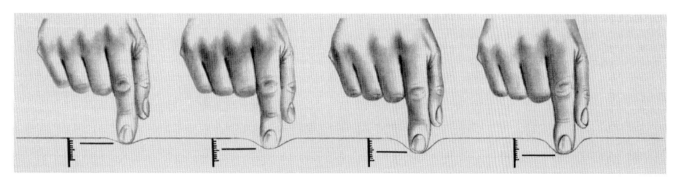

Figure 3.54 Assessment scale for pitting edema. (Source: Muscolino JE: *Kinesiology: the skeletal system and muscle function*, ed 2, St Louis, 2010, Mosby.)

Wong-Baker Faces® Pain Scale

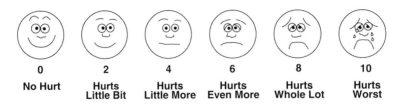

Figure 3.55 Descriptive pain intensity scale. The Wong–Baker faces pain rating scale. https://emergency.med.ufl.edu/files/2013/02/Pain-Rating-Scale.pdf.

individuals with diabetes. Caution is advised around common injection sites.

Systemic Infection: Contagious

The cause of a systemic infection are primarily bacteria or virus and occasional fungi or parasitic. The pathogen is distributed throughout the body. The most common examples of a systemic infection are cold, flu, mononucleosis, strep throat, tuberculous, and severe acute respiratory syndrome coronavirus (SARS-CoV-2/COVID-19). Main signs and symptoms are body aches, fatigue, fever, nausea as well as cough and increased mucus production if the infection is targeting the respiratory system.

Local Infection: Contagious

Bacterial Infection

Boils are superficial abscesses. A boil appears on the skin as a localized swelling that eventually ruptures and discharges pus. Folliculitis, a condition in which the hair follicles become inflamed, appears as a rash of very small blisters. Massage can break the blisters, leaving the skin open to further infection. These areas are local contraindications.

Fungal Infection

Ringworm and athlete's foot are the most common fungal infections. They can affect warm, moist areas, such as the skin between the toes, the armpits, or the area under the breast. The affected area may appear red and may have white, flaky skin. Although massage does not worsen the problem, it can cause irritation, and infection could be transmitted to the therapist's hands. For these reasons, treatment of the area is avoided.

Lymphangitis

Bacteria can invade the lymphatic system through open wounds. The wound itself may be minor, but the area around it appears red and swollen. Sometimes a dark line can be seen running up the limb toward the lymph nodes, which also may be swollen and tender. Massage could spread the infection. These individuals should be referred immediately for medical treatment.

Viral Infection

Herpes is a viral infection that currently has no cure. It is communicable, and the sores recur from time to time. Herpes is a local contraindication. Cold sores, the most common symptom of herpes, usually appear on the face and on or near mucous membranes in the general area. Before the sores erupt, the skin usually feels hypersensitive and tingles.

Other viral infections, such as warts and verrucae, should also be considered contraindications because the infection could be transmitted.

Open Wounds

An open wound is the most obvious contraindication. After a large wound has healed, a residual problem caused by scar tissue may be noted, which can be treated by massage.

Tumors

Undiagnosed tumors should be referred to a physician for diagnosis. Massage of a tumor, particularly by friction, should be avoided. If a tumor is diagnosed as benign, the tumor area is locally contraindicated. If the area is malignant, massage application follows the doctor's recommendation.

Massage should not be applied directly to any tumor, and the area should be avoided. Benign tumors are usually encapsulated, but malignant tumors are much less isolated and are more apt to have cells break away. If malignancy exists, contraindications to massage include patient fatigue, possible fragile bones in areas of radiation treatment, tissue damaged by radiation, fragile skin from chemotherapy, and a suppressed immune system.

Bleeding Disorders

Hemophilia is a hereditary disease that inhibits the blood's ability to clot. Several different forms of the disease exist, and it varies in severity. Males are primarily affected. Many other people take anticoagulant medication, for various reasons, that predisposes them to bleeding. In individuals with bleeding disorders, anything that could cause trauma to the tissues, on any level, must be avoided. The person's physician will be able to advise the massage therapist on what is safe and possible.

Varicose Veins

Varicose veins usually develop at the back of the leg. In this condition, the valves in the veins that prevent circulatory backflow break down and stop functioning. In minor cases,

TABLE 3.5 Stages of Tissue Healing and Appropriate Interventions

Stage 1 (Acute): Inflammatory	Stage 2 (Subacute): Repair and Healing	Stage 3 (Chronic): Maturation and Remodeling
Characteristics		
Vascular changes	Growth of capillary beds into area	Maturation and remodeling of scar
Inflammatory exudates	Collagen formation	Contracture of scar tissue
Clot formation	Granulation tissue	Alignment of collagen along lines of stress forces (tensegrity)
Phagocytosis, neutralization of irritants	Fragile, easily injured tissue	
Early fibroblastic activity		
Clinical Signs		
Inflammation	Decreased inflammation	Absence of inflammation
Pain before tissue resistance	Pain during tissue resistance	Pain after tissue resistance
Massage Intervention		
(3–7 days after injury)	(14–21 days after injury)	(3–12 months after injury)
Main goal: protection	Main goal: controlled motion	Main goal: return to function
Control and support effects of inflammation	Promote development of mobile scar	Increase strength and alignment of scar tissue
	Cautious and controlled soft tissue mobilization of scar tissue along fiber direction toward injury	Cross-fiber friction of scar tissue coupled with directional stroking along lines of tension away from injury
Promote healing and prevent compensation patterns	Active and passive, open- and closed-chain range of motion (midrange)	Progressive stretching and active and resisted range of motion (full range)
Passive movement midrange	Support for healing with full-body massage	Support for rehabilitation activities with full-body massage
General massage and lymphatic drainage with caution		
Support for rest with full-body massage		

Massage Approach During Healing

Acute Phase
Manage pain
Support sleep

Subacute Phase (Early)
Manage pain
Support sleep
Manage edema
Manage compensation patterns

Subacute Phase (Later)
Manage pain
Support sleep
Manage edema
Manage compensation patterns
Support rehabilitative activity
Support mobile scar development
Support tissue regeneration process

Remodeling Phase
Support rehabilitation activity
Encourage appropriate scar tissue development
Support tissue sliding
Restore firing patterns, gait reflexes, and neuromuscular responses
Eliminate reversible compensation patterns
Manage irreversible compensation patterns
Restore tissue pliability

Source: Fritz S: *Mosby's fundamentals of therapeutic massage*, ed 5, St Louis, 2012, Mosby.

BOX 3.5   Assessment for Fluid Imbalance and Intervention

1. Ask the client if tissue feels taut, distended, fat, or stiff. If the answer is no, palpate to confirm that edema is not present and then proceed with the general massage. If the answer is yes, then ask for the history.
2. The history would include any injury, swelling, bruising, static position, and unusual increase in physical activity followed by extended inactivity. If the client answers yes to any of these, then observe.
3. Observe for a decrease in muscle definition, bruising, tissue distension, and changes in color. If any of these are found, *palpate*, or ask for the history.
4. Palpate for increases in muscle tone, specifically tissue tautness and an increase in fluid (pitting edema) or venous congestion. If these are noted, observe and palpate for signs of inflammation.
5. Palpate for heat and observe for redness. Ask about pain.
6. If the area is swollen, hot, red, and painful, refer the client to a medical professional. If inflammation is present, massage the area only after the reason for the condition has been determined.
7. If the area is not hot or red, determine whether the tissue is congested or swollen.
8. Congested tissue has increased blood in the veins and capillaries; the tissue feels dense and stiff but does not show pitting edema. Swollen tissue has increased interstitial fluid; this tissue pits when pressure is applied.
9. If the tissue is congested, massage methods that enhance venous return are indicated. Observe cautions for thrombosis, kidney disease, and heart disease.
10. If the tissue is swollen, lymphatic drainage targeting movement of interstitial fluid into collectors is indicated. Observe cautions for infections, kidney disease, and heart disease.

Source: Fritz S: *Mosby's fundamentals of therapeutic massage*, ed 7, St Louis, 2021, Mosby.

BOX 3.6   Landmarks That Help Identify Lack of Symmetry

The following landmarks can be used to compare symmetry. Be sure to observe the client from the back, the front, and the left and right sides.

- The middle of the chin should sit directly under the tip of the nose. Check the chin alignment with the sternal notch. These two landmarks should be in a direct line.
- The shoulders and clavicles should be level with each other.
- The shoulders should not roll forward or backward or be rotated with one forward and one backward.
- The arms should hang freely and at the same rotation out of the glenohumeral (shoulder) joint.
- The elbows, wrists, and fingertips should be in the same plane.
- The skin of the thorax (chest and back) should be even and should not look as if it pulls or is puffy.
- The navel, located in the same line as the nose, chin, and sternal notch, should not look pulled.
- The ribs should be even and springy.
- The abdomen should be firm but relaxed and slightly rounded.
- The curves at the waist should be even on both sides.
- The spine should be in a direct line from the base of the skull and on the same plane as the line connecting the nose and the navel. The curves of the spine should not be exaggerated.
- The scapulae should appear even and should move freely. You should be able to draw an imaginary straight line between the tips of the scapulae.
- The gluteal muscle mass should be even.
- The tops of the iliac crests should be even.
- The greater trochanter, knees, and ankles should be level.
- The circumferences of the thigh and calf should be similar on the left and right sides.
- The legs should rotate out of the acetabulum (hip joint) evenly in a slight external rotation.
- The knees should be locked in the standing position but should not be hyperextended. The patellae (kneecaps) should be level and pointed slightly laterally.
- A line dropped from the nose should fall through the sternum and the navel and should be spaced evenly between.

Source: Fritz S: *Mosby's fundamentals of therapeutic massage*, ed 5, St Louis, 2012, Mosby.

---

light, superficial stroking over the area should do no harm and may in fact ease pressure off the vein and aid repair. Deep pressure and drag should not be applied because these can further damage the walls of the blood vessels. In advanced cases, even superficial stroking should be avoided because of the added risk of DVT. This contraindication affects only the actual location of the vein. Tissues adjacent to the area can be massaged, and this can improve circulation away from the varicose vein, relieving some of the pressure in it.

Kidney Disease

Massage moves fluid, helping it pass through the kidneys, and increased fluid movement strains the kidneys. Massage methods that target fluid movement, such as lymphatic drainage, must be used very cautiously and only with a doctor's supervision. Massage may be appropriate with impaired kidney function, depending on the severity of the impairment. It is impossible to do massage and not at least temporarily increase fluid movement. Energy-based methods that soothe and relax may be appropriate.

Cardiac Disease

The term *heart failure* seems to imply that the heart no longer works and nothing can be done. Actually, heart failure means that the heart is not pumping as well as it should be. This results in fatigue and shortness of breath. Everyday activities such as walking, climbing stairs, and carrying groceries can become difficult. Congestive heart failure (CHF) occurs when the heart is unable to pump blood efficiently throughout the body, and circulatory needs are not met. The two types of CHF are left-side damage and right-side damage. When the left side of the heart is damaged, blood backs up into the lung area, making breathing difficult. The kidneys also are damaged, and sudden weight gain can occur. With right-side damage, blood and other fluids accumulate in the ankles, bloating occurs in the abdominal area, and the person has extreme fatigue.

Symptoms of congestive heart failure include:
- Cough
- Decreased production of urine
- Trouble focusing
- Trouble sleeping
- Dizziness
- Fatigue
- Nausea and vomiting
- Protruding neck veins
- Excessive need to urinate at night
- Elevated or rapid pulse
- Shortness of breath after exertion and after lying down
- Swelling in the abdominal area
- Weight gain without a change in diet or exercise

Because massage moves the blood and changes the fluid pressure in the body, compromised cardiac function can be unduly strained. General massage typically is beneficial for those with cardiac conditions, but cautions are indicated. If CHF has been diagnosed, massage is contraindicated, except gentle palliative methods (Box 3.7).

MEDICAL EMERGENCIES

Although such situations are rare, a massage therapist may have a client who experiences a medical emergency. Massage practitioners should be especially aware of the conditions discussed in the following sections.

Venous Thromboembolism (Deep Vein Thrombosis and Pulmonary Embolism)

Venous thromboembolism (VTE) is a disease that includes both DVT and pulmonary embolism (PE). DVT is an

BOX 3.7	Indications for Referral

If any of the following conditions are present and cannot be explained logically, the client should be referred to a healthcare professional:
- Pain (local, sharp, dull, achy, deep, superficial)
- Fatigue
- Inflammation
- Lumps and tissue changes
- Rashes and changes in the skin
- Edema
- Mood alterations (e.g., depression, anxiety)
- Infection (local or general)
- Changes in habits (e.g., appetite, elimination, sleep)
- Bleeding and bruising
- Nausea, vomiting, and diarrhea
- Temperature (hot [fever] or cold)

Source: Fritz S: *Mosby's fundamentals of therapeutic massage*, ed 7, St Louis, 2021, Mosby.

underdiagnosed, serious, potentially preventable medical condition that occurs when a blood clot forms in a deep vein, such as in the lower leg, the thigh, or the pelvis. A PE occurs when part of the clot, or the entire clot, breaks off and travels through the bloodstream to the lungs. Without appropriate diagnosis and treatment, PE can be fatal. Blood clots may form when the flow of blood in the veins is slowed or changed. Risk factors include hypertension, diabetes mellitus, cigarette smoking, a high cholesterol level, immobility, sitting for extended periods, air travel, surgery, cancer treatment, giving birth within the previous 6 months, pregnancy, obesity, fractures in the pelvis or legs, and some medications, including hormone replacement, birth control, and some types of nonsteroidal antiinflammatory drugs (NSAIDs). The lower extremities are the most common site for DVT. Symptoms of DVT include pain or tenderness and swelling. Signs include increased warmth, edema, and erythema (reddening of skin). Because of the seriousness of this condition, refer the client immediately if it is suspected.

Stroke

Strokes happen when blood flow to the brain stops. Within minutes, brain cells begin to die. There are two kinds of stroke. The more common kind, called an ischemic stroke, is caused by a blood clot that blocks or plugs a blood vessel in the brain. The other kind, called a hemorrhagic stroke, is caused by a blood vessel that breaks and bleeds into the brain. "Mini-strokes," or transient ischemic attacks (TIAs), occur when the blood supply to the brain is briefly interrupted. A stroke happens quickly, and most people show two or more signs. The most common signs of a stroke are as follows:
- Sudden numbness or weakness of the face, arm, or leg (mainly on one side of the body)
- Sudden trouble seeing in one or both eyes

- Sudden trouble walking, dizziness, or loss of balance
- Sudden confusion or trouble talking or understanding speech
- Sudden bad headache with no known cause
  Women may have unique symptoms:
- Sudden face and arm or leg pain
- Sudden hiccups
- Sudden nausea
- Sudden tiredness
- Sudden chest pain
- Sudden shortness of breath
- Sudden pounding or racing heartbeat

Stroke Warning Signs

A good memory aid to help you recognize the signs of a stroke is "Spot a stroke FAST."
- Facial drooping: Does one side of the face droop or is it numb? Ask the person to smile.
- Arm weakness: Is one arm weak or numb? Ask the person to raise both arms. Does one arm drift downward?
- Speech difficulty: Is the person's speech slurred? Is he or she unable to speak or difficult to understand? Ask the person to repeat a simple sentence, such as "The sky is blue." Is the sentence repeated correctly?
- Time to call 911: If the person shows any of these symptoms, even if the symptoms go away, call 911 and get the person to the hospital immediately.

Concussion

Concussion is a brain injury. All concussions are serious and should be evaluated by a physician. Although usually not life-threatening, a delayed response to this type of brain injury may lead to bleeding in or around the brain which can be life-threatening. The medical emergency issue is that the bleeding may slowly occur over days before becoming potentially fatal. In rare cases, a dangerous blood clot may form on the brain in a person with a concussion and crowd the brain against the skull. Second impact syndrome occurs when a second concussion occurs before signs and symptoms of a first concussion have resolved and may result in rapid and usually fatal brain swelling. Persons taking blood thinners are at increased risk of bleeding. Clients who have had a head trauma may think they are fine and may seek massage for stiffness and headache at the point that the bleeding and swelling is becoming serious and life-threatening. Signs of medical emergency include the following:
- Headache that gets worse and does not go away
- Weakness, numbness, or decreased coordination
- Repeated vomiting or nausea
- Slurred speech
- Increasing drowsiness or the client cannot be awakened
- One pupil larger than the other
- Convulsions or seizures
- Inability to recognize people or places
- Growing confusion, restlessness, or agitation

- Unusual behavior
- Loss of consciousness (a brief loss of consciousness should be taken seriously, and the person should be carefully monitored)

Refer immediately to the emergency room and call 911 if necessary. Educate clients that even minor head trauma is serious and head trauma events need medical evaluation and monitoring.

Heart Attack

A heart attack occurs when the blood flow that brings oxygen to the heart muscle is severely reduced or cut off completely. This happens because coronary arteries that supply the heart muscle with blood flow can slowly become narrow from a buildup of fat, cholesterol, and other substances that together are called plaque. This slow process is known as atherosclerosis. When plaque in a heart artery breaks, a blood clot forms around the plaque. This blood clot can block the blood flow through the heart muscle. When the heart muscle is starved for oxygen and nutrients, the condition is called ischemia. When damage or death of part of the heart muscle occurs as a result of ischemia, this is called a heart attack or myocardial infarction (MI). Symptoms of heart disease that may lead to a heart attack include the following:
- Undue fatigue
- Palpitations: The sensation that the heart is skipping a beat or beating too rapidly
- Dyspnea: Difficult or labored breathing
- Chest pain: Pain or discomfort in the chest from increased activity; this is known as angina pectoris (also called stable angina or chronic stable angina)

The following are signs that can mean a heart attack is happening:
- Chest discomfort. Most heart attacks involve discomfort in the center of the chest that lasts more than a few minutes or that goes away and comes back. It can feel like uncomfortable pressure, squeezing, fullness, or pain.
- Discomfort in other areas of the upper body. Symptoms can include pain or discomfort in one or both arms or the back, neck, jaw, or stomach.
- Shortness of breath with or without chest discomfort.
- Breaking out in a cold sweat, nausea, or lightheadedness.
- Women are somewhat more likely than men to experience some of the other common symptoms, particularly shortness of breath, nausea/vomiting, and back or jaw pain. Learn about the warning signs of a heart attack in women.

If the client shows any of these symptoms, even if the symptoms go away, call 911 and get the person to the hospital immediately.

Sepsis

Sepsis is a life-threatening condition caused by an overwhelming response by the body to infection that it begins to cause injury to the body's own tissues and organs. Any infection minor or major can trigger sepsis. The infection can be bacterial, viral, fungal, or parasitic. People who have recently been hospitalized are at greater risk, as are those with an overall increased risk for infection such as the very young or very old and those with chronic diseases or a compromised immune system. The symptoms come on gradually. When there is an infection, sepsis can occur. Sepsis symptoms start off subtly and may mimic a flu or virus. It is important to look for the warning signs of sepsis. Spotting these symptoms early could prevent the body from entering septic shock and could save a life.

Symptoms include the following:

S—Shiver, fever, or extreme cold
E—Extreme pain or general discomfort ("worst ever")
P—Pale or discolored skin
S—Sleepiness, difficulty rousing, confusion
I—Statements such as "I feel like I might die"
S—Short of breath

Mortality from sepsis increases by as much as 8% for every hour that treatment is delayed. As many as 80% of sepsis deaths could be prevented with rapid diagnosis and treatment. Approximately 6% of all hospitalizations are due to sepsis, and 35% of all deaths in hospitals are due to sepsis.

Remember, sepsis is a medical emergency. If sepsis is suspected, refer the client immediately for medical attention.

Anaphylaxis

Anaphylaxis is a life-threatening type of allergic reaction. The condition is severe and involves the whole body. Tissues in different parts of the body release histamine and other substances. This causes the airways to tighten and leads to other symptoms. Anaphylaxis can occur in response to any allergen. Common causes include the following:

- Drug allergies
- Food allergies
- Insect bites or stings

Symptoms develop quickly, often within seconds or minutes, and may include any of the following:

- Abdominal pain
- Abnormal (high-pitched) breathing sounds
- Anxiety
- Chest discomfort or tightness
- Cough
- Diarrhea
- Difficulty breathing
- Difficulty swallowing
- Dizziness or lightheadedness
- Hives, itchiness
- Loss of consciousness
- Nasal congestion
- Nausea or vomiting
- Palpitations
- Skin redness
- Slurred speech

- Swelling of the face, eyes, or tongue
- Wheezing

If the client shows any of these symptoms, even if the symptoms go away, call 911 and get the person to the hospital immediately. A person with a known allergy often carries an epinephrine autoinjector, or EpiPen, with instructions on how to inject into the middle of the outer thigh.

Diabetic Emergencies

It is estimated that more than 20 million people in the United States have diabetes, and an estimated 6 million people are unaware that they have it. People with diabetes may experience life-threatening emergencies as a result of too much or too little insulin in their bodies. Too much insulin can cause a low sugar level (hypoglycemia), which can lead to insulin shock. Insufficient insulin can cause a high level of sugar (hyperglycemia), which can cause a diabetic coma.

Symptoms of insulin shock include the following:

- Weakness, drowsiness
- Rapid pulse
- Fast breathing
- Pale, sweaty skin
- Headache, trembling
- Odorless breath
- Numbness in the hands or feet
- Hunger

Symptoms of diabetic coma, or impending diabetic coma, include the following:

- Weak, rapid pulse
- Nausea
- Deep, sighing breaths
- Unsteady gait
- Confusion
- Flushed, warm, dry skin
- Breath odor of nail polish or sweet apple
- Drowsiness, gradual loss of consciousness

If the client shows any of these symptoms, even if the symptoms go away, call 911 and get the person to the hospital immediately.

Rhabdomyolysis

Rhabdomyolysis is a serious syndrome due to a direct or indirect muscle injury. It results from the death of muscle fibers and release of their contents into the bloodstream. These substances are harmful to the kidneys and often cause kidney damage. Rhabdomyolysis has many causes. Some of the common ones a massage therapist may encounter include the following:

- Muscle trauma or crush injury
- Severe muscle contractions from prolonged seizures
- Extreme physical activity (running a marathon, extreme workouts)
- Drug and alcohol use

- Low electrolytes
- Medications: most notably statins used to treat high cholesterol
- Variety of viruses and some bacteria
- Lack of blood perfusion to a limb

The following are common signs and symptoms of rhabdomyolysis:

- Muscle pain, especially in the shoulders, thighs, or lower back
- Muscle weakness or trouble moving arms or legs
- Abdominal pain
- Nausea or vomiting
- Fever, rapid heart rate
- Confusion, dehydration, fever, or lack of consciousness
- Dark red or brown urine; reduced or no urine output

There have been reports of aggressive, heavy-pressure, friction-based massage causing mild cases of rhabdomyolysis. This type of massage application for an individual with risk factors for rhabdomyolysis, such as extreme exercise, may increase the seriousness of the condition.

BASIC PHARMACOLOGY FOR THE MASSAGE THERAPIST

Any chemical that affects the physiologic processes of a living organism can broadly be defined as a drug. The study or science of drugs is known as pharmacology. Pharmacology encompasses a variety of topics, including the following:

- Absorption
- Biochemical effects
- Biotransformation (metabolism)
- Distribution
- Drug history
- Drug origin
- Drug receptor mechanisms
- Excretion
- Mechanisms of action
- Physical and chemical properties
- Physical effects
- Therapeutic (beneficial) effects
- Toxic (harmful) effects

Information to Help Clarify Medication Actions

A massage therapist must understand the reason a client is taking a medication and the action of that medication to determine the potential interaction of the drug with the physiologic effects of massage and to make the adjustments to massage that may be necessary. The following information must be gathered. Most of it can be obtained in a drug consult before the massage. The client and/or supervising medical personnel may be able to supply information regarding medication. Reputable drug resources are available online that can provide information on medications and dietary supplements. MedlinePlus is recommended. A trusted local pharmacist could also be consulted.

Consider these questions when inquiring about a medication:

- What is the name of the drug (generic name and brand name)?
- Why is the client taking the drug?
- What does the medicine do?
- When and how is the medication taken?
- What are the possible side effects (reactions of the body to the medicine)?
- Will the medicine react with any other medicines, food, or drinks?
- Should any activities be avoided?
- Are there any signs indicating that the medicine is working?

Common Medications and Possible Implications for Massage

The information in the following sections can help the massage practitioner determine what interaction, if any, massage may have with a pharmaceutical. General categories and examples are given for each classification. This is not meant to be an exhaustive list, but rather a general guide for the more commonly prescribed drugs and their brand names. It is important to research any medication, vitamin, dietary supplement, or herb a client takes for its action in the body and possible interaction with massage.

Cardiovascular Medications
Vasodilators (Including Antianginal Drugs)
Examples: nitroglycerin (Nitro-Dur, Nitrostat), isosorbide dinitrate (Isordil) or isosorbide mononitrate (Monoket), hydralazine, minoxidil

Vasodilating medications cause the blood vessels to dilate (widen). Some of the antihypertensive agents lower blood pressure by dilating the arteries or veins. Other vasodilators are used in the treatment of angina (chest pain), hypertension, heart failure, and diseases characterized by poor circulation. Nitrates, which are often used to treat angina, increase the amount of oxygen that reaches the heart muscle.

Implications for massage: Massage has a mild peripheral vasodilatory effect. The action of the medications may increase the effect of the massage. The blood pressure—lowering effect of massage may result in dizziness after the massage. Have the client contract and relax the leg muscles for 1— 2 minutes before getting off the massage table. The massage therapist must also be ready to assist the client off the table, if necessary.

Beta-Blockers
Examples: atenolol (Tenormin), bisoprolol (Zebeta), carvedilol (Coreg), labetalol (Normodyne, Trandate), metoprolol (Lopressor, Toprol-XL), propranolol (Inderal)

Beta-blocking medications block nerve stimulation of the heart and blood vessels, slowing the heart rate and reducing high blood pressure. They are used in the treatment of a wide range of diseases, including angina, hypertension, migraine headaches, heart failure, and arrhythmias.

Implications for massage: These drugs may distort the expected effect of the massage. Caution is warranted, and the massage therapist should watch for any exaggerated effects. The client may be susceptible to cold. Massage may help with the constipation that can be a side effect of these drugs. The blood pressure—lowering effect of massage may result in dizziness after the massage. Have the client contract and relax the leg muscles for 1—2 minutes before getting off the massage table. The massage therapist must also be ready to assist the client off the table, if necessary.

Calcium Channel Blockers

Examples: amlodipine (Norvasc), diltiazem (Cardizem LA, Tiazac), nifedipine (Adalat CC, Procardia XL), verapamil (Calan, Verelan, Covera HS)

Calcium channel blockers are thought to prevent angina and arrhythmias by blocking or slowing calcium flow into muscle cells, which results in vasodilation (widening of the blood vessels) and greater oxygen delivery to the heart muscle.

Implications for massage: The expected effect of the massage may be distorted. Care must be taken to watch for any exaggerated effects. Massage may help with constipation. The blood pressure—lowering effect of massage may result in dizziness after the massage. Have the client contract and relax the leg muscles for 1—2 minutes before getting off the massage table. The massage therapist must also be ready to assist the client off the table, if necessary.

Antiarrhythmics

Examples: amiodarone (Cordarone, Pacerone), digoxin (Lanoxin), dronedarone (Multaq), propafenone (Rythmol), sotalol (Betapace, Betapace AF), quinidine, and some beta-blockers or calcium channel blockers (discussed earlier)

Antiarrhythmics are prescribed when the heart does not beat rhythmically or smoothly (a condition called arrhythmia). The broad class is composed of many pharmacologically different types of agents, all with varying effects on electrical impulse conduction and the rate and force of contraction of the heart.

Implications for massage: The client may complain of joint and muscle pain and swelling in the extremities that are medication related. If this occurs, refer the client to the prescribing physician. Massage may help with constipation. The client may experience dizziness after the massage. Have the client contract and relax the leg muscles for 1—2 minutes before getting off the massage table. The massage therapist must also be ready to assist the client off the table, if necessary.

Antihypertensives and Diuretics

Examples of antihypertensives: beta-blockers, calcium channel blockers, angiotensin-converting enzyme (ACE) inhibitors (including benazepril, captopril, enalapril, lisinopril, quinapril), angiotensin receptor blockers (ARBs) (including candesartan, irbesartan, losartan, olmesartan, telmisartan, valsartan), prazosin, terazosin, clonidine, and minoxidil

Examples of diuretics: chlorothiazide, chlorthalidone, hydrochlorothiazide, budesonide, furosemide, torsemide

Examples of potassium-sparing diuretics: spironolactone, triamterene, amiloride

Combinations of antihypertensives: Patients commonly are prescribed a medication that is a combination of two antihypertensives, including diuretic combinations.

High blood pressure, or hypertension, occurs when the pressure of the blood against the walls of the blood vessels is higher than what is considered normal; this condition eventually can damage the brain, eyes, heart, and kidneys. Diuretics are used in antihypertensive therapy. Many diuretics may deplete the body of potassium unless they are the potassium-sparing kind, and the physician may recommend a potassium supplement or food source that is high in potassium.

Implications for massage: The expected effect of the massage may be distorted. Care must be taken to watch for any exaggerated effects. Massage may help with constipation. The blood pressure—lowering effect of massage may result in dizziness after the massage. Have the client contract and relax the leg muscles for 1—2 minutes before getting off the massage table. The massage therapist must also be ready to assist the client off the table, if necessary. The stress-reducing effect of massage may affect the dosage of these medications. Have clients monitor themselves carefully and ask their physicians to watch for a possible need to reduce the dosage or change the medication. Massage has the effect of increasing fluid movement and may enhance the diuretic effect temporarily.

Cardiac Glycosides (Digitalis Glycosides)

Examples: digoxin (Lanoxin)

Cardiac glycosides slow the heart rate but increase contraction force. Their uses include regulating irregular heart rhythm, increasing the volume of blood pumped by the heart, and medicating congestive heart failure.

Implications for massage: Monitor the client's heart rate because massage tends to slow the heart rate. If the rate falls below 50 beats per minute, stop the massage and refer the client immediately to the physician. Regular use of massage may affect the dosage of this medication. Have the client monitor the dose carefully with the physician.

Anticoagulants and Medications That Inhibit Platelets

Examples: warfarin (Coumadin, Jantoven), dabigatran (Pradaxa), ticagrelor (Brilinta), clopidogrel (Plavix), heparin, enoxaparin (Lovenox), dalteparin (Fragmin), aspirin

Anticoagulants and platelet inhibitors are medications that prevent blood clotting (blood thinners). They may be used in the treatment of conditions such as stroke, heart disease, embolism (blood clots), and abnormal blood clotting. Warfarin acts by preventing the liver from manufacturing the proteins responsible for blood clot formation.

Implications for massage: The response to stress levels can affect the action of anticoagulants. Massage alters the body's response to stress and may interact with the dosage of this medication. Avoid any massage methods that may cause bruising, including compression, friction, percussion, and skin rolling. Do not massage an injection site. Watch for bruising and report any bruising to the client. Joint swelling and aching may result from the use of these medications. Refer clients who have any joint symptoms to the physician.

Antihyperlipidemics

Examples: cholestyramine (Questran), colestipol, ezetimibe, atorvastatin (Lipitor), lovastatin, simvastatin (Zocor), pravastatin (Pravachol), rosuvastatin (Crestor), gemfibrozil, fenofibrate (Lipofen, Lofibra), omega-3 fatty acids (Lovaza)

Antihyperlipidemics are used to reduce the serum levels of cholesterol or triglycerides, which form plaque on the walls of arteries. The statins reduce the body's internal production of cholesterol. Some antihyperlipidemics bind to bile acids in the gastrointestinal tract, reducing the body's absorption of cholesterol.

Implications for massage: Occasional muscle pain and joint pain can occur when statin or fibrate medications are used. Refer clients who complain of these conditions to a physician. Massage may help constipation. Some people experience occasional dizziness. Watch clients carefully as they get up from the massage table, and provide assistance, if necessary.

Gastrointestinal Medications
Anticholinergics

Examples of anticholinergics: dicyclomine (Bentyl), hyoscyamine (Levsin, Levbid, NuLev, Symax)

Examples of opioid with anticholinergic: diphenoxylate, atropine (Lomotil, Lonox)

Anticholinergic medications slow or block nerve impulses at parasympathetic nerve endings, preventing muscle contraction and glandular secretion in the organs involved. Because these medications slow the action of the bowel by relaxing the muscles and relieving spasms, they are said to have an antispasmodic action. They also can help alleviate diarrhea.

Implications for massage: The client's response to relaxation effects may be altered as a result of the alteration of parasympathetic action.

Antiulcer Medications

Examples: cimetidine (Tagamet), famotidine (Pepcid), ranitidine (Zantac), omeprazole (Prilosec), lansoprazole (Prevacid), sucralfate (Carafate)

These medications relieve symptoms and promote healing of gastrointestinal ulcers. They also relieve gastrointestinal reflux of stomach acid, which may cause chronic heartburn. Most work by suppressing the production of excess stomach acid. Sucralfate works by forming a chemical barrier over an exposed ulcer, protecting the ulcer from stomach acid.

Implications for massage: The stress-reduction capacity of massage may enhance the effectiveness of these medications.

Hormones

A hormone is a substance produced and secreted by a gland. Hormones stimulate and regulate body functions. Most often

hormone medications are used to replace naturally occurring hormones that are not being produced in amounts sufficient to regulate specific body functions. This category of medication includes oral contraceptives and certain types of medications used to combat inflammatory reactions.

Antidiabetic Medications

Examples: glipizide, glyburide

The treatment of diabetes mellitus may involve the administration of insulin or oral antidiabetic medications. Glucagon is given only in emergencies (e.g., insulin shock or when blood sugar levels must be raised quickly). Oral antidiabetic medications are used for the treatment of type 2 diabetes (adult onset, insulin resistant). Early medications in this category induced the pancreas to secrete more insulin by acting on small groups of cells in the pancreas that make and store insulin. Newer oral agents often help increase the insulin sensitivity of the tissues. Individuals with insulin-dependent (juvenile onset, or type 1) diabetes must control their blood sugar levels with insulin injections.

Implications for massage: Changes in stress levels may affect the dosage. The client's physician should monitor the dosage if massage is used on a regular basis. Do not provide vigorous massage, because it may put undue stress on the system, requiring the blood sugar level to adjust. Avoid massaging over injection or infusion sites.

Sex Hormones

Examples: estrogens (Estradiol, Premarin, Cenestin), oral contraceptives, progesterones (medroxyprogesterone [Provera]), androgens (testosterone, AndroGel)

Estrogens are used as replacement therapy to treat symptoms of menopause in women whose bodies are no longer producing sufficient amounts of estrogen. Medroxyprogesterone is used to treat uterine bleeding and menstrual problems. Most oral contraceptives (birth control pills) combine estrogen and a progesterone, but some contain only a progesterone. Testosterone stimulates cells that produce male sex characteristics, replace hormone deficiencies, stimulate red blood cells, and suppress estrogen production. Athletes sometimes take medications called anabolic steroids (chemicals similar to testosterone) to reduce the elimination of protein from the body, which results in an increase in muscle size. This use of these medications is dangerous; anabolic steroids can adversely affect the heart, nervous system, and kidneys.

Implications for massage: Estrogens can change the body's blood clotting ability. Watch for bruising and adjust pressures as needed. Be aware of any symptoms of blood clots and refer the patient to the physician immediately if these are noted. Most hormones can increase fluid retention. Massage may temporarily increase fluid movement, reducing swelling. Unusual fluid retention should be referred to the prescribing physician immediately. Hormones have a widespread effect on the body and mood. Emotional states may fluctuate, and the ability to handle stress changes with the hormonal fluctuations. Massage can reduce stress levels, help even out mood, and promote a sense of well-being.

Steroids

Examples: dexamethasone (Decadron), methylprednisolone (Medrol), prednisolone (Orapred), prednisone

Examples of common steroid hormone creams or ointments: triamcinolone, hydrocortisone

Oral steroid preparations may be used to treat inflammatory diseases such as arthritis, or conditions such as poison ivy, hay fever, or insect bites. Steroids also may be applied to the skin to treat certain inflammatory skin conditions.

Implications for massage: Changes in stress levels may affect the dose. The client's physician should monitor the dosage if massage is used on a regular basis. Avoid any massage methods that may create inflammation, such as friction, skin rolling, or stretching methods that pull excessively on the tissue.

Thyroid Medications

Examples: levothyroxine (Synthroid, Levoxyl, Levoxine), thyroid (Bio-Throid)

Implications for massage: Changes in stress levels may affect the dosage. The client should monitor the dosage if massage is used on a regular basis.

Antiinfective Medications
Antibiotics

Examples: aminoglycosides, cephalosporins, macrolides (erythromycin, clarithromycin, azithromycin), penicillins (including ampicillin and amoxicillin), quinolones (ciprofloxacin, levofloxacin), tetracyclines

Antibiotics are used to treat a wide variety of bacterial infections. There are many different classes of antibiotics. Antibiotics do not destroy viruses.

Antivirals

Examples: acyclovir (Zovirax), valacyclovir (Valtrex), medications used to treat HIV infection

Antiviral medications are used to combat viral infections; however, they do not eliminate or cure viral infections. Medications for HIV may predispose an individual to the accumulation of lactic acidosis and muscle soreness; be alert to possible medication side effects, and if lactic acidosis may be present, refer the client to the physician before proceeding with the massage.

Antifungals

Examples: nystatin, fluconazole (Diflucan), itraconazole (Sporanox), ketoconazole (Nizoral)

Fungal infections are treated to prevent the growth of fungi and to cure the condition. Many topical antifungals are used to treat fungal skin conditions such as athlete's foot or groin itch.

Pediculicides and Scabicides

Examples: lindane, permethrin (Elimite), pyrethrins (Pronto Plus), benzyl alcohol (Ulesfia), spinosad (Natroba)

Pediculicides and scabicides are used to treat lice or scabies infestations. Lindane can cause serious neurotoxicity and must be carefully applied and handled.

Implications for massage for antiinfective medications: A person who is taking an antiinfective medication may have a stressed immune system or may be truly immunocompromised. The person may also have an infection that is considered contagious to others. Therefore, it is important to avoid overstressing the system when providing massage and to take care not to expose clients to contagious diseases, such as colds, the flu, or infestations. Postpone appointments if necessary. Gastrointestinal side effects are common with many antibiotics. Massage may calm symptoms temporarily. Universal precautions are required when dealing with any bacterial, viral, or other condition caused by infectious pathogens.

Antineoplastic Medications

Examples: tamoxifen (Nolvadex), flutamide, etoposide, Gleevec, Sprycel, Sutent, Tarceva, Votrient

Antineoplastic medications are used in the treatment of cancer. Most of the medications in this category prevent the growth of rapidly dividing cells, such as cancer cells. Antineoplastics are without exception extremely toxic and can cause serious side effects. Many more cancer drugs now are supplied in oral form, and the number of treatments is expanding rapidly.

Implications for massage: Individuals undergoing chemotherapy are physiologically stressed because of the toxicity of the medications. Work gently and under the direct supervision of the client's physician.

Central Nervous System Medications
Antianxiety Drugs/Sedatives

Examples: benzodiazepines diazepam (Valium), lorazepam (Ativan), alprazolam (Xanax), temazepam (Restoril); buspirone (Buspar); diphenhydramine (Unisom); hydroxyzine (Atarax); zaleplon (Sonata); zolpidem (Ambien); eszopiclone (Lunesta); barbiturates (phenobarbital, secobarbital)

Antianxiety drugs and sedatives are used in the treatment of anxiety, panic disorder, and insomnia. They selectively reduce the activity of certain chemicals in the brain.

Implications for massage: These medications generally act as central nervous system (CNS) depressants. Massage can increase or decrease the effect of these medications, depending on whether the massage is structured to have a more stimulating or relaxing effect. The dosage of these drugs needs to be carefully monitored when they are used in conjunction with massage. Watch for excessive drowsiness. The physician may be able to reduce the dosage if massage is used on a regular basis. Work in conjunction with the prescribing physician.

Antipsychotics

Examples: phenothiazines haloperidol, risperidone (Risperdal), aripiprazole (Abilify), olanzapine (Zyprexa), quetiapine (Seroquel), clozapine (Clozaril, FazaClo)

Major tranquilizers or antipsychotic agents usually are prescribed for patients with psychoses (certain types of mental disorders) or for bipolar illness. These medications calm certain areas of the brain but permit the rest of the brain to function normally.

Implications for massage: These medications generally act as CNS depressants. Massage can increase or decrease the effect of these medications, depending on whether the massage is structured to have a more stimulating or relaxing effect. Because of the potential effects on blood pressure or dizziness, the client should avoid sudden positional changes after the massage. The dosage of these drugs needs to be monitored carefully when they are used in conjunction with massage. These medications are used to treat severe mental disorders. Work only with direct supervision from the prescribing physician. Abdominal massage may help with constipation.

Antidepressants

Examples: tricyclic antidepressants (amitriptyline), selective serotonin reuptake inhibitors (SSRIs; e.g., fluoxetine [Prozac, Sarafem], sertraline [Zoloft], paroxetine [Paxil]), serotonin/norepinephrine reuptake inhibitors (SNRIs; e.g., venlafaxine [Effexor]), and monoamine oxidase inhibitors (MAOIs; e.g., phenelzine)

Antidepressants are used to combat depression. They also are used as preventive therapy for migraine headaches, severe premenstrual syndrome, and neuropathic types of pain, although the manner in which they help relieve pain is not clearly understood. They work mostly by increasing the concentration of certain chemicals necessary for proper nerve transmission in the brain.

Implications for massage: Massage nonspecifically causes a shift in neurotransmitters and other brain chemicals. Massage has a stimulating effect on the CNS even when used for relaxation. The relaxation effect is a secondary result of the nervous system stimulation. Massage can increase serotonin levels. Watch carefully for any increase or decrease in the effect of the medications. Work with the supervision of the prescribing physician to adjust the dosage when massage is used as part of therapy. Abdominal massage may help with constipation.

Amphetamines and Related Stimulants

Examples: methylphenidate (Ritalin, Concerta, Metadate, Daytrana), dexmethylphenidate (Focalin), amphetamine salts (Adderall)

Amphetamines are adrenergic medications that are nervous system stimulants. They commonly are used to treat attention deficit disorders and occasionally may be used as anorectics (medications used to reduce the appetite). These medications temporarily quiet the part of the brain that causes hunger, but they also keep a person awake, speed up the heart, and raise blood pressure. After 2–3 weeks, these medications begin to lose their effectiveness as appetite suppressants. They also are used to treat narcolepsy. Amphetamines stimulate most people, but they have the opposite effect on hyperkinetic children and adults. When hyperkinetic children and adults take amphetamines or adrenergic medications, their level of activity is reduced. Most likely, amphetamines selectively stimulate parts of the brain that control activity.

Implications for massage: Massage nonspecifically causes a shift in neurotransmitters and other brain chemicals. Massage has a stimulating effect on the CNS even when used for relaxation. The relaxation effect is a secondary result of the nervous system stimulation. Watch carefully for any increase or decrease in the effect of the medications. Work with supervision from the prescribing physician, who may need to adjust the dosage when massage is used as part of therapy. Abdominal massage may help with constipation.

Anticonvulsants

Examples: phenobarbital, phenytoin (Dilantin), carbamazepine (Tegretol), lamotrigine (Lamictal), levetiracetam (Keppra), divalproex (Depakote), gabapentin (Neurontin), pregabalin (Lyrica)

Anticonvulsants are used to control seizures and other symptoms of epilepsy. They selectively reduce excessive stimulation in the brain. Some of these medications are used as mood stabilizers for bipolar illness or to treat neuropathic pain syndromes.

Implications for massage: Massage has a stimulating effect on the CNS even when used for relaxation. The relaxation effect is a secondary result of the nervous system stimulation. Watch carefully for any increase or decrease in the effect of the medications. Work with supervision from the prescribing physician when massage is used as part of therapy.

Antiparkinsonism Agents

Examples: carbidopa-levodopa (Sinemet), bromocriptine (Parlodel), benztropine (Cogentin), trihexyphenidyl, ropinirole (Requip), pramipexole (Mirapex), entacapone (Comtan)

Parkinson disease is a progressive disorder that is caused by a chemical imbalance of dopamine in the brain. Antiparkinsonism drugs are used to correct the chemical imbalance, thereby relieving the symptoms of the disease. Benztropine and trihexyphenidyl also are used to relieve tremors caused by other medications. Ropinirole and pramipexole may be used to treat restless leg syndrome at night.

Implications for massage: Massage nonspecifically causes a shift in neurotransmitters and other brain chemicals, including dopamine. Massage has a stimulating effect on the CNS even when used for relaxation. The relaxation effect is a secondary result of the nervous system stimulation. Watch carefully for any increase or decrease in the effect of the medications. Watch for excessive drowsiness. Work with supervision from the prescribing physician, who may adjust the dosage when massage is used as part of therapy. Abdominal massage may help with constipation.

Analgesics

Analgesics are used to relieve pain. They may be either narcotic or nonnarcotic. Narcotics act on the brain to cause deep analgesia and often drowsiness. Narcotics relieve pain and give the patient a feeling of well-being. They also are addictive.

A number of analgesics contain codeine or other narcotics combined with nonnarcotic analgesics (e.g., aspirin or acetaminophen). Tylenol #3 and Vicodin are examples.

Nonnarcotic pain relievers include the following:

- Salicylates, such as aspirin (relieve pain, antiinflammatory, and treat fever)
- Acetaminophen (relieves pain and fever but does not reduce inflammation)
- Nonsteroidal antiinflammatory drugs (NSAIDs; e.g., celecoxib, ibuprofen, naproxen, oxaprozin) (inhibit prostaglandins, reducing pain and inflammation; some agents [ibuprofen] also relieve fever)

Implications for massage: Massage reduces pain perception in several ways: through gate control hyperstimulation analgesia and counterirritation, and by stimulating the release of pain-inhibiting or pain-modifying chemicals in the body. Massage supports analgesics and has the potential to reduce the drug dosage and the duration of treatment. Aspirin thins the blood. Watch for bruising. Timing of the massage in relation to the analgesic dosage may be important. Pain perception is inhibited when a person is taking analgesics. Feedback mechanisms for pressure and massage intensity are not accurate. Reduce the intensity of massage and avoid methods that cause inflammation. Narcotics are constipating, and massage can help with constipation. Dizziness may result with the use of these medications. Have the client relax and contract the muscles of the legs for a few minutes before getting off the table. The massage therapist must also be ready to assist the client off the table, if necessary.

Antiinflammatory Medications

Antiinflammatory medications reduce the body's inflammatory response. Inflammation is the body's response to injury, and it causes swelling, pain, fever, redness, and itching. Examples of antiinflammatory medications include the following:

- NSAIDs: see Analgesics.
  - Steroids: corticosteroids (e.g., prednisone, methylprednisolone, prednisolone, dexamethasone)

Note: Skeletal muscle relaxants often are given in combination with an antiinflammatory medication such as aspirin. However, some doctors believe that aspirin and rest are better for alleviating the pain and the inflammation of muscle strain than are skeletal muscle relaxants. When sore muscles tense, increasing muscle tone, they cause pain, inflammation, and spasm. Skeletal muscle relaxants (e.g., orphenadrine, cyclobenzaprine, meprobamate, and chlorzoxazone) can relieve pain and these symptoms.

Implications for massage: Massage therapists should not perform any techniques that create inflammation or damage tissue. Mood may be altered in addition to pain perception. Feedback mechanisms for pressure and massage intensity are not accurate. The intensity of the massage should be reduced. Massage can decrease muscle spasm, reducing the need for muscle relaxants. Muscle spasm often is a protective response acting to immobilize an injured area. Use massage to reduce but not remove these protective spasms. Many antiinflammatory

medications are available over the counter (OTC), and the client may neglect to report his or her use to the massage therapist. Ask clients whether they are taking any OTC medications.

Respiratory Medications

Antitussives

Examples: dextromethorphan, codeine, hydrocodone

Antitussives control coughs. Dextromethorphan is available in OTC products; narcotic antitussives are available by prescription.

Expectorants

Examples: guaifenesin

Expectorants are used to change a nonproductive cough to a productive one (one that brings up phlegm). Expectorants are supposed to increase the amount of mucus produced. However, drinking water or using a vaporizer or humidifier is probably as effective for increasing the production of mucus.

Decongestants

Examples: phenylephrine; restricted sale: pseudoephedrine; removed from US market: ephedrine, phenylpropanolamine hydrochloride

Decongestants constrict blood vessels in the nose and sinuses to open air passages. Adrenergic agents (decongestants) are available as oral preparations, nose drops, and nose sprays. Oral decongestants are slow-acting but do not interfere with the production of mucus or the movement of the cilia (special hairlike structures) of the respiratory tract. They can increase blood pressure; therefore, patients with high blood pressure should use them cautiously. Topical decongestants (nose drops or sprays) provide fast relief. They do not increase blood pressure as much as oral decongestants, but they do slow cilia movement. Topical decongestants should not be used for more than a few days at a time.

Implications for massage: Avoid the prone position because it increases congestion.

Bronchodilators

Examples: theophylline, aminophylline, albuterol, salmeterol, formoterol

Bronchodilators (agents that open the airways in the lungs) and agents that relax smooth muscle tissue, such as that found in the lungs, are used to improve breathing. Inhalant bronchodilators are most commonly prescribed for asthma and chronic obstructive pulmonary disease (COPD; e.g., emphysema) and act directly on the muscles of the breathing tubes. Theophylline and aminophylline have limited use.

Antihistamines

Examples: Nonsedating or low sedating: loratadine (Claritin), fexofenadine (Allegra), cetirizine (Zyrtec)

Traditional (sedating): diphenhydramine (Benadryl), clemastine (Tavist-1), dimenhydrinate (Dramamine)

Histamine is a body chemical that, when released, typically causes swelling and itching. Release of histamine is often a response to exposure to an allergen. Antihistamines counteract these symptoms of allergy by blocking the effects of histamine. Antihistamines are commonly used for mild respiratory or skin allergies, such as hay fever (seasonal allergies) or hives. Some types of antihistamines are also used to prevent or treat the symptoms of motion sickness.

Implications for massage for respiratory medications: Bronchodilators are sympathomimetic and act on sympathetic nerve stimulation. Because some respiratory agents can reduce sweating, heat hydrotherapy should be avoided. Antihistamines can excite or depress the CNS. Most of these medications can cause drowsiness. Because they act on the CNS, the expected results of the massage can be distorted. The client may be unable to relax or may be excessively drowsy and dizzy after the massage. Many massage methods produce reddening of the skin caused by the release of histamine. This reaction may be altered and feedback may be inaccurate in clients taking antihistamines. Avoid this type of work with such clients. Codeine can cause constipation. Abdominal massage may prove beneficial. Many of these medications are available over the counter, and clients may neglect to report their use to the therapist. Make sure to ask clients if they are taking any OTC medications.

Vitamins and Minerals

Vitamins and minerals are chemical substances that are vital to the maintenance of normal body function. Many people take supplemental vitamins and minerals. Multivitamins, calcium, vitamin C, and vitamin D supplements are especially common. A high intake of supplements, especially individual vitamins, can cause adverse reactions or may have implications for massage. The practitioner needs to investigate further to determine any suspected interaction. At this point, specific research has not been done to determine what the specific interactions might be. It is necessary to compare the effects of the vitamin or mineral with the type of massage application to determine whether the two together are inhibitory or synergistic.

Dietary Supplements and Herbs

Herbs and other dietary supplements are agents used to support certain functions of the body. These agents are not regulated in the same manner as drugs, and unlike drugs, they are not intended to be used to diagnose, treat, cure, or prevent any disease. However, their action may be similar to pharmaceutical medications. Some medications are derivatives of plants. Ask clients whether they are taking herbs or other dietary supplements and, if so, the names and their reasons for taking them. The practitioner needs to investigate further to determine any suspected interactions. At this point, specific research has not been done to determine what the specific interactions might be. It is necessary to compare the effects of the supplement with the type of massage application to determine whether the two together are inhibitory or synergistic.

Endangerment Sites

Endangerment sites are areas in which nerves and blood vessels surface close to the skin and are not well protected by muscle or connective tissue. Therefore, deep, sustained pressure into these areas could damage the vessels and nerves. Areas that have fragile bony projections that could be broken off are also considered endangerment sites (e.g., the xiphoid process). The kidney area is considered an endangerment site because the kidneys are loosely suspended in fat and connective tissue; heavy percussion is contraindicated in this area. To prevent damage, massage therapists should avoid endangerment sites or should use only light pressure in these areas. The areas shown in Figure 3.56 are commonly considered endangerment sites for massage therapists.

Other endangerment sites and activities that should be avoided include the following:
- Eyes
- Inferior to the ear (fascial nerve, styloid process, external carotid artery)
- Posterior cervical area (spinous processes, cervical plexus)
- Lymph nodes
- Medial brachium (between the biceps and triceps)
- Musculocutaneous, median, and ulnar nerves
- Brachial artery
- Basilic vein
- Cubital (anterior) area of the median nerve, radial and ulnar arteries, and median cubital vein
- Deep stripping over a vein in a direction away from the heart (contraindicated because of possible damage to the valve system)
- Application of lateral pressure to the knees

Medical and Assistive Devices

A device is an apparatus, such as a machine or an object, that performs some sort of function. Examples include cervical collars, intravenous lines, various tubes, pacemakers, ports for chemotherapy, cosmetic implants, colostomy bags, catheters, intrauterine devices, prostheses, and various types of monitoring equipment. These devices, whether temporary or permanent, create local areas of contraindication that are similar to endangerment sites. An added concern is sanitation, especially in areas where a line or catheter is located.

Medical devices must not be disturbed by the massage application. The massage therapist may be instructed to address scar tissue development around an implant, but the massage application is targeted to the area around the device, not on the device. To reduce the chance of contamination in the area of a device, the massage therapist should reduce or eliminate the use of lubrication and should stay about 6 inches away from the area. See Appendix A for extensive coverage of pathology (Figure 3.57).

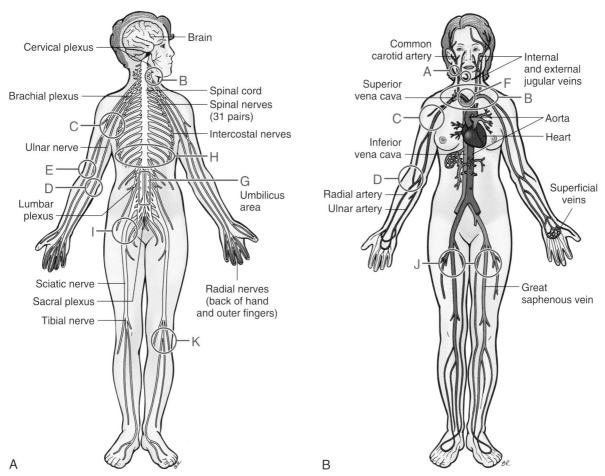

Figure 3.56 Endangerment sites of the nervous system **(A)** and the cardiovascular system **(B)**. *A,* Anterior triangle of the neck—carotid artery, jugular vein, and vagus nerve, which are located deep to the sternocleidomastoid muscle. *B,* Posterior triangle of the neck—specifically, the nerves of the brachial plexus, the brachiocephalic artery and vein superior to the clavicle, and the subclavian arteries and vein. *C,* Axillary vein—the brachial artery, axillary vein and artery, cephalic vein, and nerves of the brachial plexus. *D,* Medial epicondyle of the humerus—the ulnar nerve; also the radial and ulnar arteries. *E,* Lateral epicondyle—the radial nerve. *F,* Area of the sternal notch and anterior throat—nerves and vessels to the thyroid gland and the vagus nerve. *G,* Umbilicus area—to either side; descending aorta and abdominal aorta. *H,* 12th rib, dorsal body—location of the kidney. *I,* Sciatic notch—sciatic nerve (the sciatic nerve passes out of the pelvis through the greater sciatic foramen, under cover of the piriformis muscle). *J,* Inguinal triangle located lateral and inferior to the pubis—medial to the sartorius, external iliac artery, femoral artery, great saphenous vein, femoral vein, and femoral nerve. *K,* Popliteal fossa—popliteal artery and vein and tibial nerve.

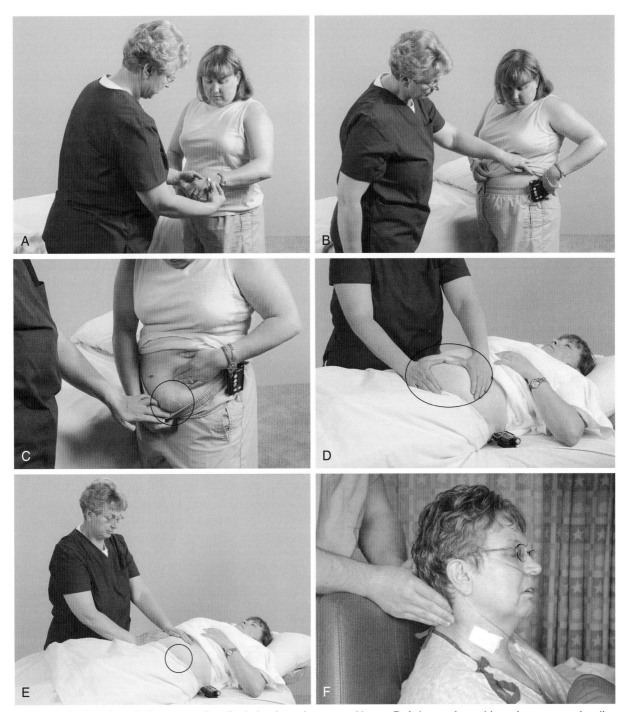

Figure 3.57 Medical devices. **A**, Be aware of medical alert bracelets or necklaces. **B**, Ask questions; this patient uses an insulin pump. **C**, Identify areas of regional contraindications. **D**, Locate areas to avoid during massage. **E**, Massage a safe distance from the area. **F**, Note the medical devices surrounding this patient, who is recovering in the hospital. (Source: Fritz S: *Mosby's fundamentals of therapeutic massage*, ed 5, St Louis, 2012, Mosby.)

ETHICS, PROFESSIONALISM, AND BUSINESS PRACTICES

The massage therapist is a professional, and professional behavior is expected. Business practices reflect ethical behavior. The massage therapist can be self-employed or may be an employee. Career pathways include the wellness setting such as many spa and massage franchise environments, sport and fitness settings such as gyms and sports teams, and healthcare settings such as hospitals, physician's offices, and long-term care facilities. It is necessary to understand what professional behavior and skills are needed to represent the massage profession in an ethical manner (Boxes 3.8 through 3.18).

BOX 3.8 The Health Insurance Portability and Accountability Act of 1996 (HIPAA)

The Health Insurance Portability and Accountability Act of 1996 is more commonly known by its acronym, HIPAA. A federal agency, the Centers for Medicare and Medicaid Services (CMS), is responsible for implementing various unrelated provisions of HIPAA, which therefore may mean different things to different people. HIPAA has had a significant impact in a number of areas of healthcare.

Health Insurance Reform
Title I of HIPAA protects health insurance coverage for workers and their families when they change or lose their jobs. This is known as the portability of health insurance coverage.

Administrative Simplification
Title II of HIPAA, the administrative simplification provision, requires the U.S. Department of Health and Human Services to establish national standards for electronic healthcare transactions and national identifiers for providers, health plans, and employers. It also addresses the security and privacy of health data. Adoption of these standards will improve the efficiency of the nation's healthcare system by encouraging widespread use of electronic data interchange in healthcare.

Preexisting Condition Exclusion
Under HIPAA regulations, a group health plan or a health insurer offering group health coverage may impose a preexisting condition exclusion with respect to a participant or beneficiary only if the following requirements are satisfied:
- The preexisting condition exclusion must relate to a condition for which medical advice, diagnosis, care, or treatment was recommended or received during the 6-month period before an individual's enrollment date.
- The preexisting condition exclusion may not last longer than 12 months (18 months for late enrollees) after an individual's enrollment date.
- The 12-month or 18-month period must be reduced by the number of days of the individual's previous creditable coverage, excluding coverage before any break in coverage of 63 days or longer.

Other HIPAA Effects
Besides limiting administrative costs by supporting the use of electronic transfer of information, HIPAA established guidelines for preventing fraud and abuse. The privacy issues arising from HIPAA have been the most discussed and debated topics related to this law. Massage therapists should receive in-service training in procedures related to HIPAA requirements and the ways they are implemented in a specific healthcare environment.

BOX 3.9 Massage Code of Ethics and Standards of Practice

Terminology
Countertransference is an inability on the part of the professional to separate the therapeutic relationship from personal feelings and expectations for the client; it is personalization of the professional relationship by the professional.

Dual role results when scopes of practice overlap (e.g., one professional provides support in more than one area of expertise) or the personal and professional relationships overlap.

Ethics is the science or study of morals, values, and principles, including the ideals of autonomy, beneficence, and justice. Ethics comprises principles of right and good conduct.

Ethical behavior is right and correct conduct based on moral and cultural standards as defined by the society in which we live.

Ethical decision-making is the application of ethical principles and professional skills to determine appropriate behavior and resolve ethical dilemmas.

Fidelity is as an ethical principle involving being loyal or faithful and exhibiting faithfulness to commitments or obligations.

Informed consent is a consumer protection process; it requires that clients be informed of the steps of treatment, that their participation be voluntary, and that they be competent to give consent. Informed consent is also an educational process that allows clients to make knowledgeable decisions about whether to receive a massage.

Jurisprudence relates to the theory and practice of the law. A jurisprudence examination is a test taken to demonstrate knowledge of a specific piece of legislation such as a massage therapy law.

Mentoring is a professional relationship in which an individual with experience and skill beyond those of the person being mentored provides support, encouragement, and career expertise.

Peer support is the interaction among those of similar skill and experience to encourage and maintain appropriate professional practice.

Principles are basic truths or rules of conduct; they are generalizations that are accepted as true and that can be used as a basis for ethical conduct.

Scope of practice is the knowledge base and practice parameters of a profession.

Standards of practice are principles that serve as specific guidelines for directing professional ethical practice and quality care, including a structure for

Continued

BOX 3.9 Massage Code of Ethics and Standards of Practice—cont'd

evaluating the quality of care. They are an attempt to define the parameters of quality care.

Standard of care is an assessment and treatment process that a clinician (massage therapist) should follow for a certain type of clinical circumstance performed at the level at which similarly qualified practitioners manage the client's care under the same or similar circumstances.

Supervision is the situation in which a person oversees others and their professional behavior. The supervisor may be from a different discipline (e.g., a nurse) or may be a massage therapist with more skill and experience than those supervised. Supervisors usually are in a position of authority. They are actively involved in such areas as the development and approval of treatment plans, review of clarity, scheduling, discipline, and teaching.

Therapeutic alliance is an interpersonal provider–client model that addresses the continuum of compliance, adherence, and collaboration in therapeutic relationships.

Therapeutic relationship is created by the interpersonal structure and professional boundaries between professionals and their clients.

Transference is the personalization of the professional relationship by the client.

Ethical Principles

The four basic concepts that constitute the code of ethics for massage professionals are as follows:

- Respect for the dignity of people. Massage professionals will maintain respect for the interests, dignity, rights, and needs of all clients, staff, and colleagues.
- Responsible caring. Competent, quality client care will be provided at the highest standard possible.
- Integrity in relationships. At all times, the professional will behave with integrity, honesty, and diligence in practice and duties.
- Responsibility to society. Massage professionals are responsible and accountable to society and shall conduct themselves in a manner that maintains high ethical standards.

Ethical Behavior

These eight principles guide professional ethical behavior:

1. Respect (esteem and regard for clients, other professionals, and oneself)
2. Client autonomy and self-determination (the freedom to decide and the right to sufficient information to make the decision)
3. Veracity (the right to the objective truth)
4. Proportionality (the principle that benefit must outweigh the burden of treatment)
5. Nonmaleficence (the principle that the professional shall do no harm and prevent harm from happening)
6. Beneficence (the principle that treatment should contribute to the client's well-being)

7. Confidentiality (respect for privacy of information)
8. Justice (the principle that ensures equality among clients)

Standards of Practice Based on Ethical Principles

In compliance with the principles of the code of ethics, massage professionals will perform the following:

1. Respect all clients, colleagues, and health professionals through nondiscrimination, regardless of age, gender, race, national origin, sexual orientation, religion, socioeconomic status, body type, political affiliation, state of health, personal habits, and life-coping skills.
2. Perform only those services for which they are qualified and honestly represent their education, certification, professional affiliations, and other qualifications. The massage professional will apply treatment only when a reasonable expectation exists that it will be advantageous to the client's condition. The massage professional, in consultation with the client, will continually evaluate the effectiveness of treatment.
3. Respect the scope of practice of other healthcare and service professionals, including physicians, chiropractors, physical therapists, podiatrists, orthopedists, psychotherapists, counselors, acupuncturists, nurses, exercise physiologists, athletic trainers, nutritionists, spiritual advisors, and cosmetologists.
4. Respect all ethical healthcare practitioners and work with them to promote health and healing.
5. Acknowledge the limitations of their personal skills, and, when necessary, refer clients to an appropriately qualified professional. The massage professional will require consultation with other knowledgeable professionals when:
   - A client requires diagnosis and opinion beyond a therapist's capabilities of assessment
   - A client's condition is beyond the therapist's scope of practice
   - A combined healthcare team is required
   - If referral to another healthcare provider is necessary, it will be done with the informed consent of the client
6. Be adequately educated and understand the physiologic effects of the specific massage techniques used to determine whether any application is contraindicated and to ensure that the most beneficial techniques are applied to a given individual.
7. Avoid false claims about the potential benefits of techniques rendered and educate the public about the actual benefits of massage.
8. Acknowledge the importance and individuality of each person, including colleagues, peers, and clients.
9. Work only with the informed consent of a client, and professionally disclose to the client any situation that may interfere with the massage professional's ability to provide the best care to serve the client's best interest.

BOX 3.9   **Massage Code of Ethics and Standards of Practice—cont'd**

10. Display respect for the client by honoring a client's process and following all recommendations by being present, listening, asking only pertinent questions, keeping agreements, being on time, draping properly, and customizing the massage to address the client's needs.
    - It is the responsibility of the massage professional to ensure the privacy and dignity of the client and to determine whether the client feels comfortable, safe, and secure with the draping provided.
    - The client may choose to be fully draped or clothed throughout the treatment.
    - The female client's breasts are not undraped unless specified by referral from a qualified healthcare professional and the massage professional is working under the supervision of such a healthcare professional.
    - The genitals, perineum, and anus are never undraped.
    - The client's consent is required for work on any part of the body, regardless of whether the client is fully clothed, fully draped, or partly draped.
11. Provide a safe, comfortable, and clean environment.
12. Maintain clear and honest communication with clients, and keep client communications confidential. Confidentiality is of the utmost importance. The massage professional must inform the client that the referring physician may be eligible to review the client's records and that records may be subpoenaed by the courts.
13. Conduct business in a professional and ethical manner in relation to clientele, business associates, acquaintances, governmental bodies, and the public.
14. Follow city, county, state, national, and international requirements.
15. Charge a fair price for the session. Gratuities are appropriate if within reasonable limits (similar to percentages for other service providers, i.e., 10%–20%). A gift, gratuity, or benefit that is intended to influence a referral, decision, or treatment may not be accepted and must be returned to the giver immediately.
16. Keep accurate records and review the records with the client.
17. Never engage in any sexual conduct, sexual conversation, or any other sexual activities involving clients.
18. Avoid affiliation with any business that uses any form of sexual suggestiveness or explicit sexuality in advertising or promoting services or in the actual practice of service.
19. Practice honesty in advertising, promoting services ethically and in good taste, and advertising only techniques for which the professional is certified or adequately trained.
20. Strive for professional excellence through regular assessment of personal strengths, limitations, and effectiveness and through continuing education and training.
21. Accept the responsibility to oneself, one's clients, and the profession to maintain physical, mental, and emotional well-being and to inform clients when the professional is not functioning at full capacity.
22. Refrain from using any mind-altering drugs, alcohol, or intoxicants before or during professional massage sessions.
23. Maintain a professional appearance and demeanor by practicing good hygiene and dressing in a professional, modest, and nonsexual manner.
24. Undergo periodic peer review.
25. Respect all pertinent reporting requirements outlined by legislation regarding abuse.
26. Report to the proper authorities any accurate knowledge and its supportive documentation regarding violations by massage professionals and other health or service professionals.
27. Avoid interests, activities, or influences that might conflict with the obligation to act in the best interest of clients and the massage therapy profession, and safeguard professional integrity by recognizing potential conflicts of interest and avoiding them.
28. Regularly self-assess for biases that influence the respect for others and ethical decision-making.

Source: Fritz S: *Mosby's fundamentals of therapeutic massage*, ed 5, St Louis, 2012, Mosby.

BOX 3.10   **Informed Consent**

The following questions should be answered at the outset of the professional relationship.
- What are the goals of the therapeutic program?
- What services will be provided?
- What behavior is expected of the client?
- What are the risks and benefits of the process?
- What are the practitioner's qualifications?
- What are the financial considerations?
- How long is the therapy expected to last?
- What are the limitations of confidentiality?
- In what areas does the professional have mandatory reporting requirements?

Source: Fritz S: *Mosby's fundamentals of therapeutic massage*, ed 7, St Louis, 2021, Mosby.

BOX 3.11	Government Credentials and Regulations

Licensing
- Requires a state or provincial board of examiners
- Requires all constituents who practice the profession to be licensed
- Legally defines and limits the scope of practice for a profession
- Requires specific educational courses or an examination
- Protects title usage (e.g., only those licensed can use the title of massage therapist)

Government Registration
- Not to be confused with private registration processes
- Administered by the state Department of Registry or other appropriate state agency

Voluntary Verification
- Does not necessarily require a specific education, such as a school diploma; often other forms of verification of professional standards, such as years in practice, are acceptable
- Does not provide title protection

Exemptions
- Means that a practitioner is not required to comply with an existing local or state regulation
- Excuses practitioners who meet specified educational requirements from meeting current regulatory requirements
- Does not provide title protection

Source: Fritz S: *Mosby's fundamentals of therapeutic massage*, ed 5, St Louis, 2012, Mosby.

BOX 3.12	Documentation Rules for Medical Records and Healthcare Professionals

Medical records must be maintained in a specific way: medical records in most situations are maintained electronically. The various software used will support proper documentation procedures.
- Each page of the record should identify the patient by name and by hospital, clinic, or private physician clinical record number.
- Each entry in the record should include the date and time the entry was made and the signature and credential of the individual making the entry.
- No blank spaces should be left between entries.
- All entries should be written in ink or produced on a printer or typewriter or recorded appropriately in an electronic format.
- The record must not be altered in any way. Erasures, use of correction fluid, and marked-out areas are not appropriate.
- Errors should be corrected in a manner that allows the reader to see and understand the error. Errors are corrected as follows:
  - A single line is drawn through the error, and the legibility of the previous entry is checked.
  - The correct information is inserted.
  - The correction is dated and initialed by the person who is recording the data.
  - If space is inadequate to allow the correction to be made legibly at the place of the error, a note should be made indicating where the corrected entry can be found; this cross-reference should be dated and initialed. The correct information should be entered in proper chronologic order for the date the error was discovered and corrected.
- All information should be recorded as soon as possible. Memories can fade, and important facts can be omitted.

- Abbreviations should be used sparingly. Only those that have been approved by the organization are appropriate. The same abbreviation can have different meanings, which can be misleading. It is always better to write out the information than to use abbreviations that can be misinterpreted.
- Health caregivers must write legibly. Because so many other clinicians and practitioners use the patient record to provide care, it is important for the quality of patient care that the record be legible. An electronic format helps in this area.
- All entries must be consistent with one another. The assessment must agree with the diagnostic testing, or an explanation must be given as to why it does not.
- Entries should be factual accounts.
- All information given to the patient before any procedures should be recorded. This ensures and verifies that the patient was properly informed of the benefits and risks before giving consent for the procedure.
- Telephone contacts should be entered into the record immediately.
- Some method of organizing entries, such as the SOAP (subjective data, objective data, assessment, and plan) format, must be used to ensure that the entries are comprehensive and reflect the thought processes involved when decisions were made about the patient's care.

These rules result in a record that is accurate, timely, specific, objective, concise, consistent, comprehensive, logical, legible, and reflective of the thought processes of the healthcare providers (including massage therapists). Not only will such a record be the best defense in a lawsuit, but it also will result in the best care for the patient.

Source: Fritz S: *Mosby's fundamentals of therapeutic massage*, ed 5, St Louis, 2012, Mosby.

BOX 3.13 Employee "Do's" and "Don'ts"

Don't
- Gossip
- Complain without providing a viable solution
- Be dishonest
- Behave unethically
- Behave irresponsibly

Do
- Get to work on time
- Look and act like a professional
- Be consistent and accurate in recording requirements of the business
- Be courteous and supportive
- Be assertive and communicate openly with your employer
- Develop a sense of commitment and loyalty to your employer
- Take your responsibilities seriously
- Improve your skills
- Own your mistakes and correct them
- Be willing to extend yourself in the short term for everyone's long-term gain
- Be a team player
- Be flexible and creative
- Use problem-solving skills to resolve potential conflict
- Commit to the job

Source: Fritz S: *Mosby's fundamentals of therapeutic massage*, ed 7, St Louis, 2021, Mosby.

BOX 3.14 Eight Keys to Employability

1. Personal Values
Valued workers
- Are honest
- Have good self-esteem and a positive self-image
- Have personal and career goals
- Demonstrate emotional stability
- Exhibit a good attitude
- Are self-motivated
- Do not limit themselves

2. Problem-Solving and Decision-Making Skills
Valued workers
- Are flexible
- Are creative and innovative
- Can adapt to the changing demands of a job
- Can reason and make objective decisions
- Can keep their mind on several parts of a job at the same time

3. Relations with Other People
Valued workers
- Work well with peers
- Accept authority and supervision
- Accept constructive criticism
- Are team members
- Are friendly
- Are consistent in their relations with people
- Are cooperative
- Accept assignments pleasantly
- Are tactful
- Accept all types of people
- Have leadership qualities

4. Communication Skills
Valued workers
- Ask relevant questions
- Seek help when needed
- Notify supervisors of absences and the reasons for the absences
- Clearly express themselves when talking
- Listen actively and communicate comprehension

5. Task-Related Skills
Valued workers
- Complete work on time
- Can follow directions
- Are not distracting or distractible
- Work neatly and leave the work environment clean and orderly
- Care for equipment and materials
- Are accurate
- Constantly improve their performance

6. Maturity
Valued workers
- Work well without supervision
- Are reliable and dependable
- Accept responsibility
- Don't let their personal problems interfere with their work
- Are willing to perform extra work and work overtime
- Are always prepared for work
- Show pride in their work
- Show initiative
- Remain calm and self-controlled
- Accept responsibility for their own behavior, including mistakes and successes
- Demonstrate maturity
- Evaluate their own work accurately
- Are patient and tolerant
- Use time wisely
- Are assertive when necessary
- Show self-confidence

7. Health and Safety Habits
Valued workers
- Observe safety and sanitation rules
- Practice good personal hygiene
- Dress appropriately and are well groomed
- Are in good health
- Practice stress management

8. Commitment to the Job
Valued workers
- Are punctual and have good attendance records
- Observe all organizational policies
- Consider work more than a job
- Are interested and enthusiastic
- Obtain relevant continuing education

BOX 3.15 **Key Constituents of a Professional Practice Model for Complementary Medicine Practitioners**

- Qualifications. Practitioners should have recognized qualifications from a training establishment that is accredited by a suitable regulatory body.
- Registration/license. Practitioners must be registered with or licensed by a recognized professional body that requires its members to abide by codes of conduct, ethics, and discipline.
- Insurance. Practitioners must have adequate professional liability insurance coverage that applies to the period of their employment.
- Consent to treatment. Patients must be fully informed about the nature of the therapy and its effects, including any side effects, and must have realistic expectations of its benefits. The informed consent of the patient or, in the case of young children, of the parent or guardian must be obtained and documented.
- Medical responsibility. Practitioners should be aware that patients referred to them for treatment remain the overall responsibility of the referring clinician. Complementary and alternative medicine (CAM) practitioners should not advise discontinuation of existing treatments without the agreement of the referring clinician.
- Documentation. Practitioners should keep a written record of the consultation and each episode of treatment. All written and oral information should be treated as confidential, in compliance with the requirements of the Health Insurance Portability and Accountability Act (HIPAA).

- Refusal to treat. Practitioners have a duty not to treat a patient if they consider the treatment unsafe or unsuitable.
- Education and training. Practitioners should take responsibility for keeping up to date on developments in the practice of their therapy.
- Quality standards. In conjunction with other healthcare professionals, practitioners should assist with the development of local standards and guidelines for practice.
- Audit. Practitioners should undertake a clinical audit and report the results to the employing or commissioning practice. They should be responsible for monitoring the outcome of therapy, and the opinions of patients should be actively sought and included in any evaluation.
- Research. Practitioners should be expected to agree to take part in research trials to support the evaluation and development of treatment programs.
- Health and safety. Practitioners should comply with the requirements of health and safety legislation and should adhere to good practice in the protection of staff, patients, and the public.
- Control of infection. Practitioners should adhere to regulations governing infection control and should follow the procedures for reporting outbreaks of infection.

Practitioners of complementary therapies, including massage, must be in compliance with these logical and attainable recommendations before a unified move can be made toward integrated medicine.

Source: Scottish Department of Health 1996 Complementary Medicine and the National Health Service: Complementary medicine information pack for primary care groups, June 2000.

BOX 3.16 **Qualities of a Professional Massage Therapist**

Professional massage therapists have knowledge of techniques and principles that include an understanding of legal and ethical issues. They also must acquire a working knowledge of and tolerance for human nature and individuals' characteristics, given that daily contact with a wide variety of individuals with a host of problems and concerns is a significant part of the work. Courtesy, compassion, and common sense are often cited as the 3 Cs most vital to the success of a massage therapist.

In fact, the first responsibility of a massage therapist is always to provide competent, courteous, and compassionate healthcare to clients. Other characteristics of a professional massage therapist include the following:
- Has an aptitude for working with his or her hands
- Is computer literate
- Has good communication skills that include writing, speaking, and listening
- Has and maintains professional boundaries and integrity
- Avoids dual relationships
- Is trustworthy and exhibits a sense of responsibility

- Prepares and maintains client records
- Keeps client information confidential
- Leaves private concerns at home
- Has patience in dealing with others and the ability to work as a member of a team
- Practices with competence and within the scope of his or her training and capabilities
- Projects a favorable professional image
- Possesses expertise that comes through three main sources: technical competence, social validation (through formal recognition of training and status), and reputation
- Has a relaxed attitude when meeting new people
- Starts and ends each session on time and lets nothing interrupt a session
- Has an understanding of and empathy for others
- Uses appropriate guidelines when releasing information
- Uses tact when resolving conflicts
- Has a willingness to learn new skills and techniques

Source: Salvo SG: *Massage therapy: principles and practice*, ed 4, St Louis, 2011, Saunders.

BOX 3.17 Accounting and Tax Terminology

Accounting: process of interpreting, measuring, and describing economic activity.

Accounts payable: money you owe to suppliers.

Accounts receivable: money owed to you or your business.

Accrual-basis accounting: charging the income and expense to the period in which they were incurred or recognized.

Assets: things that offer value to the company. Current assets are cash on hand; fixed assets are hard goods such as machines, equipment, furniture, vehicles, property, and buildings that the company owns.

Balance sheet: summary of the company's *assets, liabilities*, and owner's *equity* at an exact point in time.

Cash-based accounting: record of transactions, both monies collected and expenses, at the time they are received or paid.

Cash flow: amounts and sources of money coming into and going out of the company.

Corporation: in technical terms, it means a legal entity generally chartered by a relevant government and separate and distinct from the persons who own it.

Credits: entries made on the *right side* of an account. Credits reduce assets and expense accounts and increase liability, capital, and income accounts.

Debits: entries made on the *left side* of an account. Debits increase assets and expense accounts and reduce liability, capital, and income accounts.

Deductions: write-offs permitted to subtract from gross income to calculate taxable income. All taxpayers may claim a standard deduction, which is determined by the IRS. If qualifying expenses exceed standard deduction, you may claim the higher amount by itemizing deductions.

Depreciation: process of spreading out the deduction for the cost of an asset over time.

Equity: difference between total assets and liabilities; also called *net worth*.

Estimated tax: quarterly payments of the estimated amount needed to cover expected tax liability for the year on income that's not subject to withholding, such as investment or self-employment income.

Expenses: costs that are currently deductible, as opposed to capital expenditures, which may not be currently deducted but must be depreciated or amortized over the useful life of the property.

FICA: the Federal Insurance Contributions Act tax that pays for Social Security and Medicare is usually split 50/50 between employers and employees.

Gross income: money earned or accumulated before taxes.

Income statement: statement showing the results of a business operation for a particular period of time. The statement will show the business's revenues and expenses.

Inventory: unsold retail items on hand.

Liabilities: what the business owes, both current and long-term liabilities.

Limited Liability Company (LLC): business form that combines the flexibility and tax advantages of a partnership with the limited liability features of a joint-stock company. An LLC may be taxed as a partnership or a corporation depending on the nature of the status under which it is organized.

Net income: money left after taxes.

Partnership: association of two or more persons (individuals or companies) formed for the purpose of making a profit. A partnership can be a general partnership or a limited partnership depending on the extent of each party's liability. A general partnership is characterized by the unlimited liability of the general partners for partnership debts.

Petty cash: cash used to pay for incidental expenses, usually set up and treated as a separate account.

Profit and loss statement: statement of income that outlines revenues and expenses over a fixed period, indicating whether your business made a *profit* or a *loss*.

Proprietorship: an unincorporated business owned by a single person. The individual proprietor has the right to all the profits from the business and also the responsibility for all its liabilities.

Sales Tax: tax imposed as a percentage of the price of goods (and sometimes services). The tax is generally paid by the buyer but the seller is responsible for collecting and remitting the tax to the tax authorities.

SECA: the Self Employment Contributions Act tax that pays for Social Security and Medicare for self-employed individuals.

Self-Employed: referring to persons who work for themselves and are not employed by another. The owner-operator of a sole proprietorship or a partner is considered self-employed.

Taxable Income: it can refer to income that is taxable (such as wages, interest, and dividends) rather than tax-exempt (such as the interest on municipal bonds). On tax returns, "taxable income" is the income after subtracting all adjustments, deductions and exemptions—that is, the amount on which your tax bill is computed.

Tax identification numbers: A Taxpayer Identification Number (TIN) is an identification number used by the Internal Revenue Service (IRS) in the administration of tax laws. The Internal Revenue Service (IRS) issues a nine-digit tracking Taxpayer Identification Number (TIN) to businesses. The format of an EIN is XX-XXXXXXX. A Social Security number (SSN) is issued by the Social Security Administration. The format of an SSN is XXX-XX-XXXX.

Withholding: The amount held back from your wages each payday to pay your income and Social Security taxes for the year. The amount withheld is based on the size of your salary and the W-4 form you file with your employer.

Source: Salvo SG: *Massage therapy: principles and practice*, ed 4, St Louis, 2011, Saunders.

BOX 3.18	Business Plan

Introduction
1. Cover letter
2. Table of contents

Personal Information
1. What is my experience in this business, if any?
2. What do I love about my work?
3. What are my weaknesses and shortcomings?
4. What are my strengths and talents?
5. What is special and distinct about me as a massage therapist?
6. Why will these attributes appeal to clients?
7. What are my values?
8. What have I learned about this business from fellow therapists, teachers, trade journals, and trade suppliers?

General Description of Business
1. What is my vision statement?
2. What is my mission statement?
3. What services do I or will I offer? (Describe these services and the benefits of these services.)
4. For what purpose will people buy my service?
5. Am I willing to change what I offer, to some extent, to meet my client's changing needs?

Operating Procedures
1. What types of licenses are required for me to operate my business?
2. What will be the opening day of my business? What hours of the day and days of the week will I be in operation?
3. What will my office policies be for late clients, cancellations, out-of-date gift certificate redemption, insufficient funds, checks, and credit card sales?

Management and Personnel
1. What is my management experience?
2. What do I predict my legal structure will be?
3. Who will be the other key figures in my business? (Include an organizational chart, with a list of duties and backgrounds of key individuals, outside consultants or advisors, and board of directors.)
4. How will services be provided? Will I do all the work, or will I use employees or contract labor?
5. What are the types of support that my business may require? (Include childcare, janitorial service, lawn and garden care, and bookkeeping and accounting.)
6. What wages and benefits can I offer each type of employee and support person?

Insurance Needs
1. What are my insurance needs? (These may include professional and general liability, business personal property, automotive, life and health insurance, and disability insurance.)
2. Have I contacted an agent to discuss what types of policies the agent offers and the cost and benefit of each?

Marketing and Competition
1. What do I want my business identity to be? (Describe the image you want to project. You never get a second chance to make a first impression.)
2. What do I want people to say to others about my services?
3. Who is my target market? Who will want to buy my services? (Identify important characteristics such as age, gender, occupation, income, and so on.)
4. Who else provides a similar service? (In order of their strength in the market, list your five closest competitors by name and address. Next, describe each competitor's strengths and weaknesses.) What have I learned from my competitors' operations and from their advertising?
5. What will my fee schedule look like? How have I determined these fees? Will this price cover my material costs, labor costs, and overhead?
6. What are my competitors charging?
7. How am I different from my competitors in ways that matter to potential clients? (Refer to the previous business plan section on personal information.)

Advertising, Promotion, and Location
1. How can I get the attention of the people I want to reach? Which advertising media are appropriate for my business and targeted clients?
2. What other channels such as networking, referrals, and publicity will I use to reach clients?
3. How can I discover whether a promotion is working?
4. What is my advertising budget for 6 months? (Include specific media you will use and the cost of each.)
5. What type of location does my business require? (Describe the type of building your business needs, including office and studio space, parking, exterior lighting, security needs, and proximity to other businesses for added exposure.)
6. Where do I plan to locate my business? Is this location right for my business and me?
7. What geographic area will my business serve? Are sufficient numbers of potential clients located there?
8. What type of physical layout is needed for my business? (Include layouts for the reception area, restroom, hydrotherapy and spa room [if applicable], retail and inventory areas, and gift certificate sales.)

Financial Projections
1. How much money do I have to begin this business?
2. What is the cost of my capital equipment, supply list, and other startup items?
3. If money is to be borrowed, do I have a bank and loan officer in mind?
4. How will my business be profitable? (Produce an income projection [profit and loss statements], balance sheet, cash flow statement, and break-even analysis. The projection should cover 3 years—that is, the first year projects monthly and the next 2 years project quarterly.)
5. Based on these documents, how much money will I need to make to stay in business?
6. What are the growth opportunities?

Supporting Documents
1. Tax returns for the past 3 years
2. Personal financial statements
3. Copy of proposed lease for building space
4. Copy of licenses and other legal documents
5. Copy of your curriculum vitae

Source: Salvo SG: *Massage therapy: principles and practice*, ed 4, St Louis, 2011, Saunders.

RESEARCH LITERACY

As professionals, it is important to identify valid research and understand the implications of research for the practice of massage (Boxes 3.19 and 3.20).

BOX 3.19 **Research Vocabulary**

Absolute risk: the chance that a specific occurrence may happen over a specified time period.

Adverse effect: any effect that produces functional impairment.

Analytic study: a type of epidemiologic study in which scientists observe certain behaviors (e.g., food choices) and track whether certain outcomes (e.g., the development of disease) occur.

Bias: problems in the design of a study that can lead to effects that are not related to the variables being studied. For example, *selection bias* occurs when study subjects are chosen in a way that can misleadingly increase or decrease the strength of an association.

Blind (single or double): in a single-blind experiment, subjects do not know whether they are receiving an experimental treatment or a placebo. In a double-blind experiment, neither the researchers nor the participants are aware of which subjects receive the treatment until after the study has been completed.

Clinical trial: type of experimental research in which people are used as subjects. The effectiveness and safety of a nutrient or a medical treatment are evaluated by monitoring its effect on people participating in the clinical trial. Clinical trials may be small, involving a limited number of participants, or they may be large intervention trials that attempt to discover the outcomes of treatment on entire populations. The more participants included in a study, the greater the likelihood that the study results can be replicated in the general population.

Cohort study: an epidemiologic study in which scientists select the study population according to the participants' exposure, regardless of whether the group has the disease or the health outcome that is being studied. Researchers then determine the outcomes and compare the results on the basis of the individuals' exposure. Cohort studies often are referred to as *prospective studies* because they follow the study population forward in time.

Confounding variable (also confounding factor or hidden variable): a "hidden" variable that may cause an association that the researcher attributes to other variables. In some situations, a confounding factor may wrongly increase the effect of a substance.

Control group: the group of subjects in a study against which a comparison is made to determine whether an observation or a treatment has an effect. In an experimental study, it is the group that does not receive treatment.

Correlation: an association in which one phenomenon is found to be accompanied by another. A correlation does not prove cause and effect.

Cross-partial study: a type of epidemiologic study that is basically the same as a survey. The epidemiologist defines the population to be studied and then collects information from members of the population about their disease and exposure status. Because the data represent a point in time, completing this type of study is somewhat like taking a snapshot of the population.

Descriptive study: a type of epidemiologic study in which scientists collect information to characterize and summarize a health event or problem.

Epidemiologic study: considered the basic science of public health, this type of observational research usually focuses on the study of large groups, sometimes tens of thousands or hundreds of thousands of people. Epidemiologic studies attempt to identify possible factors that may increase the risk or probability of a disease.

Experimental group: the group of subjects in an experimental study that receives treatment.

Experimental research: research that generates data by investigating biochemical substances or biologic processes. Experimental research often is conducted in vitro, such as in test tubes. It also is conducted in vivo—that is, in both animals and humans.

Generalizability: the extent to which the results of a study can be applied to the general population.

Mechanism of action: the way in which a substance, such as a chemical, exerts its effects.

Meta-analysis: a quantitative technique in which the results of several individual studies are pooled to yield overall conclusions.

Observational research: this type of research may be used in the laboratory, but it is primarily conducted in a natural setting to study the relationship between a specific factor and some aspect of health or illness. For this reason, observational research may suggest an association but does not determine cause and effect.

Outcomes research: a type of research that provides information about the way a specific procedure or treatment regimen affects the subject (clinical safety and efficacy), the subject's physical functioning and lifestyle, and economic considerations, such as saving or prolonging life and avoiding costly complications.

Phase I study (clinical trial): researchers initially test a new treatment or intervention in a small group of people to see whether it is effective and to further

Continued

BOX 3.19   Research Vocabulary—cont'd

evaluate its safety, determine a safe dosage range, and identify side effects.

Phase II study: the treatment is given to a larger group of people to see whether it is effective and to further evaluate its safety.

Phase III study: the treatment is given to large groups of people to allow researchers to confirm its effectiveness, monitor for side effects, compare it to commonly used treatments, and collect information that will allow the drug or treatment to be used safely.

Phase IV study: a study that is done after the treatment has been marketed, to gather information about its effects in various populations and about any side effects associated with long-term use.

Placebo: sometimes casually referred to as a "sugar pill," a placebo is a "fake" treatment that seems to be identical to the real treatment. Placebo treatments are used to eliminate bias that may arise from the expectation that a treatment should produce an effect.

Prevalence: the number of existing cases of a disease in a defined population at a specified time.

Prospective study: epidemiologic research that follows a group of people over a period of time to observe the potential effects of diet, behavior, and other factors on health or the incidence of disease.

Random sampling: a method of selecting subjects to participate in a study in which all individuals in a population have an equal chance of being chosen. This process helps to ensure the generalizability of a study's results.

Randomization (or **random assignment**): the process of assigning subjects to experimental or control groups, with the subjects having an equal chance of being assigned to either group. Randomization is used to control for known variables and variables for which it is difficult to control.

Reliability: whether a test or an instrument used to collect data (e.g., a questionnaire) gives the same results if repeated with the same person several times. A reliable test gives reproducible results.

Research design: the way in which a study is set up to collect information or data. For valid results, the research design must be appropriate to answer the question or hypothesis that is being studied.

Residual confounding: the effect that remains after attempts have been made to statistically control for variables that cannot be measured perfectly. This is an important concept in epidemiologic studies because researchers' knowledge of human biology is still developing. Unknown variables may exist that could change conclusions based on epidemiologic research.

Retrospective study: research that relies on recall of past data or of previously recorded information. This type of research often is considered to have limitations because the number of variables cannot be controlled, and people's memories are fallible.

Risk: a term that encompasses a variety of measures of the probability of an outcome. It usually refers to unfavorable outcomes, such as illness or death.

Risk factor: anything statistically shown to have a relationship with the incidence of a disease. It does not necessarily imply cause and effect.

Statistical power: a mathematical quantity that indicates the probability that a study will obtain a statistically significant effect. A high power of 80% (or 0.8) indicates that the study would produce a statistically significant effect 80% of the time if conducted repeatedly. A power of 0.1 means that a 90% chance exists that the research will miss any effect or effects.

Statistical significance: the probability of obtaining an effect or association in a study sample that is as or more extreme than the effect or association observed if there was actually no effect.

Validity: the extent to which a study or study instrument or instruments measure that which the study is intended to measure. *Validity* refers to the accuracy or truthfulness of a study's conclusion or conclusions.

Variable: any characteristic that may vary in study subjects, including gender, age, body weight, diet, behavior, attitude, or other attribute. In an experiment, the treatment being investigated is called the *independent variable*. The variable that is influenced by the treatment is the *dependent variable*, which may change as a result of the effect of the independent variable.

Source: Hymel GM: *Research methods for massage and holistic strategies*, St Louis, 2005, Mosby and www.realmercuryfacts.com. Center for Food, Nutrition, and Agriculture Policy, University of Maryland, College Park, Maryland, 2006.

BOX 3.20   Criteria for Critiquing a Research Study

Preliminary Part

1. Does the title of the study provide a basis for identifying the type of study, major variables, and participants?
2. Does the abstract synthesize the main body of the report (i.e., the introduction, method, results, and discussion) with a particular focus on the research question, research hypothesis, participants, research method and design, major variables, instruments, statistical techniques, principal findings, and conclusions?

Introductory Part

3. Is the reader introduced to the relevant professional literature bearing on the study being reported by way of a general overview of the research problem area, as well as more specific coverage of individual studies?
4. Is the purpose of the study identified by means of formulation of the research question at an operational level?
5. Is a rationale or justification that is based on various features of the professional literature presented as a context or framework for the study's research hypothesis?
6. Do the authors state the study's research hypothesis in such a way that the predicted answer to the research question is clear and unambiguous?

Method Part

7. Are the study's participants clearly characterized, along with the inclusion and exclusion criteria used to identify them?
8. Did the researchers justify the number of participants constituting the sample size by means of a power analysis?
9. Was an accessible population of potential participants acknowledged and an indication given of how the sample was derived from such a population—through random selection or some other procedure?
10. Did the authors specify the manner in which the participants were assigned to the two or more comparison groups—whether through random assignment or some other means?
11. Was any clarification provided as to how the ethical aspects of the study were governed, particularly in reference to the protection of participants, the overall integrity of the research, and the earlier approval of the study by an institutional review board?
12. Was the nature of the research effort adequately characterized in terms of its position in the research continuum (i.e., its position regarding research category, strategy, method, design, and defining procedures)?
13. Were the study's variables operationalized in a comprehensive fashion so that their manipulation or measurement could be replicated?
14. Did the authors clearly specify the equipment and instruments used in the study for variable manipulation or measurement purposes, along with documentation of the technical characteristic of such, including validity and reliability?

Results Part

15. Were the data analysis techniques used identified and justified?
16. Were the results of the study communicated by an appeal to descriptive and inferential statistics consistent with the nature of the research question and the research method and measurement scales used?
17. Were the results of the data analysis related to an appropriate decision regarding the study's null (statistical) hypothesis?
18. Was the decision on the null hypothesis acknowledged as a basis for inferring decisions concerning the alternative and research hypotheses?
19. If hypothesis testing was performed, were the analyses augmented with other statistical techniques, such as confidence interval estimation or effect size calculations (or both)?
20. Were tables and figures used appropriately to make the data analysis more comprehensible?

Discussion Part

21. Did the researchers reflect on the manner in which the study was designed and conducted with regard to any limitations or delimitations (i.e., intentional or unintentional boundaries)?
22. Did the authors elaborate on the interpretation stated in the results part?
23. Did the researchers address the significance of the study and its findings, particularly as they relate to earlier studies in the problem area investigated?
24. Were possible intervening variables in the study addressed that might explain why the results obtained were forthcoming?
25. Were recommendations made to the reader about needed follow-up studies that might fully or partly replicate, or at least augment, the current study?

Concluding Part

26. Does the list of references accurately reflect each of the sources cited in the research report, with use of a consistent bibliographic citation style?
27. Does the research report have any appendixes that provide greater detail on information presented earlier in the article?
28. Are authors' notes included that provide insight into funding support for the study, contact directives for communicating with the authors as a follow-up, and collegial assistance in completing the study?
29. Are any footnotes provided that elaborate on one or more aspects of the study that would have been misplaced or distracting if they had been embedded in the main body of the report?

CHAPTER 4

Anatomy and Physiology

This content targets the sciences. This aspect of information provides the foundation for the validity of massage. Many, if not most, exam questions found on licensing exams contain aspects of science knowledge. It is necessary to know this language to understand what the question is asking.

MEDICAL TERMINOLOGY SIMPLIFIED

Tables 4.1 through 4.4 discuss common prefixes, root words, suffixes, and abbreviations.

TABLE 4.1 Common Prefixes

Prefix	Meaning	Prefix	Meaning
a-, an-	Without or not	intro-	Into, within
ab-	Away from	leuk-	White
ad-	Toward	macro-	Large
ante-	Before, forward	mal-	Bad, illness, disease
anti-	Against	mega-	Large
auto-	Self	micro-	Small
bi-	Double, two	mono-	One, single
circum-	Around	neo-	New
contra	Against, opposite	non-	Not
de-	Down from, away from, not	para-	Abnormal
dia-	Across, through, apart	per-	By, through
dis-	Separation, away from	peri-	Around
dys-	Bad, difficult, abnormal	poly-	Many, much
ecto-	Outer, outside	post-	After, behind
en-	In, into, within	pre-	Before, in front of, prior to
endo-	Inner, inside	pro-	Before, in front of
epi-	Over, on	re-	Again
eryth-	Red	retro-	Backward
ex-	Out, out of, from, away from	semi-	Half
hemi-	Half	sub-	Under
hyper-	Excessive, too much, high	super-	Above, over, excess
hypo-	Under, decreased, less than normal	supra-	Above, over
in-	In, into, within, not	trans-	Across
inter-	Between	uni-	One
intra-	Within		

Source: Fritz S: *Mosby's fundamentals of therapeutic massage*, ed 5, St Louis, 2012, Mosby.

TABLE 4.2 Common Root Words

Root (combining vowel)	Meaning	Root (combining vowel)	Meaning
abdomen (o)	Abdomen	neur (o)	Nerve
aden (o)	Gland	ocul (o)	Eye
adren (o)	Adrenal gland	orth (o)	Straight, normal, correct
angi (o)	Vessel	oste (o)	Bone
arterio (o)	Artery	ot (o)	Ear
arthr (o)	Joint	ped (o)	Child, foot
broncho (o)	Bronchus, bronchi	pharyng (o)	Pharynx
card, cardi (o)	Heart	phleb (o)	Vein
cephal (o)	Head	pnea	Breathing, respiration
chondr (o)	Cartilage	pneum (o)	Lung, air, gas
col (o)	Colon	proct (o)	Rectum
cost (o)	Rib	psych (o)	Mind
crani (o)	Skull	pulm (o)	Lung
cyan (o)	Blue	py (o)	Pus
cyst (o)	Bladder, cyst	rect (o)	Rectum
cyt (o)	Cell	rhin (o)	Nose
derma	Skin	sten (o)	Narrow, constriction
duoden (o)	Duodenum	stern (o)	Sternum
encephal (o)	Brain	stomat (o)	Mouth
enter (o)	Intestines	therm (o)	Heat
fibro (o)	Fiber, fibrous	thorac (o)	Chest
gastr (o)	Stomach	thromb (o)	Clot, thrombus
gyn, gyne, gyneco	Female	thyr (o)	Thyroid
hem, hema, hemo, hemat (o)	Blood	toxic (o)	Poison, poisonous
hepat (o)	Liver	trache (o)	Trachea
hydr (o)	Water	ur (o)	Urine, urinary tract, urination
hyster (o)	Uterus	urethra (o)	Urethra
ile (o), ili (o)	Ileum	urin (o)	Urine
laryng (o)	Larynx	uter (o)	Uterus
mamm (o)	Breast, mammary gland	vas (o)	Blood vessel, vas deferens
my (o)	Muscle	ven (o)	Vein
myel (o)	Spinal cord, bone marrow	vertebr (o)	Spine, vertebrae

Source: Fritz S: *Mosby's fundamentals of therapeutic massage*, ed 5, St Louis, 2012, Mosby.

TABLE 4.3 Common Suffixes

Suffix	Meaning	Suffix	Meaning
-algia	Pain	-megaly	Enlargement
-asis	Condition, usually abnormal	-oma	Tumor
-cele	Hernia, herniation, pouching	-osis	Condition
-cyte	Cell	-pathy	Disease
-ectasis	Dilation, stretching	-penia	Lack, deficiency
-ectomy	Excision, removal of	-phasia	Speaking
-emia	Blood condition	-phobia	Exaggerated fear
-genesis	Development, production, creation	-plasty	Surgical repair or reshaping
-genic	Producing, causing	-plegia	Paralysis
-gram	Record	-rrhage, -rrhagia	Excessive flow
-graph	Diagram, recording instrument	-rrhea	Profuse flow, discharge
-graphy	Making a recording	-scope	Examination instrument
-iasis	Condition of	-scopy	Examination using a scope
-ism	Condition	-stasis	Maintenance, maintaining a constant level
-itis	Inflammation	-stomy, -ostomy	Creation of an opening
-logy	Study of	-tomy, -otomy	Incision, cutting into
-lysis	Destruction of, decomposition	-uria	Condition of the urine

Source: Fritz S: *Mosby's fundamentals of therapeutic massage*, ed 5, St Louis, 2012, Mosby.

TABLE 4.4   **Common Abbreviations**

Abbreviation	Meaning	Abbreviation	Meaning
abd	Abdomen	IBW	Ideal body weight
ADL	Activities of daily living	ICT	Inflammation of connective tissue
ad lib	As desired	Id	The same
alt die	Every other day	L	Left, length, lumbar
alt hor	Alternate hours	Lig	Ligament
alt noct	Alternate nights	M	Muscle, meter, myopia
AM (AM, am)	Morning	Meds	Medications
ama	Against medical advice	ML	Midline
ANS	Autonomic nervous system	N	Normal
approx	Approximately	NA	Nonapplicable
as tol	As tolerated	OB	Obstetrics
BM	Bowel movement	OTC	Over the counter
BP	Blood pressure	P	Pulse
Ca	Cancer	PA	Postural analysis
CC	Chief complaint	PM (PM, pm)	Afternoon
c/o	Complains of	PT	Physical therapy
CPR	Cardiopulmonary resuscitation	Px	Prognosis
CSF	Cerebrospinal fluid	R	Respiration, right
CVA	Cerebrovascular accident	R/O	Rule out
DJD	Degenerative joint disease	ROM	Range of motion
DM	Diabetes mellitus	Rx	Prescription
Dx	Diagnosis	SOB	Shortness of breath
ext	Extract	SP, spir	Spirit
ft	Foot or feet	Sym	Symmetrical
fx	Fracture	T	Temperature
GI	Gastrointestinal	TLC	Tender loving care
GU	Genitourinary	Tx	Treatment
h (hr)	Hour	URI	Upper respiratory infection
H_2O	Water	WD	Well developed
Hx	History	WN	Well nourished

Source: Fritz S: *Mosby's fundamentals of therapeutic massage*, ed 5, St Louis, 2012, Mosby.

CELL ANATOMY REVIEW

The cell is the smallest unit of independent function in the body. The basic cell structure consists of a lipid-based cell wall that contains cytoplasm and various organelles that perform cellular functions. It is useful to think of the cell wall as the skin; the nucleus as the brain; the organelles as organs of the body; and the cytoplasm as body fluid (Figure 4.1).

STRUCTURAL PLAN

The structural organization of the body follows a clear plan. Each human being has a vertebral column that supports the trunk and forms the central axis of the body. The spine also supports two main body cavities: the dorsal cavity and ventral cavity. The dorsal cavity contains two additional cavities: the cranial and spinal cavities, which hold the brain inside the skull and spinal cord in the vertebral column. The ventral cavity contains three additional cavities: the thoracic, abdominal, and pelvic cavities, which hold the viscera (sometimes the abdominal and pelvic cavities are referred to as the *abdominopelvic cavity*). Human beings are bilaterally symmetrical beings, with left and

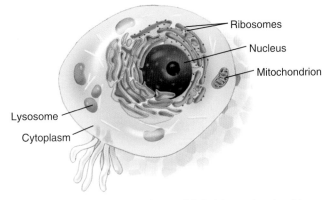

Figure 4.1 A cell. (Source: Shiland BJ: *Mastering healthcare terminology*, ed 3, St Louis, 2009, Mosby.)

right mirror images. Also, the body is segmented; this is most obvious in the vertebral column, ribs, and spinal regions of the body and surface anatomy (Figures 4.2 through 4.5).

Surface Anatomy

Regional terms are used to designate specific areas of the body (Figure 4.6).

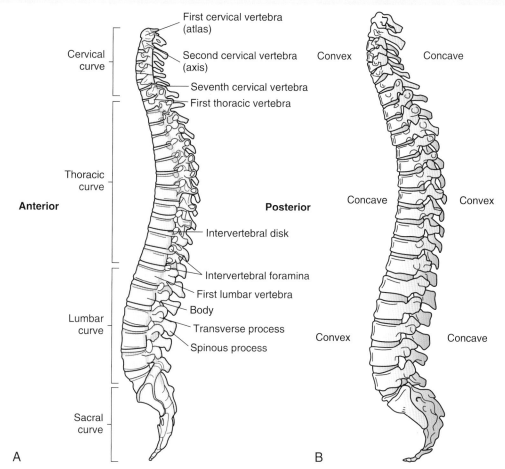

Figure 4.2 The vertebral column. **A**, The vertebral column. **B**, Convex and concave relationship of the vertebral column. (Source: Fritz S: *Mosby's essential sciences for therapeutic massage: anatomy, physiology, biomechanics, and pathology*, ed 4, St Louis, 2012, Mosby.)

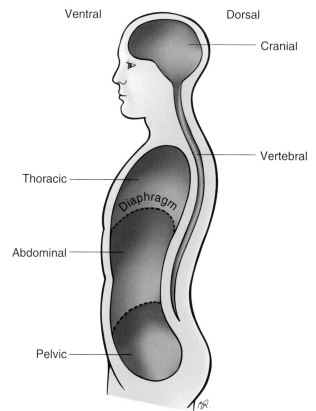

Figure 4.3 The body cavities. (Source: Fritz S: *Mosby's essential sciences for therapeutic massage: anatomy, physiology, biomechanics, and pathology*, ed 4, St Louis, 2012, Mosby.)

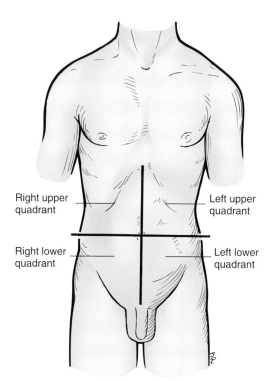

Figure 4.4 Anatomic abdominal quadrants. (Source: Fritz S: *Mosby's essential sciences for therapeutic massage: anatomy, physiology, biomechanics, and pathology*, ed 4, St Louis, 2012, Mosby.)

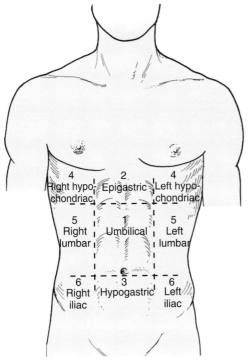

Figure 4.5 Anatomic abdominal regions. (Source: LaFleur Brooks M: *Exploring medical language: a student-directed approach*, ed 6, 2005, Elsevier.)

Terms Related to the Structural Plan

The following terms are used to describe the structural plan of the body:

- *Soma, somato:* Root words that mean "the body," as distinguished from the mind. Somatic organs and tissues are associated with the skin and the skeleton (e.g., bone and skeletal muscles, extremities, body wall) and commonly can be controlled voluntarily.
- *Axial:* Areas and organs along the central axis of the body, including the head, neck, trunk, brain, spinal cord, and abdominal organs.
- *Appendicular:* The limbs, joined to the body as lateral appendages.
- *Torso, trunk:* Structures related to the main part of the body, including the chest, abdomen, and vertebral cavity. The head and limbs are attached to the trunk.

Posterior Region of the Trunk

The two dorsal cavities are located toward the back of the body. They are as follows:

- *Cranial cavity:* Found in the skull, containing the brain and related structures.
- *Vertebral cavity:* Extending from the base of the cranial cavity and containing the spinal cord.

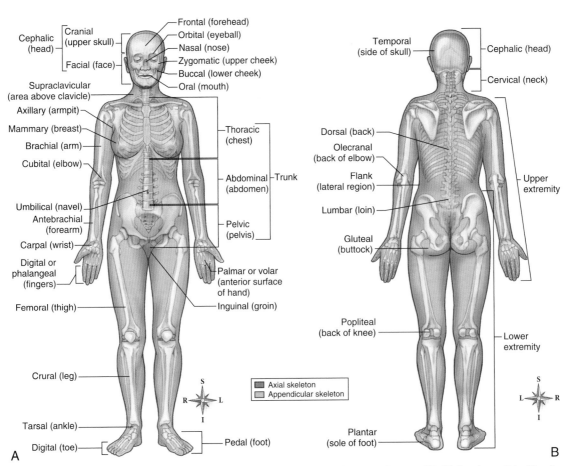

Figure 4.6 Regions of the body in anatomic position. **A,** Anterior. **B,** Posterior. (Source: Patton KT, Thibodeau GA: *The human body in health & disease*, ed 6, St Louis, 2013, Elsevier.)

The back, or posterior surface, of the trunk is divided into regions named for corresponding vertebrae in the spinal column:

- *Cervical region:* The neck (7 cervical vertebrae).
- *Thoracic region:* The chest (12 thoracic vertebrae).
- *Lumbar region:* The loin (5 lumbar vertebrae).
- *Sacral region:* The sacrum (5 sacral vertebrae fused into 1 bone).
- *Coccyx:* The tailbone (4 coccygeal vertebrae fused into 1 bone).

Anterior Region of the Trunk

Ventral cavities are located in the trunk. They include the following:

- *Thoracic cavity:* Also known as the chest; found between the neck and the diaphragm and surrounded by the ribs. The mediastinum contains the heart, lungs, thymus gland, trachea, esophagus, and other structures and divides the chest into left and right parts.
- *Abdominal cavity:* Also known as "the belly," is located below the diaphragm and enclosed within the abdominal muscles. This cavity contains the liver, kidneys, spleen, pancreas, stomach, and intestines.
- *Pelvic cavity:* Inferior to the abdomen, inside the pelvic bones; contains a portion of the large intestine, as well as the bladder and the internal reproductive organs.
- *Viscera:* Internal organs of the thoracic, abdominal, and pelvic cavities which are considered under involuntary control.
- *Membranes:* Two types, associated with the regions of the trunk: parietal membranes, lining the body cavities; and visceral membranes, covering the visceral organs.

Abdominal Quadrants and Regions

The abdomen is divided into four quadrants and nine regions, the names of which are used to describe the locations of body structures, pain, or discomfort. The four quadrants are the right upper quadrant, left upper quadrant, right lower quadrant, and left lower quadrant.

The nine regions are the right hypochondriac, epigastric, left hypochondriac, right lumbar, umbilical, left lumbar, right iliac, hypogastric, and left iliac regions.

POSITIONS OF THE BODY

Terms related to the position of the body include the following:

- *Anatomic position:* The body standing upright with the feet slightly apart, arms hanging at the sides, palms facing forward, and thumbs outward. This term is also used in Western medicine to describe the position of the body and the location of its regions and parts. The central axis of the body passes through the head and trunk.
- *Functional position:* The body standing upright with the feet slightly apart, arms hanging at the sides, palms facing the sides of body, and thumbs forward.
- *Erect position:* The body standing.
- *Supine position:* The body lying horizontally with the face up.
- *Prone position:* The body lying horizontally with the face down.
- *Lateral recumbent position:* The body lying horizontally on the right or left side.

BODY PLANES

The body can be divided into parts by imaginary lines and various planes to identify particular areas.

Movements are described as beginning in or returning to the anatomic position. Movement terms define the action as the body part passes through the various planes.

The sagittal plane is a vertical plane that divides the body into left and right parts. A midsagittal plane divides the body into equal left and right parts; a parasagittal plane divides it into unequal left and right parts. Movement in the sagittal plane consists of flexion and extension.

The frontal (coronal) plane also runs vertically but divides the body into anterior and posterior (front and back) parts. Movement in the frontal plane consists of abduction and adduction.

A transverse plane divides the body horizontally into two parts. These parts are described as superior (meaning above) and inferior (meaning below). The transverse plane runs perpendicular to the frontal and sagittal planes. Movement in the transverse plane consists of rotations—internal, external, left/right rotation, and circumduction (Figure 4.7).

Axis of movement—An axis is a straight line around which an object rotates. Movements at the joint take place in a plane about an axis. There are three axes of rotation:

- Sagittal—passes horizontally from posterior to anterior and is formed by the intersection of the sagittal and transverse planes.
- Frontal—passes horizontally from left to right and is formed by the intersection of the frontal and transverse planes.
- Vertical—passes vertically from inferior to superior and is formed by the intersection of the sagittal and frontal planes.

Examples:

- Walking forward moves on the sagittal plane along the frontal axis.
- Bending the trunk into lateral flexion occurs on the frontal plane along the sagittal axis.
- Throwing a ball occurs on the transverse plane along the vertical axis.

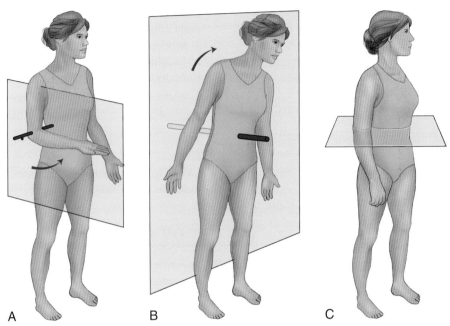

A   B   C

Figure 4.7 The corresponding axes for the three cardinal planes (the axes are shown as *red* tubes). **A**, Sagittal plane. **B**, Frontal plane. **C**, Transverse plane. (Source: **A–C**, Muscolino JE: *Kinesiology: the skeletal system and muscle function*, ed 2, St Louis, 2010, Mosby.)

TERMINOLOGY OF LOCATION AND POSITION

Kinesiology

By definition, *kinesiology* is the study of movement. Kinesiology brings together the study of anatomy, physiology, physics, and geometry to explain human movement. Kinesiology uses principles of mechanics, musculoskeletal anatomy, and neuromuscular physiology. Mechanical principles that relate directly to the human body are used in the study of biomechanics. This may involve looking at the static (nonmoving) or dynamic (moving) systems associated with various activities.

Dynamic systems can be divided into kinetics and kinematics. *Kinetics* refers to the forces that cause movement; *kinematics* consists of the aspects of time, space, and mass in a moving system.

Movement Terms
The following terms are commonly used to describe movement:
- *Flexion:* A decrease in the angle between two bones as the body part moves out of the anatomic position; flexion is a sagittal plane movement.
- *Extension:* An increase in the angle between two bones, usually moving the body part back toward the anatomic position; extension is a sagittal plane movement.
- *Hyperextension:* A term that has two definitions: (1) any extension beyond normal or healthy extension;

(2) any extension that takes the part farther in the direction of extension beyond the anatomic position.
- *Abduction:* Movement of the appendicular body part away from the midline; abduction is a frontal plane movement.
- *Adduction:* Movement of the appendicular body part toward the midline; adduction is a frontal plane movement.
- *Right lateral flexion:* Movement of the axial body part to the right; right lateral flexion is a frontal plane movement.
- *Left lateral flexion:* Movement of the axial body part to the left; left lateral flexion is a frontal plane movement.
- *Right rotation:* Partial turning or pivoting of the axial body part in an arc around a central axis to the right; right rotation is a transverse plane movement.
- *Left rotation:* Partial turning or pivoting of the axial body part in an arc around a central axis to the left; left rotation is a transverse plane movement.
- *Medial rotation:* Partial turning or pivoting of a body part of the appendicular body in an arc around a central axis toward the midline of the body; medial rotation is a transverse plane movement.
- *Lateral rotation:* Partial turning or pivoting of a body part of the appendicular body in an arc around a central axis away from the midline of the body; lateral rotation is a transverse plane movement.
- *Circumduction:* Not a movement, but a sequence of movements that turn or pivot the part through an entire arc, making a complete circle. (*Note:* Circumduction involves no rotation and is a multiplanar movement.)
- *Protraction:* Pushing of a part forward in a horizontal plane.
- *Retraction:* Pulling back of a part in a horizontal plane.

- *Elevation:* Moving a part upward (superiorly).
- *Depression:* Moving a part downward (inferiorly).
- *Supination:* Movement of the forearm (at the radioulnar joint, not the elbow joint) that turns the palm anteriorly (upward), as when cupping a bowl of soup.
- *Pronation:* Movement of the forearm (at the radioulnar joint, not the elbow joint) that turns the palm posteriorly (downward).

- *Inversion:* Movement of the sole of the foot inward, toward the midline.
- *Eversion:* Movement of the sole of the foot outward, away from the midline.
- *Plantar flexion:* Movement of the foot downward (may also be called *flexion*).
- *Dorsiflexion:* Movement of the foot upward (may also be called *extension*) (Figure 4.8).

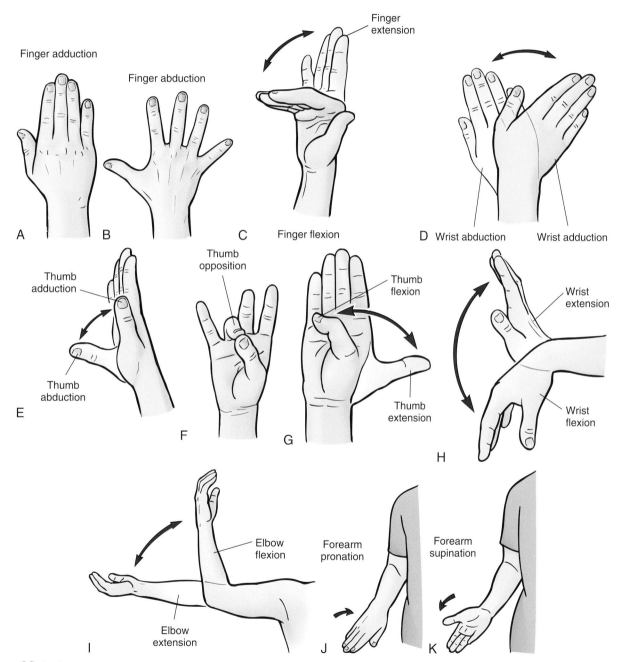

Figure 4.8 Body movements. (Source: Fritz S: *Mosby's essential sciences for therapeutic massage: anatomy, physiology, biomechanics, and pathology,* ed 4, St Louis, 2012, Mosby.)

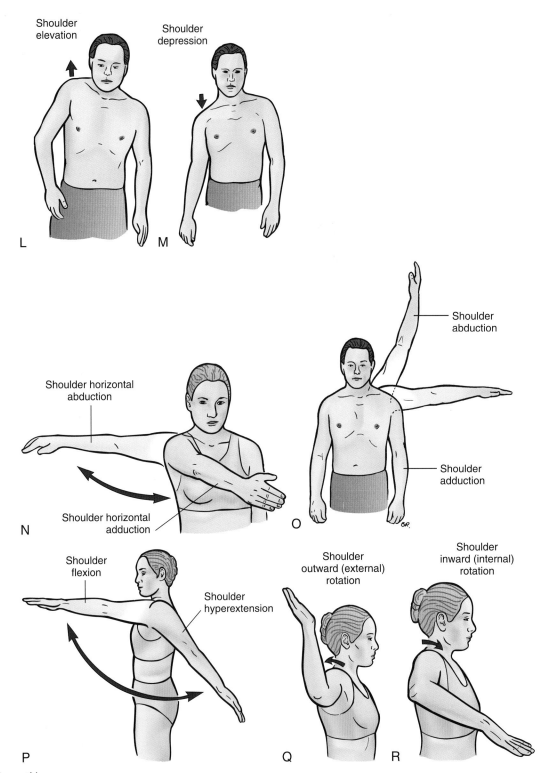

Figure 4.8, cont'd

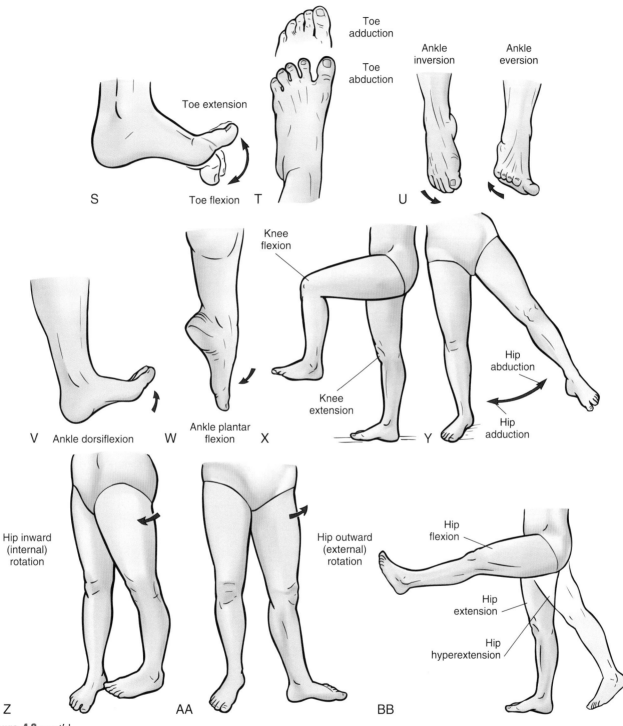

Figure 4.8 cont'd

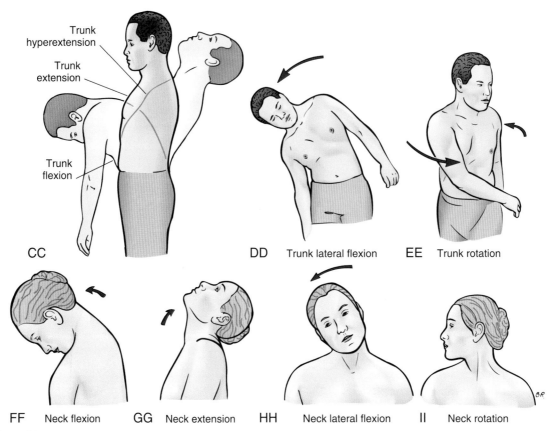

CC   **DD** Trunk lateral flexion   **EE** Trunk rotation

FF Neck flexion   **GG** Neck extension   **HH** Neck lateral flexion   **II** Neck rotation

Figure 4.8, cont'd

Directional Terms

Certain terms are used to describe the relationship of one body position to another. The following directional terms are organized in pairs of opposites:

- *Anterior (ventral):* In front of, or in or toward the front.
- *Posterior (dorsal):* Behind, in back of, or in or toward the rear.
- *Proximal:* Closer to the trunk or the point of origin (usually used on the appendicular body only).
- *Distal:* Situated away from the trunk, or midline, of the body; situated away from the origin (usually used on the appendicular body only).
- *Lateral:* On or to the side, outside, away from the midline.
- *Medial:* Relating to the middle, center, or midline.
- *Ipsilateral:* The same side.
- *Contralateral:* The opposite side.
- *Superior:* Higher than or above (usually used on the axial body only).
- *Inferior:* Lower than or below (usually used on the axial body only).
- *Volar (palmar):* The palm side of the hand.
- *Plantar:* The sole side of the foot.
- *Varus:* Ends bent inward; angulation of a part of the body such as the distal segment of a bone or joint inward toward the midline. For example, in a varus deformity of the knee, the distal part of the leg below the knee is deviated inward, resulting in a bowlegged appearance.

- *Valgus:* Ends of the distal segment of a bone or joint bent outward. For example, a valgus deformity at the knee results in a knock-kneed appearance, with the distal part of the leg deviated outward.
- *Internal:* An inside surface or the inside part of the body.
- *External:* The outside surface of the body.
- *Deep:* Inside or away from the surface.
- *Superficial:* Toward or on the surface.
- *Dextral (dextro):* Right.
- *Sinistral (sinistro):* Left; *levo* also is used to mean left.

TERMS RELATED TO DIAGNOSIS AND DISEASES

The massage practitioner must be able to understand medical terms related to diagnosis and various diseases. Two terms related to the diagnosis of a disease that massage professionals often encounter are *indication* and *contraindication*. These and other terms follow.

An *indication* is a condition for which an approach would be beneficial for health enhancement, treatment of a particular condition, or support of a treatment modality other than massage.

A *contraindication* is a condition or factor that may make an approach harmful. Contraindications may be further subdivided by severity:

- General/absolute avoidance of application—Do not massage.
- Regional avoidance of application—Do massage but avoid a particular area.
- Application with *caution*—Do massage, but carefully select the types of methods to be used, the duration of application, the frequency, and the intensity of the massage.

Most contraindications are within the regional avoidance or caution category. The massage therapist must be able to determine contraindications and respond appropriately *to protect the safety of the client*. When in doubt about the safety of massage application, the massage therapist can either refer to the appropriate healthcare professional for recommendations or provide massage in a conservative and cautious manner.

THE STRUCTURE OF THE BODY

Tissues

The body is composed of tissues. A *tissue* is a collection of specialized cells that perform a special function. *Histo* is a root word meaning "tissue." *Histology* is the study of tissue. The primary tissues of the body are the epithelial, connective, muscular, and nervous tissues (Figure 4.9).

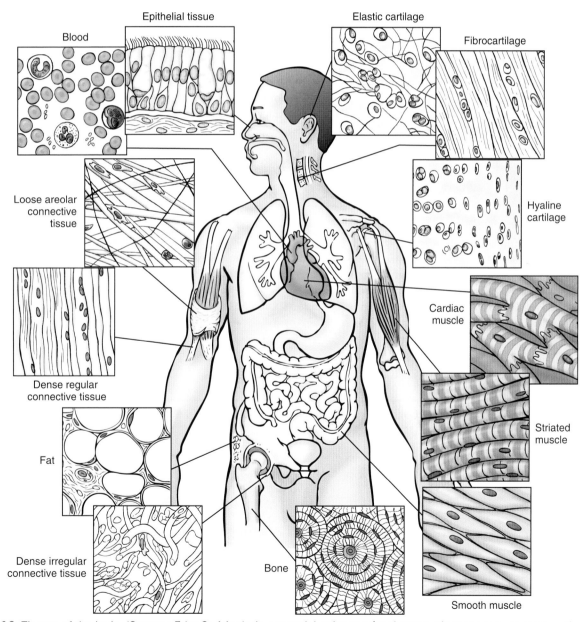

Figure 4.9 Tissues of the body. (Source: Fritz S: *Mosby's essential sciences for therapeutic massage: anatomy, physiology, biomechanics, and pathology*, ed 4, St Louis, 2012, Mosby.)

Organs and Systems

An *organ* is a collection of specialized tissues. An organ has specific functions, but it does not act independently of other organs (Table 4.5).

Organs make up systems. The body as a whole is made up of several systems. Some of these systems are concentrated in a particular part of the body (e.g., the urinary system), whereas others, such as the cardiovascular system, reach out to all parts of the body. The body consists of 10 general systems. Each system is made up of organs that collectively perform specific functions. (A more extensive description of these systems can be found in any complete anatomy and physiology textbook.)

The Skeletal System

The skeletal system consists of three types of tissues: bone, cartilage, and ligaments. *Bone* is a dense connective tissue that is composed primarily of calcium and phosphate; *os-, ossa-, oste-,* and *osteo-* are all combining forms that mean "bone." The human skeleton is composed of approximately 206 bones, and massage professionals must be familiar with most of them. Some of these bones include the skull or cranium, cervical vertebrae, thoracic vertebrae, lumbar vertebrae, sacral vertebrae, coccygeal vertebrae, ribs, sternum, manubrium, xiphoid process, clavicle, scapula, humerus, ulna, radius, carpal bones, metacarpal bones, phalanges, pelvis, ilium, ischium, pubis, femur, patella, tibia, fibula, tarsal bones, and metatarsal bones. Other terms related to bones and landmarks on bones include *malleolus, process, crest, insertion, joint, olecranon, origin, spine, trochanter,* and *tuberosity* (Figure 4.10).

The Articular System

Articulations are joints at which two or more bones meet. The articular system concerns all the anatomic and functional aspects of the joints. *Joints* are places where bones come together, where limbs are attached, and where the motion of the skeletal system occurs. Some joints are rigid, and some allow a great degree of flexibility. The joints allow motion of the musculoskeletal system; they bear weight and hold the skeleton together. Joint categories are:

- Synarthrosis (fibrous joints): Nonsynovial, fibrous, limited movement. Types: suture, gomphosis, syndesmosis.
- Amphiarthrosis (cartilaginous joints): Nonsynovial, cartilaginous, slightly movable. Types: symphysis, synchondroses.
- Diarthrosis (synovial joints): Synovial, freely movable. Features: A joint capsule with an inner synovial membrane that secretes synovial fluid to lubricate joint surfaces covered in hyaline cartilage.

Terms related to the articular system include *articulation, flexibility, synarthrodial, amphiarthrodial, diarthrodial, uniaxial symphysis pubis, sacroiliac, symphysis, articular cartilage, articular disks, ligaments, synovial fluid,* and *tendon.*

Cartilage

There are two main types of cartilage: hyaline cartilage and fibrocartilage. *Hyaline cartilage*, which is very elastic, cushiony, and slippery, makes up the articular surfaces of the joints and is the cartilage between the ribs, at the nose, larynx, and trachea, and in the fetal skeleton. It has a pearly, bluish color; the term *hyaline* means "glass." White *fibrocartilage*, which is elastic, flexible, and tough, is interarticular fibrocartilage that is found in joints such as the knee. *Connecting fibrocartilage* is cartilage that is only slightly mobile. It is found between the vertebrae (referred to as disks) and between the pubic bones (the symphysis pubis).

Ligaments

A joint or an articulation is a point at which the bones of the skeleton meet. Movable joints are covered by cartilage and are held together by *ligaments*. Ligaments are made of white fibrous tissue. They are pliant, flexible, strong, and tough.

TABLE 4.5   Systems of the Body and Their Important Organs

System	Associated organs
Musculoskeletal (can be classified separately as the skeletal, articular [joints], and muscular systems)	Bones, ligaments, skeletal muscles, tendons, joints
Nervous	Brain, spinal cord, nerves, special sense organs
Cardiovascular	Heart, arteries, veins, capillaries
Lymphatic	Lymphatic vessels, lymph nodes, spleen, tonsils, thymus gland
Digestive	Mouth, tongue, teeth, salivary glands, esophagus, stomach, small and large intestines, liver, gallbladder, pancreas
Respiratory	Nasal cavity, larynx, trachea, bronchi, lungs, diaphragm, pharynx
Urinary	Kidneys, ureters, urinary bladder, urethra
Endocrine	Endocrine glands: hypothalamus, hypophysis (pituitary), thyroid, thymus, parathyroid, pineal, adrenal, pancreas, gonads (ovary or testis)
Reproductive	Female: ovaries, uterine tubes (oviducts), uterus, vagina
	Male: testes, penis, prostate gland, seminal vesicles, spermatic ducts
Integumentary	Skin, hair, nails, sebaceous glands, sweat glands, breasts

Source: Fritz S: *Mosby's fundamentals of therapeutic massage*, ed 5, St Louis, 2012, Mosby.

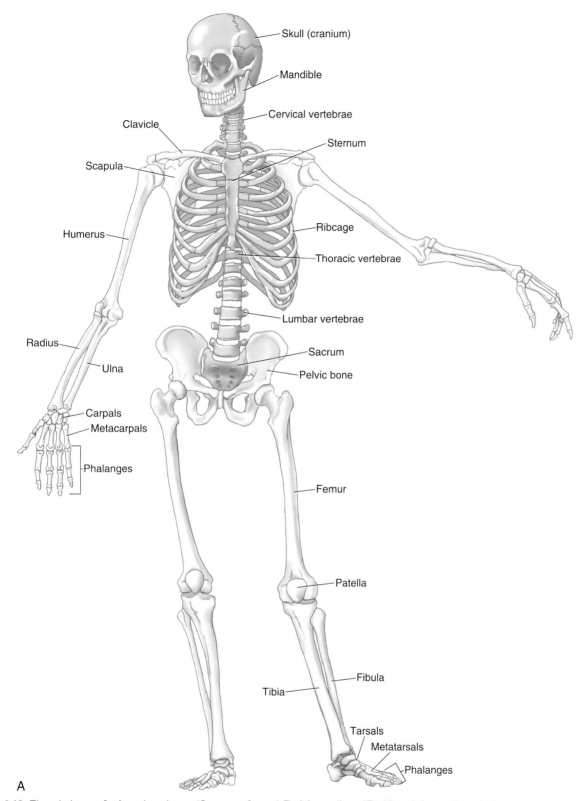

Figure 4.10 The skeleton. **A,** Anterior view. (Source: **A** and **B**, Muscolino JE: *Kinesiology: the skeletal system and muscle function*, ed 2, St Louis, 2010, Mosby.)

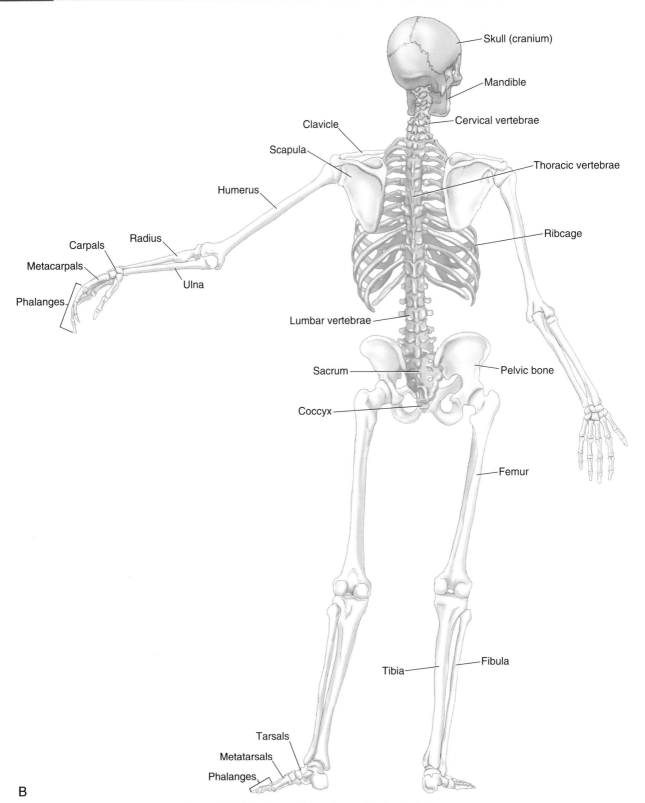

B

Figure 4.10, cont'd **B**, Posterior view. *Green,* Axial skeleton. *Beige,* Appendicular skeleton.

Diarthrodial Joints

- Uniaxial joint—joint that allows for motion within only one plane (one axis)
- Biaxial joint—joint that allows for movements within two planes (two axes)
- Multiaxial joint—a joint that allows for movements within three planes (three axes)

Types of movement permitted by *diarthrodial/synovial* (freely movable) *joints* include the following:

- *Flexion:* Bending that reduces the angle of a joint.
- *Extension:* Straightening or stretching that increases the angle of a joint.
- *Abduction:* Movement away from (*ab-*) the midline.
- *Adduction:* Movement toward (*ad-*) the midline.

- *Pronation:* Turning of the palm downward.
- *Supination:* Turning of the palm upward (you can hold a bowl of soup in a supinated hand).
- *Eversion:* Turning (*-version*) of the sole of the foot away from (*e-*) the midline (when you evert your foot, you move your little toe toward your ear).
- *Inversion:* Turning (*-version*) of the sole of the foot inward (*in-*).
- *Plantar flexion:* Bending of the plantar surface of the sole of the foot downward (plant your toes in the ground).
- *Dorsiflexion:* Bending of the top or dorsal surface of the foot toward the shin.
- *Rotation:* Rolling to the side (internal rotation: rolling toward the midline; external rotation: rolling away from the midline).
- *Circumduction:* Making a cone; the ability to move the limb in a circular manner.
- *Protraction:* Thrusting a part of the body forward (*pro-*).
- *Retraction:* Pulling a part of the body backward (*re-*).
- *Elevation:* Raising a part of the body.
- *Depression:* Lowering a part of the body.
- *Opposition:* The act of placing part of the body opposite another, as in placing the tip of the thumb opposite the tips of the fingers.

Bursae

Bursae are closed sacs or saclike structures (bursa) that usually are found close to the joint cavities. The lining of bursae often is similar to the synovial membrane lining of a true joint. Some bursae are continuous with the lining of a joint. The function of a bursa is to lubricate an area between skin, tendons, ligaments, or other structures and bones, where friction would otherwise develop (Figures 4.11 and 4.12 and Box 4.1).

The Muscular System

The *muscular system* is made up of contractile tissues. The three types of muscle tissues are cardiac muscle, smooth muscle, and skeletal muscle. Many of the body's organs contain muscle tissue. Muscle tissue also makes up the skeletal muscles, which are individual organs. These muscles give the body shape and produce movement. Muscle function is determined by the shape and location of the muscle and by the density and pliability of all fluids, fibers, and connective tissues of the muscle. The term *muscle tone* is used to describe the overall density and pliability of a muscle. The nervous system also controls how long or short a muscle is by regulating the degree of muscle fiber contraction; this is called *motor tone*.

Skeletal Muscle

Each skeletal muscle is made up of parts. Most muscles have two ends (proximal and distal), which are attached to other structures, and a belly. Muscles cause and permit motion through the actions of contraction and relaxation. Table 4.6 presents a list of terms that are used to describe the movements of different types of muscles (Figure 4.13).

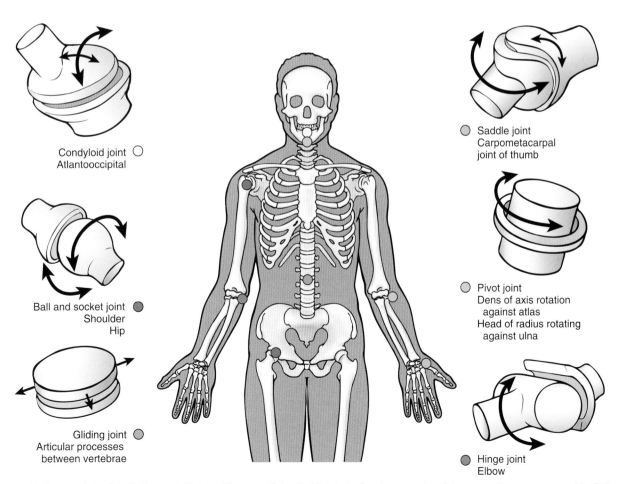

Condyloid joint ○
Atlantooccipital

Ball and socket joint ●
Shoulder
Hip

Gliding joint ●
Articular processes
between vertebrae

Saddle joint
Carpometacarpal
joint of thumb

Pivot joint
Dens of axis rotation
against atlas
Head of radius rotating
against ulna

Hinge joint
Elbow

Figure 4.11 Types of diarthrodial/synovial joints. (Source: Fritz S: *Mosby's fundamentals of therapeutic massage*, ed 5, St Louis, 2012, Mosby.)

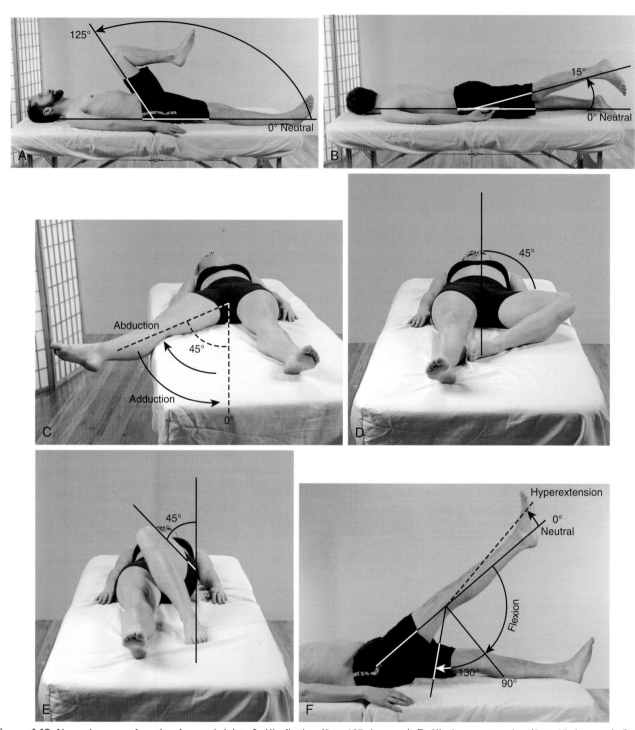

Figure 4.12 Normal range of motion for each joint. **A**, Hip flexion (0 to 125 degrees). **B**, Hip hyperextension (0 to 15 degrees). **C**, Hip abduction (0 to 45 degrees) and hip adduction (45 to 0 degrees). **D**, Hip lateral (extended rotator 0 to 45 degrees). **E**, Hip medial (internal) rotation (0 to 45 degrees). **F**, Knee flexion (0 to 130 degrees) and knee extension (120 to 0 degrees).

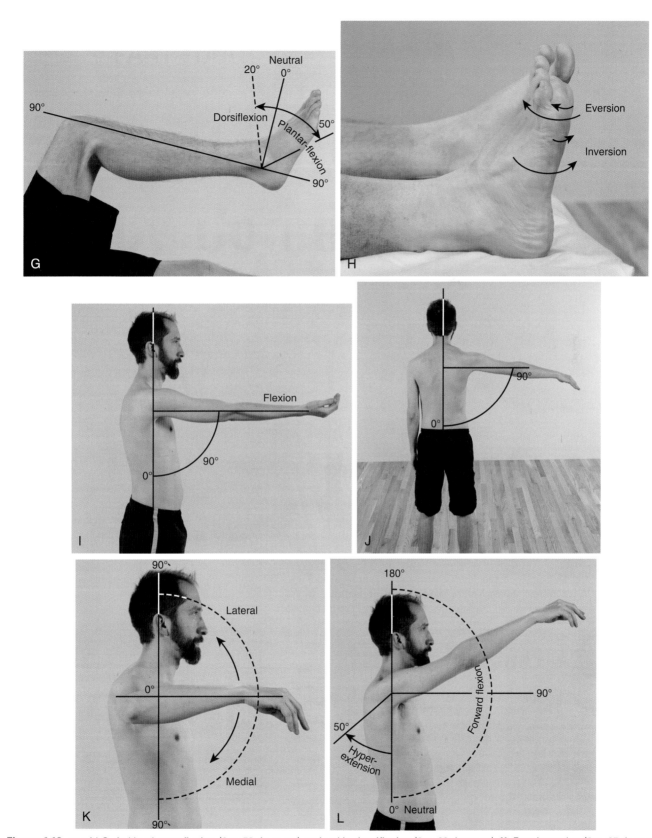

Figure 4.12, cont'd **G**, Ankle plantar flexion (0 to 50 degrees) and ankle dorsiflexion (0 to 20 degrees). **H**, Foot inversion (0 to 35 degrees) and foot eversion (0 to 25 degrees). **I**, Shoulder flexion (0 to 90 degrees) and shoulder extension (90 to 0 degrees). **J**, Shoulder abduction (0 to 90 degrees) and shoulder adduction (90 to 0 degrees). **K**, Shoulder lateral (medial) rotation (0 to 90 degrees) and shoulder medial (internal) rotation (0 to 90 degrees). **L**, Combined shoulder and scapular forward flexion (0 to 180 degrees); extension (180 to 0 degrees).

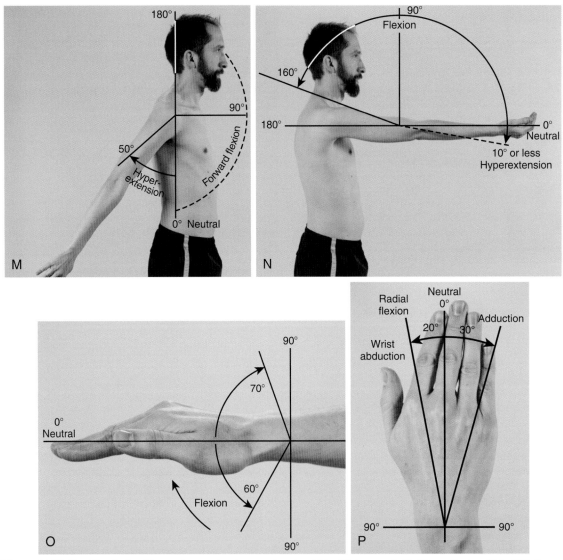

Figure 4.12, cont'd **M,** Combined shoulder and scapular hyperextension (0 to 50 degrees). **N,** Elbow flexion (0 to 160 degrees); elbow extension (160 to 0 degrees); elbow hyperextension (0 to 10 degrees). **O,** Wrist flexion (0 to 60 degrees); wrist extension (0 to 70 degrees). **P,** Wrist abduction (0 to 20 degrees); wrist adduction (0 to 30 degrees).

BOX 4.1	Joint Movement
Action	**Description**
Extension	To increase the angle of a joint
Flexion	To decrease the angle of a joint
Abduction	To move away from the midline
Abduction	To move toward the midline
Supination	To turn the palm or foot upward
Pronation	To turn the palm or foot downward
Dorsiflexion	To raise the foot, pulling the toes toward the shin
Plantar flexion	To lower the foot, pointing the toes away from the shin
Eversion	To turn outward
Inversion	To turn inward
Protraction	To move a part of the body forward
Retraction	To move a part of the body backward
Rotation	To revolve a bone around its axis

TABLE 4.6	Terms for Describing Muscle by Movement
Term	**Definition**
Adductor	Muscle that moves a part toward the midline
Abductor	Muscle that moves a part away from the midline
Flexor	Muscle that bends a part
Extensor	Muscle that straightens a part
Levator	Muscle that raises a part
Depressor	Muscle that lowers a part
Tensor	Muscle that tightens a part

Source: Fritz S: *Mosby's fundamentals of therapeutic massage,* ed 5, St Louis, 2012, Mosby.

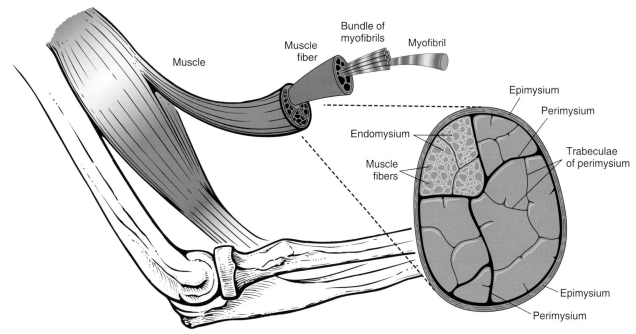

Figure 4.13 **A muscle**. (Source: Damjanov I: *Pathology for the health professions*, ed 4, St Louis, 2011, Elsevier.)

Contraction refers to a reduction in size or shortening of a muscle. When one muscle contracts, another, opposite muscle is stretched and is put in a state of tension. *Relaxation* occurs when tension is reduced, which allows the muscle to return to its normal resting length.

Muscles work in pairs of agonists and antagonists. *Agonists* are muscles that are responsible for the primary desired movement. The agonist is the prime mover, which shortens to produce movement. *Antagonists* are the muscles that oppose the action of the agonist and lengthen and control the movement produced by the agonist.

Synergists are muscles that assist the agonists by holding a part of the body steady, thereby providing leverage. In some cases, synergists also produce the same action as the prime mover.

The agonist–antagonist–synergist relationship permits the skeletal muscles to work in a purposeful manner and gives fluidity to motion. This fluid movement is called *coordination*.

Skeletal muscle: This contractile body, the muscle proper, usually is attached to two or more bony points. Attachments may be

- Tendon
- Aponeurosis
- Fleshy

Tendons are an integral part of muscle, virtually invariable in length. They are made of collagen fibers with occasional flattened fibroblasts.

Tendons take the form of cords or strips consisting of bundles (fascicles) of collagen, mainly parallel, and often are large enough to see with the naked eye; they are striated in appearance. Around the outside of the bundle is an epi-tendineum, the white fibrous sheath surrounding a tendon which obviously causes a little drag as tendons run through connective tissue. When they have to move independently of other tissues, various friction-reducing devices such as bursae are used.

A very flattened tendon often is called an *aponeurosis* (neurosis because it is white, like nervous tissue). It usually has the appearance of a flattened sheet of collagen fibers, or often of several sheets running onto each other in different directions, like plywood.

A fleshy insertion is what it sounds like—muscle joined to bone without the intervention of a collagenous tendon or aponeurosis. The collagen is still there, but it is in among the muscle fibers, or it forms a very short tendon.

ATTACHMENT TERMINOLOGY

Terminology changes occur; currently, the names of muscle attachments have multiple terms. In some circumstances, origin and insertion can be interchanged, so it is easier to talk of attachments. Proximal muscle attachments (closer to the midline and the body center) have been called *origins* but are more correctly called *proximal attachments*; insertions are now called *distal attachments*. Often a muscle arises from more than one place; it then is said to have two or more attachments (e.g., biceps brachii, triceps brachii). The terms, origin and insertion, are still used. It is understandable that the use of multiple terms for the same thing is confusing. On the MBLEx exam you may encounter any of the attachment terminology.

Forms of Muscles

Muscles exhibit wide functional variation in terms of size and shape, according to their job. The simplest is probably the *strap muscle*, which has a fleshy, wide attachment at each end. Strap muscles thus have good range but little power.

To get more power, the muscle structure becomes fusiform (three-dimensional) or produces more heads, resulting in the effect of two, three, or four muscles pulling the same tendon.

In a unipennate muscle, fibers insert along just one side of a tendon. In a bipennate or multipennate arrangement, fibers insert along two or more sides of a tendon.

Spiralized muscles are special in that they not only pull the attachments together when they contract, but they also twist or untwist the area. The twisting action often occurs because the muscle attachments are wrapped around a bone (Figure 4.14).

Actions of Muscles

Muscles undergo transition from relaxation to contraction. At any given time, some functional units (motor units, groups of fibers) will be contracting, some will be relaxing, and some will stay static to provide muscle motor tone.

When an individual fiber contracts, it tends to approximate (bring closer together) the ends, but whether or not this results in contraction depends on the force generated and the forces opposing contraction. The net result for the whole muscle may be shortening—concentric action, lengthening—eccentric action, or an increase in tension, but with no movement—isometric action.

A muscle that tries to initiate contraction is opposed by the following:

- Articular tissues
- Opposing muscles
- Opposing soft tissues
- Inertia of whatever it is trying to move
- Load
- Gravity

If the force generated exceeds the sum of all opposing factors, it is said to accelerate movement (*concentric action*); once it is moving, a smaller force will keep it moving. A muscle or muscle group that is able to move a body part (concentric action) is sometimes called a prime mover or agonist and is opposed by antagonists, which can stop the movement (*eccentric action*).

When both groups act together, nothing moves, or the movement is moderated or controlled.

Clues for identifying muscle names include the following:

- Direction of muscle fibers, named in reference to midline of body
  - Rectus (parallel, straight)
  - Transverse (right angle)
  - Oblique (slanting, not a right angle)
- Relative size of muscle
  - Major (largest)
  - Minor (smallest)
  - Longus (long)
  - Brevis (short)
- Location of muscle, named in reference to a region or nearby bone (e.g., frontalis—overlies frontal bone; abdominis—overlies abdominal region)
- Number of attachments (e.g., bi-, tri-, quad-)
- Shape of muscle
  - Deltoid—triangular
  - Trapezius—trapezoid
- Action of muscle
  - Adductor (movement toward midline); abductor (movement away from midline)
  - Extensor (increase angle between two bones); flexor (decrease angle between two bones) (Table 4.7 and Figure 4.15)

Muscles Organized as Functional Units

Muscles do not function singularly but instead are arranged in functional units. Often these functional units are bundled together by fascia into compartments, and each compartment produces the movement. For example, the thigh has four compartments: anterior, medial, posterior, and lateral. The anterior compartment consists of the muscle structures that can extend the knee and flex the hip. The posterior compartment consists of the muscle structures that can flex the knee and extend the hip. The anterior and posterior compartments are agonist and antagonist to each other. The medial compartment muscle structures adduct the hip and the lateral muscle structures (part of the anterior compartment) abduct

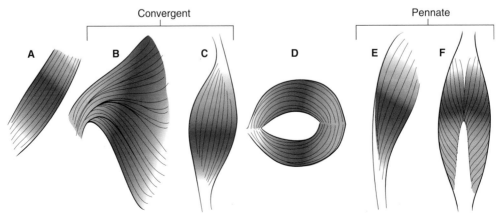

Figure 4.14 Muscle fiber arrangement. **A,** Parallel. **B,** Convergent. **C,** Fusiform. **D,** Circular. **E,** Unipennate. **F,** Bipennate. (Source: Salvo SG: *Massage therapy: principles and practice*, ed 4, St Louis, 2011, Saunders.)

TABLE 4.7 Muscle Descriptions Using Medical Word Elements

Muscle	Description
Abductor digiti minimi pedis	Little (minimi) muscle that moves the little toe (digit) away from (abductor) the midline of the foot (pedis)
Adductor longus	Long muscle that moves the leg toward (adductor) the midline
Adductor magnus	Large (magnus) muscle that moves the leg toward (adductor) the midline
Biceps brachii	Muscle with two (bi-) heads (ceps) in the arm (brachii)
Deltoid	Triangular (deltoid) muscle of the shoulder
Dilator naris posterior	Muscle of the nose (naris) that opens (dilator) the back (posterior) portion of the nostril
Extensor hallucis longus	Long (longus) muscle that extends (extensor) the great toe (hallucis)
Extensor pollicis brevis	Short (brevis) muscle that extends (extensor) the thumb (pollicis)
External oblique	Outermost (external) muscle that extends at an angle (oblique) from the ribs to the pelvis at the iliac crest
Flexor carpi radialis	Muscle that flexes (flexor) the wrist (carpi) toward the radius (radialis)
Flexor carpi ulnaris	Muscle attached to the ulna (ulnaris) that flexes (flexor) the wrist (carpi) and the hand
Frontalis	Muscle over the frontal bone
Gastrocnemius	Muscle that makes up the belly (gastroc) of the lower leg (nemius)
Gluteus maximus	Largest (maximus) muscle of the buttocks (gluteus)
Gluteus medius	Muscle of the buttocks (gluteus) that lies in the middle (medius) between the other gluteal muscles
Gracilis	Slender (gracilis) muscle of the thigh
Iliopsoas	Muscle that is formed from the iliacus and psoas major muscles; the iliacus extends from the iliac bone (iliacus), and the psoas major is the large (major) muscle of the loin (psoas)
Latissimus dorsi	Broadest (latissimus) muscle of the back (dorsi)
Masseter	Muscle of chewing (masseter) or mastication
Orbicularis oculi and oris	Muscles circling (orbicularis) the eye (oculi) or mouth (oris)
Palmaris longus	Long (longus) muscle of the palm (palmaris)
Pectineus	Muscle of the pubic (pectineus) bone
Pectoralis major	Large (major) muscle of the chest (pectoralis)
Plantaris	Muscle that flexes the foot (plantaris) and the leg
Pronator teres	Long round (teres) muscle that turns the palm downward into a prone (pronator) position
Rectus abdominis	Muscle that extends in a straight (rectus) line upward across the abdomen (abdominis); the center border of the left and right rectus abdominis muscles in the linea alba, or the white (alba) line (linea) at the midline of the abdomen
Rectus femoris	Part of the quadriceps muscle that is straight (rectus) and lies near the femur (femoris)
Sartorius	Muscle of the leg that enables a person to sit in a cross-legged tailor's (sartorial) position
Semimembranosus	Muscle made up partly (semi-) of membranous tissue; part of the hamstring group
Semitendinosus	Muscle made up partly (semi-) of tendinous tissue; this is one of the hamstring muscles
Serratus anterior	Sawtooth-shaped (serratus) muscle in front of (anterior) the shoulder and rib cage
Soleus	Muscle that resembles a flat fish (sole) located in the calf of the leg
Sternocleidomastoid	Muscle attached to the breastbone (sterno), the collarbone (cleido), and the mastoid (mastoid) process of the temporal bone
Temporalis	Muscle over the temporal (temporalis) bone
Tensor fasciae latae	Muscle that tenses (tensor) the fascia of the thigh (latae)
Teres minor	Small (minor) round (teres) muscle that moves the arm
Tibialis anterior	Muscle in front (anterior) of the tibia (tibialis)
Trapezius	Four-sided, trapezoid-shaped (trapezius) muscle of the shoulder
Triceps brachii	Three- (tri-) headed (ceps) muscle of the arm (brachii)
Vastus lateralis, medialis, intermedialis	Large (vastus) lateral (lateralis), toward the midline (medialis), and the middle (intermedialis) muscles of the quadriceps muscle group; the quadriceps has four (quadri-) heads (ceps)

Source: Fritz S: *Mosby's fundamentals of therapeutic massage*, ed 5, St Louis, 2012, Mosby.

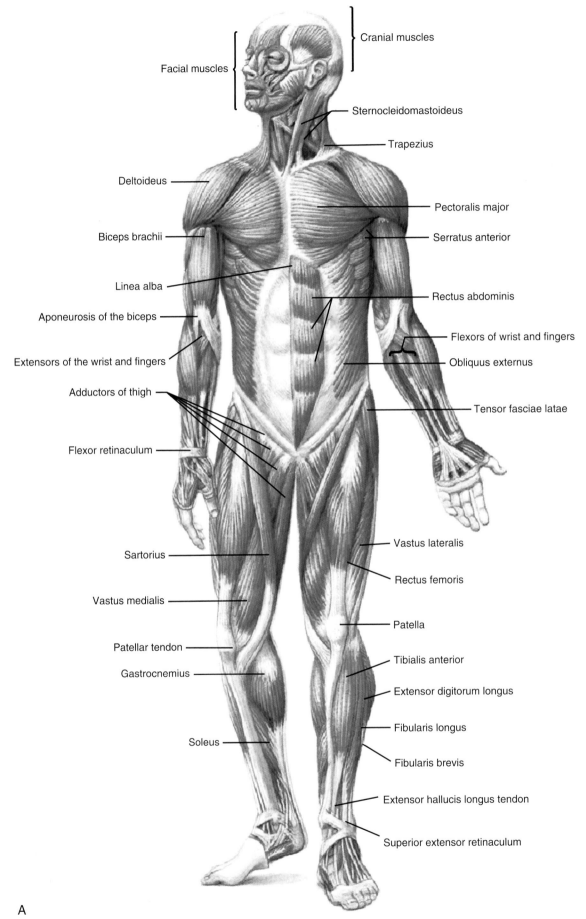

A

Figure 4.15 Skeletal muscles. **A**, Anterior view. (Source: LaFleur Brooks M: *Exploring medical language: a student-directed approach*, ed 5, St Louis, 2002, Mosby.)

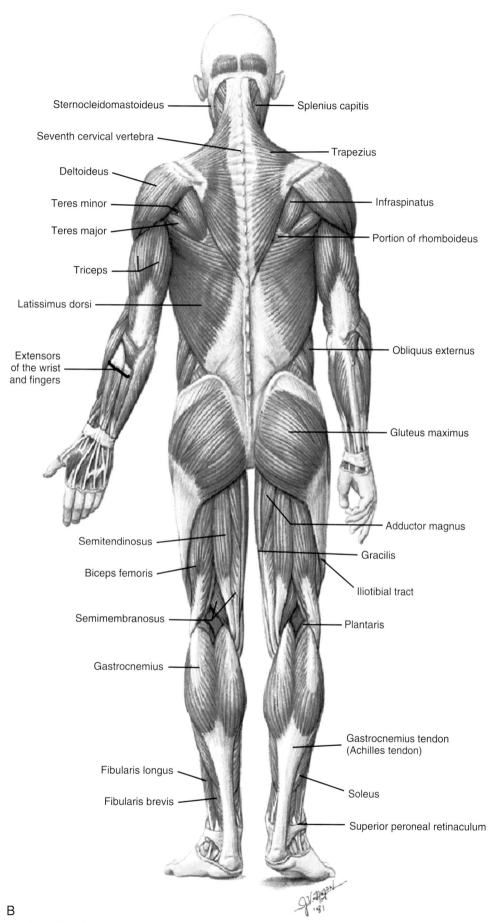

B

Figure 4.15, cont'd **B,** Posterior view.

the hip and again are agonist and antagonist to each other (Figures 4.16 and 4.17).

How to Study Muscles

To understand how muscles function, it is helpful to begin with the joint where the movement is occurring, such as the hip in this example. Because the hip is a ball and socket joint, it can move in all planes of motion: sagittal—flexion and extension; frontal—abduction and adduction; and transverse—internal and external rotation. Muscles that can create an extension movement (increase in a joint angle) are organized into functional units and bundled together by fascia. This functional unit would be called the hip extensors.

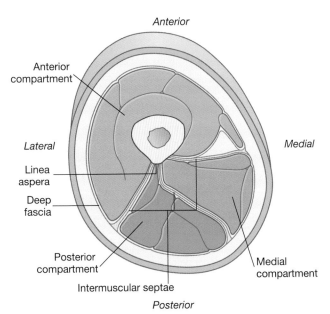

Figure 4.16 Functional muscle units. (Fritz S: *Mosby's essential sciences for therapeutic massage: anatomy, physiology, biomechanics, and pathology*, ed 4, St Louis, 2012, Mosby.)

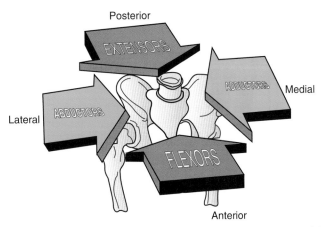

Figure 4.17 Compartmentalized functional muscle units. Example: muscle compartments of the thigh. (Source: Drake RL, Vogl W, Mitchell WM: *Gray's anatomy for students*, ed 2, Edinburgh, 2009, Churchill Livingstone.)

In order to produce hip extension, the hip extensors must attach proximally above the hip joint and distally below the hip joint. The individual muscles with attachments closest to the joint are usually deeper and initiate small movements as well as stabilize the joint. Individual muscles with attachments further from the joint are more superficial and produce larger movements. Finally, each individual muscle has its own name, specific attachments, and actions.

Hip Flexor Example

First observe the iliacus figure. This is a deep muscle that crosses the hip joint. Compare it to the figure of the psoas, which is longer and more superficial than the iliacus. This means that, although both are hip flexors, the psoas can move the joint further than the iliacus can (Figures 4.18 and 4.19).

The sartorius is the most superficial hip flexor. Notice how long it is. Also notice that it crosses above the hip joint, making it able to flex the hip when shortening. The distal attachment is below the knee, so this muscle can also move the knee (Figure 4.20).

Now look at the gluteus maximus. It crosses the hip joint on the posterior side, meaning that when shortening it can extend the hip joint (Figure 4.21).

Study the proximal and distal attachments of the semimembranosus portion of the hamstring muscle group. See how the proximal attachment on the ischial tuberosity is almost even with the hip joint; when the muscle fibers shorten, it can pull the femur into extension, which will then extend the hip joint. Notice also that this muscle is attached below the knee, like the sartorius, so it can move the knee as well (Figure 4.22).

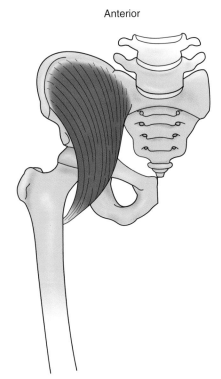

Figure 4.18 Iliacus. (Source: Fritz S: *Mosby's essential sciences for therapeutic massage: anatomy, physiology, biomechanics, and pathology*, ed 4, St Louis, 2012, Mosby.)

Anterior

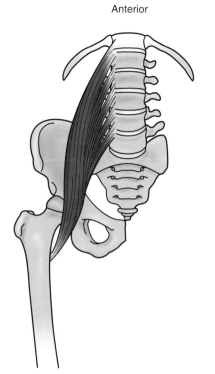

Figure 4.19 Psoas. (Source: Fritz S: *Mosby's essential sciences for therapeutic massage: anatomy, physiology, biomechanics, and pathology*, ed 4, St Louis, 2012, Mosby.)

Posterior

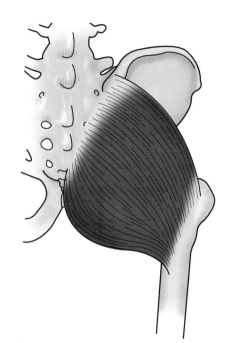

Figure 4.21 Gluteus maximus. (Source: Fritz S: *Mosby's essential sciences for therapeutic massage: anatomy, physiology, biomechanics, and pathology*, ed 4, St Louis, 2012, Mosby.)

Anterior

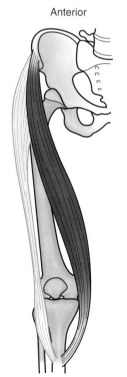

Figure 4.20 Sartorius. (Source: Fritz S: *Mosby's essential sciences for therapeutic massage: anatomy, physiology, biomechanics, and pathology*, ed 4, St Louis, 2012, Mosby.)

Posterior

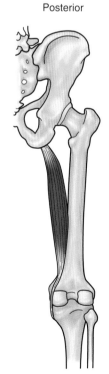

Figure 4.22 Semimembranosus. (Source: Fritz S: *Mosby's essential sciences for therapeutic massage: anatomy, physiology, biomechanics, and pathology*, ed 4, St Louis, 2012, Mosby.)

Now read the following descriptions of these muscles while continuing to view the illustrations. Notice how the individual muscles that make up functional units are similar. They share functions, synergists, and antagonists. Also notice that each muscle can perform multiple functions.

Iliacus

- Means "of the hip"

Concentric action

- Flexion and lateral rotation of the thigh at the hip joint and anterior tilt of the pelvis at the lumbosacral joint

Eccentric action

- Allows extension and medial rotation of the thigh and allows posterior tilt of the pelvis

Isometric action

- Stabilizes the pelvis and the hip joint

Origin, proximal attachment, arises from

- Internal lip of the iliac crest; anterior sacroiliac, lumbosacral, and iliolumbar ligaments; superior two-thirds of the iliac fossa; and ala of the sacrum

Insertion, distal attachment, attaches to

- Lesser trochanter of the femur, into the posterior side of the psoas major tendon

  Major synergist

  - Psoas major

  Major antagonists

  - Gluteus maximus and hamstrings

Psoas

- Means "of the loins"; major means "larger"

Concentric action

- Flexion and lateral rotation of the thigh at the hip joint, flexion and lateral flexion of the trunk at the spinal joints, and anterior tilt of the pelvis at the hip joint

Eccentric action

- Allows extension and medial rotation of the thigh and allows extension and contralateral lateral flexion of the trunk and posterior tilt of the pelvis

Isometric action

- Stabilizes the lumbar spine and the lumbosacral and hip joints

Origin, proximal attachment, arises from

- Bodies and corresponding intervertebral disks of last thoracic and all lumbar vertebrae, anterior surface of transverse processes of all lumbar vertebrae, and tendinous arches extending across the sides of the bodies of the lumbar vertebrae

- **Insertion, distal attachment, attaches to**

  Lesser trochanter of the femur

  - **Major synergists**

  Iliacus, sartorius, rectus femoris, and anterior and anterolateral abdominal wall muscles

  - **Major antagonists**

  Extensors of the thigh, extensors of the trunk, and posterior tilters of the pelvis

Sartorius

- Means "tailor"

Concentric action

- Flexion, lateral rotation, and abduction of the thigh at the hip joint; flexion and medial rotation of the leg at the knee joint (the knee joint must be semiflexed for medial rotation to occur); and anterior tilt of the pelvis at the hip joint

Eccentric action

- Restrains extension, medial rotation, and adduction of the thigh and allows extension and lateral rotation of the leg and posterior tilt of the pelvis

Isometric action

- Stabilizes the knee and hip joints

Origin, proximal attachment, arises from

- Anterior superior iliac spine

Insertion, distal attachment, attaches to

- Proximal anteromedial tibia at the pes anserinus tendon

Major synergists

- Iliopsoas, rectus femoris, lateral rotator group of the thigh, and gluteus medius

Major antagonists

Hamstrings, tensor fasciae latae, adductor group of the thigh, and quadriceps femoris group

Gluteus Maximus

- Gluteus means "buttocks"; maximus means "greatest or largest"

Concentric action

- Extends and laterally rotates the thigh at the hip joint—the upper fibers abduct the thigh at the hip joint, and the lower fibers adduct the thigh at the hip joint—and provides posterior tilt of the pelvis at the hip joint (the gluteus maximus is active primarily during strenuous activity, such as running, jumping, and climbing stairs)

Eccentric action

- Restrains flexion and medial rotation of the thigh and anterior tilt of the pelvis (the upper fibers restrain adduction of the thigh, and the lower fibers restrain abduction of the thigh)

Isometric action

- These are important postural muscles that help maintain the upright posture, stabilize the pelvis, and provide tension to the iliotibial band to keep the fascial band taut

Origin, proximal attachment, arises from

- Posterior gluteal line of the ilium, dorsal surface of the lower aspect of the sacrum and the side of the coccyx, sacrotuberous ligament and gluteal aponeurosis, and aponeurosis of the erector spinae

Insertion, distal attachment, attaches to

- Iliotibial band of the fascia lata and gluteal tuberosity of the femur

  Major synergists

  - Hamstring muscles and piriformis

  Major antagonists

- Iliopsoas, tensor fasciae latae, and gluteus medius (anterior fibers)

Semimembranosus

- Means "half membrane"

Concentric action

- Flexion and medial rotation of the leg at the knee joint (the knee joint must be semiflexed for medial rotation to occur), extension of the thigh at the hip joint, and posterior tilt of the pelvis at the hip joint; the semimembranosus also serves to move the medial meniscus posteriorly during knee flexion

Eccentric action

- Restrains extension and lateral rotation of the leg and allows flexion of the thigh and anterior tilt of the pelvis

Isometric action

- Stabilizes the knee and hip joints

Origin, proximal attachment, arises from

- Upper lateral aspect of the ischial tuberosity

Insertion, distal attachment, attaches to

- Posteromedial surface of the medial condyle of the tibia; attaches to the medial meniscus

Major synergists

- Semitendinosus, biceps femoris, and gluteus maximus

Major antagonists

- Quadriceps femoris group, iliopsoas, and tensor fasciae latae

Note: These illustrations and descriptions are taken from Fritz S and Fritz L: *Mosby's Essential Sciences for Therapeutic Massage: Anatomy, Physiology, Biomechanics, and Pathology,* ed 6, 2021, Mosby. This textbook is recommended for the study of the muscles because it provides expanded functional information about the muscles such as concentric, eccentric, and isometric actions as well as major synergists and antagonists to help you study muscles as functional units.

Muscle Descriptions Using Medical Word Elements

The muscles listed in Table 4.7 have been chosen because their names are made up of common word elements. After learning this list, you should be able to figure out the meaning of muscle names not listed.

Hints for Memorizing Muscle Names and Locations

1. Repetition is necessary. When learning muscles, the more you do it, the better you learn.
2. Think about why the muscle is named the way it is. This will help you understand its location, function, and other characteristics.
3. YouTube has extensive resources for the study of anatomy, physiology, and pathology. Many excellent websites and apps also provide study help for muscles. Just type "study muscles" within a search program to find one.
4. Be able to point to a muscle and identify it, say the muscle name, and then find the muscle on a chart.

FASCIA

The connective tissue matrix consists of the ground substance and the fibers, ranges from a fluid to a semisolid or gel, and is composed mostly of polysaccharides (protein and sugar). Aside from cells and fibers, matrix also contains many blood vessels and nerves.

Fascia is one type of connective tissue that forms in sheets. It makes up one integrated and totally connected network, from the attachments on the inner aspects of the skull to the fascia in the soles of the feet, and from the skin to the innermost center of the body. The fascia of the muscular system is as important to movement as the individual muscle cells and is an integral part of muscle structure. If any part of a fascial structure becomes deformed or distorted, adverse effects can occur to any of the interconnected structures within the network.

- Each muscle fiber is surrounded by a fine sheath of collagenic connective tissue called the *endomysium.*
- Several muscle fibers are wrapped together in side-by-side bundles, called *fascicles.*
- Fascicles are wrapped in a collagenic sheath called the *perimysium.*
- The fascicles are bound together with more dense, fibrous connective tissue called the *epimysium.*
- The epimysium surrounds the entire muscle.
- External to the epimysium is the deep fascia, an even coarser sheet of fibrous connective tissue that binds muscles into functional groups.
- The deep fascia forms partitions between muscle groups called intermuscular septa.

All these connective tissue sheaths are continuous with one another. Near the ends of muscles, the actual muscle fiber ends, but the connective tissue continues and converges to become the tendons and aponeuroses that join muscles to bones or other connective tissue structures. Tendons and aponeuroses are the continuation of the endomysium, perimysium, and epimysium, minus the muscle fibers, which attach muscle to bone. The point where the muscle fibers end and the tendon begins is called the musculotendinous junction. The difference between a tendon and an aponeurosis is one of shape. A tendon by definition is round and cordlike; an aponeurosis is a broad, flat sheet.

The tendon or aponeurosis blends and wraps into the connective tissue coverings and structures, including ligaments and other tendons, or into a seam of fibrous connective tissue, called a raphe, at the attachment site. Muscle attachments do not stick directly on bone but interweave with the periosteum around the bone.

When muscle fibers contract, they pull on the connective tissue sheaths, which transmit the force to the bone to be moved. Because the individual skeletal muscle fibers are fragile, the connective tissue supports each cell, reinforces the muscle as a whole, and gives muscle tissue its natural elasticity. These sheaths also provide entry and exit routes for the blood vessels and nerve fibers that serve the muscles, as well as a vast surface area for muscular attachment.

The entire connective tissue network is one structure. Nerve and blood vessels do not just pass through holes in the connective tissue; rather, they are contained and supported in wrappings of connective tissue that intertwine into the entire fascial network. Movement of any one body part creates a force that can be transmitted along fascial planes far and away in the body. Pulling on your big toe could transmit a force all the way to your head and every other structure in your body. No dysfunction is isolated; everything is connected.

Fascia is involved in numerous complex biochemical activities:

- Connective tissue provides a supporting matrix for more highly organized structures. It attaches extensively to and into muscles.
- The superficial fascia, which forms the adipose tissue, allows for the storage of fat and also provides a surface covering that aids in the conservation of body heat.
- Deep fascia ensheaths and preserves the characteristic contour of the extremities and promotes circulation in the veins and lymphatic vessels.
- Connective tissue sheaths cover muscle structures.
- The ensheathing layer of deep fascia, as well as intermuscular septa and interosseous membranes, provides vast surface areas for muscular attachment.
- Fascia supplies restraining mechanisms in the form of retention bands and fibrous pulleys, thereby assisting in the coordination of movement.
- In the places connective tissue has a loose texture; it allows movement between adjacent structures and, by the formation of bursal sacs, reduces the effects of pressure and friction.
- Fascia is able to contract in a smooth, musclelike manner because of the presence of myofibroblasts.
- Because connective tissue contains embryonic-like mesenchymal cells, it is capable of developing into more specialized elements.
- Connective tissue provides (by its fascial planes) pathways for nerves and blood and lymphatic vessels and structures.
- Many of the neural structures in fascia are sensory.
- Fascia has the ability to convert mechanical force into neurochemical signals forming a body-wide communication network.
- The mesh of loose connective tissue contains the tissue fluid and provides an essential medium through which the cellular elements of other tissues come into contact with blood and lymph.
- Connective tissue has a nutritive function and contains about a quarter of all body fluids.
- Chemical (nutritional) factors influence the strength of connective tissue coverings of muscles and bones.
- Because of its fibroblastic activity, connective tissue aids in the repair of injuries by generating collagenous fibers, creating scar tissue.
- Fascia is a major location of inflammatory processes.
- Fluids and infectious processes often travel along fascial planes.
- A histiocyte is a type of immune cell that ingests foreign substances in an effort to protect the body from infection.

The histiocytes of connective tissue compose part of an important defense mechanism against bacterial invasion by their phagocytic activity. Histiocytes also play a part as scavengers in removing cell debris and foreign material.

- Connective tissue represents an important neutralizer or detoxifier to endogenous toxins (those produced in the body from physiologic processes) and exogenous toxins (from outside the body).
- The mechanical barrier presented by fascia has important defensive functions in cases of infectious pathogen invasion.

Fascia is involved deeply in almost all the fundamental processes of the structure, function, and metabolism of the body. In therapeutic terms, trying to consider muscle as a separate structure from fascia is illogical because the two are related so intimately. Without connective tissue, muscle would be a jelly-like structure without form or functional ability.

Mechanical forces are important regulators of connective tissue homeostasis. This tissue is designed to move, and lack of movement creates dysfunction. Fibroblasts sense force-induced deformations (strains) in the extracellular matrix. Changes in cell shape are well-established factors regulating a wide range of cellular functions, including signal transduction, gene expression, and matrix adhesion. The extracellular matrix plays a key role in the transmission of mechanical forces generated by muscle contraction or externally applied mechanical forces such as those applied during massage.

Because muscle and fascia are anatomically inseparable, fascia moves during muscular activities acting on bone, joints, ligaments, and tendons. Sensory receptors of the nervous system exist in fascia and relate to proprioception and pain reception.

Fascia is colloidal, as is most of the soft tissue of the body. A colloid consists of particles of solid material suspended in fluid, similar to wallpaper paste; the colloid conforms to the shape of the container it is in and responds to pressure in predictable ways. The amount of resistance colloids offer to pressure applied to the tissues increases proportionally to the velocity (how fast) of force applied to them. This response makes a slow touch a fundamental requirement of massage application; it is necessary to avoid resistance when attempting to produce a change in, or release of, restricted fascial structures.

Muscle tissue has elasticity that allows it to withstand deformation when force or pressure is applied, but fascia is more plastic, and therefore these forces can be detrimental. Massage can introduce various mechanical forces to reverse the detrimental changes. Applying force is called loading, and releasing force is called unloading. Theoretically, when a mechanical force is gradually applied to fascia, it has an elastic reaction in which a degree of slack is allowed to be taken up, and then the tissue begins to creep because of its viscoelastic nature. *Creep* is the term for the slow, delayed, and continuous deformation that occurs in response to a sustained, slowly applied load. Therapeutically, the goal is to produce creep to elongate shortened and binding tissue to a more healthy position. The mechanical forces created by massage application may produce creep and must be applied with slow and appropriate pressure with sustained drag and without causing injury. Many soft-tissue methods, including massage, operate from this premise. However, the available research does not totally support the premise. Another theory is that the loading and unloading of fascia changes the water content of the tissue. According to yet another theory, myofibroblast contraction produces fascial tone as a reason for fascial changes due to manual force application.

Biomechanical Terms Relating to Fascia

- *Creep:* Continued deformation (increasing strain) of a viscoelastic material under constant load (traction, compression, twist).
- *Hysteresis:* Process of energy loss caused by friction when tissues are loaded and unloaded.
- *Load:* The degree of force (stress) applied to an area. For massage—what we do.
- *Strain:* Change in shape as a result of stress. Strain is the amount of deformation experienced by the body in the direction of force applied. Strain is the measurement of deformation induced in the object when it is subjected to the load or stress. For massage—what happens.
- *Stress:* Stress is defined as force per unit area within materials that arise from externally applied forces. Stress is developed in any object when it is subjected to load. For massage—how much intensity.
- *Stress–strain curve:* The behavior of any tissue during loading. It is used to predict safe loading conditions and failure point or facture point which would result in injury.
- *Stress–strain relationships:* The relationship between the external loads applied to a material and the resulting deformation or change in material dimensions.
- *Thixotropy:* A quality of colloids in which the more rapidly force is applied (load), the more rigid the tissue response.
- *Viscoelastic:* The potential to deform elastically when load is applied and to return to the original nondeformed state when load is removed.
- *Viscoplastic:* A permanent deformation resulting from the elastic potential having been exceeded or pressure forces sustained.

Thixotropy relates to the quality of gelatinous substances called colloids in which the more rapidly the force is applied (load), the more rigid and the less pliable the tissue response will be. Muscle tissue that is rigid or feels dense may have undergone thixotropic changes. If the practitioner gradually applies force, as described previously, the tissues absorb and store energy. To increase connective tissue pliability, massage application must not be abrupt or the tissue will respond by becoming more rigid.

Hysteresis describes the process of energy loss because of friction and tiny structural damage that occurs when tissues are loaded and unloaded repetitively. The tissues produce heat as they are loaded and unloaded, which occurs with on-and-off pressure application. Creating hysteresis reduces stiffness and improves the way the tissue responds to subsequent application of a load. The properties of hysteresis and creep provide the basis for myofascial release techniques, but, again,

new research is questioning these theories and offering new possibilities. One of the most plausible is that loading and unloading fascia changes the water content of the tissue, which in turn would change the pliability. Another is that the fascia is a communication network wherein loading and unloading the tissue changes the shape of the cells, resulting in a chemical change.

If the elastic potential of fascia has been exceeded or pressure forces are sustained for an extended period, a viscoplastic response develops and deformation can become permanent. This response results in a dysfunctional change. The same process can be used to create a therapeutic change to reverse dysfunction. Permanent deformation change depends on the uptake of water by the tissues. Elastic recoil occurs when the application of force ceases to prevent recoil, especially if released quickly. Therefore, mechanical force introduced during massage should be released gradually (Figure 4.23).

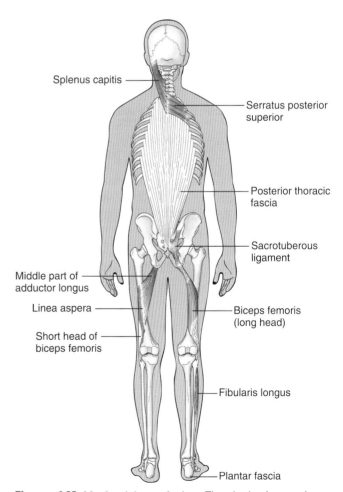

Figure 4.23 Myofascial continuity. The body is an interconnected system. This example shows an anatomic connection from the skull to the bottom of the foot. This muscle/fascia joining is necessary for the body to function as an integrated unit. (Source: Fritz S: *Mosby's essential sciences for therapeutic massage: anatomy, physiology, biomechanics, and pathology,* ed 4, St Louis, 2012, Mosby.)

NERVOUS SYSTEM

The nervous system is the most complex system in the body. Study of the nervous system is very important for the massage professional. Serious students of massage will challenge themselves to study the nervous system in depth. For purposes of study, terms related to the nervous system are presented in the following three groups:

- Central nervous system (CNS)
- Peripheral nervous system (PNS)
- Autonomic nervous system (ANS)

Central Nervous System

The CNS is the center (central) of all nervous control. It consists of the brain and spinal cord, which are located in the dorsal cavity (cranial and vertebral) (Figures 4.24 through 4.26).

Peripheral Nervous System

The PNS is composed of cranial and spinal nerves. The term *nerve* refers to a bundle of nerve fibers consisting of individual nerve cells outside the spinal cord or brain. The PNS consists of the nerves that carry impulses between the CNS and muscles, glands, skin, and other organs located outside (peripheral) the CNS. The ANS is the part of the peripheral nervous system that exerts nervous control over smooth muscle, heart muscle, and glands. Individual nerve cells are called *neurons*. The two types of nerve cells are the sensory neurons and the motor neurons (Figure 4.27).

Spinal Nerves
The 31 pairs of spinal nerves are attached to the spinal cord along almost its entire length. They are named for the region of the spinal column through which they exit. Many of the spinal nerves are located in groups called *somatic nerve plexuses*. The term *somatic* refers to the body wall; thus, these nerve plexuses contain nerves that are involved with the wall of the body, as opposed to organs within the body. A *plexus* is a network of intertwined (plexus) nerves. The four major plexuses of spinal nerves are the cervical plexus, brachial plexus, lumbar plexus, and sacral plexus (Figure 4.28).

Proprioception
Proprioception is kinesthetic sense. Sensory receptors receive information about position, rate of movement, contraction, tension, and stretch of tissues through distortion of and pressure on the sensory receptor. After proprioceptive sensory information is processed in the CNS, motor impulses carry the response message back to the muscles. The muscles then contract or relax to restore or change posture, movement, or position. Proprioception maintains motor tone in muscle. The pain-spasm-pain cycle uses proprioception as well as reflexes to maintain the feedback loop.

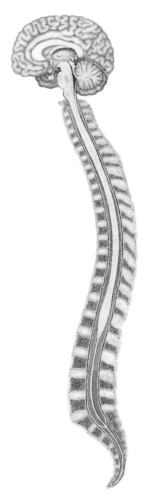

Figure 4.24 The central nervous system. (Source: Thibodeau GA, Patton KT: *Anatomy and physiology*, ed 6, St Louis, 2007, Mosby.)

Terms related to proprioception include *mechanoreceptor*, *Golgi tendon organ*, *joint kinesthetic receptors*, *kinesthetic*, and *muscle spindle cells*.

Reflex
A *reflex* is an involuntary body response to a stimulus. Important reflexes stimulated by massage are crossed, extensor thrust, flexor withdrawal, gait, intersegmental, monosynaptic, nociceptive, optical righting, ocular pelvic, pilomotor, psychogalvanic, postural, proprioceptive, righting, startle, stretch, tendon, tonic neck, vasomotor, and visceromotor reflexes.

Autonomic Nervous System

The ANS is the part of the peripheral nervous system that is an automatic, or self-governing (self [*auto*], governing [*nomic*]), system. It is also called the *involuntary system* because the effects of this system usually are not under voluntary control. The ANS is divided into two parts: the sympathetic division and the parasympathetic division.

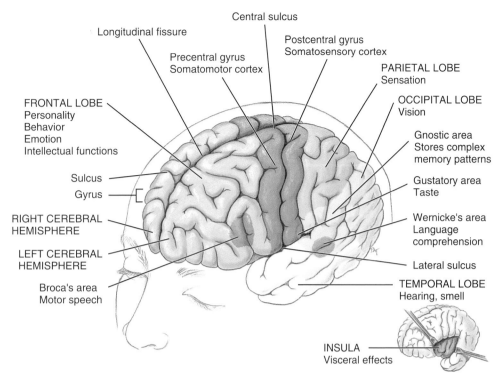

Figure 4.25 Functional organization of the cerebral cortex. (Source: Applegate E: *The anatomy and physiology learning system*, ed 4, Philadelphia, 2010, Saunders.)

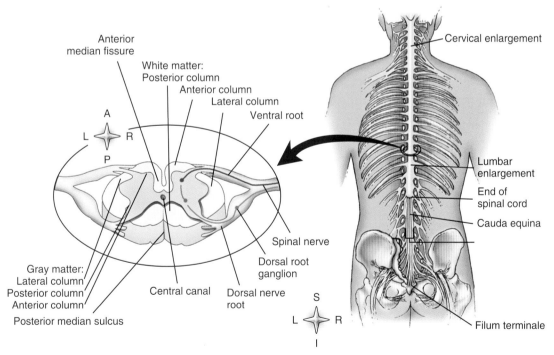

Figure 4.26 Spinal cord. The inset illustrates a transverse part of the spinal cord shown in the broader view. (Source: Thibodeau GA, Patton KT: *Anatomy and physiology*, ed 6, St Louis, 2007, Mosby.)

The *sympathetic division* controls the body's response to feelings (sympathy). Nerves in this division come off the thoracic and lumbar segments of the spinal cord; thus, this division sometimes is referred to as the *thoracolumbar division*. Actions caused by these nerves include the fight-or-flight and fear responses. The reaction of some organs includes an increase in heart rate, dilation of the pupils, and an increase in adrenaline secretion. A person sometimes may exhibit great strength as a result of a sympathetic response.

The nerves in the parasympathetic division come off the cranial and sacral segments of the spinal cord; thus, this division sometimes is called the *craniosacral division*. The

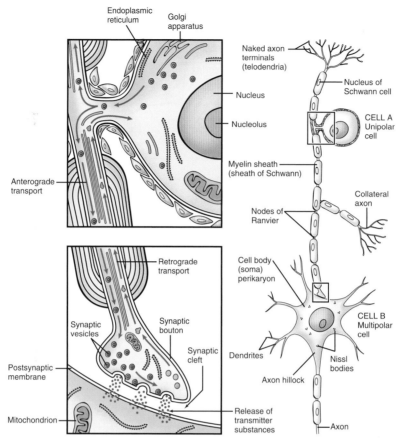

Figure 4.27 A typical neuron. An electrical pulse travels along the axon of the first neuron to the synapse. A chemical transmitter is secreted into the synaptic cleft to depolarize membranes (dendrite or cell body) of the next neuron in the pathway. (Source: Fritz S: *Mosby's essential sciences for therapeutic massage: anatomy, physiology, biomechanics, and pathology*, ed 4, St Louis, 2012, Mosby.)

parasympathetic division generally causes effects opposite (para-) to those caused by the sympathetic system. These effects include constriction of the pupils, return of the heart rate to normal, and stimulation of the lacrimal glands to produce tears.

Intertwined nerves (plexus) of the ANS are called the *autonomic plexuses*. Examples of these plexuses include the cardiac plexus, or the intertwined nerves of the heart (cardiac), and the celiac plexus, or the intertwined nerves of the organs of the abdomen (celiac). The celiac plexus sometimes is called the *solar plexus* because of the sunray (solar) fashion in which the nerves exit the plexus (Figure 4.29 and Table 4.8).

The Enteric Nervous System

The digestive system has its own, local nervous system referred to as the enteric or intrinsic nervous system. The enteric nervous system, along with the sympathetic and parasympathetic nervous systems, constitutes the autonomic nervous system. The vagus nerve is part of the gut—brain axis.

The enteric nervous system functions autonomously, but normal digestive function requires communication links between this intrinsic system and the central nervous system. These links take the form of parasympathetic and sympathetic fibers that connect either the central and enteric nervous systems or connect the central nervous system directly with the digestive tract.

In general, sympathetic stimulation causes inhibition of gastrointestinal secretion and motor activity, and contraction of gastrointestinal sphincters and blood vessels. Conversely, parasympathetic stimuli typically stimulate these digestive activities.

Function of the Nervous System

The function of the nervous system is to receive impressions from the external environment, organize the information, and provide appropriate responses. In other words, the nervous system allows the body to detect changes in and respond to outside influences (environment). Outside information enters the nervous system through nerve endings in the skin and in special sense organs. These nerve endings are referred to as *receptors*.

Nerve endings in the skin are sensitive to pain, touch, pressure, vibration, and temperature. Special sense nerve endings are responsible for taste, smell, vision, hearing, and sense of position and movement. Sensations from the environment are picked up by these receptors and are sent to the CNS by way of the PNS. The CNS sorts out the information and sends back a message, again by way of the PNS. Information is transferred from one nerve to another by chemicals called *neurotransmitters*.

The nervous system and neurotransmitters, along with the endocrine system, also maintain the internal environment, or

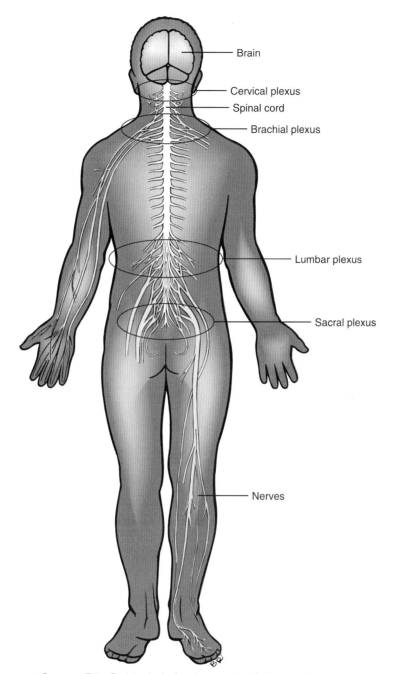

Figure 4.28 Major nerve plexuses. (Source: Fritz S: *Mosby's fundamentals of therapeutic massage*, ed 5, St Louis, 2012, Mosby.)

the balance of the many activities within the body (homeostasis). Although divisions of the nervous system may be treated independently, they do not function independently.

Terms Related to Nerves

Neuron is a nerve cell that is the basic building block of the nervous system.

- *Neuroglial cells*—usually referred to simply as glial cells or glia. There are three types of glial cells in the central nervous system:
  - Astrocytes maintain an appropriate chemical environment for neuronal signaling.

- Oligodendrocytes make myelin around some, but not all, axons. In the peripheral nervous system Schwan cells perform this function.
- Microglial cells are primarily scavenger cells that remove cellular debris from sites of injury or normal cell turnover.
- *Afferent nerves* are nerves that carry (*ferent*) messages to (*af-*, variation of *ad-*) the CNS; they are also known as *sensory nerves* because they pick up and transmit sensation (*sen*).
- *Efferent nerves* are nerves that carry (*ferent*) messages away from (*ef-*, variation of *ex-*) the brain, resulting in motion (*motor*). They are also known as *motor nerves*.
- *Cranial nerves* are the 12 pairs of nerves that arise from the brainstem in the cranium or skull (*cranial*).

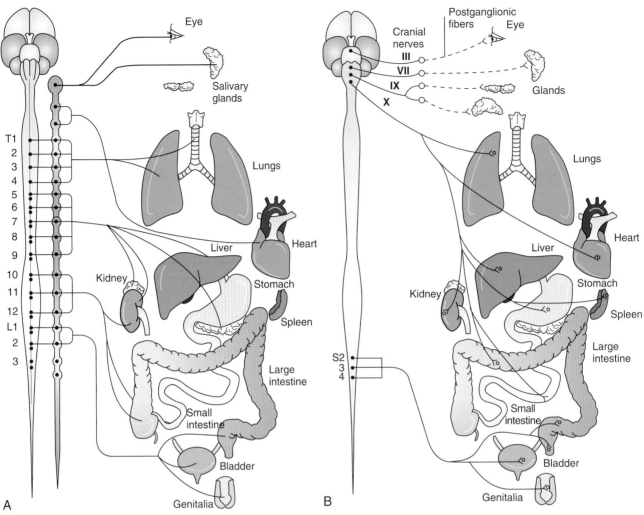

Figure 4.29 **A**, The sympathetic portions of the autonomic nervous system. **B**, The parasympathetic portions of the autonomic nervous system. (Source: **A**, Vidic B, Suarex FR: *Photographic atlas of the human body*, St Louis, 1984, Mosby. **B**, Fritz S: *Mosby's essential sciences for therapeutic massage: anatomy, physiology, biomechanics, and pathology*, ed 4, St Louis, 2012, Mosby.)

TABLE 4.8	Functions of the Autonomic Nervous System	
Component	**Sympathetic control**	**Parasympathetic control**
Viscera		
Heart	Accelerates heartbeat	Slows heartbeat
Smooth muscle		
Most blood vessels	Constricts blood vessels	None
Blood vessels of skeletal muscle	None	Dilates blood vessels
Digestive tract	Decreases peristalsis; inhibits defecation	Increases peristalsis
Anal sphincter	Stimulates (closes sphincter)	Inhibits (opens sphincter for defecation)
Urinary bladder	Inhibits (relaxes bladder)	Stimulates (contracts bladder)
Urinary sphincters	Stimulates (closes sphincters)	Inhibits (opens sphincters for urination)
Iris	Stimulates radial fibers (dilation of pupil)	Stimulates circular fibers (constriction of pupil)
Ciliary muscles	Inhibits (accommodates for far vision; flattening of lens)	Stimulates (accommodates for near vision; bulging of lens)
Hair (pilomotor muscles)	Stimulates (goose bumps)	None
Glands		
Adrenal medulla	Increases secretion of epinephrine	None
Sweat glands	Increases secretion of sweat	None
Digestive glands	Decreases secretion of digestive juices	Increases secretion of digestive juices

Source: Fritz S: *Mosby's fundamentals of therapeutic massage*, ed 5, St Louis, 2012, Mosby.

- *Spinal nerves* are the 31 pairs of nerves that branch off the spinal cord.
- A *ganglion* is a mass of nerve cell bodies located outside the CNS; *ganglia* is the plural form.

- *Neuro* is the root word meaning "nerve."
- *Dermatomes* are the distribution of spinal nerve innervations (Figures 4.30 through 4.33).

PROXIMAL

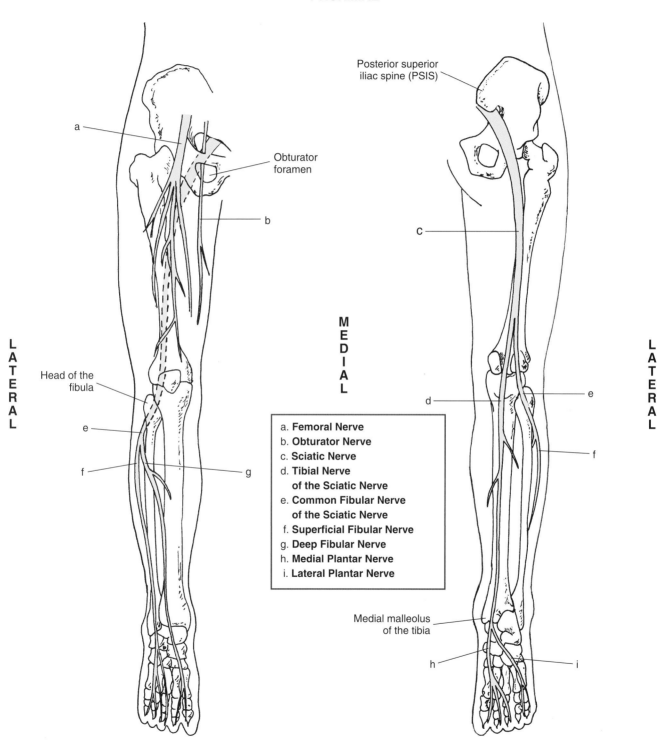

a. **Femoral Nerve**
b. **Obturator Nerve**
c. **Sciatic Nerve**
d. **Tibial Nerve**
   of the Sciatic Nerve
e. **Common Fibular Nerve**
   of the Sciatic Nerve
f. **Superficial Fibular Nerve**
g. **Deep Fibular Nerve**
h. **Medial Plantar Nerve**
i. **Lateral Plantar Nerve**

DISTAL

Figure 4.30 A, Anterior (*left*) and posterior views (*right*) of the lower extremity. (Source: Muscolino JE: *The muscular system manual: the skeletal muscles of the human body*, ed 3, St Louis, 2009, Elsevier.)

PROXIMAL

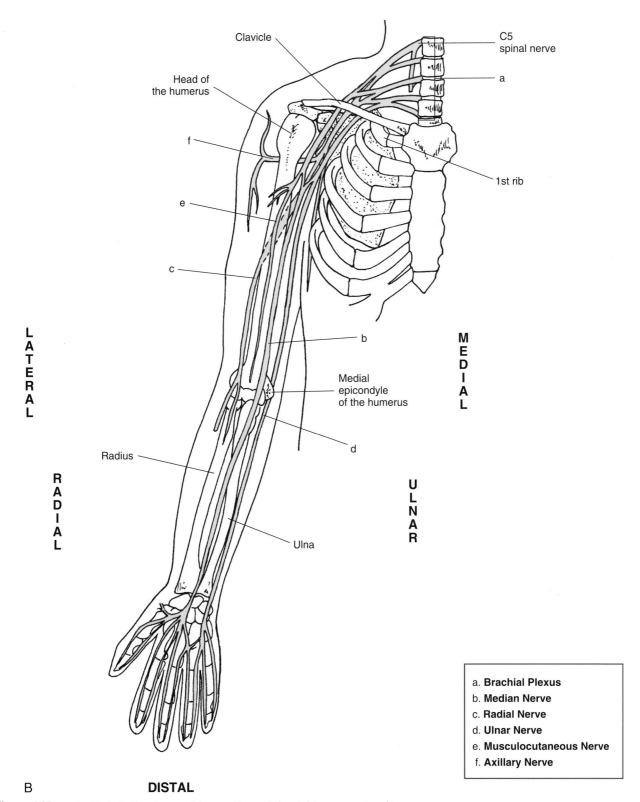

Clavicle

Head of
the humerus

f

e

c

C5
spinal nerve

a

1st rib

**L
A
T
E
R
A
L**

b

Medial
epicondyle
of the humerus

d

Radius

Ulna

**M
E
D
I
A
L**

**R
A
D
I
A
L**

**U
L
N
A
R**

| a. **Brachial Plexus** |
| b. **Median Nerve** |
| c. **Radial Nerve** |
| d. **Ulnar Nerve** |
| e. **Musculocutaneous Nerve** |
| f. **Axillary Nerve** |

B   **DISTAL**

Figure 4.30, cont'd **B,** Anterior view and innervations of the right upper extremity.

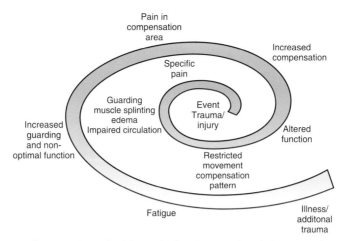

Figure 4.31 Pain-spasm-pain cycle. (Source: Fritz S: *Mosby's fundamentals of therapeutic massage*, ed 5, St Louis, 2012, Mosby.)

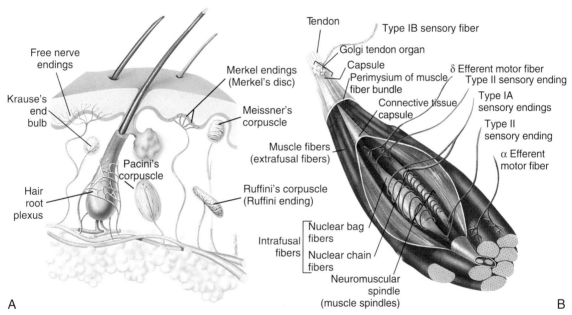

Figure 4.32 Somatic sensory receptors. **A**, Exteroreceptors. **B**, Proprioceptors. (Source: Thibodeau GA, Patton KT: *Anatomy and physiology*, ed 6, St Louis, 2007, Mosby.)

CARDIOVASCULAR SYSTEM

The cardiovascular system consists of three parts: the heart, blood, and blood vessels. The *heart* is a four-chambered pump. *Arteries* are tubes (vessels) that deliver oxygenated blood to the body. They carry blood under pressure and are located relatively deep within the body.

Veins are vessels that return blood to the heart. They are located in more superficial areas; therefore, veins are easier to palpate. Veins have a valve system that prevents the backflow of blood. Breakdown of a valve may result in a varicose vein. *Capillaries* are very small, thin (usually one-cell-thick) vessels that allow for the exchange of blood gases and nutrients. Blood vessels vasoconstrict, or become smaller inside, and vasodilate, or become larger inside.

Blood pressure is a measurement of the pressure exerted by the circulating volume of blood on the walls of the arteries, veins, and heart chambers. Blood pressure is maintained through the complex interaction of the homeostatic mechanisms of the body. Normal blood pressure varies according to age, size, and gender, but the average is approximately 120 mm Hg during systole and 70 mm Hg in diastole. High blood pressure is called *hypertension,* and low blood pressure is called *hypotension.*

Blood is composed of a clear, yellow fluid called *plasma,* blood cells, and platelets. The main function of blood is to transport oxygen and nutrients to the cells and remove carbon dioxide and other waste products. The amount of blood in muscle tissue influences the muscle tone. If muscle tissue contains too much blood, it is said to be congested, and methods to encourage blood flow are used (Figure 4.34).

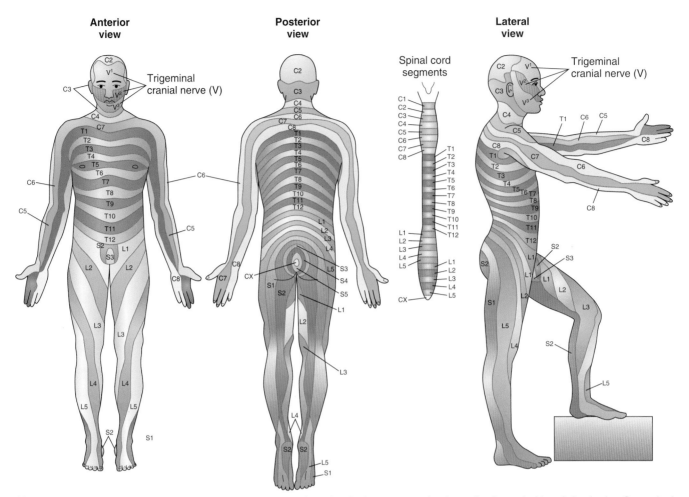

Figure 4.33 Dermatomes. Segmental dermatome distribution of spinal nerves to the front, back, and side of the body. *C*, cervical segments; *CX*, coccygeal segments; *L*, lumbar segments; *S*, sacral segments; *T*, thoracic segments.

LYMPHATIC SYSTEM

The *lymphatic system* is responsible for several functions and operates in the following ways:

1. It returns vital substances, such as plasma protein, to the bloodstream from the tissues of the body. Fluid around the cells in tissues is called *interstitial fluid.*
2. It assists in the maintenance of fluid balance by draining fluid from body tissues.
3. It helps in the body's defense against disease-producing substances.
4. It helps in the absorption of fats from the digestive system.

The lymphatic system is a network of channels and nodes in which a substance called *lymph* travels. Lymph is a clear, watery fluid similar to plasma. The system collects and drains fluid from around tissue cells from different areas of the body and carries it through the lymphatic channels back to the venous system. There, it is deposited, mixed with venous blood, and recirculated.

Lymphatic capillaries are found near and parallel to the veins that carry blood to the heart. The ends of the lymphatic capillaries meet to form larger lymph vessels. The lymph vessels in the right chest, head, and right arm join the right lymphatic duct, which drains into the right subclavian vein. Lymph vessels from all other parts of the body join to meet the thoracic duct, which drains into the left subclavian vein.

Throughout the lymph system are lymph nodes. Lymph nodes are small bodies that are present in the path of the lymph channels and that act as filters for lymph before it returns to the bloodstream. The main locations of the more superficial lymph nodes are the cervical area, the axillary region, and the groin or inguinal area.

Plexuses of lymph channels are found throughout the body:

- *Mammary plexus:* Lymphatic vessels around the breasts.
- *Palmar plexus:* Lymphatic vessels in the palm (palmar) of the hand.
- *Plantar plexus:* Lymphatic vessels in the sole (plantar) of the foot.

If soft tissue has too much interstitial fluid around the cells, or if the lymph vessels are full of fluid that is moving slowly or is stagnant, the tissue is said to be infused or edematous (relating to edema). Excess fluid in muscle tissue contributes to muscle tone problems (Figure 4.35 and Table 4.9).

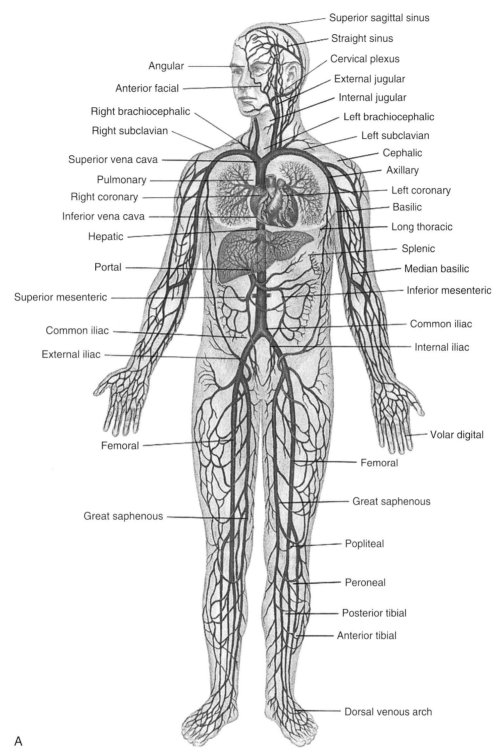

Superior sagittal sinus
Straight sinus
Cervical plexus
External jugular
Internal jugular
Left brachiocephalic
Left subclavian
Cephalic
Axillary
Left coronary
Basilic
Long thoracic
Splenic
Median basilic
Inferior mesenteric
Common iliac
Internal iliac
Volar digital
Femoral
Great saphenous
Popliteal
Peroneal
Posterior tibial
Anterior tibial
Dorsal venous arch

Angular
Anterior facial
Right brachiocephalic
Right subclavian
Superior vena cava
Pulmonary
Right coronary
Inferior vena cava
Hepatic
Portal
Superior mesenteric
Common iliac
External iliac
Femoral
Great saphenous

A

Figure 4.34 The systemic circulation. **A,** Veins. (Source: Seidel HM, et al.: *Mosby's guide to physical examination,* ed 7, St Louis, 2010, Mosby.)

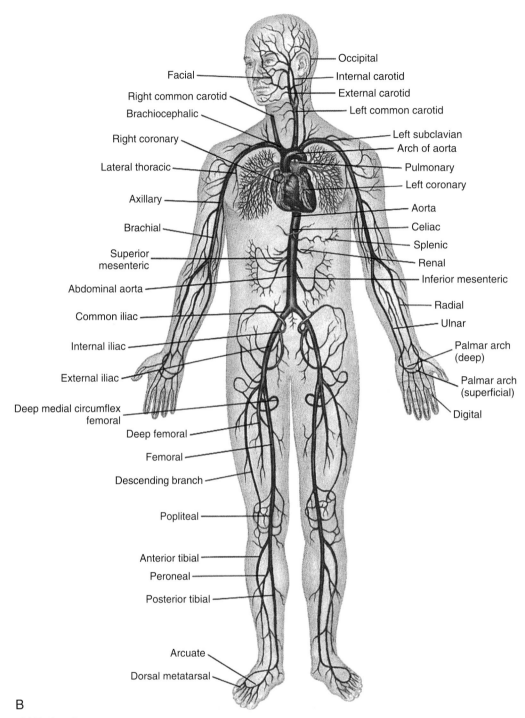

B

Figure 4.34, cont'd **B**, Arteries.

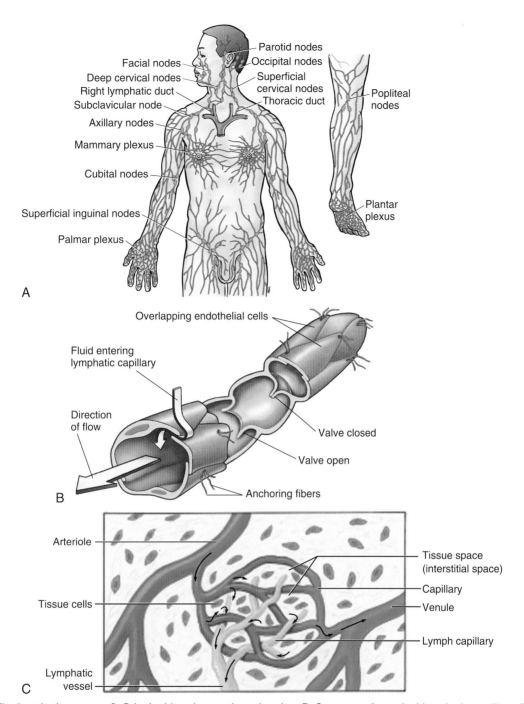

Figure 4.35 The lymphatic system. **A**, Principal lymph vessels and nodes. **B**, Structure of a typical lymphatic capillary. The interstitial fluid enters through clefts between overlapping endothelial cells that line the wall of the vessel. Semilunar valves ensure one-way flow of lymph out of the tissues. **C**, Distribution from lymphatic capillaries in the tissue. (Source: **A**, Fritz S: *Mosby's essential sciences for therapeutic massage: anatomy, physiology, biomechanics, and pathology*, ed 4, St Louis, 2012, Mosby. **B**, Thibodeau GA, Patton KT: *Anatomy and physiology*, ed 6, St Louis, 2007, Mosby. **C**, Applegate E: *The anatomy and physiology learning system*, ed 4, Philadelphia, 2010, Saunders.)

TABLE 4.9	Types of Lymph Nodes
Nodes	**Description**
Parotid	Nodes around (para-) or in front of the ear (otid)
Occipital	Nodes over the occipital bone at the back of the head
Superficial cervical	Nodes close to the surface (superficial) of the neck (cervic-)
Subclavicular	Nodes under (sub-) the collarbone (clavicular)
Hypogastric	Nodes in the area beneath (hypo-) the stomach (gastric)
Facial	Nodes draining the tissue in the face
Deep cervical	Deeply (deep) situated nodes in the neck (cervic-)
Axillary (superficial)	Nodes in the armpit (axilla)
Mediastinal	Nodes in the mediastinal part of the thoracic cavity
Cubital	Nodes of the elbow (cubit-)
Para-aortic	Nodes around (para-) the aorta (aortic)
Deep inguinal	Deeply (deep) situated nodes in the groin (inguin-)
Superficial inguinal	Nodes in the groin (inguin-) close to the surface (superficial)
Popliteal	Nodes in back of the knee (popliteal)

Source: Fritz S: *Mosby's fundamentals of therapeutic massage*, ed 5, St Louis, 2012, Mosby.

IMMUNE SYSTEM

The human body is able to resist organisms or toxins that tend to damage its tissues and organs. This ability is called *immunity* (Figure 4.36). There are natural barriers to infection, both physical and physiological, which are known collectively as *innate immunity*. The skin or mucous membranes of the respiratory tract are obvious barriers and may contain bacteriostatic or bactericidal agents that delay widespread infection until other defenses can be activated. The effects of macrophages, neutrophils, natural killer cells, and substances such as serum proteins, cytokines, complement, lectins, and lipid-binding proteins are part of the innate immunity.

Naturally acquired active immunity occurs when the person is exposed to a live pathogen, develops the disease, and becomes immune as a result of the primary immune response.

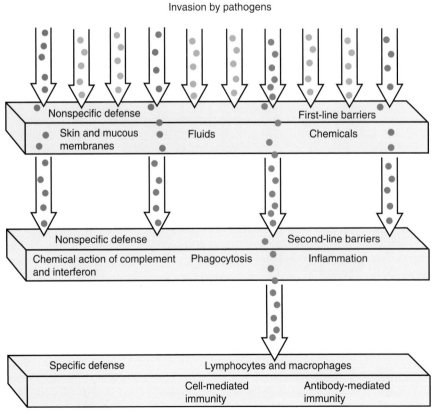

Figure 4.36 Overview of defense mechanisms of the immune system. (Source: Applegate E: *The anatomy and physiology learning system*, ed 4, Philadelphia, 2010, Saunders.)

Artificially acquired active immunity can be induced by a vaccine, a substance that contains the antigen. A vaccine stimulates a primary response against the antigen without causing symptoms of the disease.

Selected Terms Related to Immunology

- *Acquired immunity:* Resistance (immunity) to a particular disease developed by people who have acquired the disease.
- *Acquired immunodeficiency:* A group of symptoms (syndrome) caused by the transmission (acquired) of a virus that causes a breakdown (deficiency) in the immune system (AIDS).
- *Active immunity:* Resistance (immunity) resulting from antibodies the body has produced.
- *Allergy:* A state of hypersensitivity to a particular substance; the immune system overreacts (over [hyper-], reacts [sensitive]) to foreign substances, and physical changes occur.
- *Antibody:* An immune protein produced by the body in response to a specific antigen.
- *Antigen:* A substance that stimulates the immune response; the body recognizes it as foreign.
- *Innate immunity:* Natural barriers to infection, both physical and physiological.
- *Susceptible:* An individual who is capable (-ible) of acquiring (suscept-) a particular disease.

RESPIRATORY SYSTEM

The respiratory system supplies oxygen to and removes carbon dioxide from the cells of the body. Respiration is divided into two phases: external and internal. *External respiration* involves the absorption of oxygen from the air by the lungs and the transport of carbon dioxide from the lungs back into the air. *Internal respiration* involves the exchange of oxygen and carbon dioxide within the cells of the body.

Terms and combining forms related to the respiratory system include *alveoli*, *lungs*, *nares*, *nostrils*, *olfactory cells*, *pneumo-*, *rhino-*, and *trachea* (Figure 4.37).

DIGESTIVE SYSTEM

The anatomy of the digestive system is basically a long muscular tube that travels through the body. The organs of the digestive system transport food through this muscular tube. The wavelike contraction of the smooth muscles of the digestive tube is called *peristalsis*. Accessory organs carry out functions directly related to digestion and are connected to the system by means of ducts. Understanding the flow of contents through the large intestine is important for the massage professional because methods of massage can be used to enhance this process (Figures 4.38 and 4.39 and Table 4.10).

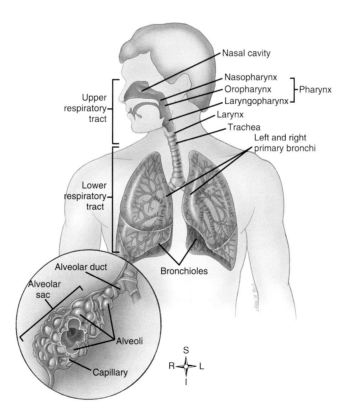

Figure 4.37 Structural plan of the respiratory system. The inset shows the alveolar sacs where the interchange of oxygen and carbon dioxide takes place through the walls of the grapelike alveoli. Capillaries surround the alveoli. (Source: Fritz S: *Mosby's fundamentals of therapeutic massage*, ed 5, St Louis, 2012, Mosby.)

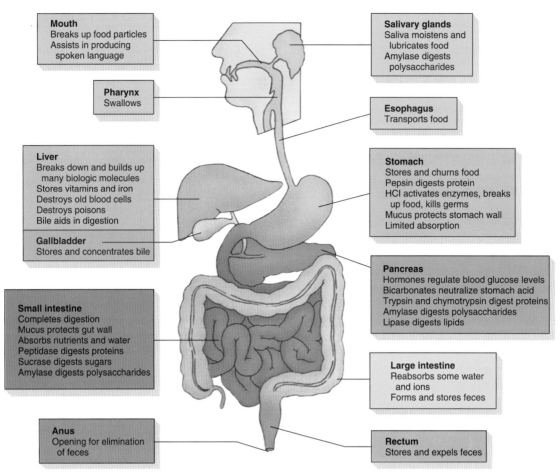

Mouth
Breaks up food particles
Assists in producing
spoken language

Pharynx
Swallows

Liver
Breaks down and builds up
many biologic molecules
Stores vitamins and iron
Destroys old blood cells
Destroys poisons
Bile aids in digestion

Gallbladder
Stores and concentrates bile

Small intestine
Completes digestion
Mucus protects gut wall
Absorbs nutrients and water
Peptidase digests proteins
Sucrase digests sugars
Amylase digests polysaccharides

Anus
Opening for elimination
of feces

Salivary glands
Saliva moistens and
lubricates food
Amylase digests
polysaccharides

Esophagus
Transports food

Stomach
Stores and churns food
Pepsin digests protein
HCl activates enzymes, breaks
up food, kills germs
Mucus protects stomach wall
Limited absorption

Pancreas
Hormones regulate blood glucose levels
Bicarbonates neutralize stomach acid
Trypsin and chymotrypsin digest proteins
Amylase digests polysaccharides
Lipase digests lipids

Large intestine
Reabsorbs some water
and ions
Forms and stores feces

Rectum
Stores and expels feces

Figure 4.38 The organs of the digestive system with a summary of digestive function. (Source: Fritz S: *Mosby's essential sciences for therapeutic massage: anatomy, physiology, biomechanics, and pathology*, ed 4, St Louis, 2012, Mosby; and Fritz S: *Mosby's fundamentals of therapeutic massage*, ed 5, St Louis, 2012, Mosby.)

GENERAL NUTRITIONAL INFORMATION

This information is designed to help adults make informed decisions about their health and is intended for general nutritional information and educational purposes only. It is not intended to prescribe, treat, cure, diagnose, or prevent any particular medical problem or disease, or to promote any particular product. Women who are pregnant or nursing should always consult with their doctors before taking any supplements. You should always consult your healthcare professional for individual guidance regarding specific health concerns. Persons with medical conditions should seek professional medical care. Massage therapists are not able to diagnose conditions, make recommendations, or prescribe vitamins, minerals, supplements, herbs, or other medicinal products.

ENDOCRINE SYSTEM

The endocrine system is composed of glands that produce hormones, which are secreted directly into the bloodstream to stimulate cells in a specific way, to stimulate a body function, or to inhibit a body function.

Hormone Systems

Hormones produced by target glands are regulated by pituitary hormones, which in turn are controlled by hypothalamic hormones that create hormone systems. Examples of such regulatory hormonal cascades include the hypothalamic–pituitary–adrenal (HPA) axis, the hypothalamic–pituitary–gonadal (HPG) axis, and the hypothalamic–pituitary–thyroidal (HPT) axis.

The endocrine system is complex and important because it serves as a control and regulation system for the body. As with the nervous system, the massage professional should commit to an in-depth study of the endocrine system, its relationship to the nervous system, and its connection to mind/body processes. Information from research on the mind/body phenomenon is being released too quickly to stay current in any textbook. The massage professional must read medical and scientific research to remain current. The implications for

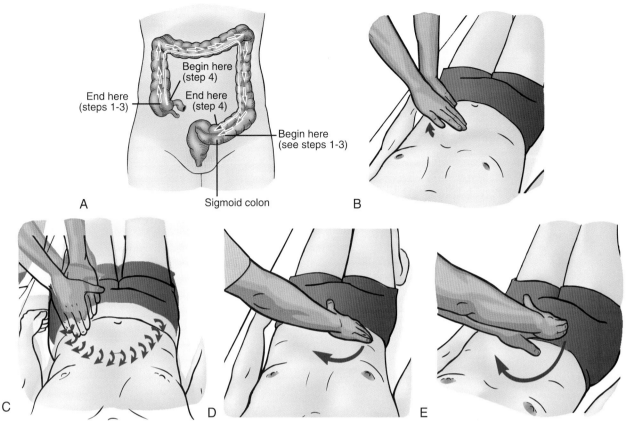

Figure 4.39 A, Colon (the *arrows* indicate the flow pattern). All massage manipulations are directed in a clockwise fashion. The manipulations begin in the lower left quadrant (on the *right side* as you view the illustration) at the sigmoid colon. The methods progressively contact all of the large intestine and eventually end up covering the entire colon area. **B**, Abdominal sequence shows the direction of flow for emptying of the large intestine and colon. Massage down the left side of the descending colon using short strokes directed toward the sigmoid colon. **C**, Massage across the transverse colon to the left side using short strokes directed toward the sigmoid colon. **D**, Massage up the ascending colon to the left side using short strokes directed toward the sigmoid colon. End at the right side ileocecal valve, which is located in the lower right quadrant of the abdomen. **E**, Massage the entire flow pattern of the abdominal sequence using long, light to moderate strokes, from the ileocecal valve to the sigmoid colon. Then repeat the sequence. (Source: Fritz S: *Mosby's fundamentals of therapeutic massage*, ed 5, St Louis, 2012, Mosby.)

massage are very important because the effects of massage are connected with the nervous system and endocrine body control functions (Figures 4.40 and 4.41).

URINARY AND REPRODUCTIVE SYSTEMS

The urinary system consists of two kidneys, two ureters, one bladder, and one urethra. The kidneys maintain homeostasis by filtering waste products from the blood and keeping the proper quantities of water and nutrients in the blood. Urine passes out of the kidneys and down through the ureters to the bladder for storage. When the bladder reaches a certain volume, one has the urge to void. The bladder expels urine through the urethra (Figures 4.42 and 4.43 and Box 4.2).

Functions of the Urinary System

Important functions of the urinary system include the following:
- Conservation of water

- Maintenance of the normal concentration of electrolytes
- Regulation of the acid–base balance
- Regulation of blood pressure
- Activation of vitamin D

The kidneys filter and eliminate most waste. In the average person, the kidneys filter about 100 L of blood, reabsorbing 99 L of filtrate and leaving about 1 L of urine. Substances secreted from the capillaries into the tubular filtrate include hydrogen, potassium, and ammonia.

Micturition (voiding, urination) is a parasympathetic action that is modified by voluntary control. It is initiated when afferent impulses from stretch receptors in the bladder stimulate the sacral portion of the spinal cord. The detrusor muscle contracts, and the sphincter relaxes.

Functions of the Reproductive System

The male reproductive system consists of the testicles, epididymis, vas deferens, ejaculatory duct, urethra, penis, and scrotum. The two testicles are enclosed in the scrotum, which is an external sac. Tiny seminiferous tubules in the testicles produce sperm. Sperm cells travel from the testicles into the

| TABLE 4.10 | Functions and Sources of Vitamins | | |

Vitamin	Function	Food source	Adult RDA
Fat soluble			
Vitamin A	Healthy mucous membranes, skin, hair; essential for bone development and growth; component of pigments for night vision in the retina	Yellow, orange, green vegetables; milk and cheese	800–1000 µg
Vitamin D	Formation and development of bones and teeth; assists in absorption of calcium	Fortified milk, fish oils; made in the skin when exposed to sunlight	5–10 µg
Vitamin E	Conserves certain fatty acids; aids in protection against cell membrane damage	Whole grains, wheat germ, vegetable oils, nuts, green leafy vegetables	8–10 µg
Vitamin K	Needed for synthesis of factors essential in blood clotting	Green leafy vegetables, cabbage; synthesized by bacteria in intestine	65–80 µg
Water soluble			
Thiamine (B$_1$)	Release of energy from carbohydrates and amino acids; growth; proper functioning of nervous system	Whole grains, legumes, nuts	1.5 mg
Riboflavin (B$_2$)	Helps transform nutrients into energy; involved in citric acid cycle	Whole grains, milk, green vegetables, nuts	1.7 mg
Niacin (B$_3$)	Helps transform nutrients into energy; involved in glycolysis and citric acid cycle	Whole grains, nuts, legumes, fish, liver	20 mg
Pyridoxine (B$_6$)	Involved in amino acid metabolism	Legumes, poultry, nuts, dried fruit, green vegetables	2 mg
Cyanocobalamin (B$_{12}$)	Aids in formation of red blood cells; helps in nervous system function	Dairy products, eggs, fish, poultry	2 µg
Pantothenic acid	Part of coenzyme A; functions in steroid synthesis; helps in nutrient metabolism	Legumes, nuts, green vegetables, milk, poultry	7 mg
Folic acid	Aids in formation of hemoglobin and nucleic acids	Green vegetables, legumes, nuts, fruit juices, whole grains	200 µg
Biotin	Fatty acid synthesis; movement of pyruvic acid into citric acid cycle	Eggs; made by intestinal bacteria	0.3 mg
Ascorbic acid (C)	Important in collagen synthesis; helps maintain capillaries; aids in absorption of iron	Citrus fruits, tomatoes, green vegetables, berries	60 mg

µg, microgram; *mg,* milligram.
Source: Applegate E: *The anatomy and physiology learning system,* ed 4, Philadelphia, 2010, Saunders.

epididymis, where they mature. Sperm then moves into the vas deferens, which extends upward into the body cavity, over the symphysis pubis, and around the urinary bladder to connect with the two seminal vesicles.

The female reproductive system is designed for childbearing. This system consists of two ovaries, two fallopian tubes, a uterus, and a vagina. Also included in the system are the external genitalia and the mammary glands. The ovaries are solid glands that produce the hormones estrogen and progesterone. The uterus receives the fertilized ovum and allows the embryo to grow and develop into a fetus. The inner lining is a soft, spongy layer, the endometrium, the surface of which is shed each month during menstruation (Figures 4.44 and 4.45).

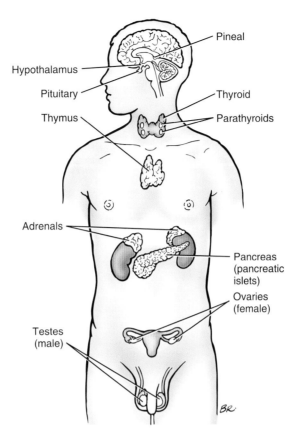

Figure 4.40 The locations of the endocrine glands. (Source: Fritz S: *Mosby's fundamentals of therapeutic massage*, ed 5, St Louis, 2012, Mosby.)

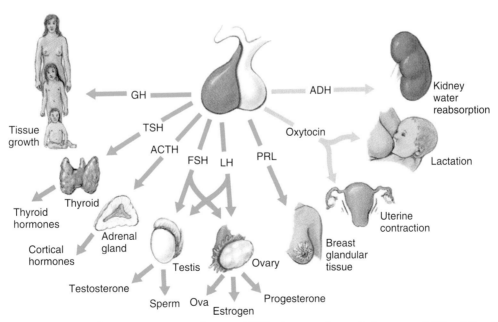

Figure 4.41 The effects of pituitary hormones on target tissues. *ACTH*, adrenocorticotropic hormone; *ADH*, antidiuretic hormone; *FSH*, follicle-stimulating hormone; *GH*, growth hormone; *LH*, luteinizing hormone; *PRL*, prolactin; *TSH*, thyroid-stimulating hormone. (Source: Applegate E: *The anatomy and physiology learning system*, ed 4, Philadelphia, 2010, Saunders.)

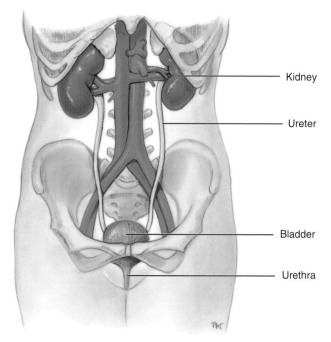

Figure 4.42 Urinary system. (Source: Applegate E: *The anatomy and physiology learning system*, ed 4, Philadelphia, 2010, Saunders.)

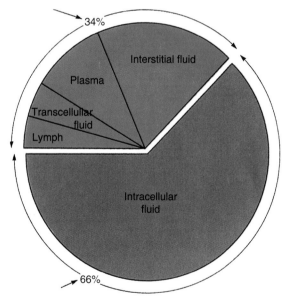

Figure 4.43 Distribution of total body water. (Source: Thibodeau GA, Patton KT: *Anatomy and physiology*, ed 6, St Louis, 2007, Mosby.)

INTEGUMENTARY SYSTEM

The integumentary system consists of the skin and its appendages, including the hair and nails.

The Skin

The skin is the largest organ of the body. It is composed of three layers of tissue: the epidermis, the dermis, and the

---

> **BOX 4.2** | **Functions of Water in Human Physiology**
>
> - Water provides a medium for chemical reactions.
> - Water is crucial for the regulation of chemical and bioelectrical distributions within cells.
> - Water transports substances such as hormones and nutrients.
> - Water aids oxygen transport from lungs to body cells.
> - Water aids carbon dioxide transport from body cells to lungs.
> - Water dilutes toxic substances and waste products and transports them to the kidneys and the liver.
> - Water distributes heat around the body.

subcutaneous tissue. The *epidermis*, the outer layer of skin, contains many layers of tissue and melanocytes, the cells that give skin color. The *dermis*, or dermal layer, lies directly under the epidermis and often is called "the true skin." It is made of connective tissue. Embedded in the dermis are the blood vessels, lymphatic vessels, hair follicles, and sweat glands. *Subcutaneous tissue* attaches the dermis to the underlying structures. This fatty tissue contains varying amounts of adipose tissue and acts as insulation for the body.

The functions of the fascial network of the skin include protection; control and maintenance of body temperature; detection of the sensations of touch, temperature, pain, and pressure; secretion of sweat and sebum; and production of vitamin D when the skin is exposed to the sun.

Many disease signs (particularly color changes) may be noticed first in the skin. Terms related to skin color changes include *cyanosis* (bluish), *erythema* (red), *jaundice* (yellow-orange), and *pallor* (a decrease in color).

Sebaceous Glands

Sebaceous glands are located in the skin. They secrete an oily substance called *sebum*, which gives the skin and hair a glossy appearance. Most of these glands open into the walls of hair follicles. Other sebaceous glands are located at the corners of the mouth and around the external sex organs that open directly onto the surface of the skin.

Sudoriferous Glands

Sudoriferous glands are sweat glands and are found in most areas of the body. They function to cool the body through evaporation of perspiration (sweat). The most abundant type is the eccrine sweat gland. The palms of the hands and the soles of the feet contain large numbers of these glands. Sweat from these glands is odorless. Another type of sweat gland is the apocrine sweat gland, which is connected to

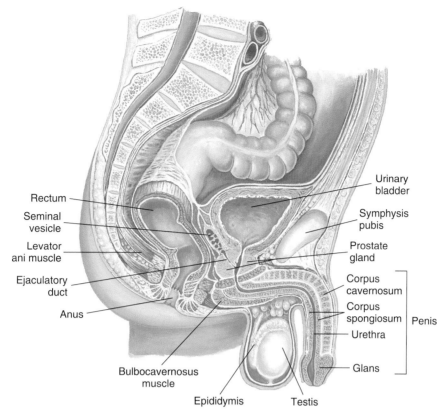

Figure 4.44 Male pelvic organs. (Source: Seidel HM, et al.: *Mosby's guide to physical examination*, ed 7, St Louis, 2010, Mosby.)

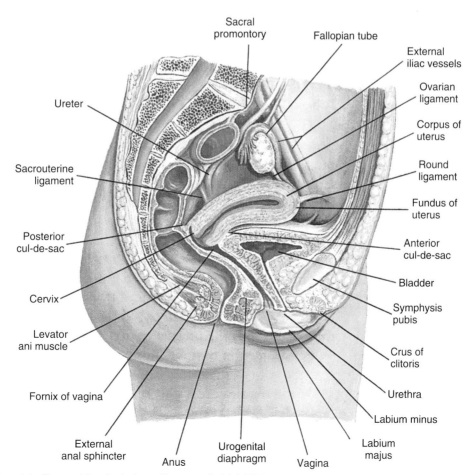

Figure 4.45 Female pelvic floor, midsagittal view. (Source: Seidel HM, et al.: *Mosby's guide to physical examination*, ed 7, St Louis, 2010, Mosby.)

hair follicles in the armpits and the pubic area and is found at the navel and nipples. Secretions from these sweat glands increase in response to sexual stimulation. They function to lubricate the genital area, and they play a part in sexual arousal by producing a mild odor (Figures 4.46 and 4.47).

REVIEW OF SYSTEMS OF THE BODY AND THEIR IMPORTANT ORGANS

System = Associated Organs

- Musculoskeletal (can be classified separately as the skeletal, articular [joints], and muscular systems) = Bones, ligaments, skeletal muscles, tendons, joints
- Nervous = Brain, spinal cord, nerves, special sense organs
- Cardiovascular = Heart, arteries, veins, capillaries

- Lymphatic = Lymphatic vessels, lymph nodes, spleen, tonsils, thymus gland
- Digestive = Mouth, tongue, teeth, salivary glands, esophagus, stomach, small and large intestines, liver, gallbladder, pancreas
- Respiratory = Nasal cavity, larynx, trachea, bronchi, lungs, diaphragm, pharynx
- Urinary = Kidneys, ureters, urinary bladder, urethra
- Endocrine = Endocrine glands: Hypothalamus, hypophysis (pituitary), thyroid, thymus, parathyroid, pineal, adrenal, pancreas, gonads (ovary or testis)
- Reproductive = Female: Ovaries, uterine tubes (oviducts), uterus, vagina
- Reproductive = Male: Testes, penis, prostate gland, seminal vesicles, spermatic ducts
- Integumentary = Skin, hair, nails, sebaceous glands, sweat glands, breasts

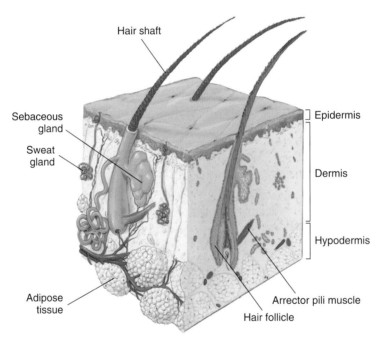

Figure 4.46 The structure of the skin. (Source: Jarvis C: *Physical examination and health assessment,* ed 6, Philadelphia, 2011, Saunders.)

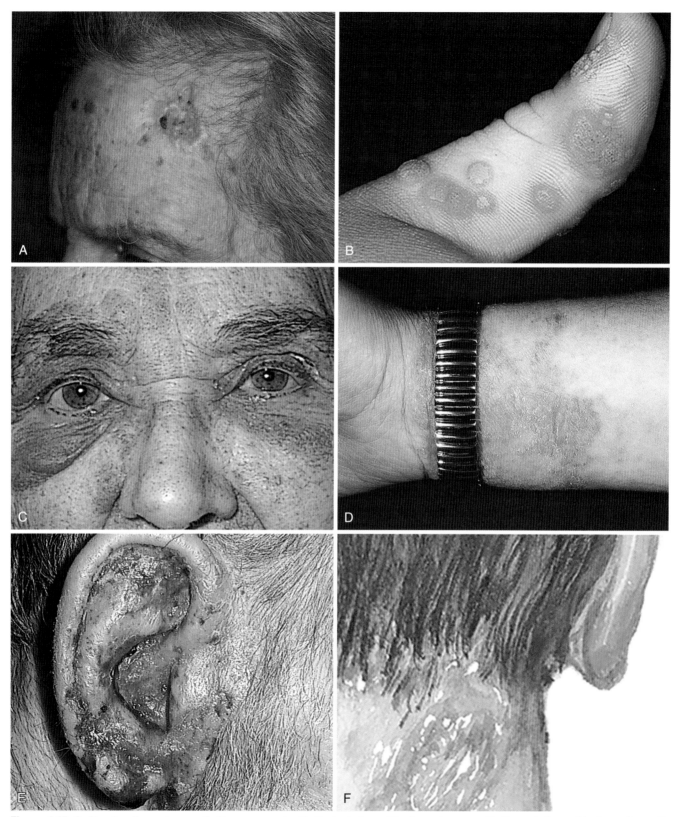

Figure 4.47 A, Basal cell carcinoma. **B**, Common warts. **C**, Contact dermatitis from shampoo. **D**, Contact dermatitis from shoes. **E**, Contact dermatitis from application of Lanacane. **F**, Dermatitis. (Source: **A**, Swartz M: *Textbook of physical diagnosis: history and examination*, ed 6, Philadelphia, 2009, Saunders. **B**, Habif TP: *Clinical dermatology: a color guide to diagnosis and therapy*, ed 2, St Louis, Mosby. **C**, Cox NH, Lawrence CM: *Diagnostic problems in dermatology*, St Louis, 1998, Mosby. **D**, Habif TP, Campbell J, Quitadamo M, Zug K: *Skin disease: diagnosis and treatment*, ed 3, St Louis, 2011, Mosby. **E**, Cox NH, Lawrence CM: *Diagnostic problems in dermatology*, St Louis, 1998, Mosby. **F**, Bork K, Brauniger W: *Skin diseases in clinical practice*, Philadelphia, 1998, Saunders.)

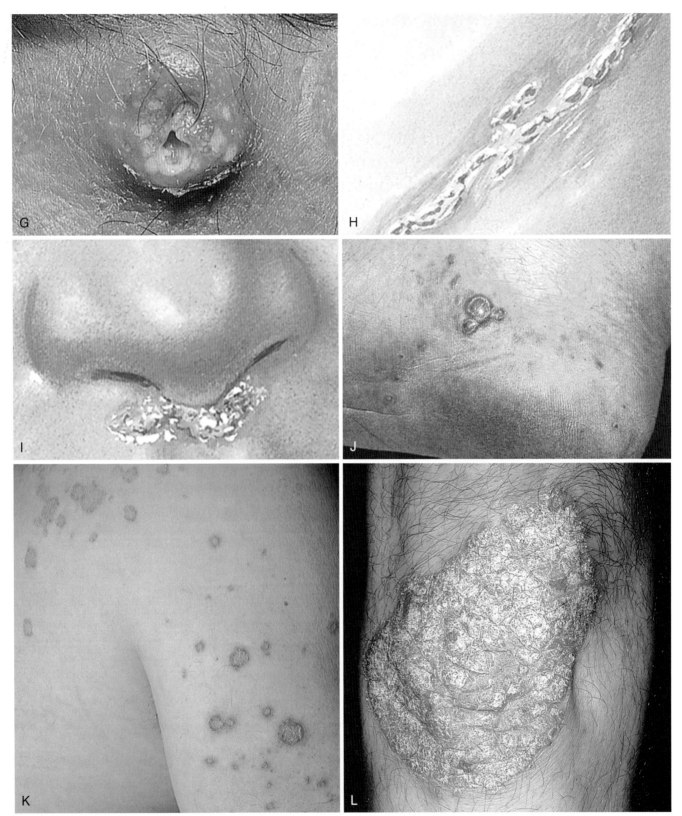

Figure 4.47, cont'd **G**, Furuncle (boil). **H**, Herpes zoster (shingles). **I**, Impetigo contagiosa. **J**, Kaposi's sarcoma. **K**, Nummular eczema. **L**, Psoriasis. (**G**, Courtesy of Jaime Tschen, Baylor College. **H**, Bork K, Brauniger W: *Skin diseases in clinical practice*, Philadelphia, 1998, Saunders. **I**, Bork K, Brauniger W: *Skin diseases in clinical practice*, Philadelphia, 1998, Saunders. **J**, Habif TP: *Clinical dermatology: a color guide to diagnosis and therapy*, ed 3, St Louis, 1996, Mosby. **K**, Habif TP: *Clinical dermatology: a color guide to diagnosis and therapy*, ed 4, St Louis, 2005, Mosby. **L**, Habif TP, Campbell J, Quitadamo M, Zug K: *Skin disease: diagnosis and treatment*, ed 3, St Louis, 2011, Mosby.)

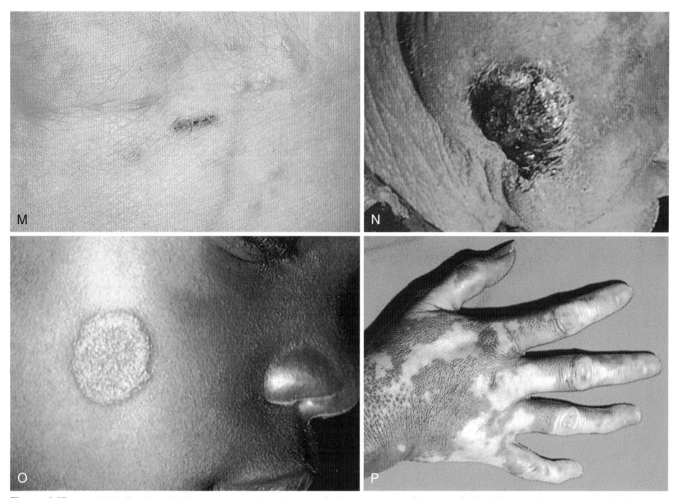

Figure 4.47, cont'd **M**, Scabies. **N**, Squamous cell carcinoma. **O**, Tinea corporis (ringworm). **P**, Vitiligo. **A**, Anterior view. **B**, Posterior view. **A**, Rib cage. **B**, Typical rib. **C**, Sternum. **A**, Anterior view. **B**, Posterior view. (**M**, Habif TP: *Clinical dermatology: a color guide to diagnosis and therapy*, ed 2, St Louis, Mosby. **N**, Lookingbill DP, Marks JG: *Lookingbill and Marks' principles of dermatology*, ed 4, Philadelphia, 2006, Saunders. **O**, Hurwitz S: *Clinical pediatric dermatology: a textbook of skin disorders of childhood and adolescence*, ed 4, Philadelphia, 2011, Saunders. **P**, Lookingbill DP, Marks JG: *Lookingbill and Marks' principles of dermatology*, ed 4, Philadelphia, 2006, Saunders.)

LABELING EXERCISES

Labeling Exercise 1: Generalized Cell

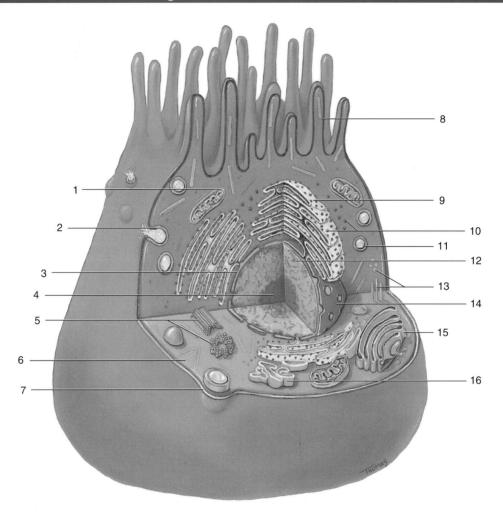

Choices

Fill in the blank in front of each term with the correct corresponding label number.

_____ Cell membrane
_____ Centrioles
_____ Chromatin
_____ Cilia
_____ Cytoplasm
_____ Golgi apparatus

_____ Lysosome
_____ Microtubules
_____ Mitochondrion
_____ Nuclear membrane
_____ Nucleus

_____ Nucleolus
_____ Ribosomes
_____ Rough endoplasmic reticulum
_____ Secretory vesicle
_____ Smooth endoplasmic reticulum

Labeling Exercise 2: Vertebral Column

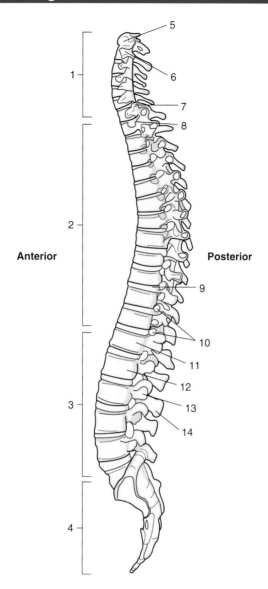

Choices

Fill in the blank in front of each term with the correct corresponding label number.

_____ Body
_____ Cervical lordotic curve
_____ First cervical vertebra (atlas)
_____ First lumbar vertebra
_____ First thoracic vertebra

_____ Intervertebral disk
_____ Intervertebral foramina
_____ Lumbar lordotic curve
_____ Sacral kyphotic curve
_____ Second cervical vertebra (axis)

_____ Seventh cervical vertebra
_____ Spinous process
_____ Thoracic kyphotic curve
_____ Transverse process

Labeling Exercise 3: Skeleton

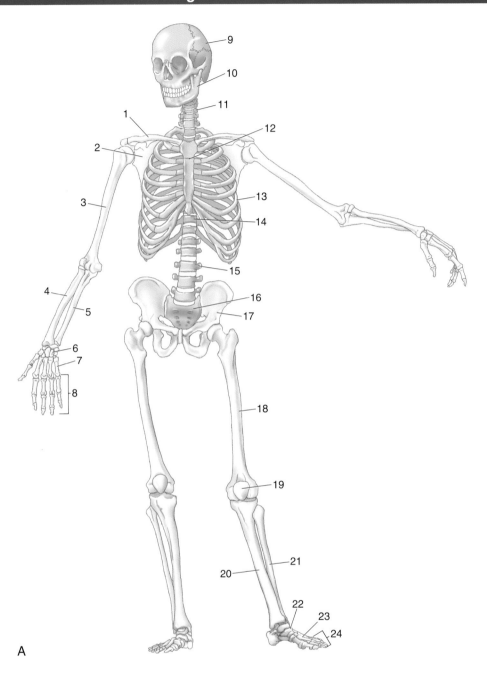

A

Choices

Fill in the blank in front of each term with the correct corresponding label number.

_____ Carpals
_____ Cervical vertebrae
_____ Clavicle
_____ Femur
_____ Fibula
_____ Humerus
_____ Lumbar vertebrae
_____ Mandible

_____ Metacarpals
_____ Metatarsals
_____ Patella
_____ Pelvic bone
_____ Phalanges (two times)
_____ Radius
_____ Rib cage
_____ Sacrum

_____ Scapula
_____ Skull (cranium)
_____ Sternum
_____ Thoracic vertebrae
_____ Tarsals
_____ Tibia
_____ Ulna

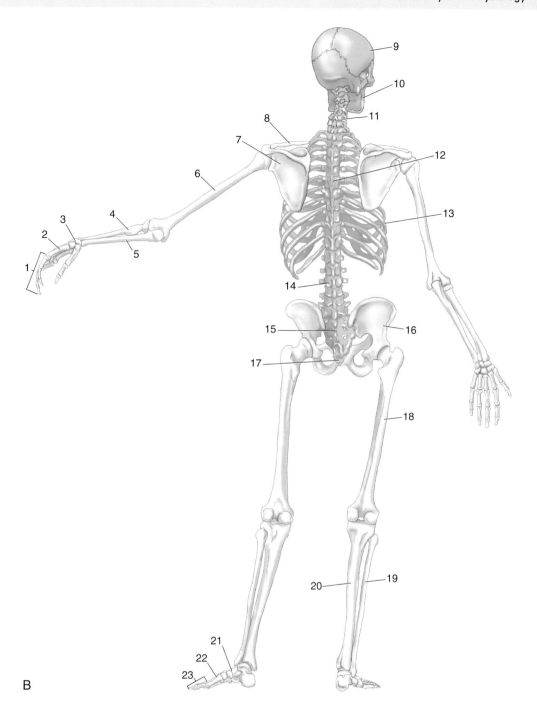

B

Choices

Fill in the blank in front of each term with the correct corresponding label number.

_____ Carpals
_____ Cervical vertebrae
_____ Clavicle
_____ Coccyx
_____ Femur
_____ Fibula
_____ Humerus
_____ Lumbar vertebrae

_____ Mandible
_____ Metacarpals
_____ Metatarsals
_____ Pelvic bone
_____ Phalanges (two times)
_____ Radius
_____ Rib cage
_____ Sacrum

_____ Scapula
_____ Skull (cranium)
_____ Thoracic vertebrae
_____ Tarsals
_____ Tibia
_____ Ulna

Labeling Exercise 4: Ribs

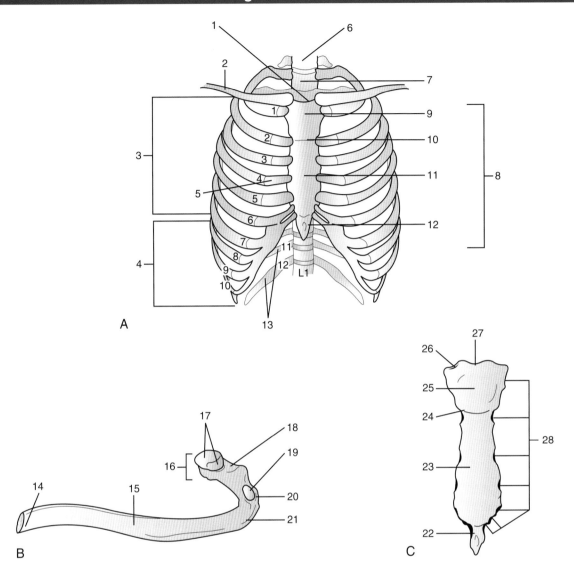

A

B

C

Choices

Fill in the blank in front of each term with the correct corresponding label number.

_____ Angle
_____ Articular facets for body of vertebrae
_____ Articular facet for transverse process of vertebrae
_____ Body (three times)
_____ Clavicle
_____ Clavicular notch
_____ Costal cartilage
_____ Facets for attachment of costal cartilages 1 to 7
_____ False ribs
_____ First thoracic vertebra
_____ Floating ribs
_____ Head

_____ Jugular notch (two times)
_____ Manubrium (two times)
_____ Neck
_____ Seventh cervical vertebra
_____ Sternal angle (two times)
_____ Sternal end
_____ Sternum
_____ True ribs
_____ Tubercle
_____ Xiphoid process (two times)

Labeling Exercise 5: Clavicle

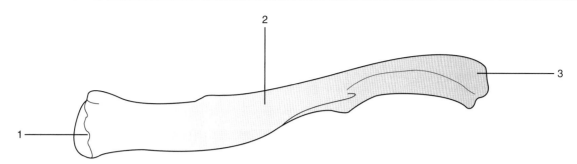

Choices

Fill in the blank in front of each term with the correct corresponding label number.

_____ Acromial end　　　　　　_____ Sternal end
_____ Body

Labeling Exercise 6: Scapula: Three Views

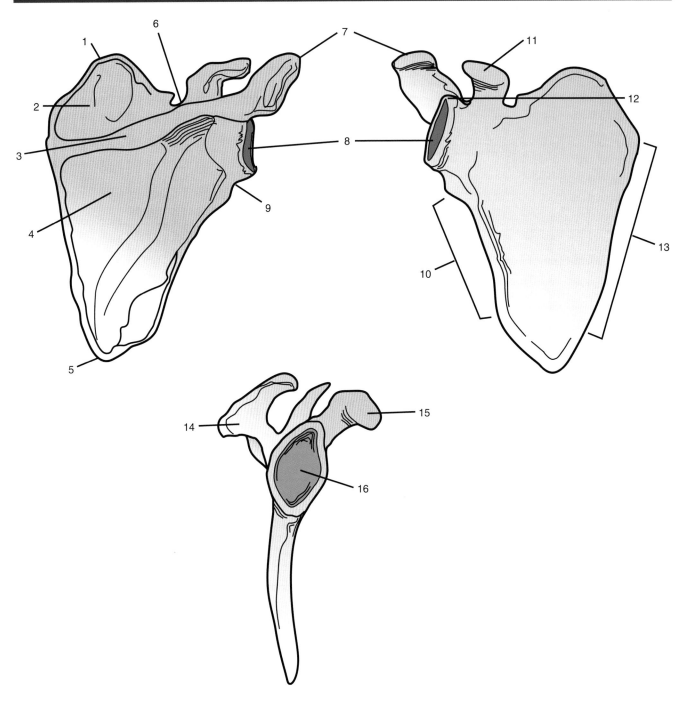

Choices

Fill in the blank in front of each term with the correct corresponding label number.

_____ Acromion
_____ Coracoid fossa
_____ Coracoid process
_____ Glenoid fossa
_____ Inferior angle

_____ Infraglenoid tubercle
_____ Infraspinous fossa
_____ Lateral border
_____ Medial border
_____ Scapular spine (two times)

_____ Superior angle
_____ Supraglenoid tubercle
_____ Suprascapular notch
_____ Supraspinous fossa
_____ Vertebral border

Labeling Exercise 7: Humerus: Anterior and Posterior Views

Anterior view

Posterior view

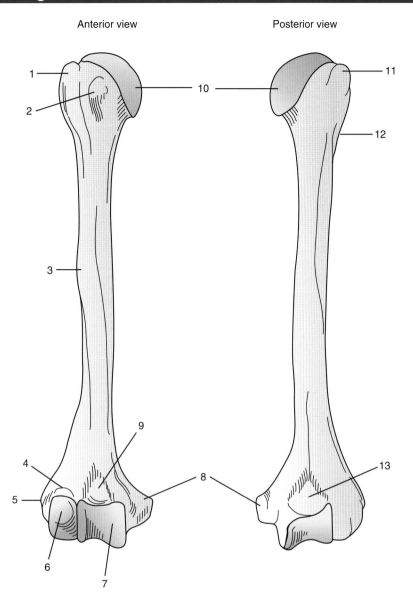

Choices

Fill in the blank in front of each term with the correct corresponding label number.

_____ Capitulum	_____ Head	_____ Olecranon fossa
_____ Coronoid fossa	_____ Lateral epicondyle	_____ Radial fossa
_____ Deltoid tuberosity	_____ Lesser tubercle	_____ Surgical neck
_____ Greater tubercle (two times)	_____ Medial epicondyle	_____ Trochlea

Labeling Exercise 8: Forearm Bones

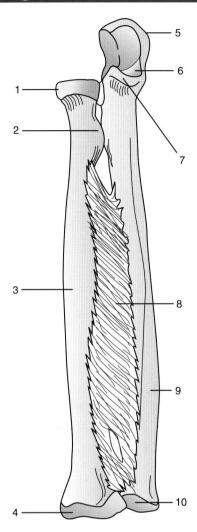

Choices

Fill in the blank in front of each term with the correct corresponding label number.

_____ Coronoid process   _____ Radial tuberosity   _____ Ulna

_____ Interosseous membrane   _____ Radius   _____ Ulnar styloid

_____ Olecranon process of ulna _____ Radial styloid

_____ Radial head   _____ Trochlear notch

Labeling Exercise 9: Hand Skeleton: Volar View

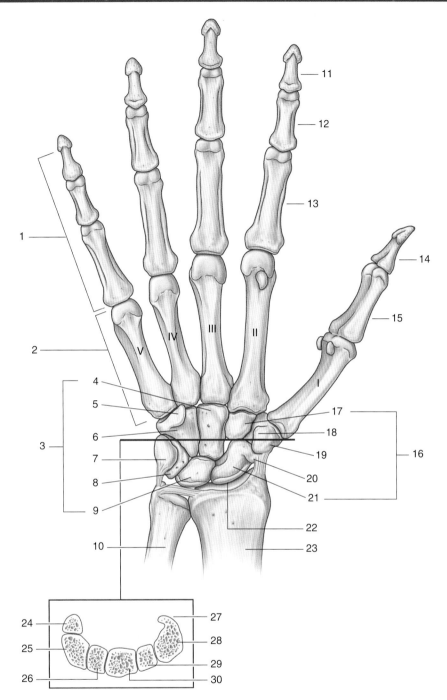

Choices

Fill in the blank in front of each term with the correct corresponding label number.

_____ Capitate (two times)
_____ Carpal bones (two times)
_____ Distal (two times)
_____ Hamate (two times)
_____ Hook of hamate
_____ Lunate
_____ Metacarpals

_____ Middle
_____ Phalanges
_____ Pisiform (two times)
_____ Proximal (two times)
_____ Radius
_____ Scaphoid
_____ Trapezium (two times)

_____ Trapezoid (two times)
_____ Triquetrum (two times)
_____ Tubercle
_____ Tubercle of scaphoid
_____ Tubercle of trapezium
_____ Ulna
_____ Wrist joint

Labeling Exercise 10: Pelvis

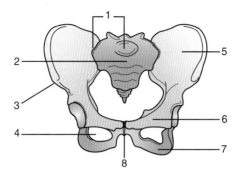

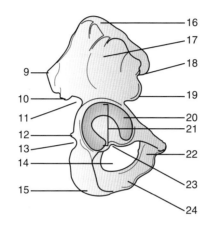

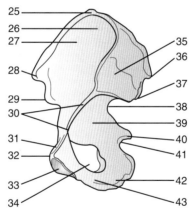

Choices

Fill in the blank in front of each term with the correct corresponding label number.

_____ Acetabular notch
_____ Acetabulum
_____ Anterior superior iliac spine (three times)
_____ Anterior inferior iliac spine (two times)
_____ Articular surface
_____ Body of ischium
_____ Greater sciatic notch (two times)
_____ Iliac crest (two times)
_____ Iliac fossa
_____ Iliopectineal line
_____ Ilium (three times)
_____ Inferior pubic ramus (two times)
_____ Ischial ramus (two times)
_____ Ischial spine (two times)

_____ Ischial tuberosity
_____ Ischium
_____ Lesser sciatic notch (two times)
_____ Lunate surface
_____ Obturator foramen (three times)
_____ Posterior inferior iliac spine (two times)
_____ Posterior superior iliac spine (two times)
_____ Pubic crest
_____ Pubis
_____ Sacral promontory
_____ Sacroiliac joint
_____ Sacrum
_____ Superior pubic ramus
_____ Symphysis pubis (two times)

Labeling Exercise 11: Right Femur: Anterior and Posterior Views

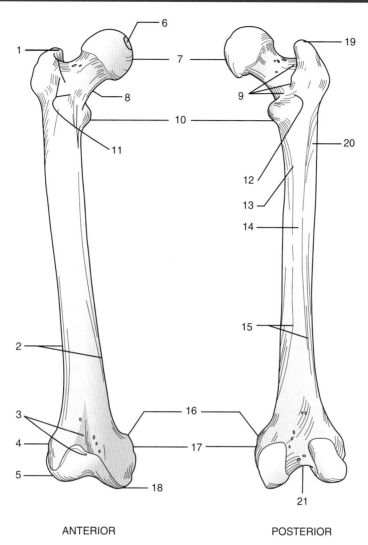

ANTERIOR   POSTERIOR

Choices

Fill in the blank in front of each term with the correct corresponding label number.

_____ Adductor tubercle
_____ Fovea capitis
_____ Gluteal tuberosity
_____ Greater trochanter (two times)
_____ Head of femur
_____ Intercondylar fossa
_____ Intertrochanteric crest
_____ Intertrochanteric fossa
_____ Intertrochanteric line
_____ Lateral and medial supracondylar ridges
_____ Lateral condyle

_____ Lateral epicondyle
_____ Lesser trochanter
_____ Linea aspera
_____ Medial and lateral supracondylar lines
_____ Medial condyle
_____ Medial epicondyle
_____ Neck
_____ Patellar groove
_____ Pectineal line

Labeling Exercise 12: Tibia and Fibula

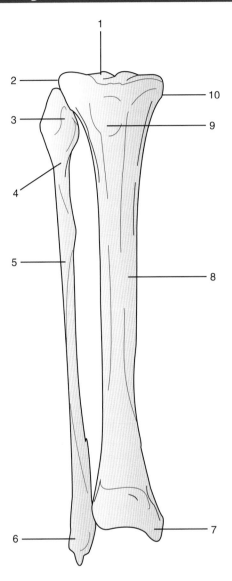

Choices

Fill in the blank in front of each term with the correct corresponding label number.

_____ Fibula

_____ Head

_____ Intercondylar eminence

_____ Lateral condyle

_____ Lateral malleolus

_____ Medial condyle

_____ Medial malleolus

_____ Neck of fibula

_____ Tibia

_____ Tibial tuberosity

Labeling Exercise 13: Bones of Foot and Ankle

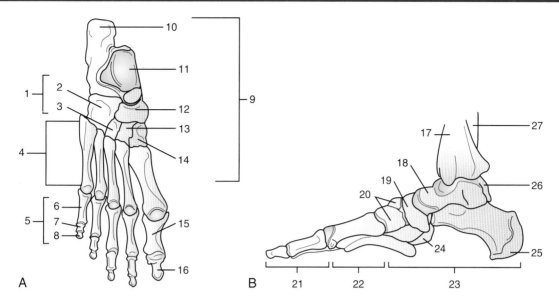

Choices

Fill in the blank in front of each term with the correct corresponding label number.

_____ Calcaneus (two times)
_____ Cuboid (two times)
_____ Cuneiforms
_____ Distal phalanx
_____ Distal phalanx of great toe
_____ Fibula
_____ Intermediate cuneiform
_____ Lateral cuneiform
_____ Medial cuneiform
_____ Metatarsals (two times)

_____ Middle phalanx
_____ Navicular (two times)
_____ Phalanges (two times)
_____ Proximal phalanx
_____ Proximal phalanx of great toe
_____ Talus (three times)
_____ Tarsals (three times)
_____ Tibia

Labeling Exercise 14: Skull: Top View

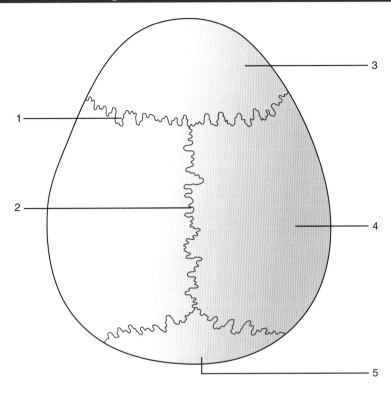

Choices

Fill in the blank in front of each term with the correct corresponding label number.

_____ Coronal suture

_____ Frontal bone

_____ Occipital bone

_____ Parietal bone

_____ Sagittal suture

Labeling Exercise 15: Temporomandibular Joint

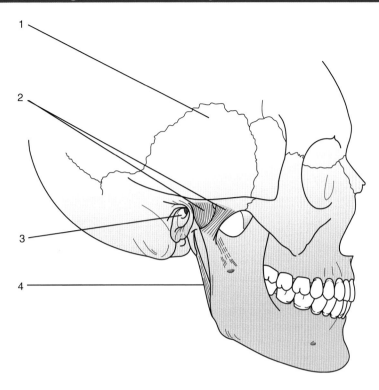

Choices

Fill in the blank in front of each term with the correct corresponding label number.

_____ External auditory meatus

_____ Lateral temporomandibular ligament

_____ Stylomandibular ligament

_____ Temporal bone, squamous part

Labeling Exercise 16: Ligaments of Shoulder: Anterior and Posterior Views

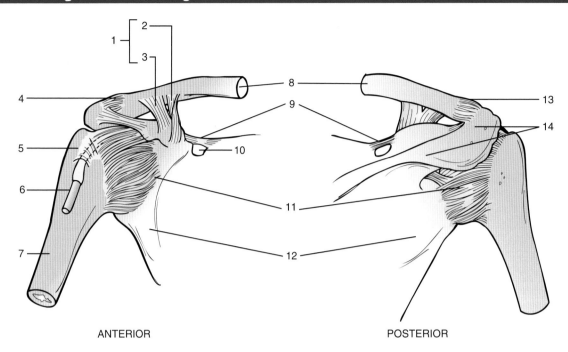

ANTERIOR   POSTERIOR

Choices

Fill in the blank in front of each term with the correct corresponding label number.

_____ Acromioclavicular ligament (two times)
_____ Clavicle
_____ Conoid ligament
_____ Coracoclavicular ligament
_____ Glenohumeral ligament
_____ Humerus
_____ Long head of biceps muscle

_____ Scapula
_____ Scapular spine and acromion
_____ Suprascapular notch
_____ Transverse humeral ligament
_____ Transverse scapular ligament
_____ Trapezoid ligament

Labeling Exercise 17: Joints of Sternum

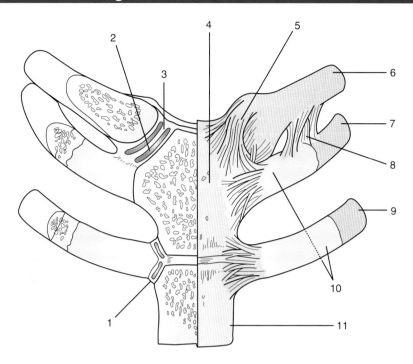

Choices

Fill in the blank in front of each term with the correct corresponding label number.

_____ Articular disk
_____ Body of sternum
_____ Clavicle
_____ Costal cartilages

_____ Costoclavicular ligament
_____ First rib
_____ Manubrium of sternum
_____ Second rib

_____ Sternoclavicular joint
_____ Sternoclavicular ligament
_____ Synovial chondrosternal joint

Labeling Exercise 18: Acromioclavicular Joint of Shoulder Girdle: Superior View

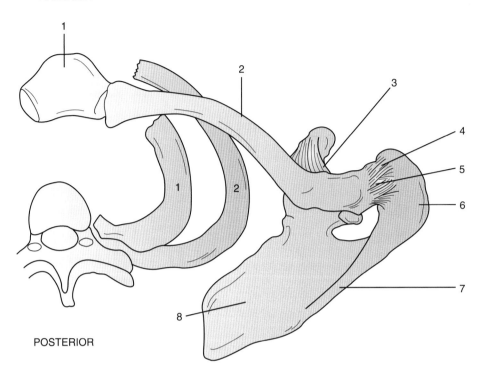

ANTERIOR

POSTERIOR

Choices

Fill in the blank in front of each term with the correct corresponding label number.

_____ Acromioclavicular joint   _____ Clavicle   _____ Sternum
_____ Acromioclavicular ligament   _____ Coracoclavicular ligament   _____ Supraspinous fossa
_____ Acromion   _____ Scapular spine

Labeling Exercise 19: Ligaments of Elbow Joint: Anteroposterior and Lateral Views

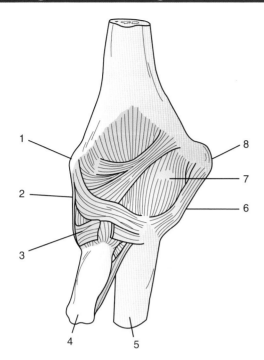

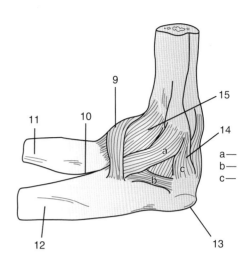

Choices

Fill in the blank in front of each term with the correct corresponding label number.

_____ Annular ligament
_____ Annular ligament of radius
_____ Anterior band
_____ Anterior elbow capsule
_____ Elbow joint capsule
_____ Lateral epicondyle
_____ Medial epicondyle
_____ Medial (ulnar) collateral ligament
_____ Olecranon of ulna

_____ Posterior band
_____ Radial collateral ligament
_____ Radial tuberosity
_____ Radius (two times)
_____ Transverse band
_____ Ulna (two times)
_____ Ulnar collateral ligament

Labeling Exercise 20: Joints of Hand

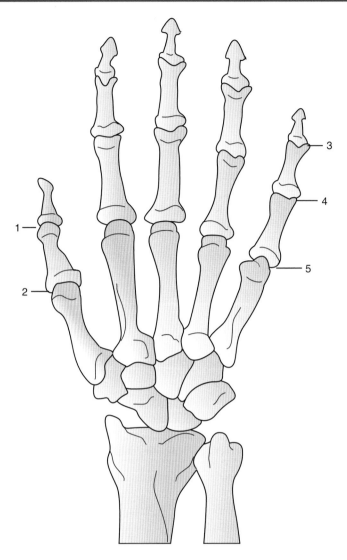

Choices

Fill in the blank in front of each term with the correct corresponding label number.

_____ Distal interphalangeal joint (DIP)

_____ Interphalangeal joint (IP)

_____ Metacarpophalangeal joint (MCP) (twice)

_____ Proximal interphalangeal joint (PIP)

Labeling Exercise 21: Pelvic Ligaments: Superoanterior View

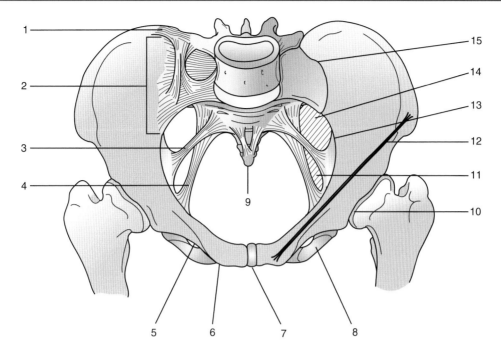

Choices

Fill in the blank in front of each term with the correct corresponding label number.

_____ Acetabulum
_____ Arcuate line
_____ Coccyx
_____ Greater sciatic foramen
_____ Iliolumbar ligament

_____ Inguinal ligament
_____ Ischium
_____ Lesser sciatic foramen
_____ Pectineal line
_____ Pubic symphysis

_____ Pubic tubercle
_____ Sacroiliac joint
_____ Sacroiliac ligament
_____ Sacrospinous ligament
_____ Sacrotuberous ligament

Labeling Exercise 22: Ligaments of Hip Joint

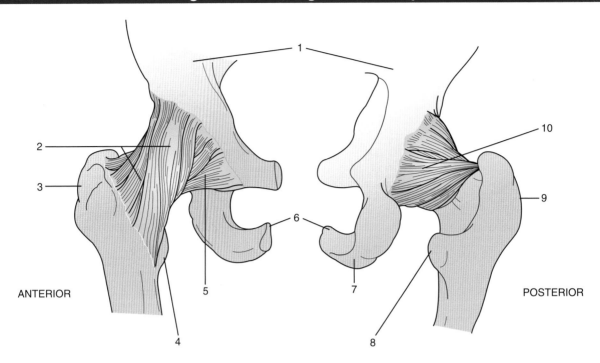

ANTERIOR

POSTERIOR

Choices

Fill in the blank in front of each term with the correct corresponding label number.

_____ Greater trochanter (two times)
_____ Iliofemoral ligament
_____ Ilium
_____ Inferior pubic ramus
_____ Ischial tuberosity

_____ Ischiofemoral ligament
_____ Lesser trochanter (two times)
_____ Pubofemoral ligament

Labeling Exercise 23: Knee Joint, Opened

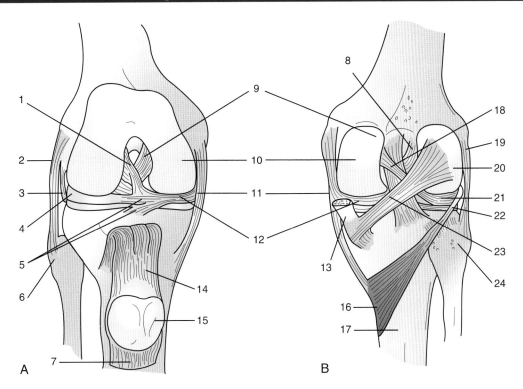

Choices

Fill in the blank in front of each term with the correct corresponding label number.

_____ Anterior cruciate ligament (two times)
_____ Fibular head (two times)
_____ Fibular (lateral) collateral ligament (two times)
_____ Lateral condyle
_____ Lateral meniscus (two times)
_____ Medial condyle
_____ Medial meniscus
_____ Oblique popliteal ligament
_____ Patella
_____ Patellar ligament

_____ Patellar tendon
_____ Popliteus muscle
_____ Popliteus tendon
_____ Posterior cruciate ligament
_____ Posterior meniscus femoral ligament
_____ Semimembranous tendon
_____ Tendon of popliteus muscle
_____ Tibia
_____ Tibial (medial) collateral ligament
_____ Transverse ligament

Labeling Exercise 24: Ankle

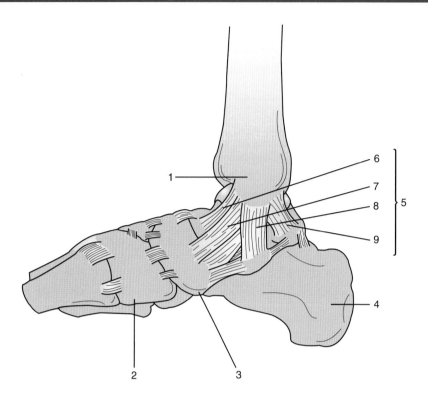

Choices

Fill in the blank in front of each term with the correct corresponding label number.

_____ Anterior tibiotalar   _____ Medial cuneiform   _____ Posterior tibiotalar
_____ Calcaneus   _____ Medial malleolus   _____ Tibiocalcaneal
_____ Deltoid ligament   _____ Navicular   _____ Tibionavicular

Labeling Exercise 25: Structures of a Synovial Joint (Knee)

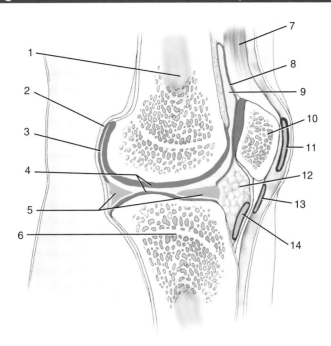

Choices

Fill in the blank in front of each term with the correct corresponding label number.

_____ Articular cartilage
_____ Femur
_____ Fibrous capsule
_____ Infrapatellar bursa
_____ Menisci
_____ Patella
_____ Prepatellar bursa

_____ Quadriceps femoris muscle
_____ Subcutaneous infrapatellar bursa
_____ Suprapatellar bursa
_____ Suprapatellar fat
_____ Synovial membrane (two times)
_____ Tibia

Labeling Exercise 26: Section of Skeletal Muscle With Contractile and Noncontractile Connective Tissue

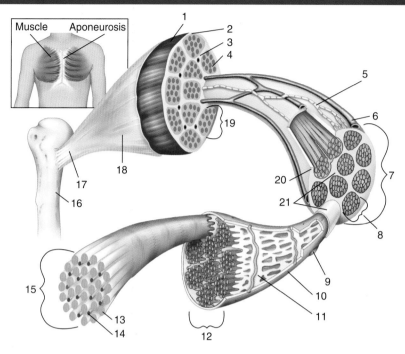

Choices

Fill in the blank in front of each term with the correct corresponding label number.

_____ Aponeurosis	_____ Myofibril
_____ Axon of motor neuron	_____ Nucleus
_____ Blood vessel	_____ Perimysium (two times)
_____ Bone	_____ Sarcolemma
_____ Endomysium (two times)	_____ Sarcoplasmic reticulum
_____ Epimysium	_____ Tendon
_____ Fascia	_____ Thick filaments
_____ Fascicle (two times)	_____ Thin filaments
_____ Muscle (two times)	
_____ Muscle fiber (muscle cell) (two times)	

Labeling Exercise 27: Muscular System: Anterior View

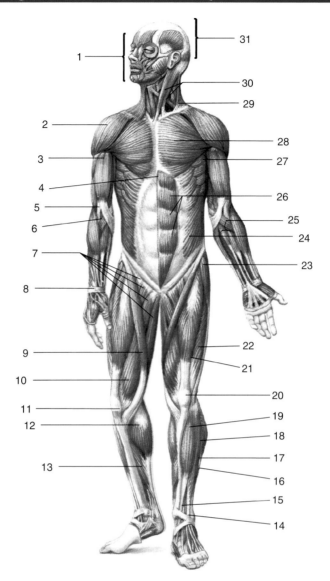

Choices

Fill in the blank in front of each term with the correct corresponding label number.

_____ Adductors of thigh
_____ Aponeurosis of the biceps
_____ Biceps brachii
_____ Cranial muscles
_____ Deltoid
_____ Extensor digitorum longus
_____ Extensor hallucis longus tendon
_____ Extensors of wrist and fingers
_____ External obliques
_____ Facial muscles
_____ Flexor retinaculum
_____ Flexors of wrist and fingers
_____ Gastrocnemius
_____ Linea alba
_____ Patella
_____ Patellar tendon

_____ Pectoralis major
_____ Peroneus brevis fibularis
_____ Peroneus longus fibularis
_____ Rectus abdominis
_____ Rectus femoris
_____ Sartorius
_____ Serratus anterior
_____ Soleus
_____ Sternocleidomastoid
_____ Superior extensor retinaculum
_____ Tensor fasciae latae
_____ Tibialis anterior
_____ Trapezius
_____ Vastus lateralis
_____ Vastus medialis

Labeling Exercise 28: Muscular System: Posterior View

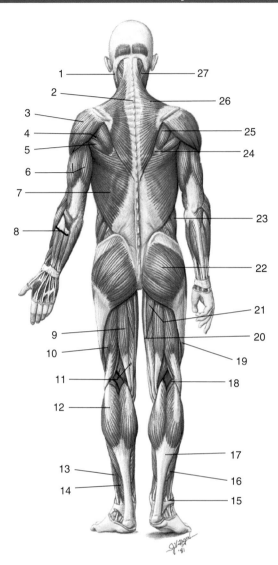

Choices

Fill in the blank in front of each term with the correct corresponding label number.

_____ Adductor magnus
_____ Biceps femoris
_____ Deltoid
_____ Extensors of the wrist and fingers
_____ External obliques
_____ Gastrocnemius
_____ Gastrocnemius tendon (Achilles tendon)
_____ Gluteus maximus
_____ Gracilis
_____ Iliotibial tract
_____ Infraspinatus
_____ Latissimus dorsi
_____ Peroneus brevis fibularis
_____ Peroneus longus fibularis

_____ Plantaris
_____ Portion of rhomboid
_____ Semimembranosus
_____ Semitendinosus
_____ Seventh cervical vertebra
_____ Soleus
_____ Splenius capitis
_____ Sternocleidomastoideus
_____ Superior peroneal retinaculum
_____ Teres major
_____ Teres minor
_____ Trapezius
_____ Triceps

Labeling Exercise 29: Facial Muscles: Lateral View

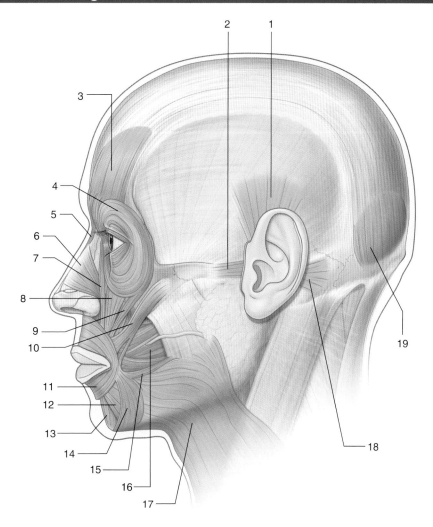

Choices

Fill in the blank in front of each term with the correct corresponding label number.

_____ Anterior auricular
_____ Buccinator muscle
_____ Depressor anguli oris
_____ Depressor labii inferioris
_____ Frontal belly of occipitofrontalis
_____ Levator labii superioris
_____ Levator labii superioris alaeque nasi muscle
_____ Mentalis
_____ Nasalis
_____ Occipital belly of occipitofrontalis

_____ Orbicularis oculi muscle
_____ Orbicularis oris muscle
_____ Platysma
_____ Posterior auricular
_____ Procerus muscle
_____ Risorius
_____ Superior auricular
_____ Zygomaticus major muscle
_____ Zygomaticus minor muscle

Labeling Exercise 30: Back Muscles: First (Left) and Second (Right) Layers

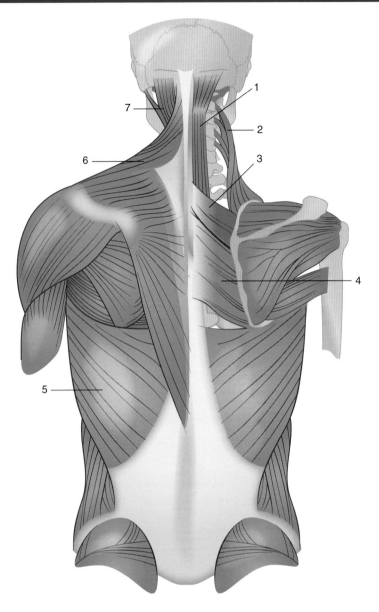

Choices

Fill in the blank in front of each term with the correct corresponding label number.

_____ Latissimus dorsi muscle   _____ Rhomboid minor muscle   _____ Trapezius muscle

_____ Levator scapulae muscle   _____ Semispinalis capitis muscle

_____ Rhomboid major muscle   _____ Splenius capitis muscle

Labeling Exercise 31A: Muscles of the Shoulder

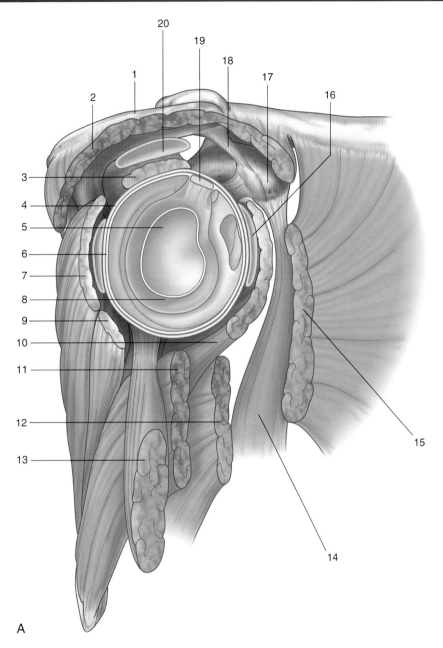

A

Choices

Fill in the blank in front of each term with the correct corresponding label number.

_____ Acromion
_____ Coracoacromial ligament
_____ Coracoid process
_____ Deltoid
_____ Fibrous membrane
_____ Glenoid cavity
_____ Glenoid labrum
_____ Infraspinatus
_____ Latissimus dorsi
_____ Long head of biceps brachii tendon

_____ Long head of triceps brachii
_____ Pectoralis major
_____ Short head of biceps brachii and coracobrachialis
_____ Subacromial bursa (subdeltoid)
_____ Subscapular bursae
_____ Subscapularis
_____ Supraspinatus tendon
_____ Synovial membrane
_____ Teres major
_____ Teres minor

Labeling Exercise 31B: Muscles of the Arm

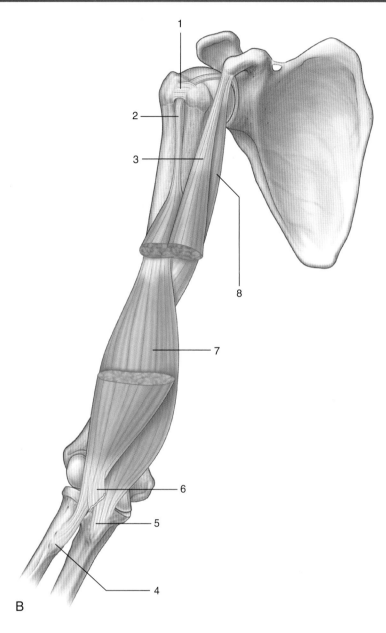

B

Choices

Fill in the blank in front of each term with the correct corresponding label number.

_____ Bicipital aponeurosis (cut)
_____ Brachialis muscle
_____ Coracobrachialis muscle
_____ Long head of biceps brachii muscle
_____ Radial tuberosity

_____ Short head of biceps brachii muscle
_____ Transverse humeral ligament
_____ Tuberosity of ulna

Labeling Exercise 32: Muscles of the Forearm

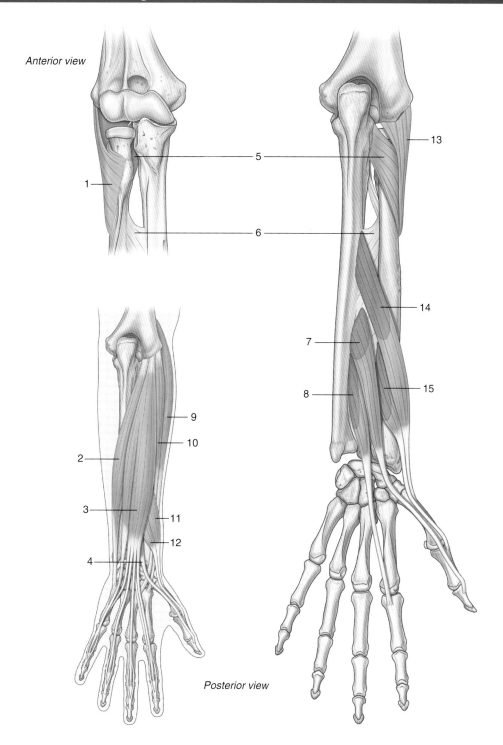

Anterior view

Posterior view

Choices

Fill in the blank in front of each term with the correct corresponding label number.

_____ Abductor pollicis longus (two times)
_____ Extensor carpi radialis brevis
_____ Extensor carpi radialis longus
_____ Extensor carpi ulnaris
_____ Extensor digitorum
_____ Extensor indicis

_____ Extensor pollicis brevis (two times)
_____ Extensor pollicis longus (three times)
_____ Interosseous membrane
_____ Supinator (deep head)
_____ Supinator (superficial head) (two times)

Labeling Exercise 33: Deeper Muscles of Palm: Anterior View

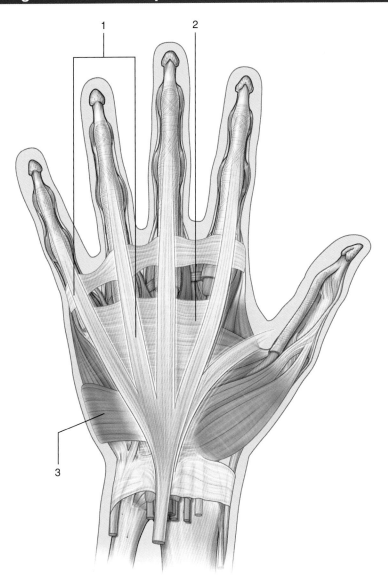

Choices

Fill in the blank in front of each term with the correct corresponding label number.

_____ Longitudinal fibers of palmar aponeurosis
_____ Palmar brevis muscle
_____ Transverse fibers of palmar aponeurosis

Labeling Exercise 34: Muscles of Leg

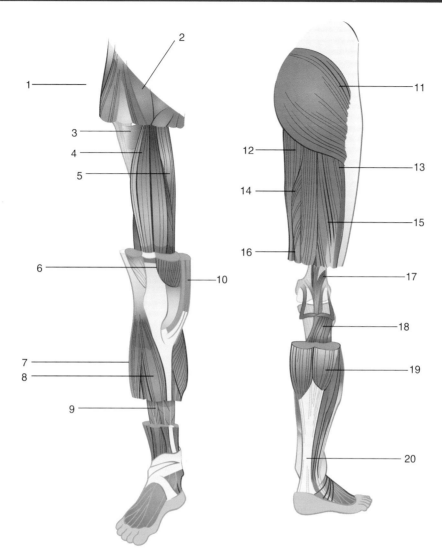

Choices

Fill in the blank in front of each term with the correct corresponding label number.

_____ Adductor longus
_____ Adductor magnus
_____ Biceps femoris
_____ Calcaneal tendon (Achilles tendon)
_____ Extensor digitorum longus
_____ Fibularis longus
_____ Gastrocnemius
_____ Gluteus maximus
_____ Pectineus
_____ Plantaris
_____ Rectus femoris

_____ Sartorius
_____ Semimembranosus
_____ Semitendinosus
_____ Soleus
_____ Tensor fasciae latae
_____ Tibialis anterior
_____ Vastus intermedius
_____ Vastus lateralis
_____ Vastus medialis

Labeling Exercise 35: Peripheral Nerve Trunk and Coverings

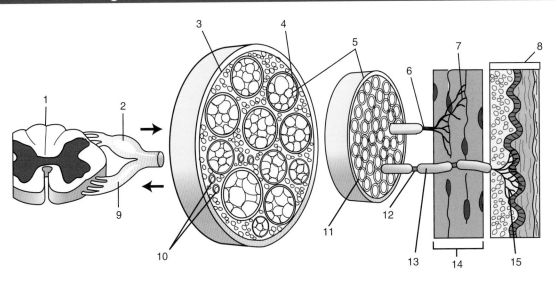

Choices

Fill in the blank in front of each term with the correct corresponding label number.

_____ Axon

_____ Blood vessels

_____ Dorsal root ganglion

_____ Endoneurium

_____ Epineurium

_____ Motor end plate

_____ Muscle

_____ Myelin sheath

_____ Nerve bundle (fasciculus)

_____ Node of Ranvier

_____ Pain receptors

_____ Perineurium

_____ Skin

_____ Spinal cord

_____ Ventral root

Labeling Exercise 36: Nervous System: Simplified View

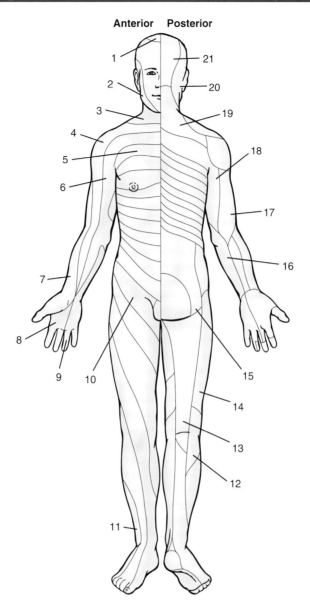

Anterior   **Posterior**

Choices

Fill in the blank in front of each term with the correct corresponding label number.

_____ C2
_____ C3
_____ C4
_____ C5
_____ T2
_____ T1
_____ C6
_____ C7

_____ C8
_____ L1
_____ S1
_____ Dorsal rami (C3 to C5)
_____ Dorsal rami (L1 to L3)
_____ Dorsal rami (S1 to S3)
_____ Greater occipital (C2, C3)

_____ Lateral femoral cutaneous (L2, L3)
_____ Lesser occipital (C2)
_____ Medial antebrachial cutaneous (C8, T1)
_____ Medial brachial cutaneous (C8, T1) and intercostobrachial (T2)
_____ Posterior brachial cutaneous (radial C5 to C8)
_____ Posterior femoral cutaneous (S1 to S3)

Labeling Exercise 37: Pulse Points

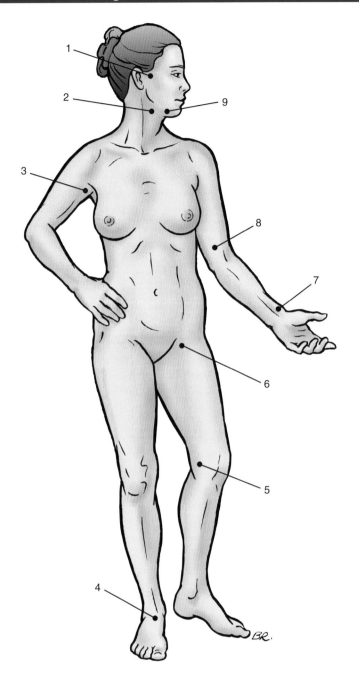

Choices

Fill in the blank in front of each term with the correct corresponding label number.

_____ Axillary artery

_____ Brachial artery

_____ Carotid artery

_____ Dorsalis pedis artery

_____ Facial artery

_____ Femoral artery

_____ Popliteal (posterior to patella) artery

_____ Radial artery

_____ Superficial temporal artery

Labeling Exercise 38: Major Organs and Vessels of Lymphatic System

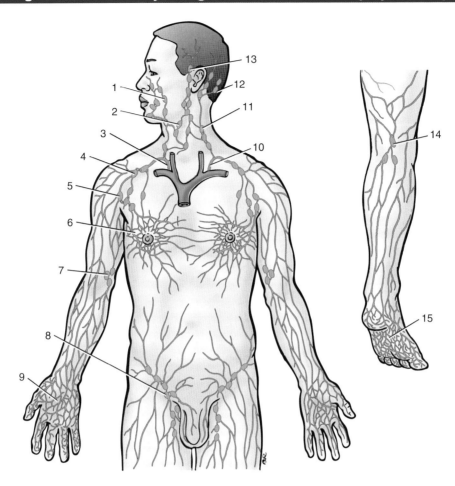

Choices

Fill in the blank in front of each term with the correct corresponding label number.

_____ Axillary lymph node
_____ Cervical lymph node
_____ Entrance of thoracic duct into subclavian vein
_____ Inguinal lymph node
_____ Peyer's patches
_____ Red bone marrow
_____ Right lymphatic duct
_____ Right lymphatic duct

_____ Spleen
_____ Thoracic duct
_____ Thoracic duct
_____ Thymus gland
_____ Thymus gland
_____ Tonsils

Labeling Exercise 39: Pharynx, Trachea, and Lungs, With Alveolar Sacs in Inset

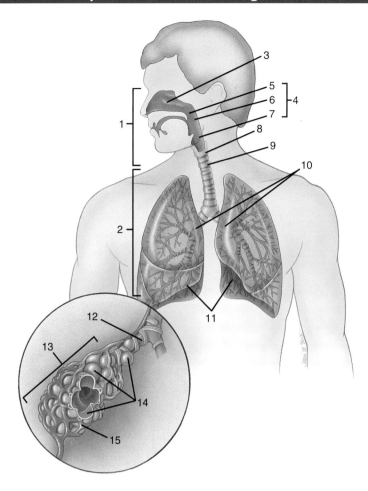

Choices

Fill in the blank in front of each term with the correct corresponding label number.

_____ Alveoli	_____ Larynx	_____ Pharynx
_____ Alveolar duct	_____ Left and right primary bronchi	_____ Trachea
_____ Alveolar sac	_____ Lower respiratory tract	_____ Upper respiratory tract
_____ Bronchioles	_____ Nasal cavity	
_____ Capillary	_____ Nasopharynx	
_____ Laryngopharynx	_____ Oropharynx	

Labeling Exercise 40: Male Pelvic Organs

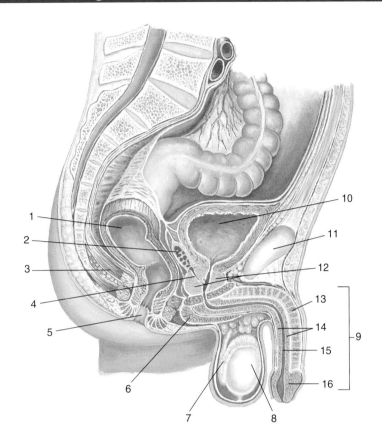

Choices

Fill in the blank in front of each term with the correct corresponding label number.

_____ Anus
_____ Bulbocavernosus muscle
_____ Corpus cavernosum
_____ Corpus spongiosum
_____ Ejaculatory duct
_____ Epididymis

_____ Glans
_____ Levator ani muscle
_____ Penis
_____ Prostate gland
_____ Rectum
_____ Seminal vesicle

_____ Symphysis pubis
_____ Testis
_____ Urethra
_____ Urinary bladder

Labeling Exercise 41: Female Pelvic Floor: Midsagittal View

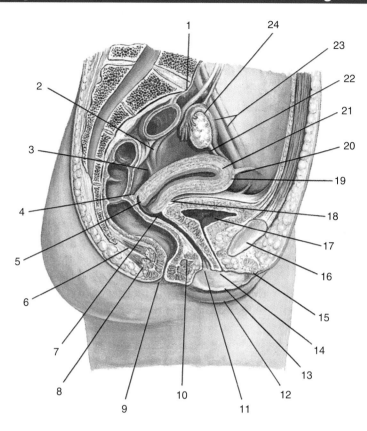

Choices

Fill in the blank in front of each term with the correct corresponding label number.

_____ Anterior cul-de-sac
_____ Anus
_____ Bladder
_____ Cervix
_____ Corpus of uterus
_____ Crus of clitoris
_____ External anal sphincter
_____ External iliac vessels
_____ Fallopian tube

_____ Fornix of vagina
_____ Fundus of uterus
_____ Labium majus
_____ Labium minus
_____ Levator ani muscle
_____ Ovarian ligament
_____ Posterior cul-de-sac
_____ Round ligament
_____ Sacral promontory

_____ Sacrouterine ligament
_____ Symphysis pubis
_____ Ureter
_____ Urethra
_____ Urogenital diaphragm
_____ Vagina

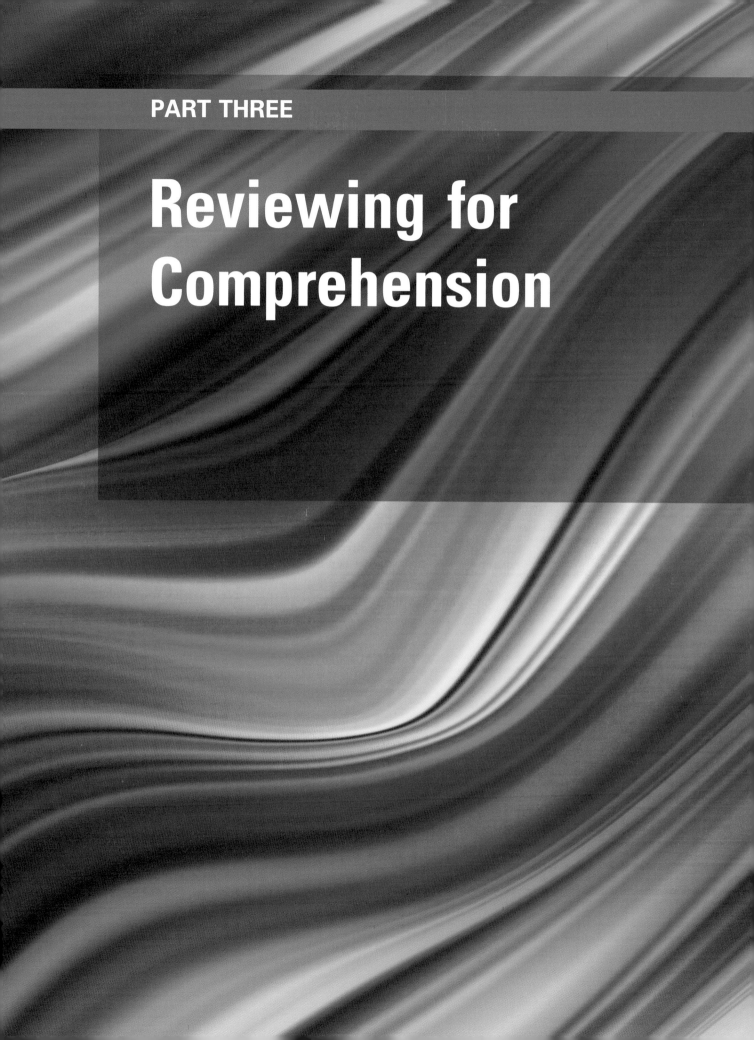

PART THREE

Reviewing for Comprehension

INTRODUCTION

This part of the review process begins to integrate terminology from Part 2 to produce a level of comprehension that extends beyond definition of terminology and anatomic location. Factual content is now presented in a narrative form, primarily using written content instead of visual content. Because licensing exams are reading exams, it is important to be able to convert the facts and figures into concepts presented in written form. Careful and repetitive reading (not memorizing) will help you connect the terminology "dots" to gain a better understanding of the effects of massage on the body. This part supports the understanding of Part 2 and explains the next phase of study in Part 4.

TAKE 5 Remember: Repetition is the key (i.e., the same information, just in a different format).

The brain naturally processes data in about 15-minute segments. The following symbol will let you know when you have been reading and studying for about 15 minutes. When you see it, please take a break for about 30 minutes, and do something different. Do something that does not require brainpower but does involve movement, such as going for a walk or folding laundry. Even a stretch break or looking out the window at nature for 5 minutes is helpful. Your brain will use the time to process the content. After your break has ended, continue reading where you left off.

Remember: The study strategy for this part is to read the content multiple times and in multiple ways over a period of days or weeks. Do not attempt to memorize. Instead, allow yourself time to understand the material. Read silently, read out loud, have someone read to you, read, then restate the information, record yourself or someone else reading the content, and then listen to it over and over. Use Part 2, along with the glossary in the appendix, to define terminology that you do not understand.

BRIDGING THE GAP: FROM MEMORIZATION TO COMPREHENSION

Know these terms. (Additional defined terms are found in the glossary in Appendix B.) *Study tip:* It may be helpful to place the key terms onto flash cards.

Acidosis the condition that occurs when the hydrogen ion concentration of the arterial blood increases and, therefore, pH decreases.

Adhesions abnormal joining of connective tissue between gliding surfaces.

Agonists muscles that contract concentrically to perform a certain movement.

Alkalosis the condition that occurs when the hydrogen ion concentration in arterial blood decreases and pH increases as a major and rapid effect of overbreathing.

Amygdala a brain region that plays a special role in aversive or negative emotions such as fear and is involved in determining the emotional meaning of events and objects.

Antagonists muscles that perform movement opposite to movement of the agonists and provide control through deceleration during eccentric function.

Apnea cessation of breathing.

Arteries carry oxygenated blood from the heart to the tissues of the body.

Arterioles the smallest arteries.

Atria two small, thin-walled upper chambers of the heart; receive blood coming into the heart.

Autonomic nervous system (ANS) the part of the nervous system that innervates the heart, blood vessels, diaphragm, internal organs, and endocrine glands; it influences every other part of the body, including the muscular system.

Axon the single branch of a neuron that conducts an impulse away from the cell body.

Basal ganglia the part of the brain that is involved in the initiation of motion and the integration of motivational states; it can become dysfunctional with addictive disorders.

Best practice evidence-informed and evidence-based recommendations for massage application.

Blood pressure amount of pressure exerted by the blood on the walls of the blood vessels.

Blood vessels vessels that transport blood throughout the body.

Bradycardia a heart rate less than 50 or 60 beats per minute.

Bradypnea slow breathing that occurs in alcohol or other depressant drug intoxications.

Brainstem the center for the automatic control of respiration and heart rate.

Breathing the mechanical action of inhalation and exhalation that draws oxygen into the lungs and releases carbon dioxide into the atmosphere.

Breathing pattern disorder chronic overbreathing or acute hyperventilation.

Bursae synovial fluid-filled sacs lined with a synovial membrane that cushion in areas of increased friction.

Capillary a small-diameter blood vessel with partly permeable thin walls; specialize in diffusion of substances through their walls.

Cardiac cycle one heartbeat; consists of diastole, which is the relaxation of the ventricles as they fill with blood, and systole, the contraction of the ventricles as they push blood out.

Cardiovascular system a transport system composed of the heart, blood, and blood vessels.

Cartilage a dense, fibrous connective tissue composed of collagen, chondrocytes (cartilage cells), and ground substance.

Cartilaginous joints united by fibrocartilage; permit only slight movement.

Central nervous system (CNS) consists of the brain and spinal cord.

Cerebellum controls muscle coordination, motor tone, and posture.

Cerebrum the largest portion of the brain, which is generally responsible for higher mental functions and personality.

Chemoreceptors sensory receptors that are sensitive to the acid–base balance, oxygen, and other factors.

Chiropractic a therapy that focuses primarily on manipulation or adjustment of the human skeletal structure.

Chondrocyte a type of cartilage cell found in the collagen matrix of cartilage.

Co-contraction occurs when the agonist and the antagonist are working together.

Collagen a protein fiber that forms approximately 80% of tendons, ligaments, and joint capsules, and a large percentage of cartilage and bone, giving shape to the soft tissue.

Computer-based client record a method of documentation that uses electronic systems.

Concentric function occurs when a muscle shortens while it contracts. The main outcome is movement/acceleration.

Confidentiality a professional responsibility of not sharing or divulging to another party client personal information or matters discussed in confidence.

Core the lumbo–pelvic–hip complex, thoracic spine, and cervical spine; the core operates as an integrated functional unit to dynamically stabilize the body during functional movements.

Cortisol glucocorticoid stress hormone produced by the adrenal glands during prolonged stress.

TAKE 5 **Counterirritation** a superficial irritation that relieves some irritation of deeper structures.

Dehydration water loss or lack of fluid intake or relative dehydration in which the body loses no overall water content but rather gains sodium ions and stimulates osmoreceptors.

Dendrites branches of neuron that receive an impulse and conduct it toward the cell body.

Diastolic pressure pressure of blood against the walls of arteries when the ventricles relax.

Documentation written records, and the way of using various information forms.

Dopamine a neuroendocrine chemical that influences motor activity involved with movement (especially learned, fine movement such as handwriting), conscious selection (the ability to focus attention), and mood (in terms of inspiration, intuition, joy, and enthusiasm); dopamine is involved in pleasure states, seeking behavior, and the internal record system; low levels of dopamine produce the opposite effects, such as lack of motor control, clumsiness, inability to focus attention, and boredom.

Dynorphin a neuroendocrine chemical that is a mood lifter; it supports satiety and modulates pain.

Eccentric eccentric function occurs when the proximal and distal attachments move apart; the main outcomes are control of movement and deceleration.

Edema excess interstitial fluid.

Elasticity the ability of soft tissue to return to its resting length after passive stretch.

Elastin fibers the more elastic connective tissue fibers found in ligaments and the linings of arteries.

Electrolyte any chemical that dissociates into ions when dissolved in a solution.

Endocardium the smooth, thin, inner lining of the heart.

Endocannabinoid the natural cannabis-like molecules produced by the human body. The endocannabinoid system helps maintain bodily homeostasis.

Endorphin a neuroendocrine chemical that is a mood lifter; it supports satiety and modulates pain.

Enkephalin a neuroendocrine chemical that is a mood lifter; it supports satiety and modulates pain.

Entrainment coordination or synchronization to a rhythm.

Epicardium outer membrane of the heart.

Epinephrine a neuroendocrine chemical that activates arousal mechanisms in the body; it is one of the activation, arousal, alertness, and alarm chemicals of the fight-or-flight response and of all sympathetic arousal functions and behaviors.

Ethical dilemma a professional issue that, for resolution, requires clinical reasoning regarding moral principles and obligations.

Ethical distress the feeling experienced when ethical dilemma is not resolved.

Ethics a system of principles and a moral obligation to provide the best service and use the best conduct.

Etiquette social manners and behavior.

Expiratory reserve volume the amount of air that can be TAKE 5 exhaled forcefully after a normal exhalation.

Fascia fibrous connective tissue arranged as sheets or tubes.

Fibrosis a connective tissue condition in which fibers pack closer together, lubrication is decreased, and water content of ground substance is reduced.

Fibrous joints joints united by fibrous tissues that have little movement.

Force couples integrated muscle groups that provide neuromuscular control during functional movements.

Force stability dynamic stability provided by the muscles.

Form stability joint stability created by the shape of bones that make up the joint.

Frontal plane movement motions that occur only in the frontal plane such as adduction and abduction.

Full-body protonation in a closed kinetic chain, multiplanar (frontal, sagittal, and transverse) synchronized joint motion that occurs with eccentric muscle function.

Full-body supination in a closed kinetic chain, multiplanar (frontal, sagittal, and transverse) synchronized joint motion that occurs with concentric muscle function.

Functional movement patterns acceleration, stabilization, and deceleration motions that occur at every joint.

Gate control theory a gating mechanism that functions at the level of the spinal cord; pain impulses pass through a "gate" to reach the lateral spinothalamic system; pain impulses are transmitted by large-diameter and small-diameter nerve fibers; stimulation of large-diameter fibers interferes with the transmission of impulses in small-diameter fibers because they travel to the "gate of the spinal cord" first; stimulation (e.g., rubbing, massage) of large-diameter fibers helps suppress the sensation of pain, especially sharp or visceral pain. Some aspects of the theory are being disputed.

Global muscles muscles that cross multiple joints and form the outer unit.

Golgi tendon organs sensory receptors in the form of a slender capsule located within the musculotendinous junction; sense changes in muscle tension and fire during minute changes in muscle tension.

Growth hormone promotes cell division and, in adults, has been implicated in tissue repair and regeneration; this hormone is necessary for healing and is most active during sleep.

Guarding irritation and injury to the joint capsule that create muscle contractions designed to protect the joint.

Heart rate the number of cardiac cycles that occur in 1 minute.

Hippocampus brain region that initially encodes and consolidates specific memories of persons, places, and things.

Hyaline or articular cartilage covers the ends of bones and provides a smooth gliding surface for opposing joint surfaces.

Hydrostatic pressure force that a liquid exerts against the walls of its container.

Hyperpnea fast breathing.

Hyperstimulation analgesia stimulating techniques, such as percussion or vibration, performed on painful areas to decrease pain sensations.

Hypertension blood pressure above 140/90.

Hypotension blood pressure under 100/60.

Hypothalamus brain region that integrates emotional states, visceral responses, and the muscular system through endocrine and neurotransmitter chemicals.

Informed consent information used to educate the client about making choices regarding care.

Inspiratory reserve volume the amount of air inhaled forcefully after normal tidal volume inspiration.

Isometric muscle function muscle contraction in which its length stays constant whereas muscle tone increases; the main purpose is stabilization.

Isotonic muscle function muscle contraction in which the muscle changes length, either shortening or lengthening.

Joint arthrokinematics refers to roll, slide, glide, and translation that occur between two articular surfaces.

Joint play involuntary movement that occurs between articular surfaces that are separate from the range of motion of a joint produced by muscles.

Length–tension relationship the concept that muscle develops its maximum strength or tension at its resting length, or just short of its resting length, because the actin and myosin filaments are positioned to form the maximum number of cross bridges; when a muscle is excessively shortened or lengthened, the amount of tension that the muscle is able to generate decreases.

Ligaments composed of dense, white, short bands of nearly parallel bundles of collagen fibers embedded in a matrix of ground substance and a small number of fibroblasts; they contain some elastic fibers and a "crimp" structure. Ligaments attach bones at joints, help stabilize joints, help guide joint motion, prevent excessive motion, and act as sensory receptors.

Ligand-gated channel a class of neurotransmitter receptor; when neurotransmitters interact with this type of receptor, a pore within the receptor molecule itself is opened, and positive or negative charges enter the cell; receptors that admit positive charge are excitatory neurotransmitter receptors; inhibitory neurotransmitters act by permitting negative charges into the cell, taking the cell farther away from firing.

Limbic system brain region that integrates emotional states, visceral responses, and the muscular system through endocrine and neurotransmitter chemicals.

Local muscles muscles that cross only one joint.

Mechanoreceptors sensory receptors that respond to touch, pressure, and movement.

Modulating system neurotransmitters in the brain that use norepinephrine, serotonin, and dopamine to influence postsynaptic neuron activity.

Muscle spindles specialized muscle fibers called *intrafusal fibers* that are surrounded by a fluid-filled capsule embedded within the muscle belly; they detect changes in muscle length.

Muscle tone a combination of fluid pressure, tension, and density in the connective tissue elements of the myofascial structure of muscle. Low-level muscle contraction modulated by the nervous system.

Musculotendinous junction the junction of muscle fibers and connective tissue where the tendon begins.

Myocardium cardiac muscle that makes up the thickest part of the heart; generates the contractions.

Neuron nerve cell that conducts impulses.

Nociceptors sensory receptors that detect irritation or pain.

Norepinephrine a neuroendocrine chemical that functions in the brain and is one of the activation, arousal, alertness, and alarm chemicals of sympathetic functions.

Osteocytes bone cells that transport materials to maintain the structure of bones; they are active in the repair of bone.

Oxytocin hormone that has been implicated in pair or couple bonding, parental bonding, feelings of attachment, and care taking, along with its more clinical functions during pregnancy, delivery, and lactation.

Pain subjective experience of physical or emotional distress.

Parasympathetic nervous system responsible for energy building, food digestion, and assimilation; functions to restore homeostasis and is active when the body is at rest and recuperating.

Pericardium sac that surrounds and protects the heart; secretes a lubricating fluid that prevents friction caused by movement of the heart.

Peripheral nervous system outside of the central nervous system; contains 12 pairs of cranial nerves and 31 pairs of spinal nerves.

pH measurement of the hydrogen concentration of a solution; lower pH values indicate a higher hydrogen concentration or higher acidity. Higher pH values indicate a lower hydrogen concentration or higher alkalinity.

Phasic (moving) muscles primary role is quick movement.

Piezoelectricity   ability of a tissue to generate electrical impulses in response to the pressure of mechanical deformation.

Plasma   straw-colored liquid found in blood; it is about 90% water and 10% nutrients, gases, and waste products.

Plasticity   tendency of soft tissue to assume a new and greater length after the stretch force has been removed.

Platelets   also called *thrombocytes*; cellular blood cell fragments that clot blood.

Proprioceptors   sensory receptors that respond to changes in position and movement.

Pulse   pressure wave that travels along the arteries and expands the arterial wall when the ventricles contract.

Pus   buildup of neutrophils and the debris they collect.

Red blood cells   also known as *erythrocytes* or *red blood corpuscles*; responsible for transporting oxygen to the cells.

Reserve volume   amount of air that remains in the lungs and respiratory passageways after maximal expiration.

Resistance   measure of the friction between fluid molecules and the tube wall.

Respiration   movement of air into and out of the lungs; the exchange of oxygen and carbon dioxide between the lungs and blood, and between blood and body cells.

Reticular fibers   mesh network of connective tissue fibers that supports organs and glands.

Rights   expectations and privileges in the healthcare setting.

Sagittal plane movement   Motions that occur within the sagittal plane; examples are flexion and extension.

Serial distortion pattern   state in which the functional and structural integrity of the kinetic chain is altered, and in which compensations and adaptations occur.

Serotonin   neuroendocrine chemical that allows context-appropriate behavior, which means doing the appropriate thing at the appropriate time; it regulates mood in terms of appropriate emotions, attention to thoughts, and calming, quieting, comforting effects; it also subdues irritability and regulates drive states so that the urge to talk, touch, and be involved in power struggles can be suppressed; serotonin is also involved in satiety, adequate levels of which reduce the sense of hunger and craving, such as for food or sex; it also modulates the sleep–wake cycle; a low serotonin level has been implicated in depression, eating disorders, pain disorders, and obsessive–compulsive disorders.

Skin   an extension of the nervous system, the body's largest organ; it contains blood vessels, glands, muscles, connective tissue, and nerve endings.

Somatic motor nerves   relay information from the brain, through the spinal cord, and to the skeletal muscles.

Somatic sensory nerves   relay information to the central nervous system (CNS) concerning pain, temperature, touch, and pressure from the skin; these nerves also convey pain, proprioceptive information, movement about position, and mechanoreceptor information from the muscles, tendons, ligaments, joint capsules, and periosteum.

Spinal cord   a continuation of the medulla oblongata of the brain; it relays sensory impulses from the periphery up to the brain, and motor impulses from the brain out to the periphery; also, certain reflexes are processed within the spinal cord.

Spurs   bone outgrowths.

Strain   overstretching or tearing of muscle fibers and associated connective tissue.

Synapses   gaps between a neuron and another neuron, muscle cell, or gland.

Synergist   a muscle that works with another muscle to accomplish a certain motion.

Synergistic dominance   when synergists compensate for weak or inhibited prime mover patterns.

Synovial joints   joints with a joint cavity that is filled with synovial fluid and surrounded by a joint capsule; this structure allows the joint to move freely.

Systolic pressure   pressure of blood against the walls of arteries when the ventricles contract.

Tachycardia   resting heart rate greater than 100 beats per minute.

Tachypnea   rapid, shallow breathing.

Tendons   a continuation of the connective tissue within the muscle; they connect muscle to bone; tendons consist of long, spiraling bundles of parallel collagen fibers, oriented in a longitudinal pattern along the line of force stress, and are embedded in ground substance with a small number of fibroblasts; tendons have a microscopic "crimp," or wave-like structure, that acts like a spring, enabling them to withstand large internal forces.

Tenoperiosteal junction   where the periosteum blends with the tendons.

Tidal volume   the amount of air taken in or exhaled in a single breath during normal breathing, usually during rest.

Tonic/postural/stabilizing muscles   play a primary role in posture maintenance and joint stability.

Transverse plane rotational movement   motion that occurs within the transverse plane; examples are internal and external rotation/spinal rotation.

Vascular system   part of the cardiovascular system that consists of blood vessels; transports blood throughout the body.

Venous system   veins that return deoxygenated blood from the capillary networks to the heart.

Ventricles   two large, lower heart chambers; have thick walls that pump blood out of the heart.

Venules   the smallest veins.

Vestibular apparatus   a complex system composed of sensors in the inner ear (vestibular labyrinth), upper neck (cervical proprioception), eyes (visual motion and three-dimensional orientation), and body (somatic proprioception); sensations from these areas are processed in several areas of the brain (brainstem, cerebellum, and parietal and temporal cortex).

Viscosity   measure of the tendency of a liquid to resist flow.

Vital capacity   total of the tidal volume, inspiratory reserve volume, and expiratory reserve volume.

White blood cells   *leukocytes* or *white blood corpuscles*; protect the body from pathogens and remove dead cells and substances.

TAKE 5

TAKE 5

Now that the terminology has been reviewed, this chapter uses this terminology to describe the relationship between massage therapy and the sciences. Although all anatomy and physiology and pathology information is important, there are areas of concentration in this material that are most relevant to massage therapy. This part of the review guide provides targeted content that is most likely to serve as the basis of questions for exams. For study purposes, read this part multiple times to reinforce the content. Do not attempt to memorize it, but you should be able to restate the information and to understand what it means and how it relates to massage. If you do not know the definition of a particular word, refer to the comprehensive glossary in Appendix B and the list of key terms for this part.

CHAPTER 5

Massage Theory and Application

This chapter reviews massage application. Expert opinion and some research evidence appear to indicate that basic massage methods exert mechanical force to alter tissue structures or to stimulate responses in the nervous system with the intent of creating beneficial structural and physiologic changes in the body. Even though massage can be explained in this simple way, the actual application is seldom simple. Expert application of massage is a complex intentional interaction of the subtle influences of pressure changes, drag, duration, rhythm, and speed. Study strategies for multiple-choice exams prepare for the ability to read and problem-solve each question using accumulated knowledge. This chapter involves comprehesion in written form of the acculmulated knowledge needed for professional massage therapy practice. Memorization is not the goal. Understanding what you read it the focus.

THE COMPONENTS OF MASSAGE APPLICATION

Qualities of Touch

Massage is the manual manipulation of the soft tissues. Analysis of the various aspects of manual manipulation involves a massage therapist using some part of their body (i.e., hands, arms, legs, feet) to alter the soft tissue of the person receiving the massage. Obviously, massage involves physical contact. However, some methods are thought to apply a stimulus to the body without touching it. Typically called *energy-based modalities*, these methods are not massage, even though they are easily incorporated into a massage as an adjunct method. All massage consists of a combination of the following aspects of touch.

- Depth of pressure (compressive load), which can be light, moderate, firm/deep, or variable. Most soft tissue areas of the body consist of three to seven layers of tissue, which include the skin; the superficial fascia; the superficial, middle, and deep layers of muscle; and the various fascial

sheaths and connective tissue structures. Pressure must be delivered through each successive layer to reach deeper tissue layers without causing damage and discomfort to the more superficial tissues. The deeper the pressure, the broader the base of contact required with the surface of the client's body. Otherwise, the surface tissue tightens and guards against compression injury. It takes more pressure to address thick, dense tissue compared to delicate or thin tissue.

- Drag is the amount of pull (stretch) on the tissue (tensile load). Many structural and functional tissue changes depend on the amount of drag on the tissue. Connective tissue changes, in particular, appear to be attained during massage applied with drag on the tissues.

- Direction can move outward from the center of the body (centrifugal) or inward from the extremities toward the center of the body (centripetal). It can proceed from proximal to distal attachment (or vice versa) of the muscle, following the muscle fibers, transverse to the tissue fibers, or in circular motions. Direction is particularly useful when addressing fluid movement in the body and stretching/elongation methods.

- Speed of manipulation can be fast, slow, or variable.

- Rhythm is the regularity of application of a technique. If the method is applied at regular intervals, it is considered even, or rhythmic. If the method is disjointed or irregular, it is considered uneven, or nonrhythmic. Massage usually is applied in a rhythmic fashion, especially if fluid movement and relaxation are the goals.

- Frequency is the rate at which a method repeats itself within a given time frame. Typically, the massage therapist repeats each method about three times before moving or switching to a different approach. In general, the first application is assessment, the second is treatment/intervention, and the third is post-assessment. If the first application assesses normal tissue, the next two applications are typically slightly slower and slightly deeper to maintain the continuity of the general massage. If post-assessment indicates remaining dysfunction, the frequency is increased to repeat the treatment and post-assessment until desired results have been achieved or it is evident that the tissue will not change at this time.

- Duration is the length of time a method lasts or a manipulation stays in the same location. Typically, the duration should not be longer than 30–60 seconds if the nervous system is being targeted. A connective tissue application may be sustained longer but usually not longer than 2 or 3 minutes.

Through these varied qualities of touch, basic massage methods are adapted to the client's desired outcomes. The qualities of touch provide the therapeutic benefit. The mode of application (e.g., gliding, kneading) provides the most efficient application. Mode of application can be varied, depending on the desired outcome, by adjusting depth, drag, direction, speed, rhythm, frequency, and duration. In perfecting massage application, the quality of touch is more important than the method. Quality of touch is altered when a contraindication or a caution exists for massage. For example, when a client is fatigued, the duration of the application often is reduced; if a client has a fragile bone structure, the depth of pressure is altered.

TAKE 5

Mechanical Forces

All massage manipulations introduce mechanical forces into the soft tissues. The application of a force to an object is known as loading. These forces are able to stimulate various physiologic responses. Force may be perceived as mechanical, which is discussed in relationship to massage, or as a field force, such as gravity or magnetism, which is not part of massage application. Examples of actions that create mechanical forces are those that involve pushing, pulling, twisting, friction, or sudden loading (e.g., a direct blow). Mechanical forces can act on the body in a variety of ways. They can cause injury, or they can be beneficial if applied appropriately.

It is helpful to identify the different types of mechanical force loads which comprise massage techniques. The response of tissues to various loads relates directly to the therapeutic effects of massage on the body.

Variations in depth of pressure, drag on the tissue, speed of application, direction of movement, frequency of application, duration of application, and rhythm allow for extensive application options related to the therapeutic outcomes identified for the client in the individual session plan and long-term treatment plan.

Mechanical force loads tissues in the following ways.

- Tension loading
- Compression loading
- Bending loading
- Shear loading
- Rotational or torsion loading
- Combined loading

How mechanical force loads are applied during massage becomes the mode of application. The historical/classical/Swedish terms used to describe the mode of application are *effleurage*, *pétrissage*, *tapotement*, and so forth. Because massage therapy has expanded to include multiple manual therapy approaches, these terms are being replaced with more generic terms such as *stroking*, *gliding*, *kneading*, *percussion*, and *oscillation*. When studying for exams, it is necessary to be able to recognize multiple terms that describe the same application.

Mechanical and Neurological Effects

Manual methods of massage that most specifically affect body structure involve the application of mechanical forces to the body to load the tissue. For example, the pumping mechanisms of the heart, arteries, veins, lymphatic vessels, muscles, respiratory system, and digestive tract can be supported by applying massage methods with a rhythmic pumping action. Mechanical forces influence the nervous system in multiple ways such as interacting with muscle tone. Muscle tone is the interaction between the skeletal muscles and the nervous system. This process activates few motor units at a time causing a continuous and passive partial contraction of the muscles, or the muscle's resistance to passive stretch during resting state.

Tension Loading

Tension (also called *tensile*) occurs when two ends of a structure are pulled apart from one another. This is different from muscle tension. Muscle tension is created by excessive nervous system driven muscular contraction or by an increase in fluid pressure, not by strong levels of pulling force applied to the tissue. Tissues elongate under tension loading during massage, which fulfills the intent of lengthening shortened tissues. Tension is created by methods such as traction, longitudinal stretching, and stroking with tissue drag. Tensile loading improves the direction of connective tissue fiber development, stiffness, and strength. Tension loading is effective during the secondary phase of injury healing, after the acute inflammatory stage has begun to dissipate supporting mobile and pliable scar tissue development. It also is thought to be effective in moving body fluids. Tension loads are applied during massage applications that drag, glide, lengthen, elongate, and stretch tissue.

Certain tissues, such as bone, are highly resistant to tensile loading and resulting stress in the tissue. An extreme amount of force is needed to break or damage a bone by pulling its two ends apart. However, soft tissues are very susceptible to tension injuries. In fact, tensile stress injuries are the most common soft tissue injuries. Examples of such injuries include muscle strains, ligament sprains, tendonitis, fascial pulling or tearing, and nerve traction injuries (i.e., sudden stretching of nerves, such as occurs in whiplash). Muscles and other soft tissues that are long and taut are being pulled apart by tensile loading. However, this taut condition is often mistaken for short, contracted tissue because it is palpated as "tight," when actually the tissue is excessively elongated, much like an overstretched rubber band. Typically tension loads should not be applied to tissues that are long and taut; this will result in further stretching and exaggerated dysfunction.

Compression Loading

Compressive loading occurs when two structures are pressed together. This kind of force may be sudden and strong, as with a direct blow (tapotement/percussion), or it may be slow and gradual, as with gliding methods combined with compression. The magnitude and duration of the applied force are important in determining the outcome of the application of compression. Some tissues are resilient to compressive loads, whereas others are more susceptible. Nerve tissue is an interesting example. Nerve tissue can withstand a moderately strong compressive load if the force does not last long (e.g., a sudden blow to the back of your elbow that hits your "funny bone"). However, even slight compressive load applied for a long time (as occurs with carpal tunnel syndrome) can cause severe nerve damage. The massage therapist needs to consider this when determining the duration of a massage application that uses compression, especially over areas of nerves.

Ligaments and tendons are sturdy and resistant to strong compressive loads. Muscle tissue, on the other hand, with its extensive vascular structure, is not as resistant to compressive load stresses. Excessive compressive loading will rupture or tear muscle tissue, causing bruising and connective tissue damage. This is a matter of concern when pressure is applied to deeper layers of tissue. To avoid tissue damage, the massage therapist must distribute the compressive load over a broad contact area on the body. The greater the compressive load that is used, the broader should be the base of contact with the tissue.

Compressive loading is used therapeutically to affect circulation, nerve stimulation, and connective tissue pliability. Compression is effective because it acts as a rhythmic, pumplike method of facilitating fluid dynamics. With this technique, tissue shortens and widens, increasing pressure within the tissue and affecting fluid flow. Sustained compression, especially with a drag component, seems to result in more pliable connective tissue structures and is effective in reducing tissue density and binding.

Bending Loading

Bending is a combination of compression and tension loading. One side of a structure is exposed to compressive stress, whereas the other side is exposed to tensile stress. Bending occurs during many massage applications. Pressure is applied to the tissue, or force is applied across the fiber or across the direction of the muscles, tendons or ligaments, and fascial sheaths. Bending rarely damages soft tissues; however, it is a common cause of bone fracture. Bending loads are used therapeutically to increase connective tissue pliability and affect proprioceptors in the tendons and belly of the muscles.

To create bend load on the tissue, the massage therapist applies a combination of tension to the convex side and compression to the concave side of the tissue. Bending is used when the combined effects of lengthening, shortening, and increased pliability are desired.

Shear Loading

Shear loading moves tissue back and forth, creating a combined pattern of compression and elongation of tissue. Shearing is a sliding application; as a result, significant friction often is created between the structures that slide against each other. Excessive friction (shear loading) may result in inflammatory irritation and cause many soft tissue problems. The massage method of friction uses shear loads (1) to generate physiologic change by increasing tissue temperature and creating therapeutic inflammation and (2) to ensure that tissue layers can slide over one another instead of adhering to underlying layers, creating bind.

Rotational (Torsion) Loading

Torsion loading refers to the combined application of compression and wringing that elongates tissue along the axis of rotation. Torsion involves a twisting application. It is used when a combined effect of fluid dynamics and connective tissue pliability is desired. Massage methods that use kneading introduce torsion loads. Torsion loading is not often applied to a single soft tissue structure and is rarely the cause of significant tissue injury. However, torsion loads applied to a group of structures (e.g., a joint) have a much higher likelihood of causing significant injury. For example, when the foot is on the floor and the person turns the body, the knee as a whole is exposed to significant torsion force.

Combined Loading

Combined loading blends two or more forces to effectively load tissues. The more forces are applied to tissue, the more intense is the response. Tension and compression underlie all the different modes of loading; therefore, any form of manipulation occurs as tension, compression, or a combination of the two. Oscillation (vibration, rocking, and shaking) of tissue can be considered combined loading.

TAKE 5

THE METHODS OF MASSAGE

Terminology for massage methods is not consistent. This part of the textbook presents the multiple terms used to name massage. While studying for exams, it is important to become familiar with terminology variations.

The Mode of Application

Holding/Resting Position
Initial contact with the client must be made with respect and with a client-centered focus that includes a clear intention and understanding of the outcome of the massage. The body needs time to process all the sensory information it receives

during a massage. Holding is achieved by stopping the motions and simply resting the hands on the body to provide moments of integration.

Gliding/Stroking/Effleurage

The distinguishing characteristic of gliding strokes is that they are applied horizontally in relation to the tissues, thus generating tensile loads. The amount of drag on the tissues is modified by the lubricant type and amount used during application. When lubricant is not used, drag during gliding is maximized.

During a gliding method, light pressure remains on the skin, and moderate pressure extends through the subcutaneous layer to reach muscle tissue but does not penetrate deeply enough to compress the tissue against the underlying bony structure. Moderate to heavy pressure that puts sufficient drag on the tissue mechanically affects connective tissue and the proprioceptors (spindle cells and Golgi tendon organs) found in the muscle. Heavy pressure produces a distinctive compressive load of soft tissue against bone.

Methods that use moderate pressure from the fingers and toes toward the heart, in keeping with the muscle fiber direction, supports normal fluid circulation, particularly venous blood return and lymphatics. Light to moderate pressure with short, repetitive gliding with a drag component, consistent with the patterns for lymph vessels, forms the basis for manual lymph drainage, which encourages interstitial fluid to move into lymphatic cavities. Light stroking over nerve pathways can be called a nerve stroke.

Kneading/Pétrissage/Pulling/Skin Rolling

Kneading is a technique in which the soft tissue is lifted, rolled, and squeezed. Terms related to knead/petrissage methods are pulling, wringing, and rolling.

The main purpose of this manipulation is to lift tissue by applying bending, shear, and torsion loads. Kneading is effective for reducing muscle tension. The lifting, rolling, and squeezing action affects muscle spindles in the muscle belly. As the belly of the muscle is squeezed (thus squeezing the muscle spindles), the muscle becomes less tense. When lifted, the tendons are stretched, thus increasing tension in both the tendons and the Golgi tendon organs.

Kneading is effective for mechanically softening the superficial fascia. Kneading methods support circulation by squeezing the capillary beds in tissues and helping fluid exchange. Kneading may incorporate a wringing or twisting component (torsion) after the tissue is lifted. Changes in depth of pressure and drag determine whether the client perceives the manipulation as superficial or deep. By the nature of the manipulation, pressure and pull peak when the tissue is lifted to its maximum and then decrease at the beginning and end of the manipulation. Skin rolling is a variation of the lifting manipulation. Whereas deep kneading attempts to lift the muscular component away from the bone, skin rolling lifts only the skin and superficial fascia from the underlying muscle layer. It has a warming and softening effect on the superficial fascia, causes reflexive stimulation of the

spinal nerves, and is an excellent assessment method. Areas of "stuck, bound, dense, thick" tissue often suggest underlying problems.

Skin rolling is one of the few massage methods that is safe to use directly over the spine. Because only the skin and superficial fascia are accessed and the direction of pull to the tissue is up and away from the underlying bones, risk of injury to the spine is minimal, unlike when any type of downward pressure is used.

Sometimes a client's superficial tissue does not lift. This may be caused by excessive edema (swollen tissue), a heavy fat layer, scarring that extends into the deeper body layers, or thickened areas of connective tissue, especially over aponeuroses (flat sheets of connective tissue). If these conditions exist, applications of kneading or skin rolling are uncomfortable for the client. Shifting to gliding and compression with drag may soften the tissue enough that kneading can be used more effectively later in the massage session.

Compression

Compression moves down into the tissues, with varying depths of pressure adding bending and compressive loading. The manipulations of compression usually penetrate the subcutaneous layer, whereas in the resting position, the forces stay on the skin surface. Much of the effect of compression is caused by tissue that is pressing against underlying structures, causing it to spread. This can be called *tissue displacement.*

Compression used in the belly of the muscle spreads the muscle spindles, causing the muscle to sense that it is stretching. The theory of benefit is that to protect the muscle from overstretching, the muscle spindles signal for the muscle to contract. The lift-press application stimulates muscle and nerve tissue. The combination of these two effects makes compression a good method for stimulating muscles and the nervous system. However, because of this stimulation, compression is a little less desirable for a relaxing or soothing massage.

Compression is a method for enhancing circulation. Pressure against the capillary beds changes pressure inside the vessels, which encourages fluid exchange. Compression appropriately applied to arteries allows back pressure to build, and the release of compression promotes arterial flow.

Compression can be done with the point of the thumb or with a stabilized finger; with the palm and heel of the hand, the fist, the knuckles, and the forearm; and, in some systems, with the knee and the heel of the foot. Even though compressive pressure is exerted perpendicular to the tissue, the position of the forearm in relation to the wrist allows the wrist to remain within the acceptable position of less than 60 degrees of extension. Application against a 45-degree angle of the body plus the 45-degree angle of the therapist's hand and forearm results in 90-degree contact on the tissue. If you are using your knuckles or fist, make sure the forearm is in a direct line with the wrist. Use of the thumb should be avoided if possible because the thumb joints can be damaged by extensive use, especially on large muscle masses.

Compression proceeds downward into the tissues; the depth is determined by what is to be accomplished, where compression is to be applied, and how broad or specific the contact with the individual's body. Deep compression presses tissue against underlying bone. Because of the diagonal pattern of the muscles, the massage therapist should stay perpendicular (i.e., at a 90-degree angle) to the bone, with actual compression somewhere between a 60- and 90-degree angle to the body. Beyond those angles, the stroke may slip and turn into a glide.

Oscillation: Shaking, Vibration, and Rocking

Oscillation is the rhythmic or dysrhythmic movement of tissues on a body part. Oscillation is one of the most effective methods of normalizing the tone of muscles. Shaking is a massage method that is effective for relaxing muscle groups or an entire limb. Shaking manipulations seem to confuse the positional proprioceptors because the sensory input is too disorganized for the integrating systems of the brain to interpret; muscle relaxation is the natural response in such situations.

Shaking warms and prepares the body for deeper bodywork and addresses the joints in a nonspecific manner. Shaking is effective when the muscles seem extremely tight because tone has increased. This technique is reflexive in effect, but a small mechanical influence may be exerted on the connective tissue as well as a result of the lift-and-pull component of the method. Shaking begins with a lift-and-pull component. Either a muscle group or a limb is grasped, lifted, and shaken.

Shaking is not a manipulation to be used on the skin or superficial fascia, nor is it effective for use on the entire body. Rather, it is best applied to any large muscle groups that can be grasped and to the synovial joints of the limbs. Good areas for shaking are the upper trapezius and shoulder area, biceps and triceps groups, hamstrings, quadriceps, gastrocnemius, and, in some cases, the abdominals and the pectoralis muscles close to the axilla. The joints of the shoulders, hips, and extremities also respond well to shaking.

The larger the muscle or joint, the more intense the method must be to be effective. If the movements are performed with all the slack out of the tissue, the focus point of the shake is very small, and the technique is extremely effective. The more purposeful the approach, the smaller is the focus of the applied shaking. Always stay within the limits of both range of motion of a joint and elastic give of the tissue.

Vibration is a smaller, more focused oscillation that involves very fast, small movements. When applied it can have a stimulatory effect such as increased muscle tone.

Rocking is a soothing, rhythmic method. Rocking also works through the vestibular system of the inner ear and feeds sensory input directly into the cerebellum. Other reflex mechanisms are most likely affected as well. For this reason, rocking is one of the most productive massage methods for achieving entrainment. Recall that entrainment is the tendency for synchronizing of rhythms. During massage, external rhythms such as the pace of the massage, music, and rhythmic stroke application can support the inherent trend for the client's physiology to respond beneficially.

Rocking is rhythmic and should be applied with a deliberate, full body movement. The easiest way to do this is to take the client's pulse and match the rhythm to that of the pulse. Work within the rhythm to maintain and amplify it by attempting to gently extend the limits of movement or by slowing the rhythm if it is too fast. Clients seem to relax more easily when a subtle rocking movement which matches their innate rhythm is incorporated during the generalized massage. This can further guide the pacing of all techniques used such as gliding, kneading, compression, joint movement, and especially passive movement.

Percussion (Tapotement)

Percussion, also called *tapotement*, is classified as light or heavy (i.e., surface or deep). The difference between light and heavy tapotement involves whether the compressive force of the blows penetrates only to the superficial tissue of the skin and subcutaneous layers (light) or more deeply into the muscles, tendons, and visceral structures, such as the pleura in the chest cavity (heavy).

Percussion is a stimulating manipulation that involves nerve responses. Because of its intense stimulating effect on the nervous system, percussion initiates or enhances sympathetic activity of the autonomic nervous system. The effects of the manipulations are neurologic except for the mechanical results of percussion in loosening and moving mucus in the chest. When applied to the joints, percussion affects the joint kinesthetic receptors responsible for determining the position and movement of the body. The quick blows confuse the system, similar to the effect of joint-focused rocking and shaking, but the response is muscle tone facilitation instead of inhibition. Therefore, this method is useful for stimulating weak muscles. The intensity of application when used over joints should be modified to avoid causing injury. For example, one finger may be used over the carpal joints, whereas the fist may be used over the sacroiliac joint.

Percussion is very effective when used at motor points that usually are located in the same area as traditional acupuncture points. Repetitive stimulation causes the nerve to fire repeatedly, thus stimulating the nerve pathway.

Percussion that is focused primarily on the skin affects the superficial blood vessels of the skin, initially causing them to contract. Heavy percussion or prolonged lighter application dilates the vessels as a result of the release of histamine, a vasodilator. Although prolonged percussion seems to increase blood flow, surface application enhances the effect of cold application used in hydrotherapy.

Heavy percussion should not be done over the kidneys or other endangerment site areas, or anywhere that pain or discomfort is present. Terms related to tapotement/percussion are slapping, tapping, hacking, cupping, beating, and pincement.

Friction

Friction can be superficial, such as fast back-and-forth movement on the skin. Deep friction consists of small, deep movements performed in a local area. It creates shear loads to the tissue. Friction burns may result if the fingers are allowed to slide back and forth over the skin.

Modified use of friction post the acute phase or after a scar has stabilized may promote a more normal healing process. This application also reduces pain through the mechanisms of counterirritation and hyperstimulation analgesia.

Movement in deep friction usually is transverse to the fiber direction, and the technique generally is applied for 30 seconds to 10 minutes. This type of friction initiates a small, controlled inflammatory response. The chemicals released during inflammation activate tissue repair mechanisms and reorganize connective tissue. This type of work, coupled with proper healing and rehabilitation, is valuable therapeutically.

Friction is a mechanical approach that is best applied to areas of high connective tissue concentration, such as the musculotendinous junction. Microtrauma caused by repetitive movement and overstretching is common in this area. Microtrauma predisposes the musculotendinous junction to inflammatory problems, connective tissue changes, and adhesion.

Experts disagree on whether an area that is to receive friction should be stretched or relaxed. Because both methods have merit, both positions should be included in frictioning. Another use for friction is to combine it with compression, thereby adding a small stretch component, but with movement that includes no slide. This application has mechanical, chemical, and reflexive effects and is the most common approach for the use of friction.

Remember that the main focus when deep friction is used is to move tissue under the skin. Do not use lubricant because the tissues must not slide. Place the area to be frictioned in a soft or slack position. Begin with a specific and moderate to deep compression using the fingers, the palm, or the flat part of the forearm near the elbow. After reaching the depth of pressure required to contact the target tissue, move the upper tissue repeatedly across the underlying tissue. Back-and-forth movement perpendicular to the grain or fiber direction of the underlying tissue creates transverse or cross-fiber friction. Circular movement creates circular friction.

 TAKE 5

Joint Movement Methods

Joint movement is effective because it provides a means of controlled stimulation to the joint mechanoreceptors. Movement initiates muscle tone readjustment through the reflex center of the spinal cord and lower brain centers. As positions change, supported movement gives the nervous system an entirely different set of signals to process. Joint sensory receptors are able to learn not to be so hypersensitive. As a result, protective spasm and movement restriction may lessen.

Joint movement also encourages lubrication of the joint and contributes an important enhancement to the lymphatic and venous circulatory systems. Much of the pumping action that moves these fluids within the vessels results from compression of the lymph and blood vessels during joint movement and muscle contraction. Also, movement loads the tendons, ligaments, and joint capsule. This mechanical effect helps keep these tissues pliable.

Types of Joint Movement Methods

Joint movement involves moving jointed areas within the physiologic limits of the client's range of motion. The two types of joint movement are active movement and passive movement.

In *active joint movement*, the client moves the joint by means of active contraction of muscle groups. Active joint movement is subcategorized as active-assisted movement, which occurs when both the client and the massage therapist move the area, and active resistive movement, which occurs when the client actively moves the joint against a resistance provided by the massage therapist.

In *passive joint movement*, the client's muscles remain relaxed and the massage therapist moves the joint with no assistance from the client. For example, joint oscillation is a passive joint movement.

Joint movements are used to assess the range of motion of an individual joint. Available range of motion is measured from the neutral anatomic position (0). If the 0 appears first (hip abduction, 0-45), this means that the joint movement begins at anatomic position and moves away. If the number appears first (hip adduction, 45-0), this mean that the joint position is beginning outside of the anatomic position and is moving back into anatomic position.

Normal Range of Motion for Each Joint
Normal values (in degrees):
- Hip flexion, 0-125
- Hip extension, 105-0
- Hip hyperextension, 0-15
- Hip abduction, 0-45
- Hip adduction, 45-0
- Hip lateral (external) rotation, 0-45
- Hip medial (internal) rotation, 0-45
- Knee flexion, 0-130
- Knee extension, 120-0
- Ankle plantar flexion (movement downward), 0-50
- Ankle dorsiflexion (movement upward), 0-20
- Foot inversion (turned inward), 0-35
- Foot eversion (turned outward), 0-25
- Shoulder flexion with scapular movement, 0-180
- Shoulder (glenohumeral joint only) flexion, 0-90
- Shoulder extension, 0-50
- Shoulder abduction with scapular movement, 0-180
- Shoulder (glenohumeral joint only) abduction, 0-90
- Shoulder (glenohumeral joint only) adduction, 90-0
- Shoulder lateral (external) rotation, 0-90
- Shoulder medial (internal) rotation, 0-70
- Elbow flexion, 0-160
- Elbow extension, 145-0
- Elbow pronation, 0-90
- Elbow supination, 0-90
- Wrist flexion, 0-90
- Wrist extension, 0-70
- Wrist abduction, 0-25
- Wrist adduction, 0-65

Stretching/Elongation

Stretching is a mechanical method of introducing various forces into connective tissue to elongate areas of connective tissue shortening. Stretching affects the fiber component of connective tissue by elongating the fibers past their normal give to engage elastic range past the existing bind or resistance barrier.

Stretching is an intervention that is used purposefully to cause an adaptation in the soft tissues, including tissue around joints of the body. Joint movement and palpation are the assessments used to determine if stretching should be used to address areas of tissue shortening and increased density involved in a lack of flexibility.

Stretching methods can be passive or active. Passive stretching occurs when a second person applies the force to stretch the tissue. Active stretching occurs when the person stretches themselves. Stretching of both types can also be included into the massage session. During massage, each jointed area should be moved actively, passively, or both as part of an assessment to determine the range of motion available. It is important not to confuse joint movement with stretching. Joint movement assesses for the limits of movement as indicated by the palpation of the resistance barrier. If assessment indicates hypomobility in the joint, then stretching begins when the joint is taken to bind, then through bind. The goal is to increase the amount of movement available, which is called flexibility. Using muscle energy methods before stretching enhances the effect by increasing the client's tolerance to the stretch sensation.

Because stretching is an intervention that requires adaptation, it is important to determine if:

- The current condition is resourceful compensation that is productive and should not be changed
- The client has sufficient adaptive capacity and time to respond to the change
- The change positively affects function

Stretching as an intervention method must be used carefully to avoid adverse outcomes. Joints should not be stretched beyond the normal range of motion. Stretching should not be painful. If an increase in flexibility is indicated, stretching methods should be introduced gently and progressively over a period of time over multiple sessions. Hypermobile joints should not be stretched; however, direct elongation of tissues between the joints can be effective.

MUSCLE ENERGY TECHNIQUES

Muscle energy techniques (METs) involve a voluntary contraction of the client's muscles in a specific and controlled direction, at varying levels of intensity, against a specific counterforce applied by the massage therapist. Muscle energy procedures have a variety of applications and are considered active techniques in which the client contributes the corrective force. The exact mechanisms of action are not understood, but when used in conjunction with stretching METs help by increasing the client's tolerance to the stretch sensation.

Postisometric Relaxation

Postisometric relaxation (also called tense and relax, and contract relax) occurs after isometric contraction of a muscle.

Combined Methods: Contract–Relax–Antagonist–Contract

Combined methods use contraction of target muscles and their antagonists to support stretching. First the target (short tissue) contracts and then relaxes. Next the antagonist muscles contract, taking the short tissues into the lengthened position.

Pulsed Muscle Energy

Pulsed muscle energy procedures involve engaging the comfort barrier where tissues begin to bind and using small, resisted contractions (usually 20 in 10 seconds); this introduces mechanical pumping. The contraction direction can be toward the restriction or away from the restriction (or combined). Pulsed muscle energy methods can be used to support stretching or without stretching to stimulate inhibited (assesses as weak) muscle function.

TAKE 5

Body Mechanics

Effective body mechanics is essential for the massage therapist. The profession does not agree on what constitutes proper body mechanics. However, the following basic concepts appear to provide the foundation for body mechanics—type questions. Four basic concepts pertaining to body mechanics are common to all techniques used to apply compressive force to body tissues during massage application:

- Weight transfer
- Perpendicularity
- Stacking of the joints in close-packed position
- Keeping the back straight

Weight transfer allows the massage therapist to transfer their body weight by shifting the center of gravity forward to achieve a pressure that is comfortable for the client.

Perpendicularity is necessary to ensure that the pressure exerted sinks straight into the tissues. The line from the shoulders to the point of contact (e.g., forearm, heel of the hand) must be 90 degrees to the plane of the contact point on the client's body. The client should be positioned in such a way that pressure is applied against a 45-degree incline whenever possible.

Stacking of the joints one atop another is essential to the concepts of perpendicularity and weight transfer. The therapist's body must be in a straight line from the heel of the weight-bearing rear foot through the knee, hip, and shoulder, and then from the shoulder to the forearm, or through the elbow, which acts as an extension of the shoulder, to the heels of the hands. The ankle, knee, hip of the back leg, and spine are stacked and stable in a close-packed joint position. The pelvic girdle and the shoulder girdle are lined up. The shoulder is stacked over the elbow, which in turn is stacked over the wrist. Stacking the joints in this way allows the pressure exerted by the massage therapist to travel straight and effortlessly into the client's body as the therapist's center of gravity moves forward.

Keeping the back straight involves the ability to stack the joints and then provide stability using the core muscles involved in upright posture. Trunk flexion at the hip is maintained at 20 degrees and not to exceed 30 degrees.

TAKE 5

SANITATION/STANDARD PRECAUTIONS

Massage therapists should always be meticulous about hygiene and sanitation. However, this behavior is even more important in the medical setting, in which exposure to disease is increased and clients are more susceptible to pathogens. The concepts of disease transmission and response to infection are the basis for understanding the importance of the first line of defense in preventing disease. Infectious diseases can spread only under certain circumstances. Infection starts with the infectious agent. The five groups of potentially pathogenic organisms are viruses, bacteria, protozoa, fungi, and rickettsiae, as well as parasites such as lice and mites. For infection to occur, an infectious microorganism must be present. Any disease caused by the growth of pathogenic microorganisms in the body falls into the category of infectious (communicable) diseases. The goal of sanitation is to prevent the spread of infectious disease. Pathogens can be spread by direct and indirect contact, through food or liquids that are ingested (vehicle transmission), and from other insects or animals that carry the pathogen. Infection from the bites of insects or animals or exposure to their waste products is called vector transmission.

The best way to prevent the spread of disease is to use adequate infection control procedures; these include consistent hand washing, washing up past the elbow since forearms are used during massage application, proper use of antiseptics, and disinfection and sterilization methods. The Occupational Safety and Health Administration has established guidelines for sanitation. Because these standards are written to cover employees in all health fields, only some of the regulations apply to the practice of therapeutic massage. The information presented here is what applies most to massage therapists. There is a difference between cleaning and sanitation. Cleaning activities revolve around general housekeeping needs and can be accomplished with specialized cleaning products or common household products such as soap, vinegar, or baking soda, whereas sanitation goes a step further to address pathogenic organisms. Sanitation involves use of a method or product that will kill pathogens and reduce the exposed to infection. High heat is a form of sterilization, the intent being to kill all pathogens. Bleach and other approved disinfecting products such as quaternary ammonium compounds may also be used.

Hand Washing

One of the simplest and most effective techniques for preventing the spread of disease is hand washing. In medical practice, every procedure begins and ends with hand washing. Normally, two types of bacteria can be found on the skin: transient bacteria, which are surface bacteria that remain a short time, and resident bacteria, which are found under the fingernails, in hair follicles, in the openings of sebaceous glands, and in the deeper layers of the skin. The goal of thorough hand washing is to eliminate or reduce the number of transient bacteria on the skin surface, thus preventing transient bacteria from becoming resident bacteria. The most effective barrier against infection is unbroken skin.

It is impossible to sterilize hands; therefore, the goal of hand washing is to reduce the number of bacteria on the skin by using mechanical friction, antimicrobial soaps, and warm running water. Each sink should be equipped with a liquid soap dispenser.

The water should be warm because water that is too hot or too cold causes the skin to become chapped. Friction involves firmly rubbing all surfaces of the hands, wrists, and forearms. Remember that fingers have four sides, and fingernails have two sides. All jewelry is removed for hand washing. The hands and forearms are washed under running water, with the fingertips pointing downward. Soap and friction are applied to the hands, wrists, and forearms because these areas are used for massage application. Allow the water to wash away debris from the elbows down toward the fingertips.

A water-soluble lotion may be rubbed into the hands after they have been washed and dried. Dry, cracked, chapped skin is an interruption of the skin's integrity and can result in the transmission of disease. An antiseptic can be used on the skin.

Personal Protective Equipment

Personal protective equipment (PPE) refers to protective clothing, gloves, face shields, goggles, facemasks, and/or respirators or other equipment designed to protect the wearer from injury or the spread of infection or illness. Effective use of PPE includes properly removing and disposing of contaminated PPE to prevent exposing both the wearer and other people to infection. The process to put on (don) and take off (doff) PPE is of great importance to protect from infections, especially in the steps taken to dispose of used PPE. To start, should wash hands, then follow these PPE steps as directed by the CDC:
- Don apron, gown, or other protective clothing.
- Don surgical mask or respirator.
- Don face shield on for eye protection.
- Don protective gloves.

When removing PPE, the correct sequence is as follows:
- Doff gloves first and decontaminate your hands after removing.
- Doff gown, apron, or other protective clothing.
- Doff the face shield.

- Doff surgical mask or respirator.
- Decontaminate hands again.

Lubricants

Lubricants serve only one purpose for massage application: they reduce drag on the skin during gliding-type strokes. Medicinal and cosmetic use of lubricants is out of the scope of practice for therapeutic massage.

Oils, and creams can be vegetable, mineral, or petroleum-based. Gels consist of cellulose, water, and alcohol. If possible, use the most natural products available, and avoid using petrochemicals and talc, because many people are allergic to these substances. All lubricants must be dispensed from a contamination-free container.

Positioning

Positioning is placing a client into the position that best enhances the benefits of the massage. The four basic massage positions are supine (face up), prone (face down), side lying, and seated, which includes a semireclined position. A client may be placed in all four positions during a massage session.

Pillows or other supports, such as folded towels, blankets, or specially designed pieces of foam, are used to make the client comfortable. These supports fill any gaps in contour when the client is positioned and provide soft areas against which the client can lean. Supports generally are used under the knees, ankles, and neck.

Draping

Draping has two purposes:
- To maintain the client's privacy and sense of security. The drape becomes a boundary between the practitioner and the client. It is also a way to establish touch as professional. Skillfully undraping an area to be massaged and purposefully redraping the area is much more professional and less invasive than is sliding the hands under the draping materials. Respect for the client's personal privacy and boundaries fosters an environment in which the client's welfare is safeguarded.
- To provide warmth.

Principles of Draping
Draping can be done in many ways, although certain primary principles apply:
- All reusable (multiple use) draping material must have been freshly laundered with bleach or other approved solution for each client. Disposable (single-use) linens if used must be fresh for each client and then disposed of properly.
- Only the area that is being massaged is undraped.

- The genital area is never undraped. The breast area of women is not undraped during routine wellness massage. Specific massage that targets the breast under the supervision of a licensed medical professional may require special draping procedures for the breast area of females. Breast massage for medical purposes follows a specific method and a consent process. These methods are out of the scope of practice for the wellness massage practitioner.
- Draping methods should keep the client covered in all positions, including the seated position.

TAKE 5

EFFECTIVE AND INTELLIGENT APPLICATION OF MASSAGE

There are basically two approaches to the delivery of massage. One approach can be considered a routine or protocol-based method. The client's intent is to experience the method rather than achieve a specific change in a body condition or behavior. Examples might include a signature spa massage or a general relaxation massage. There is a general therapeutic value in this approach, and it provides an important service for clients.

The other is considered outcome based and consists of a comprehensive, integrated process to assess client needs, determination of goals for the massage, a plan of massage application to achieve the goals, and measurement of treatment outcomes at regular intervals based on changes in the condition or behavior of the client resulting from specific interventions or actions. No one massage type is used exclusively. Instead, methods are used together to achieve client goals. Common outcomes include relaxation, stress management, pain management, and support of mobility and physical function.

Regardless of approach, the effective and intelligent application of massage is dependent on knowledge of anatomy, physiology, kinesiology, biomechanics, pathology, and pharmacology and considers the following.
- Structure can be thought of as anatomy, and function as physiology. Most massage outcomes influence physiology through neurologic and mechanical applications.
- The massage therapist most often works with the structural fluid and fiber aspects of the body, and with the functional interplay of body system function coordinated by chemicals and electrical signals.
- Chemicals and electrical signals control the body, and fluid and fibers make up the bone and soft tissue.
- Soft tissue includes the skin, fascia and other connective tissues, muscles, tendons, ligaments, cartilage, bursae, joint capsules, nerves, and vascular and lymphatic tubes.
- The various body fluids include blood, lymph, interstitial fluid, synovial fluid, mucus, cranial sacral fluid, digestive fluid, and various fluids produced by membranes in the body.

- All massage methods introduce mechanical forces into the soft tissues. These forces mimic and stimulate various physiologic responses.
- Neuroendocrine stimulation occurs when forces are applied during massage that generate various shifts in physiology.
- Massage causes the release of vasodilator substances that then promote circulation in a particular area.
- Forces applied during massage stimulate proprioceptors, which alter tone in muscles. Some of the listed benefits are supported by valid research and some by less rigorous forms of evidence such as consensus of expert opinion.

ASSESSMENT AND CARE/TREATMENT PLAN DEVELOPMENT

Assessment identifies the structures that need to be addressed, establishes clear intentions for treatment goals, provides a baseline of objective information for measuring the effectiveness of treatment, and helps identify conditions in which a particular treatment may be contraindicated. The massage therapist must gather specific information about treatment goals, both long term and short term, as well as data that are pertinent to the massage treatment.

The Clinical Reasoning Process

Similarities in application occur, but there is no one-size-fits-all "massage recipe" to follow. *Clinical reasoning* is the process of collecting data, analyzing the data, and developing appropriate treatment plans based on required outcomes relative to the data. *Justification* is the process of explaining the validity of a particular method of treatment. Justification describes the expected benefits of massage versus the potential harm (i.e., the harm vs. benefit ratio).

Assessment is fact gathering. Fact gathering is the first part of the clinical reasoning process. Massage therapists typically use history taking and physical assessment, which includes observation, palpation, and muscle tests.

Outcome Goals and the Care or Treatment Plan

Outcome goals are the targeted objectives that should be achieved as a result of massage application. Treatment plans (also called *care plans*) are the "maps" that direct the approach to care that is selected to achieve outcome goals. Outcome goals need to be quantifiable. This means that they must be able to be measured according to objective criteria, such as time, frequency, a scale of 1–10, an increase or decrease in the ability to perform an activity, or an increase or decrease in a sensation (e.g., relaxation, pain).

Goals also must be qualifiable. How will the client and the massage therapist know when a goal is achieved? After a goal has been reached, what will the person be able to do that they are not able to do now?

Short-Term and Long-Term Outcome Goals

Outcome goals are divided into short-term and long-term goals. Short-term goals typically support a session-by-session process and depend on the client's current status and are addressed by session planning. Long-term goals typically support recovery, performance, or healing and rehabilitation. Long-term goals focus on the result toward which treatment is targeted. Short-term goals work on the client's current status and serve as incremental steps toward achieving long-term goals. Short-term goals should not conflict with long-term goals.

Each and every session is uniquely developed and applied on the basis of multiple factors. Assessment is the identification of all these influences. Clinical reasoning is the sorting of this information and the development of an appropriate treatment session that is based on the assessment. Effective charting (discussed later) records the session-by-session massage application and the results.

Assessment and Development of the Initial Treatment Plan

First, the client's goals and desired outcomes for the massage sessions are identified. The client agrees to proceed with the next part of the session, which consists of history taking (with the use of a client information form) and a physical assessment (with an assessment form). Gathered information is evaluated so that a care plan can be developed for the client. Care plans usually envision a series of sessions.

A care/treatment plan is developed that spells out the following:
- Specific outcomes (i.e., therapeutic goals)
- Frequency of visits (number of appointments per week or month) and duration of visits (e.g., 30, 45, 60 minutes)
- Estimated number of appointments needed to achieve therapeutic goals (e.g., 10 sessions, 15 sessions, ongoing with no time limit)
- General methods to be used (e.g., classical massage, muscle energy methods, neuromuscular methods, myofascial methods)
- Objective progress measurements (e.g., pain decreased on a scale of 1–10, 50% increase in range of motion, sleep improved by increasing 1 hour per night, episodes of tension headache reduced from four per week to one per week, feelings of relaxation maintained for 24 hours)

The client provides (informed) consent for the care/treatment plan by signing the appropriate form.

Indications/Contraindications

Therapeutic massage is indicated for both illness and injury. Massage approaches for illness involve a general application of massage to support the body's healing responses (e.g., stress management, pain control, restorative sleep). This approach to massage, sometimes called *general constitutional application*, is neurological in nature primarily affecting neurochemical mechanisms and is used to reduce the stress load so that the body can heal or cope more effectively. Massage for injury incorporates aspects of general constitutional massage because healing is necessary for tissue repair. In addition, the more mechanical application of targeting fluid movement from the interstitial spaces into the lymphatic capillarity is used to control edema. Gliding methods are used to approximate (bring close together) the ends of some types of tissue injuries (e.g., minor muscle tears, strains, sprains), which supports healing. Hyperstimulation analgesia and counterirritation can reduce acute pain perception. Methods used to support local circulation to the injured area support tissue healing. Connective tissue applications are used to manage scar tissue formation. With proper training and supervision, massage therapists can use their skills to aid recovery or maintenance (or both) for most health concerns.

Cautions and Contraindications: Yellow and Red Flags

Contraindications and cautions are unique to each situation. The ability to reason clinically is essential for making appropriate decisions about modifying or forgoing massage interventions.

Contraindication means that some element of the client's condition makes a type of treatment more harmful than beneficial; therefore, the treatment should not be used, or referral is necessary before massage. Contraindication can be considered a red flag. *Cautions* mean that a treatment (e.g., massage application) must be adjusted to provide benefit without doing harm. Cautions are considered yellow flags. Modifications typically involve the following:

- Avoiding an area.
- Altering the mode of application, some aspects of qualities of touch (usually depth of pressure and duration), and type of mechanical force loading applied.
- Avoiding or altering an adjunct method such as essential oil use.

Massage may be totally/absolutely contraindicated if the client's condition is critical or acute, or if the body could be damaged by the results of the massage. Few situations are totally contraindicated, but many conditions will mandate caution and require a change in the massage application rather than the elimination of massage. The massage therapist must adjust the technique or avoid a particular area to apply methods safely.

Contraindications and cautions can be categorized as regional (local) or general (systemic). Regional contraindications pertain to a specific area of the body. For our purposes, the existence of a regional contraindication means that massage may be provided, but the application must be altered or the problematic area must be avoided. Examples of situations involving regional contraindications include a skin wound, a fracture, and a tumor site at which some sort of medical device is used.

In a few conditions, the contraindications are significant. Extreme caution and medical supervision are necessary. These include the following:

- Advanced kidney disease
- Congestive heart failure
- Advanced liver failure
- Systemic infection with high fever

Caution in any situation that raises concern is prudent. Trust your intuition.

TAKE 5

TREATMENT GOAL PATTERNS FOR THERAPEUTIC MASSAGE

The typical outcomes of massage application are to influence the adaptive, restorative, and healing capacities of the body. Wellness massage that targets prevention can stand on its own or become the platform for addressing more specific client outcomes. All outcomes can be applied appropriately for wellness and preventive healthcare or can be used to support the healing and rehabilitation of a pathologic condition, especially within a multidisciplinary environment. The four general outcomes described are based on current research evidence and can be considered evidence informed:

- Healing and rehabilitation/therapeutic change (fix)
- Condition management (contain and cope)
- Restorative care (rest and renew)
- Palliative care (pleasurable sensation, reduce suffering, and provide compassionate support)

Each of the four common outcomes for massage supports wellness, healing, rehabilitation, and recovery, as well as condition management and reduction of suffering. The four generalized outcomes provide a combination of the following massage benefits:

- Local tissue repair, such as a sprain or contusion
- Connective tissue normalization, which affects elasticity, stiffness, strength, pliability, and overall flexibility, as well as the neurologic influence of various mechanoreceptors in the fascia
- Shifts in pressure gradients to influence body fluid movement
- Neuromuscular function interfacing with muscle tension–length relationships; motor tone of muscles; concentric, eccentric, and isometric functions; and contraction–activation patterns of muscles working together to support efficient movement
- Mood and pain modulation through shifts in autonomic nervous system function, resulting in neurochemical and neuroendocrine responses
- Increased immune response to support systemic health and healing

Healing and Rehabilitation/Therapeutic Change

Healing and rehabilitation together result in the return to normal function from a state of illness or injury. Massage for this goal is complex and requires the most extensive training.

Also, the benefit of massage in this context is limited. Massage cannot "fix" things, as surgery can, but it can support the healing process.

Specific massage applications are integrated into the general massage application. Massage can support physical rehabilitation by managing postexercise soreness, reducing pain awareness, and supporting sleep. If the condition is primarily of soft tissue origin (which is rare), massage may be suggested as a primary care modality.

Condition Management

Unfortunately, many health conditions are chronic. In these cases, the goals for healthcare professionals, including massage therapists, are to manage symptoms, stabilize the condition, stop or slow its progression, and increase functioning (i.e., contain and cope). This approach is used for disorders such as diabetes, depression, migraine headache, arthritis, fibromyalgia, chronic pain syndrome, irritable bowel syndrome, and conditions of aging.

Restorative Care

A restorative care approach to massage supports normal rest and restorative function. It helps restore the body to a state of calm and allows it to relax and repair. Daily living, work and recreational activities, and maintenance of homeostasis require energy. It is necessary to regularly replenish resources with health-promoting behaviors, nutritious food, and restorative sleep. The parasympathetic autonomic nervous system (ANS) response is responsible for maintaining the "rest and digest" homeostasis. The massage approach supports parasympathetic and enteric ANS function. With a restorative approach, the client is generally healthy and has adaptive capacity. A restorative care plan functions from the premise that capacity to adapt exists for a return to the current functional state after demand. This care approach can be considered preventive and part of health maintenance. It is a very important care approach. Regular massage sessions are needed to best benefit from a restorative approach to care. An ongoing weekly or biweekly appointment schedule is recommended.

Palliative Care

Palliative care massage reduces suffering and provides pleasurable, soothing sensations. These may be the most important outcomes of massage. Comfort, support, nurturing, pleasure, and soothing are essential in the care of people, regardless of their condition. Attention to creating a warm and inviting environment, atmosphere, and ambience is part of the caring experience.

The massage application is slow, painless, rhythmic, and general, with sufficient pressure to produce relaxation (remember, light touch is arousing). History taking and assessment should reveal any contraindications and cautions, including areas to avoid and changes that should be made in the massage application. Palliative care massage is different from massage provided to achieve therapeutic change, condition management, or restorative function which requires specific treatment plans. In palliative care massage, palliative care is the treatment plan, and it involves methods to ease suffering and produce pleasurable sensations.

Patience, flexibility, and commitment are necessary when palliative care is the goal in a medical environment. Injured, ill, fragile, or elderly clients may be tired, discouraged, and in pain. Periods of exhilaration and disappointment occur within complex life experiences; reducing suffering and offering pleasurable sensations are invaluable for supporting beneficial psychological and physical responses to these stresses.

During healing and rehabilitation, a client's progress can plateau. The satisfaction of seeing ongoing change is diminished, and palliative care may help support the client during these times. Clients who receive medical care can experience diminished progress or setbacks. These individuals can be comforted temporarily by a nurturing touch. Sometimes there is just too much pain and discomfort to endure, regardless of the outcome goals, and palliative massage is the recommended approach when a "vacation" from treatment would be beneficial.

Massage Sequence Based on Clinical Reasoning to Achieve Specific Outcomes

1. Massage application intent (outcome) determines mode of application and variation on quality of touch:
   - Mode of application—influenced by type/mode of application (e.g., glide, knead, oscillation compression, percussion, movement)
   - Quality of touch—location of application, depth of pressure (light to deep), tissue drag, rate (speed) of application, rhythm, direction, frequency (number of repetitions), and duration of application of the method
2. Mode of application with variations in quality of touch generates the following:
   - Mechanical force application to affect tissue changes from physical loading (tension, compression, bend, shear, torsion) leading to the following:
   - Influence on physiology
   - Mechanical changes (tissue repair, connective tissue viscosity and pliability, fluid dynamics)
   - Neurologic changes (stimulus-response motor system, neuromuscular, pain reflexes, mechanoreceptors)
   - Psychophysiologic changes (changes in mood, pain perception, sympathetic and parasympathetic balance)

- Interplay with unknown pathways and physiology (e.g., energetic, meridians, chakras)

3. Mode of massage contributes to the development of a treatment approach.
4. Desired outcomes are achieved.

Documentation

Problem-Oriented Medical Record

The problem-oriented medical record (POMR) focuses on specific client problems. It was originally developed by doctors and later was adapted by nurses. The POMR is most effective in acute care or long-term care and home care settings. The massage community tends to use the POMR method.

SOAP, SOAPIE, SOAPIER Charting

SOAP

To use the SOAP format in POMR charting, document the following information for each problem:

- *Subjective data:* Information that the client, family members, or healthcare professionals tell the massage therapist, such as the chief complaint and other impressions.
- *Objective data:* Factual, measurable data gathered during assessment, such as observed signs and symptoms, vital signs, laboratory test values, and interventions used.
- *Assessment (analysis) data:* Conclusions based on collected subjective and objective data and formulated as client problems or nursing diagnoses. This dynamic and ongoing process changes as more or different subjective and objective information becomes known. This area also includes analysis of the effectiveness of interventions used.
- *Plan:* The massage therapist's strategy for relieving the client's problem. This plan should include both immediate or short-term actions and long-term measures.

SOAPIE

This modification to the SOAP method adds two areas. This content was moved out of the objective area to its own part: labeled intervention and evaluation.

- *Intervention:* Measures taken to achieve an expected outcome. As the client's health status changes, it may be necessary to modify the intervention plan. Be sure to document the client's understanding and acceptance of the initial plan in this part of the notes.
- *Evaluation:* An analysis of the effectiveness of interventions used. This content was moved out of the assessment part.

SOAPIER

The SOAPIER format adds a revision part for the documentation of alternative interventions. If the client's outcomes fall short of expectations, use the evaluation process called for in SOAPIE as a basis for developing revised interventions, then document these changes.

- *Revision:* Document any changes from the original plan of care in this part. Interventions, outcomes, or target dates may have to be adjusted to reach a previous goal.

TAKE 5

ETHICS, PROFESSIONALISM, CAREER, AND BUSINESS DEVELOPMENT

Ethics and professionalism have a unique language. The following definitions clarify some common terminology:

- *Ethics* is the science or study of morals, values, and principles, including the ideals of autonomy, beneficence, and justice. Ethics comprises principles of right and good conduct.
- *Ethical behavior* is right and correct conduct that is based on moral and cultural standards as defined by the society in which we live.
- *Ethical decision-making* is the application of ethical principles and professional skills to determine appropriate behavior and resolve ethical dilemmas.
- A *principle* is a basic truth or rule of conduct.
- A *therapeutic relationship* is created by the interpersonal structure and professional boundaries between professionals and their clients.
- *Transference* is the personalization of the professional relationship by the client.
- *Countertransference* is an inability on the part of the professional to separate the therapeutic relationship from personal feelings and expectations for the client; it is personalization of the professional relationship by the professional.
- A *dual role* results when scopes of practice overlap, with one professional providing support in more than one area of expertise.
- The *scope of practice* is the knowledge base and practice parameters of a profession.
- *Standards of practice* are principles that serve as specific guidelines for directing professional ethical practice and quality care, including a structure for evaluating the quality of care. They represent an attempt to define the parameters of quality care.
- *Informed consent* is a consumer protection process; it requires that clients be informed of the steps of treatment, that their participation be voluntary, and that they be competent to give consent. Informed consent is also an educational process that allows clients to make knowledgeable decisions about whether to receive a massage.
- *Mentoring* is a professional relationship in which an individual with experience and skill beyond those of the person being mentored provides support, encouragement, and career expertise.
- *Peer support* is the interaction among those of similar skill and experience to encourage and maintain appropriate professional practice.
- *Supervision* involves a person who oversees others and their professional behavior. The supervisor may have come from a different discipline (e.g., nursing) or may be a massage

therapist who has more skill and experience than those supervised. Supervisors usually are in a position of authority.
They are actively involved in areas such as the development
and approval of treatment plans, review of clarity, scheduling, discipline, and teaching.

Definitions of Therapeutic Massage and the Scope of Practice for Massage

Currently there is no formally agreed-upon definition of
massage therapy. This is difficult, since the definition and
scope of practice are linked. Scope of practice is determined
by licensing. Commonly used definitions included:
- Massage: Massage is a patterned and purposeful soft tissue
  manipulation accomplished by use of digits, hands, forearms, elbows, knees, and/or feet, with or without the use
  of emollients, liniments, heat and cold, handheld tools,
  or other external apparatus, for the intent of therapeutic
  change.
- Massage therapy: Massage therapy consists of the application of massage and non–hands-on components,
  including health promotion and education messages, for
  self-care and health maintenance; therapy, as well as outcomes, which can be influenced by: therapeutic relationships and communication; the therapist's education, skill
  level, and experience; and the therapeutic setting.
- Massage therapy practice: Massage therapy practice is a
  client-centered framework for providing massage therapy
  through a process of assessment and evaluation, plan of
  care, treatment, reassessment and reevaluation, health
  messages, documentation, and closure in an effort to
  improve health and/or well-being. Massage therapy practice is influenced by scope of practice and professional
  standards and ethics.

Definition Derived From Licensing, Certification, and Professional Organizations

Therapeutic massage is the scientific art and system of
assessment and systematic, manual application of a technique
to the superficial soft tissue of the skin, muscles, tendons,
ligaments, and fascia (and to the structures that lie within the
superficial tissue) using the hand, foot, knee, arm, elbow, and
forearm. The manual technique involves systematic application of touch, gliding/stroking (effleurage), friction, vibration,
percussion, kneading (pétrissage), stretching/elongation,
compression, or passive and active joint movements within
the normal physiologic range of motion. Included are
adjunctive external applications of water, heat, and cold for
the purposes of establishing and maintaining good physical
condition and health by normalizing and improving muscle
tone, promoting relaxation, stimulating circulation, and
producing therapeutic effects on the respiratory and nervous
systems and the subtle interactions among all body systems.
These intended effects are accomplished through the

physiologic, energetic, and mind/body connections in a safe,
nonsexual environment that respects the client's self-
determined outcome for the session.

Entry-Level Analysis Projects Definitions

Bodywork: A broad term that refers to many forms, methods,
and styles, including massage, that positively influence the
body through various methods that may or may not include
soft tissue deformation, energy manipulation, movement
reeducation, and postural reeducation.

Massage: The ethical and professional application of
structured, therapeutic touch to benefit soft tissue health,
movement, posture, and neurologic patterns.

Wellness-oriented massage: Massage performed in well-
ness- or relaxation-oriented environments to facilitate stress
reduction, relaxation, or wellness.

Healthcare-oriented massage: Massage performed in
medical or healthcare-oriented environments to facilitate
therapeutic change, condition management, or symptom
management.

Federation of State Massage Therapy Boards Practice of Massage Therapy

The practice of Massage Therapy means the manual application of a system of structured touch to the soft tissues of the
human body, including but not limited to: (1) Assessment,
evaluation, or treatment; (2) Pressure, friction, stroking,
rocking, gliding, kneading, percussion, or vibration; (3)
Active or passive stretching of the body within the normal
anatomic range of movement; (4) Use of manual methods or
mechanical or electrical devices or tools that mimic or
enhance the action of human hands; (5) Use of topical applications such as lubricants, scrubs, or herbal preparations;
(6) Use of hot or cold applications; (7) Use of hydrotherapy;
(8) Client education.

The National Center for Complementary and Integrative Health

Massage therapy encompasses many techniques. In general,
therapists press, rub, and otherwise manipulate the muscles
and other soft tissues of the body. They most often use their
hands and fingers but may use their forearms, elbows, or feet.
The term *massage therapy* (also called massage, for short;
massage also refers to an individual treatment session) covers
a group of practices and techniques. More than 80 types of
massage therapies exist. In all of them, the therapist presses,
rubs, and otherwise manipulates the muscles and other soft
tissues of the body, often varying pressure and movement.
The hands and fingers most often are used for this purpose,
but the forearms, elbows, or feet also may be used. Typically,
the intent is to relax the soft tissues, increase the delivery of
blood and oxygen to the massaged areas, warm them, and
reduce pain.

American Massage Therapy Association

The American Massage Therapy Association defines massage or massage therapy as any skilled manipulation of soft tissue, connective tissue, or body energy fields with the intention of maintaining or improving health by effecting change in relaxation, circulation, nerve responses, or patterns of energy flow. Massage or massage therapy may be accomplished manually with or without the use of the following: movement, superficial heat or cold, electrical or mechanical devices, water, lubricants, or salts.

Associated Bodywork and Massage Professionals

Massage, bodywork, and somatic therapies are defined by the Associated Bodywork and Massage Professionals as the application of various techniques to the muscular structure and soft tissues of the human body. *Massage* is defined as the application of soft tissue manipulation techniques to the body; these generally are intended to reduce stress and fatigue while improving circulation. The many variations of massage account for several different techniques. *Bodywork* refers to the various forms of touch therapies that may use manipulation, movement, or repatterning to effect structural changes in the body.

Somatic (meaning "of the body") therapy usually denotes a body/mind or whole-body approach as distinguished from a physiology-only or environmental perspective.

There are more than 250 variations of massage, bodywork, and somatic therapies, and many practitioners use multiple techniques. The application of these techniques may include, but is not limited to, stroking, kneading, tapping, compression, vibration, rocking, friction, and pressure to the muscular structure or soft tissues of the human body. This may also include nonforceful passive or active movement or the application of techniques intended to affect the energy systems of the body. The use of oils, lotions, and powders may be included to reduce friction on the skin.

Note: Massage, bodywork, and somatic therapies specifically exclude diagnosis, prescription, manipulation, or adjustments of the human skeletal structure, or any other service, procedure, or therapy that requires a license to practice orthopedics, physical therapy, podiatry, chiropractic, osteopathy, psychotherapy, acupuncture, or any other profession or branch of medicine.

Standards of Practice

All standards of practice provide a guide to the knowledge, skills, judgment, and attitudes that are needed to practice safely. The standards are based on the premise that the massage therapist is responsible for and accountable to the individual client for the quality of massage care he or she receives.

Federal and state laws, rules and regulations, and other professional agencies/organizations help define standards of practice. The Standard of Practice document from the *National Certification Board for Therapeutic Massage and Bodywork* is available on its website Standards of Practice | NCBTMB.

Informed Consent

Informed consent is information used to educate the client about making choices regarding care. To receive informed consent, the following questions should be answered at the outset of the professional relationship between the client and the massage therapist:
- What are the goals of the therapeutic program?
- What services will be provided?
- What behavior is expected of the client?
- What are the risks and benefits of the process?
- What are the practitioner's qualifications?
- What are the financial considerations?
- How long is the therapy expected to last?
- What are the limitations of confidentiality?
- In what areas does the professional have mandatory reporting requirements?

The Health Insurance Portability and Accountability Act

The Health Insurance Portability and Accountability Act (HIPAA) requires that the transactions on all client healthcare information should be formatted in a standardized electronic style; this law sets standards for maintaining confidentiality of client information in the healthcare environment. In addition to protecting the privacy and security of client information, HIPAA includes legislation on the formation of medical savings accounts, the authorization of a fraud and abuse control program, the easy transport of health insurance coverage, and the simplification of administrative terms and conditions.

Who Must Follow These Laws?
- Health plans, including health insurance companies, HMOs, company health plans, and certain government programs that pay for healthcare, such as Medicare and Medicaid
- Most healthcare providers—those that conduct certain business electronically, such as electronically billing your health insurance—including most doctors, clinics, hospitals, psychologists, chiropractors, nursing homes, pharmacies, and dentists

Credentialing

The following list highlights important distinctions for various credentialing processes:
- LICENSING
- Requires a state or provincial board of examiners

- Requires all constituents who practice the profession to be licensed
- Legally defines and limits the scope of practice for a profession
- Requires specific educational courses or an examination
- Protects title usage (e.g., only those licensed can use the title of massage therapist)
- GOVENRMENTAL CERTIFICATION
- Administered by an independent board
- Voluntary but required for anyone who uses the protected title (e.g., massage therapist); others can provide the service but cannot call themselves *massage therapists*
- Requires specific educational courses and an examination
- GOVERNMENTAL REGISTRATION
- Should not be confused with private registration processes
- Administered by the state Department of Registry or other appropriate state agency
- Voluntary verification
- Does not necessarily require a specific education, such as a school diploma; often other forms of verification of professional standards, such as years in practice, are acceptable
- Does not provide title protection
- EXEMPTION
- Means that a practitioner is not required to comply with an existing local or state regulation
- Excuses practitioners who meet specified educational requirements from meeting current regulatory requirements
- Does not provide title protection
- PROFESSIONAL CERTIFICATION
- Self-regulation by a profession
- Voluntary, not required of individuals prior to practice and without governmental oversight
- Private organizations recognize individuals for meeting certain criteria established by the private organization
- Individuals recognized for advanced knowledge and skills

Licensing of the Massage Therapist

Most states now require massage therapists to be licensed in order to protect the health, safety, and welfare of the public. Licensing is the entry-level point for career practice. Each state has its own individual licensing law. Some states require a jurisprudence exam, which is written to ensure that the licensed professional understands the legislation that governs their practice.

MASSAGE THERAPY CAREERS

In massage therapy, two main categories of practice have emerged, with six distinct practice settings:
1. Wellness and health promotion
   - Spa setting
   - Massage franchise/wellness center
   - Sports and fitness setting
   - Independent massage practice
2. Medical care
   - Clinical/medical/rehabilitation settings
   - Independent massage practice with clients who have medical conditions

Career Success

A career in massage can be developed as an employee or as a self-employed individual.

Those who will be successful have the following characteristics:
- Honest
- Motivated
- Flexible
- Able to adapt to change
- Able to plan and organize work
- Friendly
- Cooperative
- Tactful
- Work well without supervision
- Observe safety rules
- Enthusiastic
- Punctual and maintain good attendance

Successful massage therapists will do the following:
- Have personal and career goals
- Have a positive self-image
- Exhibit a good attitude
- Reason and make objective judgments
- Have leadership qualities
- Respect the rights and property of others
- Respect constructive criticism
- Respect diversity
- Ask questions and listen well
- Express themselves clearly
- Seek help when needed
- Maintain schedules
- Follow directions
- Stick with a task
- Work to improve their performance
- Accept responsibility
- Have good health habits
- Dress appropriately
- Practice good personal hygiene
- Give their best efforts

Emotional Intelligence

Successful massage therapists develop emotional intelligence. Emotional intelligence is a relatively new concept in psychology and involves the knowledge, skills, abilities, attitudes, and self-awareness to support productive and beneficial interpersonal relationships. Since massage is a service profession and the delivery of massage is client-centered, it is necessary to monitor and reflect on the meaning of individual and client emotions and behavior and to use that information to create productive therapeutic relationships.

Characteristics of a Successful Employee

- Respectful
- Patient
- Loyal
- Professional
- A positive mental attitude
- Organized
- Has up-to-date skills and the ability to learn new skills and procedures with ease
- Presents a professional appearance and attitude at all times
- Does not bring personal problems to work

Characteristics of the Self-Employed

Being self-employed takes discipline and self-sufficiency because those who are self-employed need to rely on themselves in the job market. For many, however, the benefits of being self-employed outweigh the sacrifices—and all the stress that goes with them. Those who are self-employed spend the most of their days doing all the tasks necessary to make their businesses a success.

According to the U.S. Small Business Administration, two of the core questions that prospective business owners need to ask themselves are these:

1. What service or product does my business provide, and what needs does it fill?
2. Who are the potential customers for my product or service, and why will they purchase it from me?

Business Plan

A business plan is a great place to start when one is in the beginning stages of starting a business. A business plan is a summary of the business and the objectives and activities needed for it to succeed. Components may include the following:

- Executive summary
- Company summary
- List of products or services
- Market analysis
- Strategy and implementation
- Management summary
- Financial plan
- Marketing plan
- Business cards
- Website

Marketing and Advertising

The business needs a marketing and advertising plan. The following are a few marketing or advertising concepts:

- Become a part of the local business and civic community.
- Develop and prepare press releases for local newspapers.
- Budget an affordable amount for advertising. This may include advertising in the Yellow Pages, local newspapers, and business directories.

TAKE 5

POPULAR METHODS OF MASSAGE AND ADJUNCT METHODS

Some questions on exams may require general knowledge of bodywork methods other than therapeutic massage or may include some sort of specialized name or trademark. This list of styles, systems, founders, and developers is not meant to be all-inclusive because the information changes almost daily, but it should be sufficient to address exam questions that include this information.

Asian Massage Approaches

Amma, Acupressure, Shiatsu, Jin Shin Do, Do-In, Tui-Na, Watsu, Thai Massage

These methods derive from original Chinese concepts and from offshoots of traditional Chinese methods. The philosophy of these systems is grounded in ancient concepts involving the energetic, physical, mental, emotional, and spiritual aspects of the body. The effects are both reflexive and mechanical. These approaches use compressive manipulations and stretches that focus on specific areas of the body and elicit responses in the nervous and cardiovascular systems. Efficient use of the therapist's body and the performance of these techniques on a clothed client provide many benefits.

Structural and Postural Integration Approaches

Bindegewebs Massage, Rolfing, Soma, Bowen Therapy, Myofascial Release, Soft Tissue Mobilization, Deep Tissue Massage, and Connective Tissue Massage

These techniques focus specifically on the connective tissue structure to influence posture and biomechanics. The approaches are systematic and effective because they are grounded in the fundamentals of physiology and biomechanics. Practitioners of these styles have received an extensive education. These systems focus specifically on various aspects of mechanical and reflexive connective tissue functions. Dr. William Garner Sutherland was the first to formalize the concept of minute movement of the cranium and dura. Dr. John Upledger and John Barnes, physical therapist, have expanded upon and formalized his work. Both light and deep touch may be used, depending on the method selected. Dr. James Cyriax's cross-fiber friction methods fall into this category.

Neuromuscular Approaches

Neuromuscular techniques, METs, strain/counterstrain, ortho-bionomy, Trager, myotherapy, proprioceptive neuromuscular facilitation, reflexology, and trigger points—these are the European approaches based on the work of Dr. Stanley Leif and Dr. Boris Chaitow and the Western methods based on the work of Dr. Janet Travell, Dr. John Mennell, Dr. Raymond Nimmo, Dr. Lawrence Jones, Dr. Milton Trager, Eunice Ingham, William Fitzgerald, Arthur Lincoln Pauls, Bonnie Prudden, and others. Dr. Leon Chaitow wrote extensively on these concepts. Many of these techniques are similar to those found in Rolfing, Asian methods, and Swedish massage and gymnastics. As the name implies, the approach is a nervous or reflexive method. Observation of the systems reveals that connective tissue also is affected. Common threads running through all these styles include the basic concepts of activation of the tonus receptor mechanism, reflex arc stimulation, positional receptors, and applications of stretching and lengthening.

Manual Lymphatic Drainage

Vodder Lymphatic Drainage

Emil Vodder developed an excellent system that uses the anatomy and physiology of lymphatic movement along with both mechanical and reflexive techniques to stimulate the flow of lymphatic fluid. Others, including Brian Chickly and Lyle Lederman, have contributed to the understanding of lymphatic drain procedures. Variations of this system sometimes are referred to as systemic massage.

Energetic (Biofield) Approaches

Polarity, Therapeutic Touch, Reiki, and Zero Balancing

These systems, which are based on ancient concepts of body energy patterns, were formalized by Dr. Randolph Stone, Dr. Dolores Krieger, Dr. Fritz Smith, and others. Subtle energy medicine is under study by Dr. Elmer Green at the Menninger Foundation in Topeka, Kansas, and elsewhere by other researchers. Polarity and similar energetic approaches use near touch or light touch to initiate reflexive responses, often with highly effective results.

Applied Kinesiology

Touch for Health, Applied Physiology, Educational Kinesiology, and Three-in-One Concepts

Dr. George Goodheart formalized the system of applied kinesiology within the chiropractic discipline. The approach blends many techniques but works primarily with reflexive mechanisms. A specific muscle testing procedure is used for evaluation; this process acts somewhat like a biofeedback mechanism. Some of the corrective measures use Asian channels (meridians) and acupressure; others rely on the osteopathic reflex mechanisms defined by Chapman, Bennett, and McKenzie that seem to correspond to traditional Chinese acupuncture points. Dr. John Thie and others have modified these techniques for use by massage professionals and the public.

Integrated Approaches

Sports Massage, Infant Massage, Equine/Animal Massage, On-Site or Seated Massage, Prenatal Massage, Geriatric Massage, Massage for Abuse Survivors, Russian Massage, Oncology Massage

Many styles of massage that focus on a specific type of population use combinations of methods that are based on physiologic interventions. Founders and teachers of integrated methods include every massage professional who designs a massage specifically for an individual client and every devoted massage instructor who attempts to combine and explain methods to students.

TAKE 5

Hydrotherapy

Water is unique in that it is universally available, readily accessible, and is applied with relatively simple and inexpensive equipment. The therapeutic properties of hydrotherapy are based on its mechanical or thermal effects and the body's reaction to hot and cold stimuli. Therapeutic effects also occur in response to the hydrostatic pressure exerted by water on the body (or body part) when immersed in (surrounded by) water. The peripheral nerves are stimulated by the temperature or pressure of the water, and impulses from the sensation on the skin are carried deeper into the body, stimulating the central nervous system, the autonomic nervous system, and, indirectly, all other systems in the body.

Generally, heat quiets and soothes the body, slowing the activity of internal organs. Cold, in contrast, stimulates and invigorates, increasing internal activity. When the body is submerged in water, such as a bath, a pool, or a whirlpool, the constant pull of gravity is reduced. Water also has a hydrostatic pressure effect, and it has a massage-like effect because water in motion stimulates touch receptors on the skin.

Water is effective as a therapeutic agent for several reasons:

- It has the ability to store and transmit heat.
- It is a good conductor of heat.
- It has solvent properties.
- It is nontoxic and therefore can be used both internally and externally.
- It can change states within a narrow, easily attainable temperature range.
- In its solid form (ice), it is an effective cooling agent.

- In its liquid form (water), it may be applied with the use of many pressures and temperatures, as well as methods ranging from total immersion to local compression.
- In its gaseous form (steam), it may be used in vapor or steam baths or for inhalation treatments.
- The density of water is near that of the human body; therefore, it supports exercise for clients with joint disease, paralysis, or atrophy.
- The hydrostatic pressure exerted on the body surface during immersion increases urine output, as well as venous and lymphatic flow from the periphery.

Water may be applied to the human body in a variety of ways to achieve a therapeutic effect. To apply hydrotherapy successfully, the practitioner must be familiar enough with the procedure to use it efficiently and competently. For example, the equipment required for techniques must be sanitized and maintained properly. However, it is the comfort of the client that increases the effectiveness of treatments.

Rest and relaxation are potential benefits of hydrotherapy; it is useful for some anxious clients because it promotes general relaxation of the nervous system. Hydrotherapy usually is one component of an overall health and wellness program. It also can offer specific relief to individuals with various conditions, such as:

- Arthritis problems
- Back and neck pain
- Sports injuries
- Work-related injuries

Physiologic Effects

The physiologic effects of hydrotherapy are classified as thermal, mechanical, and chemical. Thermal effects are produced by the application of water at temperatures above or below the body's temperature. The greater the variation from body temperature, the greater is the effect. Mechanical effects are produced by the impact of water on the body surface in the form of sprays, douches, frictions, whirlpools, and hydrostatic pressure forces. Chemical effects are produced when water is ingested and when it is used to irrigate a body cavity, such as the colon.

Heat is transferred from one object to another in several ways, including conduction, convection, and conversion. In hydrotherapy, heating and cooling effects are produced through the conduction of heat from the water to the body, or vice versa.

The normal or usual temperature of the human body in a state of health is considered to be around 98.6°F (when taken orally), although it varies throughout the day and from person to person. Body temperature also reflects a number of other factors, such as exercise, fasting, ovulation, and so on. When a person has a fever, body temperature is elevated as a result of any of several factors, such as the following:

- Dehydration
- Foreign proteins in the blood
- Hormonal imbalance
- Infection
- Malignancy
- Muscular or chemical activity
- Tissue destruction

When water temperature is considered, the terms *hot* and *cold* are related to body temperature. The temperatures used in hydrotherapy applications range from very cold to very hot.

Effects of Cold Applications

In the skin, cold receptors are more numerous than heat receptors. The temperature-regulating mechanism in the hypothalamus responds to signals by attempting to prevent cooling or overheating. Cold applications consist of one or more of the following: ice, cold water, cold air, or evaporation of water or other liquids from the surface of the body. Although the applications may vary, the principles and effects remain consistent. Cold water may cause shivering, goose bumps, increased pulse and respirations, dilation of blood vessels, and increased muscle tone and metabolism. This may be called a *tonic*—a stimulating reaction to cold. The response to hot or cold water varies with the length of application.

The primary or direct effect of cold application is depressant in nature, leading to a decrease in function, either locally or systemically, depending on the application. The longer and colder the application, the longer and more intense is the depressant effect. However, as the body responds to the cold application, a return to normal function occurs that may lead to a state of increased activity; this is known as the secondary, or indirect, effect of cold, also called the *reaction*. The secondary effect, or reaction, occurs only when the body has the vitality to respond to the cold, either after its removal (e.g., in such applications as showers, sprays, baths, and so on) or after the body has warmed the application (e.g., as with cold compresses or packs). In general, the colder the application, the greater is the reaction. Many hydrotherapy techniques are directed at producing the reaction to the cold application.

Effects of Hot Applications

All hot applications produce definite physiologic responses; these are the body's attempts to eliminate heat to prevent a rise in local and systemic temperatures. The effects produced by hot applications depend on the method, temperature, duration of the application, and on the client's condition. A water temperature of 98°F or higher generally is perceived as hot; a temperature over 104°F is considered very hot. The mucous membranes, unlike the skin, may endure temperatures as high as 135°F, which accounts for our ability to drink very hot liquids, such as tea or coffee. Hot air may be tolerated by many individuals for fairly long periods, such as in a sauna, in which the temperature may reach as high as 200°F. Caution is required. The young, elderly, or pregnant and those who are fragile should avoid temperature extremes and long exposure duration.

Heat may be applied to the body in a variety of ways, including hot packs, hydrocollator therapy packs, fomentations, steam, hot air, baths, and showers. Although exposure to the high temperatures of hot tubs and saunas has become popular, prolonged use may weaken the individual, unless this practice is counteracted by frequent cold applications, such as showers.

Risks, Cautions, and Contraindications

Persons with impaired temperature sensation run the risk of scalding or frostbite at temperature extremes. If the client has diabetes, avoid hot applications to the feet or legs and full body heating treatments, such as body wraps. Avoid cold applications if the client has been diagnosed with Raynaud disease. Elderly individuals and young children may be exhausted by too much heat and should avoid long, full-body hot treatments such as immersion baths and saunas. Hot immersion baths and long, hot saunas are not recommended for individuals with diabetes or multiple sclerosis, women who are pregnant, or anyone with abnormally high or low blood pressure or a cardiac condition. Temperatures higher than 106–110°F should not be used because such temperatures can raise the body temperature very quickly, inducing an artificial fever.

Effects of Hydrotherapy Using Heat, Cold, and Ice Applications

Effects of Heat

- Increases circulation
- Increases metabolism
- Increases inflammation
- Increases respiration
- Increases perspiration
- Decreases pain
- Decreases muscle spasm
- Decreases tissue stiffness
- Decreases white blood cell production

Applications of Heat

- As a *sedative:* Water is an efficient, nontoxic, calming substance. It soothes the body and promotes sleep.
- *Techniques:* Use hot and warm baths to quiet and relax the entire body. Salt baths, neutral showers, or damp sheet packs can be used to relax certain areas.
- For *elimination:* The skin is the largest organ of the body, and simple immersion in a long, hot bath or a session in a sauna or steam room can stimulate the excretion of toxins through the skin. Inducing perspiration is useful for treating acute diseases and many chronic health problems.
- *Techniques:* Use hot baths, Epsom salts or common salt baths, hot packs, hydrocollator therapy packs, dry blanket packs, and hot herbal drinks.
- As an *antispasmodic:* Water effectively reduces cramps and muscle spasm.
- *Techniques:* Use hot compresses (depending on the problem), herbal teas, and abdominal compresses.

Effects of Cold and Ice

The effects of cold are as follows:
- Increases stimulation
- Increases muscle tone
- Increases tissue stiffness
- Increases white blood cell production
- Increases red blood cell production
- Decreases circulation (primary effect); increases circulation (secondary effect)
- Decreases inflammation
- Decreases pain
- Decreases respiration
- Decreases digestive processes

The effects of ice are as follows:
- Increases tissue stiffness
- Decreases circulation
- Decreases metabolism
- Decreases inflammation
- Decreases pain
- Decreases muscle spasm

Types of Applications

- Ice packs
- Ice immersion (ice water)
- Ice massage
- Cold whirlpool
- Chemical cold packs
- Cold gel packs (use with caution)
- Hydrocollator therapy packs

Contraindications to Use of Ice

- Vasospastic disease (spasm of blood vessels)
- Cold hypersensitivity; signs include the following:
  - *Skin:* Itching, sweating
  - *Respiratory:* Hoarseness, sneezing, chest pain
  - *Gastrointestinal:* Abdominal pain, diarrhea, vomiting
  - *Eyes:* Puffy eyelids
  - *General:* Headache, discomfort, uneasiness
- Cardiac disorder
- Compromised local circulation

Precautions for Use of Ice

- Do not use frozen gel packs directly on the skin.
- Do not use ice applications (cryotherapy) for longer than 20 minutes continuously.
- Do not do exercises that cause pain after cold applications.
- Do not use cryotherapy on individuals with certain rheumatoid conditions or on those who are paralyzed or have coronary artery disease.

Applications of Cold

Ice is a primary therapy for strains, sprains, contusions, hematomas, and fractures. It has a numbing, anesthetic effect and helps control internal hemorrhaging by reducing circulation to and metabolic processes within the area:

- For *restoring and increasing muscle strength and increasing the body's resistance to disease:* Cold water boosts vigor, adds energy and tone, and aids in digestion.

- *Techniques:* Use cold-water treading (standing or walking in cold water), whirlpool baths, cold sprays, alternate hot and cold contrast baths, showers and compresses, salt rubs, apple cider vinegar baths, and partial packs.
- For *injuries:* The application of an ice pack controls the flow of blood and reduces tissue swelling.
- *Technique:* Use an ice bag in addition to compression and elevation.
- As an *anesthetic:* Water can dull the sense of pain or sensation.
- *Technique:* Use ice to chill the tissue.
- For *minor burns:* Water, particularly cold and ice water, has been rediscovered as a primary healing agent.
- *Technique:* Use ice water immersion or saline water immersion.
- To *reduce fever:* Water is nature's best cooling agent. Unlike medications, which usually only diminish internal heat, water both lowers temperature and removes heat by conduction.
- *Techniques:* Use ice bags at the base of the neck and on the forehead and feet, as well as cold-water sponge baths and drinking of cold water.

Rules of Hydrotherapy

Hydrotherapy has a powerful effect on the body. The following rules, taken from the Ontario, Canada, curriculum guidelines for massage therapy, should be followed when hydrotherapy is used in the massage setting:

1. Always take a thorough case history to check for possible contraindications. Contraindications include various circulatory and kidney problems, as well as skin conditions.
2. Always adapt the method to the individual, not vice versa. Time, temperatures, and other variables selected in procedures should be considered guidelines, not absolutes.
3. Have the client go to the bathroom before treatment begins.
4. Stay with the client during treatment, or have some way for the client to contact you, such as by using a bell.
5. Explain the complete treatment to the client beforehand so that he or she knows what to expect and what is expected.
6. Make sure the room is draft-free, clean, and quiet. All equipment should be sanitary and in good working condition. Each client should have clean towels and sheets.
7. Keep the client from becoming chilled during or after the treatment.
8. For cold-water treatments, the water should be as cold as possible, within the client's tolerance. A 10-degree difference is the minimum needed to produce stimulation and change in the circulation.
9. For warm-water treatments, the water should be as warm as necessary, within the client's tolerance. A temperature that is too hot can be debilitating.

10. More is not better. It is not always more effective to use greater extremes in temperature or greater lengths of time. The aim is to achieve a positive change, and too much can overtax, damage, or set back the condition.
11. Ask pertinent questions during the treatment, including questions about comfort level and thirst, but keep talking to a minimum to allow the client to relax.
12. Check the client's respiratory rate and pulse before, during, and after treatments as required, especially with prolonged hot treatments. The pulse should stay fairly even.
13. Watch for discomfort or negative reactions to the treatment.
14. Stop the treatment if a negative reaction occurs.
15. Generally, short cold treatments are followed by active exercise. Prolonged cold and hot treatments are followed by bed rest and then exercise.
16. Apply cold compresses to the head with hot treatments and prolonged cold treatments.
17. Never give a cold treatment to a cold body. Always warm the body first. The easiest method for this is a warm foot-bath (Table 5.1).

Hot and Cold Stones and Other Thermal Applications

The use of stones is an ancient healing art that has been rediscovered, particularly in the spa setting. Its modern form came in the early 1990s, when massage therapist Mary Hannigan of Tucson, Arizona, trademarked her particular style and called it LaStone Therapy. Stone therapy is a type of thermotherapy. It uses deep penetrating heat from smooth, heated stones and alternating cold from chilled stones. As is shown in the hydrotherapy part of this textbook, the physiologic benefits of applying alternating temperatures to the body have long been scientifically investigated and validated. The weight of the stones also has value for providing a sustained compressive force against the tissue while the stone is in place. It is important to note safety concerns from hot stone application. It is important to protect the client from burns and avoid static placement of stones directly on the skin.

Procedures for Using Stones During Massage

1. Before the client arrives, sanitize the stones by boiling or soaking in a 10% bleach solution. Cool stones from 100 to 110°F.

TABLE 5.1	**Classifying Water Temperatures**	
Very cold	32–56°F	Painful
Cold	56–65°F	Uncomfortable
Cool	65–92°F	Goose bumps
Neutral	92–98°F	Normal skin temperature
Warm to hot	98–104°F	Comfortable
Very hot	104–110°F	Reddened skin

Temperatures higher than 110°F should not be used.

2. Use gliding strokes while holding a heated stone. As the stone cools, replace it with another. Observe precautions for body mechanics.

3. Preferably, use the warm stone to heat your hands. Use your hands for massage, and place the stone as described in the next step.

4. Place heated stones at specific points along the body meridians, along the spine, in the palms of the hand, or between the toes (anywhere they will stay) to improve the flow of energy in the body.

5. For pain management use cold stones.

6. Instruct the client to speak up if the stones are too warm or if the pressure is too intense.

7. Cover the area with a sheet, and then place the stones on the sheet rather than directly on the skin; this is the safest and most sanitary method. With direct application to the skin, the most serious concern is burning the client if the stone is too hot for the individual's skin or if it is left on too long. *Always use warm, not hot, stones.*

8. Apply the stones with an intentional, centered approach.

9. Placement of stones can be combined with general massage.

TAKE 5

Aromatherapy/Essential Oils

Essential oils are subtle, volatile chemicals distilled from plants, shrubs, flowers, trees, roots, bushes, and seeds. They have hormone-like properties and are natural antiseptics. Each oil is thought to have a unique power on the body and mind, but the oils also can be classified easily as antiseptic, analgesic, antiinflammatory, detoxifying, regenerating, stimulating, or sedating.

Massage can be combined with aromatherapy. This combination is based on the idea that essential oils, because they are lipids, are absorbed readily through the skin. Topical application allows the client to inhale the aroma molecules as they are absorbed through the mucous membranes. Essential oils are also beneficial through inhalation of the scent, which affects the limbic system.

Aromatherapy is an extensive study, and care and caution are advised in the use of essential oils. Pure essential oils should be used, and these should be diluted in a carrier oil (e.g., olive, jojoba, grape seed, or almond) before they are applied to the skin. Only three or four drops of essential oil are needed in 2 ounces of carrier oil. When a drop of oil is mixed with a small amount of salt ($\frac{1}{4}$ cup), it can be dissolved in a warm-water immersion, such as a bath. Essential oils in the pure state should *never* be applied directly to the skin.

Safety Guidelines for the Use of Essential Oils
Essential oils are highly concentrated substances that can be beneficial if used correctly. However, some oils are not safe to use at all. Even though essential oils should *never* be used undiluted on the skin, an experienced aromatherapist may make exceptions to this precaution. A large number of aromatherapy sources list lavender and tea tree oil as oils that can be used undiluted. However, this should be done only rarely because severe sensitivity still could occur in some individuals. The safest rule of thumb is to *never* use any essential oil undiluted.

Some oils can cause sensitization or allergic reactions in some individuals. When using new oil for the first time, do a patch test on a small area of skin. Place a small amount of the diluted essential oil on the inside of the elbow, and apply a bandage. Wait 24 hours to see whether any type of reaction occurs. Even if a particular essential oil is not known to cause irritation, this step should *never* be ignored. Some essential oils should be avoided during pregnancy and by those with asthma, epilepsy, or other health conditions.

Less is more—When using essential oils, use the smallest amount that will get the job done. If one drop is sufficient, for example, do not use two drops.

Not all essential oils are suitable for use in aromatherapy. Wormwood, pennyroyal, onion, camphor, horseradish, wintergreen, rue, bitter almond, and sassafras are some of the essential oils that should be used only by qualified aromatherapy practitioners, if at all.

Children should never be allowed to use essential oils unless supervised by an adult who is knowledgeable in their use. Most essential oils smell wonderful, and many of them, such as citrus oils, smell like they are safe to drink. Keep essential oils away from children. Treat the oils like medicines that are poison in unknowing hands. Keep essential oils away from animals.

Essential oils should not be taken internally.

Essential oils are flammable. Keep them out of the way of fire hazards. Keep oils away from the eyes. If a drop or so of oil accidently gets into the eye, put some vegetable oil (e.g., almond oil) into the eye, which will absorb the essential oil; then use a tissue to remove the oil. Do not use water, which will spread the oil. If burning or itching occurs, seek medical treatment. Do not use the same oils for a prolonged period.

Use photosensitizing oils (i.e., bergamot, verbena, lime, angelica root, bitter orange, lemon, and grapefruit) cautiously. Avoid sun exposure and the use of tanning beds for 12 hours after application of these oils. Store essential oils away from light and heat, and keep the cap tightly closed. Essential oils are volatile and evaporate readily.

Carrier Oils
As mentioned, essential oils are mixed with a carrier oil. Carrier oils are high-quality, fresh vegetable oils that are used to dilute essential oils. Carrier oils also have their own therapeutic properties.

TAKE 5

Asian Bodywork Methods

The richness of Asian health theory and the unity of its body/mind/spirit connection are based on the energy of life. Life force, called *chi*, or Qi/Ri energy, flows through the body through interconnected pathways as water flows through the streams, rivers, lakes, and oceans of the earth. When *chi* energy flows through the body like pure water, all of the processes of life are balanced. However, if obstruction or stagnation develops in the life force, it becomes the basis for disease.

The Tao, or "the Way," supports the balanced function of all the senses and teaches a lifestyle of moderation that avoids deprivation and excess. *Chi* energy is the vital force of life, and Tao is the path or the way to sustain *chi* energy.

Some are concerned about the taking of pieces from the totality as expressed in the Tao. Western science has lifted techniques from this simultaneously simple but complex and all-encompassing system. This is called appropiation. Often, a technique separated from its theoretic basis is less effective. Although a technique can stimulate physiologic functions, it cannot support the human experience. This small part presented in this textbook is based on a limited part of the total Asian medicine system commonly found on exams. As you begin to develop an understanding of these methods, be mindful and respectful concerning the larger structure of the body of knowledge from which this information has been taken.

Midline Meridians (Channels)

The body has two midline meridians. The conception or central vessel (yin) meridian starts in the center of the perineum and runs up the midline of the anterior aspect of the body to terminate just below the lower lip; it is responsible for all yin meridians (24 points). The governing vessel (yang) meridian starts at the coccyx and runs up the center of the spine and over the midline of the head; it terminates on the front of the upper gum and is responsible for all yang meridians (28 points). If the concepts of yin and yang and of vital energy or life force (Qi) are removed from the acupuncture/meridian phenomenon, the explanation provided by neuroanatomy and neurophysiology remains partial. Western research so far has produced no great breakthrough in understanding acupuncture. Sufficient evidence has been acquired regarding acupuncture to explain many of the effects as neurohumoral chemical mechanisms.

Yin—Yang Theory

Yin—yang theory is one of the oldest doctrines in Chinese culture. The words *yin* and *yang* were originally representations of the shady and sunny sides, respectively, of a mountain or a hill. They came to represent two primordial forces that were the fundamental constituents of the universe and everything in it.

When yin and yang were separated from the singularity at the beginning of existence, the resulting potential gave rise to Qi. To the Chinese, Qi is a vital component of everything, and everything is sensed or experienced in a manifestation of Qi.

Yin and yang frequently are described as opposites or complementary opposites. In terms of Western science, the notion of opposing forces is a powerful one, echoing in religious, moral, and ethical concepts of right and wrong and good and evil. However, in Chinese theory, yin and yang are conceived of as being in opposition, but not in conflict. Yin and yang nourish and foster the growth of each other; they restrain each other; they support each other; they penetrate each other; they coexist.

TAKE 5

Myofascial Massage Methods

Adapting massage application to influence connective tissues, particularity fascial layer gliding, is often called myofascial release. In most cases, a lubricant is not used with myofascial approaches because the drag quality on the tissue is necessary to produce results, and lubricant reduces drag. Methods that primarily affect the ground substance require a quality of slow, sustained pressure and agitation. Most massage methods can soften the ground substance to reduce stiffness as long as the application is not abrupt. Tapotement and abrupt compression are less effective than slow gliding methods that have a drag quality. Kneading and skin rolling that incorporate a slow pulling action are effective as well. The appropriate application introduces one or a combination of the mechanical force loading of tension, compression, bind, shear, and torsion to achieve results.

The fiber component is affected by stretching methods that elongate the natural crimp of the fiber. This creates a freeing or unraveling of fibers.

The important consideration for all connective tissue focused massage methods is that the pressure exerted vertically and horizontally must actually move the tissue to create tension, torsion, shear, or bend loads. In addition, these forces must alter the ground substance long enough for energy to build up, soften the ground substance, and influence the smooth muscle bundles. The development of connective tissue patterns is highly individualized; therefore, systems that follow a precise protocol and sequence often are less effective for dealing with these complex patterns.

Trigger Points

There is contradiction regarding the exact nature of a trigger point. There is also controversy surrounding the existence of the trigger point phenomena. The concept of trigger points remains part of manual therapy and so is described in this section. A *trigger point* (also called *myofascial trigger point*) has been defined as an area of local nerve facilitation of a muscle that is aggravated by stress of any sort that affects the body or mind. Trigger points are small areas of hyperirritability within muscles. If these areas are located near motor nerve points, the person may experience referred pain caused by nerve stimulation. The area of the trigger point often is the motor point at which nerve stimulation initiates a contraction in a small, sensitive bundle of muscle fibers that in turn activates the entire muscle. The tissue fluid surrounding the area of a trigger point is slightly acidic, which may contribute to the phenomenon.

A trigger point area often is located in a tight band of muscle fibers. Palpation across the band may elicit a twitch response, which is a slight jump in the muscle fibers. This is difficult to detect when the trigger point is in the deeper muscle layers. The development of trigger points is accompanied by the characteristic referred pain pattern and the restriction of motion associated with myofascial pain. With classic trigger points, the referred pain pattern can be traced to its site of origin.

Trigger points in the muscle belly usually are found in short, concentrically contracted muscles. Trigger points located near the attachments usually are found in eccentric patterns and in long, inhibited muscles that act as antagonists to concentrically contracted muscles. Muscle contractions may serve as a response for compensation purposes. The best course is to address the trigger point activity in the short tissues first and wait to see whether the trigger points in the long muscles and at the attachments resolve as the posture of muscle interaction normalizes. The sequence for addressing trigger points is as follows:

1. Those that are most painful and that reproduce familiar symptoms
2. Those that are most medial
3. Those in the short tissue
4. Those in the muscle belly

Trigger point treatment with manual therapy such as massage is a good example of the integration of multiple methods because effective intervention involves the use of several treatment protocols, massage manipulations, muscle energy methods, stretching methods, and hydrotherapy methods.

Implement Assisted

An **implement** is some sort of device that is used to augment the massage application. The device can roll and press, scrape or suction. The two main reasons for using an implement are as follows:

- The device reduces the effort required to apply massage, making massage application easier for the massage therapist.
- The device can apply mechanical force to the soft tissue more effectively than the massage therapist's hands, forearms, or other part of the body used to apply massage methods.

Remember that massage methods apply mechanical forces to deform soft tissue and that mechanical forces are a push or a pull. Any devices incorporated into massage should assist this process. There are many implements that can be used to push into tissue. In general, these devices are used to create compression stress. Rollers, balls, knobs, and so forth in a variety of designs are made from different types of material including plastic and wood. The stones used in hot and cold stone massage are implements.

The main safety concerns are compression injury to soft tissue and sanitation. The various tools must be disinfected after every use. Compression injury is called a contusion. A contusion (bruise) is an injury to the soft tissue often produced by a blunt force resulting in pain, swelling, and discoloration. Nerves are especially susceptible to compression injury.

Implements can also be used for percussion and vibration. Bundled sticks, usually bamboo or rattan, and soft head mallets are examples of tools that can be used to replace the hands when performing percussion methods. The main implement that can apply vibrations is a tuning fork. When the tuning fork is hit with a rubber hammer, the tines begin to vibrate. The end of the tuning fork is placed on the body.

The main safety concern is the tissue damage that could occur with aggressive percussion. The tissue can be bruised, and depending on the implement (e.g., bundled sticks), the skin could be cut. Tuning forks present a low risk of harm, and because vibration performed by the massage therapist is fatiguing, they may be a valuable tool.

Electric devices can create percussion and vibration to augment massage application. A percussion device moves in-out and up-down like hammers or pistons. A vibration device moves back and forth.

The main safety concern for electrical devices is for the massage therapist being exposed to hand-arm vibration, which causes damage to hands and fingers. The resulting condition is known as white finger disease, Raynaud phenomenon, or hand-arm vibration syndrome. One of the symptoms is that affected fingers may turn white, especially when exposed to cold. Caution is required. As always, the tools must be disinfected after each use.

Traction devices pull. Traction is the act of applying a mild stretch at constant pressure to the body tissues, especially muscles and ligaments, around jointed areas. Most often implements that assist the massage therapist in performing traction are straps and bands.

The main safety concern from straps is skin damage. There is also a potential for traction application to be too aggressive when a strap is used to assist with the traction method.

Vacuum manual therapy is performed by applying a suction device to selected skin points and creating a subatmospheric pressure by suction. Often this method is called cupping. The term vacuum manual therapy accurately describes these methods.

Various adverse effects may occur but are rare and related to too much suction and leaving the suction devise in one place for too long resulting in capillary damage. Because of the capillary breakage caused by the suction, the skin can become marked with dark red or purplish areas in the shape of the suction devise. These areas are not bruising which is tissue damage caused by compression. The discoloration can be significantly reduced or avoided by moving the suction devise or only leaving it stationary for short periods such as 15 seconds.

Elastic Therapeutic Tape

Elastic therapeutic tape, also called kinesiology tape or kinesiology therapeutic tape, Kinesio tape, k-tape, or KT tape, is an elastic cotton strip with an acrylic adhesive. Kinesiology tape may improve circulation, support muscles, and help heal and prevent muscle injury. However, supporting research is scant. The main safety issue is sensitivity to the adhesive and potential skin irritation when removing the tape. Suggested removal of tape incorporates warm water.

Ayurveda

Ayurveda is a system of health and medicine developed in India. The foundation of its theory base is similar to that of Asian systems. The language of Ayurveda is being used more often in Western society, and massage professionals should be familiar with some of the terms that describe ayurvedic principles of thought.

The word *Ayurveda* means life knowledge or right living. Ayurveda is grounded as a body/mind/spirit system in the Vedic scriptures. The *tridosha* theory is unique to this system. A *dosha* is a body chemical pattern. When doshas combine, they constitute the nature of every living organism. The three doshas are *Vata* (wind), *Pitta* (bile), and *Kapha* (mucus). These three combine to form the five elements (similar to Asian theory) of ether, air, fire, water, and earth.

Bones, flesh, skin, and nerves belong to the *earth element.* Semen, blood, fat, urine, mucus, saliva, and lymph belong to the *water element.* Hunger, thirst, temperature, sleep, intelligence, anger, hate, jealousy, and radiance belong to the *fire element.* All movement, breathing, natural urges, sensory and motor functions, secretions, excretions, and transformation of tissues belong to the *air element.* Love, shyness, fear, and attachment belong to the *ether element.*

The points connected with this system are called *marmas.* There are about 100 marmas, which are concentrated at the junctions of muscles, vessels, ligaments, bones, and joints. These junctions form the seat of vital life force (in Hindi, *Prana*). Marmas have a strong correlation to common trigger points and the locations of the traditional meridians.

In Ayurveda, *chakras* are considered the seven centers of the Prana. They are located along the spinal column, interrelated with the nervous system and endocrine glands. These subtle centers of consciousness serve as the link between the universal source of intelligence and the human body. Chakras are wheels of energy that govern various physical organs, as well as etheric bodies, such as the emotional body (the feelings). Within every living body, although on the subtle rather than the gross or the physical level, there are said to be a series of energy fields or centers of consciousness, which in traditional Tantric teachings are called *chakras* (wheels) or *padmas* (lotuses). These are said to be located along, or just in front of, the vertebral column, even though they might express themselves externally at points along the front of the body (e.g., navel, heart, throat). Associated with the chakras is a latent subtle energy, called *kundalini* in Shaktism and *tumo* in Tibetan Buddhist Tantra. Massage methods of Ayurveda include tapping, kneading, rubbing, and squeezing. The use of specialized oil preparations is integral to the systems.

Reflexology

In the bodywork community, **reflexology** means the stimulation of areas beneath the skin to improve the function of the whole body or of specific body areas away from the site of stimulation. Eunice Ingham has been credited with formalizing the system, which is based on the theory that certain points in the foot and hand affect other body organs and areas. Historically, the approach seems to have originated in China. Foot reflexology is the most popular type of reflexology.

Another approach to reflexology is referred to as *zone therapy*. It is postulated that 10 zones run through the body. Reflex points for stimulation can be located within these zones.

Reflexology applies the stimulus/response principle to healing the body. The foot has been mapped to show the areas of contact that affect different parts of the body. Charts that map these areas vary somewhat. Typically, the large toe represents the head, and the junction of the large toe and the foot represents the neck. The next toes represent the eyes, ears, and sinuses. The waist is about midway on the arch of the foot, with various organs above and below the line. The reflex points for the spine are along the medial longitudinal arch. It is thought that this stimulus-response reflex is conducted through neural pathways in the body that activate the body's electrical and biochemical activities.

Energy Systems

The more subtle energetic approaches have not yet been researched enough to be scientifically validated. Energy medicine includes all energetic and informational interactions that result from self-regulation or are brought about through other energy linkages to mind and body. In addition to various therapeutic energies that we may use, energy pulses from the environment may influence humans and animals in a variety of ways. For instance, low-level changes in magnetic, electrical, electromagnetic, acoustic, and gravitational fields often have profound effects on both biology and psychology.

Subtle energy, compared with "energy medicine," is a concept that is more difficult to define within the current scientific paradigm. Ancient and modern wisdom traditions describe human bioenergies, referred to by many names (e.g., chi, ki, Prana, etheric energy, fohat, orgone, odic force, mana, homeopathic resonance), that are believed to move throughout the so-called etheric (or subtle) energy body and thus are difficult to measure with the use of conventional instrumentation.

Various individuals and cultures have developed energy-based healing systems. These systems overlap when applied to support energy flow, balance, and harmony. Depending on which energy-based healing system is used, the methods may include tapping, massaging, pinching, or twisting, or energy may be influenced by connecting specific energetic points on the skin through tracing or swirling the hand over the skin along specific energy pathways. Some systems use exercises or postures designed for specific energetic effects. Most use focus of the mind to move specific energies.

The key to effectiveness in all systems is intention. It would be prudent to be clear about the intention of the massage provided and to realize that it is likely that some interaction among the various energy mechanisms is at work when a compassionate and skilled massage therapist touches in a therapeutic way.

Polarity

Polarity is a holistic health practice that encompasses some of the theory bases of Asian medicine and Ayurveda. Polarity therapy was developed by Dr. Randolph Stone in the middle 1900s. It is an eclectic, multifaceted system. Life force energy (e.g., chi, Qi, Prana) has not been a popular subject of Western scientific research. The abstract quality and esoteric nature of the concepts are still primarily held in the knowledge base of "spiritual truth." Many spiritual disciplines practice the "laying on of hands." Polarity therapy is a respectful, compassionate, and intentional laying of the hands on the body.

Principles and Applications of Polarity Therapy

The purpose of polarity therapy is to locate blocked energy and release it, using the principles outlined here. When blocked energy is released, body systems and organs can function normally, and healing can take place naturally. Polarity therapy does not treat illness or disease; it affects body (life) energy, which flows in invisible electromagnetic currents through the body's organs and tissues. It stimulates the energy that is inactive in a diseased body part.

Remember to read this chapter over and over. Only read—do not attempt to memorize. Strive for comprehension.

CHAPTER 6

Functional Anatomy and Physiology

NEUROENDOCRINE STRUCTURE AND FUNCTION

The nervous system is anatomically and functionally connected throughout the entire body. Structurally, it is divided into the central nervous system (CNS) and the peripheral nervous system (PNS). Functionally, the PNS is divided into the somatic (or motor) nervous system, and the autonomic nervous system. Endocrine hormone and neurotransmitter functions are interrelated because they work together to regulate homeostasis. Any demand for response affects homeostasis, including injury and disease. Since massage application also creates demand upon the body to respond, it generally affects every part of nervous and endocrine system function, thus influencing injury and disease.

Massage can affect the nervous system in several ways. It alters CNS processing of cognitive perception, including pain perception, and influences the peripheral somatic and autonomic nervous system (ANS), including fluctuations in neurotransmitters and hormones. Sensory input causes the body to respond, creating the necessity for homeostasis to be restored. Massage stimulates nerve receptors in the tissues. On a sensory level, the mechanoreceptors that respond to touch, pressure, warmth, etc., are stimulated. Generally, the effect leads to relaxation of the tissues and a reduction in pain, although the opposite can also happen.

Central Nervous System

The CNS consists of the brain and the spinal cord. The brain is divided into three parts—the cerebrum, brainstem, and cerebellum. The cerebrum, which is the largest portion of the brain, is generally responsible for higher mental functions and personality. The frontal lobe area of the cerebrum also contains the motor cortex, which controls voluntary movement. The parietal lobe of the cerebrum contains the sensory cortex, which receives information about touch and proprioception.

The brainstem is the center for the automatic control of respiration and heart rate. The cerebellum controls muscle coordination, motor tone, and posture.

The limbic system and the hypothalamus integrate emotional states, visceral responses, and the muscular system through endocrine and neurotransmitter chemicals. Emotions can alter muscle tension by increasing motor tone, primarily through increased sympathetic dominance in ANS. States of anxiety and depression commonly create sustained increase in muscle tension.

The typical neuron has a cell body, which contains the genetic material and much of the cell's energy-producing machinery. Extending from the cell body are dendrites, branches that are the most important receptive surface of the cell for communication. The dendrites of neurons can assume a great many shapes and sizes, all relevant to the way in which incoming messages are processed. The output of neurons is carried along what is usually a single branch called the *axon.* It is in this part of the neuron that signals are transmitted out to the next neuron. At its end, the axon may branch into many terminals.

The workings of the brain depend on the ability of nerve cells to communicate with each other. Communication occurs at small, specialized gaps called *synapses.* The synapse typically has two parts. One is a specialized presynaptic structure on a terminal portion of the sending neuron that contains packets of signaling chemicals, or neurotransmitters. The second is a postsynaptic structure on the dendrites of the receiving neuron that has receptors for the neurotransmitter molecules.

The usual form of communication involves electrical signals that travel within neurons, giving rise to chemical signals that cross synapses, which, in turn, give rise to new electrical signals in the postsynaptic neuron. The complexity of the brain is such that a single neuron may be part of more than one circuit. The organization of circuits within the brain reveals that the brain is a massive information processor.

TAKE 5

Some places in the brain are specialized for particular functions. The cerebral cortex, which is the layer of neurons with its surface area increased by outpouchings, called *gyri*, and indentations, called *sulci*, can be functionally subdivided into four lobes. The posterior portion of the cerebral cortex (i.e., the occipital lobe) is involved in the initial stages of visual processing. Anterior and superior to the occipital lobe is the parietal lobe, which is involved in processing tactile information. Lateral and inferior to the parietal lobe is the temporal lobe, which is involved in processing auditory information. Anterior to the parietal lobe is the frontal lobe, which is involved in motor behavior. The central sulcus is a lateral line which divides the frontal lobe from the parietal lobe.

The anterior region of the frontal lobe is called the *prefrontal cortex*, which is involved in some of the highest functions of the human being, including the ability to plan and the ability to integrate cognitive and emotional streams of information.

Beneath the cortex are enormous numbers of axons sheathed in the insulating substance, myelin. This subcortical "white matter" (because of its appearance on freshly cut brain parts) surrounds groups of neurons, or "gray matter," which, like the cortex, appears gray because of the presence of neuronal cell bodies.

The white matter can be thought of as the wiring that conveys information from one region to another. It is within gray matter that the brain processes information. Gray matter regions include the basal ganglia, the part of the brain that is involved in the initiation of motion (affected in Parkinson's disease), but that is also involved in the integration of motivational states and becomes dysfunctional with addictive disorders. Other important gray matter structures in the brain include the amygdala and the hippocampus. The amygdala appears to play a special role in aversive or negative emotions such as fear and is involved in determining the emotional meaning of events and objects. The hippocampus initially encodes and consolidates specific memories of persons, places, and things.

The brain is chemically and structurally complex. As previously described, electrical signals within neurons are converted at synapses into chemical signals, or neurotransmitters, which then create electrical signals on the other side of the synapse. Two major types of molecules serve the function of neurotransmitters: small molecules, some well known, with names such as *dopamine*, *serotonin*, and *norepinephrine*, and larger molecules, which are essentially protein chains, called *peptides*. These include the endogenous opiates, substance P, and corticotropin-releasing factor, among others. A neurotransmitter can cause a biologic effect in the postsynaptic neuron by binding to a protein called a *neurotransmitter receptor*. Its job is to pass the information contained in the neurotransmitter message from the synapse to the inside of the receiving cell.

It appears that almost every known neurotransmitter has multiple receptors that can stimulate different signals on the receiving neuron. By definition, therefore, receptors that admit positive charge are excitatory neurotransmitter receptors. The classic excitatory neurotransmitter receptors in the brain use the excitatory amino acids glutamate and, to a lesser degree, aspartate as neurotransmitters. Inhibitory neurotransmitters act by permitting negative charges into the cell, taking the cell farther away from firing. Classic inhibitory neurotransmitters in the brain include the amino acids gamma aminobutyric acid, or GABA, and, to a lesser degree, glycine.

Most of the neurotransmitters in the brain, such as dopamine, serotonin, and norepinephrine, are not only excitatory or inhibitory but produce complex biochemical changes in the receiving cell that alter the way in which receiving neurons can process signals from glutamate (excitatory) or GABA (inhibitory). These neurotransmitters are responsible for brain states such as degree of arousal, ability to pay attention, and identification of the emotional significance of cognitive information. The effects of neurotransmitters influenced during massage may explain and validate the use of sensory stimulation methods for treating clients with chronic pain, anxiety, and depression. Some of the main neuroendocrine chemicals that may be influenced by massage include the following:

- Dopamine
- Serotonin
- Epinephrine/adrenaline
- Norepinephrine/noradrenaline
- Enkephalins/endorphins/dynorphins
- Endocannabinoids
- Oxytocin
- Cortisol
- Growth hormone

It is unlikely that massage sensation targets a specific chemical. Instead, a more general influence on neuroendocrine function is more logical.

Dopamine

Dopamine influences motor activity that involves movement (especially learned fine movement, such as handwriting), conscious selection (the ability to focus attention), and mood (in terms of inspiration, intuition, joy, and enthusiasm). Dopamine is involved in pleasure states, seeking behavior, and the internal record system. Low levels of dopamine produce the opposite effects, such as lack of motor control, clumsiness, inability to focus attention, and boredom. Massage seems to increase the availability of dopamine in the body, which can explain the pleasure and satisfaction experienced during and after massage.

Serotonin

Serotonin allows a person to maintain context-appropriate behavior—that is, to do the appropriate thing at the appropriate time. It regulates mood in terms of appropriate emotions, attention to thoughts, and calming, quieting, comforting effects; it also subdues irritability and regulates drive states so that we can suppress the urge to talk, touch, and be involved in power struggles. Serotonin is also involved in satiety; adequate levels reduce the sense of hunger and craving, such as for food or sex. It also modulates the sleep/

wake cycle. A low serotonin level has been implicated in depression, eating disorders, pain disorders, and obsessive–compulsive disorders. A balancing effect has been noted between dopamine and serotonin, much like those seen in agonist and antagonist muscles. Aggressive and impulsive behavior of individuals can be connected to imbalances in this area. Massage seems to increase the available level of serotonin. Massage may support the optimal ratio of these chemicals.

Epinephrine/Adrenaline and Norepinephrine/Noradrenaline

The terms *epinephrine/adrenaline* and *norepinephrine/noradrenaline* are used interchangeably in scientific texts. Epinephrine activates arousal mechanisms in the body, whereas norepinephrine functions more in the brain. These are the activation, arousal, alertness, and alarm chemicals of the fight-or-flight response and of all sympathetic arousal functions and behaviors. If the levels of these chemicals are too high, or if they are released at an inappropriate time, a person feels as though something very important is demanding their attention and reacts with the basic survival drive of fight or flight (hypervigilance and hyperactivity). The person might have a disturbed sleep pattern, particularly a lack of rapid eye movement sleep, which is restorative sleep. With low levels of epinephrine and norepinephrine, the individual is sluggish, drowsy, fatigued, and under aroused.

Massage seems to have a regulating effect on epinephrine and norepinephrine through stimulation or inhibition of the sympathetic and parasympathetic nervous system. This generalized balancing function of massage seems to recalibrate the appropriate adrenaline and noradrenaline levels. Depending on the response of the ANS, then, massage can just as easily wake a person up and relieve fatigue as it can calm down a person who is anxious.

It should be noted that initially, touch stimulates the sympathetic nervous system, whereas it seems to take 15 minutes or so of sustained stimulation for the parasympathetic functions to be engaged. Therefore, it makes sense that a 15-minute chair massage tends to increase production of epinephrine and norepinephrine, which can help people become more attentive, whereas a 45–60 minute slow, rhythmic massage engages the parasympathetic functions, reducing epinephrine and norepinephrine levels and encouraging a good night's sleep, which is necessary for recovery and healing.

Enkephalins/Endorphins/Dynorphins

Enkephalins/endorphins/dynorphins are mood lifters that support satiety and modulate pain. Massage seems to increase the available levels of enkephalins and endorphins. The massage effect appears to be delayed until the enkephalin level rises, which usually takes about 15 minutes. Appropriate availability of these pain-modulating chemicals is essential for individuals who deal with pain.

Endocannabinoids

Endocannabinoids are a group of neuromodulatory chemicals involved in a variety of physiologic processes, including appetite, pain sensation, mood, memory, motor coordination, blood pressure regulation, and combating cancer. Endocannabinoids, which are endogenous, stimulate the same receptors as cannabis. Endocannabinoids are synthesized on demand, but the question is: What triggers the process?

The endocannabinoid system modulates anxiety-like behaviors and stress adaptation. Most research studies suggest that acute stress triggers the release of the endocannabinoid chemicals, which then bind to cells' receptors. This causes changes in cell function, which causes changes in emotional behavior, reversing the stress response. The endocannabinoid system functions as a neuromodulator of the CNS.

Oxytocin

Oxytocin is a hormone that has been implicated in pair or couple bonding, parental bonding, feelings of attachment, and caretaking, along with its more clinical functions during pregnancy, delivery, and lactation. Massage tends to increase the available level of oxytocin, which could explain the connected and intimate feeling of massage.

Cortisol

Cortisol and other glucocorticoids are stress hormones produced by the adrenal glands during prolonged stress. Elevated levels of these hormones indicate increased sympathetic arousal. Cortisol and other glucocorticoids have been implicated in many stress-related symptoms and diseases, including suppressed immunity states, sleep disturbances, and increases in the level of substance P. Individuals with medical concerns are particularly susceptible to increased and sustained cortisol levels. Massage may affect levels of cortisol and substance P secondary to reduction of sympathetic autonomic dominance by supporting relaxation.

Growth Hormone

Growth hormone promotes cell division and in adults has been implicated in the functions of tissue repair and regeneration. This hormone is necessary for healing and is most active during sleep. Massage indirectly increases the availability of growth hormone through increased vagal stimulation, parasympathetic dominance, restorative sleep, and reduction of cortisol.

Spinal Cord

The spinal cord, which is a continuation of the medulla oblongata of the brain, travels through the vertebral canal from the foramen magnum to the lumbar spine. It relays sensory impulses from the periphery up to the brain, and motor impulses from the brain out to the periphery.

Information from all four classes of sensory receptors—the mechanoreceptors, proprioceptors, chemoreceptors, and nociceptors—send information to the spinal cord, which stimulates countless reflexive adjustments in the body to maintain homeostasis, without any active thought from the person.

The spinal cord becomes individual spinal nerves as they exit the vertebral column through openings between the sides of the vertebra called the *intervertebral foramina*. Anatomically, this is where the peripheral nervous system begins.

Peripheral Nervous System

The PNS consists of 12 pairs of cranial nerves and 31 pairs of spinal nerves. These nerves carry sensory impulses from the periphery into the brain and spinal cord, and motor impulses from the brain and spinal cord out to the periphery. The peripheral nerves are vulnerable to compression and irritation at the nerve roots in the area of the intervertebral foramen, as well as entrapment, irritation, or compression in the extremities. They can become restricted or entrapped by adhesions in the connective tissue spaces or hypertonic muscles through which they travel. Nerve pain tends to radiate and follow traceable pathways in the body.

TAKE 5

The peripheral nervous system is divided into the somatic nervous system and the autonomic nervous system.

Somatic Nervous System

The somatic sensory nerves relay information to the CNS regarding pain, temperature, touch, and pressure from the skin. These nerves also convey pain signals, proprioceptive information about movement, and position and mechanoreceptor information from the muscles, tendons, ligaments, joint capsules, and periosteum.

Epithelial Tissue
The epithelium and the nervous system are derived from the same embryologic tissue, the ectoderm. Therefore, our skin is an extension of the nervous system. The skin is the body's largest organ and contains blood vessels, glands, muscles, connective tissue, and nerve endings.

The skin contains sensory nerve receptors called *mechanoreceptors*, which communicate with every other part of the body. The mechanoreceptors are sensitive to touch, pressure, movement, superficial proprioception, pain, and temperature. Skin provides sensation, information, and protection; assists with water balance; and regulates temperature.

Sensory information from the skin communicates with the spinal cord, where reflex connections are made to muscles, internal organs, and blood vessels. Skin pain can cause a contraction in the skeletal muscle or internal organ symptoms, and vice versa, with skeletal muscle and internal organs referring pain to the skin. Massage accesses the body through the skin and sends signals of pressure, movement, stimulation, etc., for the body to process.

Somatic Sensory Nerves
The somatic motor nerves relay information from the brain, through the spinal cord, and then to the skeletal muscles. The somatic sensory nerves are the principal means by which the massage therapist communicates with the body. Each touch and movement sends messages to the CNS (spinal cord and brain), which, in turn, communicates with every other part of the body. Soft tissue consists of five basic categories of sensory nerves, including the following:

- Mechanoreceptors: respond to touch, pressure, and movement
- Proprioceptors: respond to changes in position and movement
- Thermoreceptors: located inside the skin, specialized neurons which detect changes in environmental temperatures
- Chemoreceptors: sensitive to acid—base balance, oxygen, etc.
- Nociceptors: detect noxious stimuli and alert the brain when an injury is likely or imminent

The main proprioceptors influenced by massage are the muscle spindle and the Golgi tendon organ. Also influenced are the mechanoreceptors of the skin and connective tissue because of stretching, compression, rubbing, and vibration. Stimulation of joint mechanoreceptors affects adjacent muscles. Stimulation of the skin overlying muscle and joint structures has beneficial effects caused by shared innervations.

Somatic sensory nerves are specialized receptors that relay information to the CNS about touch, pressure, position, and movement. Touch and pressure originate from the skin sensory nerve endings located in the superficial and deep layers of the skin, which communicate light touch, deep pressure, temperature, and pain. These nerve endings respond to external information from the environment. Massage stimulation of the skin and superficial fascia provides effective communication with these sensors.

Proprioceptors and mechanoreceptors are located in fascia, muscles, tendons, and joints and communicate information about body position and movement. Massage interacts with these receptors through active and passive movement, and the various mechanical forces applied.

TAKE 5

Muscle Tone

Muscle tone is a low level of continuous contraction in muscle. It is produced by motor neuron excitability and is influenced by massage application that inhibits or stimulates motor neuron activity. The most common reason for increased muscle tone is the increase in sympathetic arousal and sustained sympathetic dominance. Another cause is proactive muscle guarding/splinting after injury and nervous system damage.

Sensory Nerve Receptors of Muscle
Five types of sensory nerve receptors supply each muscle. These sensory nerves respond to pain, chemical stimuli, temperature, deep pressure, muscle length, the rate of muscle

length changes, muscle tension, and the rate of change in tension.

- Type 1a is a primary muscle spindle.
- Type 1b is a Golgi tendon organ (GTO).
- Type 2, a secondary muscle spindle, includes paciniform and pacinian corpuscles, which are sensitive to deep pressure.
- Type 3 consists of free nerve endings that are sensitive to pain, chemicals, and temperature.
- Type 4 is made up of nociceptors.

The two classes of sensory receptors that have particular significance for the massage therapist are the muscle spindles and the Golgi tendon organs. They detect length and tension in the muscle and tendon, set the resting motor tone of the muscle, adjust the motor tone in a muscle for coordination and fine muscular control, and protect the muscles and joints through reflexes that contract or inhibit the muscle automatically.

Muscle spindles are specialized muscle fibers called *intrafusal fibers*, which are located in a fluid-filled capsule embedded within the muscle belly. These muscle spindles respond to slow and rapid changes in muscle length; the secondary endings respond to slow changes in muscle length and are sensitive to deep pressure. The spindles also play a role in joint position, muscle coordination, muscular control, and muscle tone. Because muscle spindles detect changes in muscle length, stretching a muscle will increase its rate of signal discharge.

The more refined the muscle's function, the greater is the concentration of spindles. The greatest concentration of spindles is found in the lumbrical muscles of the hand, the suboccipital muscles, and the muscles that move the eyes.

States of anxiety or emotional or psychological tension can cause an increase in the firing rate of muscle spindles. This increase causes the muscle tone to be "set" to high, creating hypertonicity and stiffness. If the muscle spindles are set too high, the firing rate can be decreased in three ways, causing the muscle to relax (decrease in tone):

- Decrease muscle length by bringing the proximal and distal attachments toward each other.
- Contract a muscle isometrically, as is done for contract-and-relax methods. This method causes the spindle activity to stop temporarily, allowing the muscle to be set to a new, more relaxed length.
- Use inhibiting compression in the belly of the muscle to decrease firing.

Golgi tendon organs are sensory receptors that take the form of a slender capsule located along the muscle fiber at the musculotendinous junction. They sense changes in muscle tension and fire during minute changes in muscle tension. They perform the protective function of preventing damage to a muscle that is being contracted forcefully. Discharge of the Golgi tendon organ stimulates nerves at the spinal cord, called *inhibitory interneurons*, causing the muscle to relax. Abnormal firing of the Golgi tendon organ can set the resting tone of the muscle too high, creating hypertonicity.

The Golgi tendon organs can be influenced in three ways:

- Muscle energy methods can reset the muscle to its resting length and tone, but the exact mechanism is not fully understood.
- When a muscle voluntarily contracts isometrically, the Golgi tendon organ increases its discharges, which has an inhibiting effect on the muscle, causing it to relax.
- Inhibiting compression at the tendons can also decrease Golgi tendon organ activity.

When these methods are used in combination with stretching, the tissue seems to better tolerate the stretching process.

Massage Application

Dysfunction of soft tissue (muscle and connective tissue) without proprioceptive hyperactivity or hypoactivity is uncommon. It is believed that proprioceptive hyperactivity causes tense or spastic muscles and hypoactivity of opposing muscle groups.

Deep, nonpainful broad-based massage has a minimal and short-term inhibitory effect on the tone of muscle as the result of motor neuron activity. It is used primarily to support a muscle reeducation process such as therapeutic exercise, to temporarily reduce motor tone so that muscle firing patterns can be reset, or to reduce muscle spasm associated with other mechanical methods which address tissue shortening. Active movements of the body, including techniques such as active-assisted joint movement or application of muscle energy methods that utilize active muscle contraction and release (contract and relax, contract/relax/antagonist/contract, positional release, etc.), seem to improve motor function by interacting with proprioceptive function.

Chemoreceptors

As mentioned previously, chemoreceptors are sensory receptors that respond to changes in acid—base balance, oxygen, etc. Chemoreceptors may be irritated, for example, when the body is inflamed or when a muscle is in a sustained contraction, thus decreasing the amount of oxygen in the tissue. These chemicals interact with fibroblasts, mast cells, and other cells to create a neurogenic inflammatory response.

Massage may purposefully use controlled focused pain, such as pressure on acupuncture points to release pain-inhibiting chemicals. Tension in the soft tissues or the stress response can cause overactivity in the sympathetic nervous system. By reducing soft tissue tension, massage can help restore balance and can stimulate the parasympathetic system, resulting in a positive effect on minor and sometimes major medical conditions, such as high blood pressure, migraine, insomnia, and digestive disorders.

The usual outcome of massage targeting neural chemical mechanisms is inhibitory and anti-arousal. Anti-arousal massage (relaxation massage) may influence muscle tone activity in the same way that pharmaceutical muscle relaxers do because the main reason for tone difficulties is sympathetic arousal.

Vestibular Apparatus and Cerebellum

The vestibular apparatus is a complex system composed of sensors in the inner ear (vestibular labyrinth), upper neck (cervical proprioception), eyes (visual motion and three-dimensional orientation), and body (somatic proprioception) that are processed in several areas of the brain (brainstem, cerebellum, parietal and temporal lobes). These reflexes affect the eyes (vestibulo-ocular reflexes), the neck (vestibulocollic reflexes), and balance (vestibulospinal reflexes) by sending and receiving information all at the same time about orientation to the surrounding environment. Many amusement park rides create disorienting sensations that contribute to the effects of the ride.

The vestibular apparatus and the cerebellum are interrelated. Output from the cerebellum goes to the motor cortex and brainstem. Stimulating the cerebellum by altering muscle tone, position, and vestibular balance stimulates the hypothalamus to adjust functions to restore homeostasis. This is a very complex process, which makes it difficult to determine the exact mode of effect created by mechanical and neurological stimulation massage methods.

Massage Application

The techniques that most strongly affect the vestibular apparatus and therefore the cerebellum are those that produce rhythmic oscillation, including rocking during the application of massage. Rocking produces movement at the neck and head that influences the sense of equilibrium. Rocking stimulates inner ear balance mechanisms, including the vestibular nuclear complex and the labyrinthine righting reflexes, to keep the head level. Stimulation of these reflexes produces a body-wide effect involving muscle contraction patterns throughout the body.

Massage can alter body positional sense and the position of the eyes in response to postural change. It can initiate a specific movement pattern that changes sensory input from muscles, tendons, joints, and the skin and stimulates various vestibular reflexes. This feedback information, which adjusts and coordinates movement, is relayed directly to the motor cortex and the cerebellum, allowing the body to integrate the sensory data and adjust to more efficient postural balance and optimal movement strategies.

If massage application involves vestibular influences, short-term nausea and dizziness can occur while the mechanisms rebalance. Using massage to restore appropriate muscle activation pattern sequences and gait reflexes is valuable. By influencing balance massage can shift the relationship of the eyes, neck, hips, etc., and may affect posture, mobility, and agility.

TAKE 5

Nerve Impingement/Compression/Entrapment

Soft tissue often impinges nerves. Tissues that can bind include skin, fascia, muscles, ligaments, joint structures, and bones. An increase in fluid in a particular area can impinge nerves. Shortened muscles and stiff and dense connective tissue (fascia) often impinge on major and minor nerves, causing discomfort. Tissues that are long and taut can also impinge. The specific nerve root, trunk, or division affected determines the condition, such as thoracic outlet syndrome, sciatica, or carpal tunnel syndrome.

Major nerves and general innervations include:

- Musculocutaneous—anterior arm muscles
- Medial cutaneous—arm and forearm
- Ulnar—forearm and hand
- Median—forearm and hand
- Radial—forearm and hand
- Sciatic—thigh and leg
- Femoral—hip and thigh
- Obturator—medial thigh adductors
- Popliteal—leg and foot
- Fibular—leg and foot

Cervical Plexus

The cervical plexus is formed by the ventral rami of the upper four cervical nerves. The phrenic nerve is part of this plexus. It innervates the diaphragm, and any disruption to this nerve affects breathing. Many cutaneous (skin) branches of the cervical plexus transmit sensory impulses from the skin of the neck, ear, and shoulder. The motor branches innervate muscles of the anterior neck.

Symptoms of cervical plexus impingement include headache, neck pain, and breathing difficulties. The muscles most responsible for pressure on the cervical plexus are the suboccipital and sternocleidomastoid muscles. Shortened connective tissues at the cranial base also press on these nerves.

Brachial Plexus

The brachial plexus, situated partly in the neck and partly in the axilla, provides virtually all the nerves that innervate the upper extremity. Any imbalance that brings pressure on this complex of nerves results in shoulder pain, chest pain, arm pain, wrist pain, and hand pain. A person may also experience numbness or tingling in the upper extremity as well.

The muscles most often responsible for impingement of the brachial plexus are the scalenes, pectoralis minor, and subclavius. Muscles of the arm occasionally impinge branches of the brachial plexus. Brachial plexus impingement is responsible for thoracic outlet symptoms, which often are misdiagnosed as carpal tunnel syndrome. Whiplash injury involves the brachial plexus.

Lumbar Plexus

Lumbar plexus nerve impingement may cause low back discomfort with a belt-like distribution of pain, as well as pain in the lower abdomen, genitals, thigh, and medial lower leg. The main muscles that impinge the lumbar plexus are the quadratus lumborum and the psoas. Shortening of the lumbar dorsal fascia exaggerates lordosis and causes vertebral impingement of the lumbar plexus.

Sacral Plexus

The sacral plexus has approximately a dozen named branches. Almost half of these serve the buttock and lower limb; the others innervate pelvic structures. The main branch is the sciatic nerve. Impingement of this nerve by the piriformis muscle can cause sciatica. Ligaments that stabilize the sacroiliac joint can affect the sacral plexus. Pressure on the sacral plexus can cause gluteal pain, leg pain, genital pain, and foot pain.

Therapeutic massage techniques work in many ways to reduce pressure on nerves. These techniques can be used to do the following:

- Neurologically change the tension pattern and lengthen the short muscles
- Mechanically soften connective tissue and increase tissue pliability
- Reduce localized edema
- Interrupt the pain-spasm-pain cycle caused by protective muscle spasm that occurs in response to pain
- Support the effectiveness of therapeutic exercise to shift posture and function
- Complement the use of medications such as antispasmodics, analgesics, antiinflammatories, and circulation enhancers such as vasodilators

TAKE 5

Autonomic Nervous System

The ANS is the part of the nervous system that innervates the heart, blood vessels, diaphragm, internal organs, and endocrine glands. It influences every other part of the body, including the muscular system, and has two main divisions: the sympathetic and the parasympathetic nervous systems.

Visceral Sensation

Visceral sensory nerves are part of the ANS and send pain and pressure information from the internal organs to the CNS. The visceral motor nerves transmit impulses from the ANS to the involuntary muscles, such as those found in internal organs, and glandular tissue.

Sympathetic Nervous System

The sympathetic nervous system is responsible for the "fight-flight-freeze" response, excitement, anticipation, and performance, and it is active when a person is under stress. It releases adrenaline into the blood, causes constriction of the peripheral blood vessels, increases the heart rate, and inhibits normal movement of the intestines, so that blood is available to the skeletal muscles. When a person is under stress, tone of muscles is increased because of the effects of the sympathetic nervous system. This process uses energy, and if the pattern is not reversed, fatigue may occur. Stress can lead to sympathetic dominance and a collection of problems such as breathing disorder, slowed healing, emotional agitation, digestive upset, sleep disturbance, and more.

Parasympathetic Nervous System

The parasympathetic nervous system is responsible for energy building, food digestion, and assimilation. It restores

homeostasis and is active when the body is at rest and recuperating. It causes a decrease in heart rate, stimulates the normal peristaltic smooth muscle movement of the intestines, and promotes the secretion of all digestive juices and tropic (tissue-building) hormones. A person can be in parasympathetic override (dominance), which contributes to lethargy, loss of normal motivation, and depression.

Many individuals have an underactive parasympathetic nervous system and an overactive sympathetic nervous system. One of the primary benefits of massage delivered in a soothing way is stimulation of the parasympathetic nervous system. This induces a state of relaxation and promotes the parasympathetic nervous system functions of healing and rejuvenation, which supports homeostasis.

Enteric Nervous System

The enteric portion of the ANS is a meshwork of nerve fibers that innervate the gastrointestinal tract, pancreas, and gallbladder. The ENS is sometimes called the "belly brain."

Traumatic Stress Syndrome and State-Dependent Memory

Sensory input during massage may trigger a memory pattern of an emotionally charged event. Each memory—including all sensory information, nervous system functions, and endocrine functions involved at the time of the experience—is stored in a multidimensional way.

Compassion is required to support the client during these times. No verbal interaction is necessary. Referral to a psychiatrist or a psychologist may be necessary. The neurochemical aspect of the body-mind interaction is necessary for physical and emotional healing.

Stress Response and Effects of Massage on the Stress Response

Excessive sympathetic output causes most stress-related diseases and dysfunction. Examples include headache, gastrointestinal difficulties, high blood pressure, anxiety, muscle tension and aches, and sexual dysfunction. Long-term stress (i.e., stress that cannot be resolved by fleeing or fighting) also may trigger the release of cortisol, a cortisone manufactured by the body. Long-term high blood levels of cortisol cause side effects similar to those of the drug cortisone, including fluid retention, hypertension, muscle weakness, osteoporosis, breakdown of connective tissue, peptic ulcer, impaired wound healing, vertigo, headache, reduced ability to deal with stress, hypersensitivity, weight gain, nausea, fatigue, and psychic disturbances.

Physical and tactile measures which result in the perception of comfort are associated with reduction of arousal and promotion of self-regulation (homeostasis). Pleasure is an important experience in health and healing. Pain causes muscular contraction, withdrawal, abrupt movement, breath holding, increased heart rate, and increased generalized stress. Pain perception is heightened according to psychological states, especially anxiety or depression. Pain tolerance is lowered in cases such as low self-esteem and apprehension. Since pleasure can counteract the pain response, massage providing pleasurable sensation affects both pain hypersensitivity and decreased pain tolerance.

Emotional states such as anticipation, anxiety, anger, depression, and tension usually result in increased tone of muscles; relaxed states supported by pleasure sensation seem to reduce muscular tone. The limbic system modulates these responses. Applications of touch that are perceived as pleasurable are usually sedative and parasympathetic in nature. Initial adaptation to touch, as well as touch perceived as uncomfortable, aggressive, and nonproductive, increases sympathetic arousal. The importance of these pleasurable factors during massage is evident in palliative care. Because of its generalized effect on the ANS and associated functions, massage can cause changes in mood and excitation, inducing the relaxation/restorative response. Massage seems to be a gentle, pleasure producing modulator, thus supporting the outcomes of well-being and comfort.

Initially, massage stimulates sympathetic functions. The increase in autonomic, sympathetic arousal is followed by a decrease if the massage is slowed and sustained with sufficient pleasurable pressure and lasts about 45–60 minutes. Pressure levels must be relatively firm and broad based but not painful. Slow, moderate pressure, repetitive stroking, broad-based compression, rhythmic oscillation, and movement all seem to initiate relaxation responses. Superficial stroking stimulates the itch and tickle response. Painful compression, and fast-paced applications stimulate sympathetic responses. Although not usually indicated, stimulation of the sympathetic nervous system may temporarily benefit symptoms of lethargy and depression.

TAKE 5

Environmental Influences

The sympathetic ANS supports the client's ability to monitor the environment for danger. Called vigilance, this normal survival response can be overactive. The environment the massage is conducted in can affect the response to massage. If relaxation is the goal, then the environment needs to feel safe for the client. A quiet, pleasant atmosphere of comfortable temperature with soft lighting and pleasurable music will support relaxation.

Entrainment is the process of synchronization to rhythms. The body entrains to external rhythms such as music in the environment. Any activity that uses a repetitive motion or sound, depending on its rhythmic speed or pace, quiets or excites the nervous system through entrainment and thereby alters the physiology of the body. Sometimes the body rhythms are disrupted. Multiple rhythms and noise out of sync in the same environment are disruptive.

Gate Control Theory

In 1965, Melzack and Wall proposed the gate control theory. Although some aspects of the original theory have been modified over the years, the basic premise remains viable.

According to this theory, a gating mechanism functions at the level of the spinal cord. Pain impulses pass through a "gate" to reach the lateral spinothalamic system. Pain impulses are transmitted by large-diameter and small-diameter nerve fibers. Stimulation of large-diameter fibers prevents the small-diameter fibers from transmitting signals because they travel to the "gate of the spinal cord" first. Stimulation (e.g., rubbing, massage) of large-diameter fibers helps suppress the sensation of pain, especially sharp or visceral pain.

Hyperstimulation Analgesia

Various massage methods, including pressure, positioning, and elongation, provide this stimulation to the large-diameter nerve fibers at sufficient intensity to activate the gating mechanism and produce hyperstimulation analgesia.

Tactile stimulation produced by massage travels through the large-diameter fibers. These fibers also carry a faster signal. In essence, massage sensations win the race to the brain, and pain sensations are blocked because the gate is closed. Stimulating techniques, such as percussion or vibration of painful areas to activate "stimulation-produced analgesia," and hyperstimulation analgesia also are effective. The benefits of reflexology (foot massage) and various manual techniques seem to be mediated by hyperstimulation analgesia. Since pain management is a common massage outcome, these methods are beneficial.

Counterirritation

Counterirritation is a superficial irritation that relieves some irritation of deeper structures. Counterirritation may be explained by the gate control theory. Inhibition in central sensory pathways, produced by rubbing or oscillating (shaking) an area, may explain counterirritation. All methods of massage can be used to produce counterirritation. Any massage method that introduces a controlled sensory stimulation intense enough to be interpreted by the client as a "good pain" signal will work to create counterirritation.

Massage therapy in many forms stimulates the skin over an area of discomfort. Techniques that use friction to the skin and underlying tissue to cause reddening are effective. Many therapeutic ointments contain cooling and warming agents and mild caustic substances (capsicum), which are useful for muscle and joint pain. This is also a form of counterirritation.

NEUROMATRIX THEORY OF PAIN

The neuromatrix theory of pain is an expanded understanding of the pain experience and particularly relevant to chronic pain. It provides a conceptual framework for understanding that the experience of pain is in the brain. Pain perceptions are produced by the output of a widely distributed neural network in the brain, rather than directly by sensory input evoked by injury, inflammation, or other pathology. General massage can be helpful in reeducating the neuromatrix response, thus easing chronic pain sensations.

TAKE 5

FLUID DYNAMICS

The human body consists of approximately 70% water. Water is a constituent of all living things and often is referred to as the universal biologic solvent. The water content of body tissues varies. Adipose tissue (fat) has the lowest percentage of water; the skeleton has the second lowest water content. Skeletal muscle, skin, and the blood include tissues with the highest content of water.

The total water content of the body decreases most dramatically during the first 10 years and continues to decline through old age, at which time water content may account for only 45% of total body weight. Men tend to have higher percentages of water (about 65%) than women (about 55%), mainly because of their increased muscle mass and lower amount of subcutaneous fat.

Water is continuously lost from, and taken into, the body. In a normal healthy human, water input equals water output. Maintaining this equivalence is of prime importance in maintaining health. Approximately 90% of water intake occurs via the gastrointestinal tract (food and liquids). The remaining 10% is called *metabolic water* and is produced as the result of various chemical reactions in the cells of the tissues.

The amount of water lost via the kidneys is under hormonal control. The average amount of water lost and consumed per day is around 2.5 L (approximately 4 1/4 pints) in a healthy adult. Perspiration lost during exercise increases water loss and requires increased water consumption.

The body's water, or fluid, is named for the tubes or compartments that contain it. These fluids include the blood in the vessels and heart, lymph in the lymph vessels, synovial fluid in the joint capsules and bursa sacs, cerebrospinal fluid in the nervous system, and interstitial fluid which surrounds all soft tissue cells. Water is found inside all cells (intracellular fluid). Water is bound by glycoproteins in connective tissue ground substance. The amount of water in connective tissue helps determine its consistency and pliability.

The fluids in the body are moved in waves by pumps, which include the heart, the respiratory diaphragm, the smooth muscle of the vascular and lymph systems, and rhythmic movement of muscles, fascia, and joints. Fluid moves along paths of least resistance from high pressure to low pressure and flows downhill with gravity. Fluid also moves at differing speeds according to other variables present. Therefore, the properties of water must be considered when massage methods are applied. The goal of massage to influence fluid dynamics should attempt to mimic normal physiological function.

Water is in a constant state of motion inside the body, shifting between the two major fluid compartments, which are the lymphatic and circulatory systems. The walls of the blood vessels form a barrier to the free passage of fluid between interstitial areas and blood plasma. In the capillaries, these walls are only 1 cell thick. These capillary walls generally are permeable to water and small solutes but impermeable to large organic molecules such as proteins. Blood plasma tends

to have a higher concentration of these molecules compared with interstitial fluid. Water from the blood moves through the capillary walls into spaces around the cells, thereby becoming interstitial fluid. Much of the interstitial fluid is taken up by the lymphatic system and eventually finds its way back into the bloodstream. Increased interstitial fluid is a common form of edema. Lymphatic drain massage methods support movement of interstitial fluid into the lymph capillaries.

Water and small solutes such as sodium, potassium, and calcium can be exchanged freely between the blood plasma and the interstitial fluid. The action of the kidneys on the blood regulates these electrolytes. This exchange depends mainly on the hydrostatic and osmotic forces of these fluid compartments.

Water can exert a force called *hydrostatic pressure. The force is created* by the weight of water pushing against a surface, as in a dam or in a river or the wall of a blood vessel. The pressure of blood in the capillaries serves as a major hydrostatic force in the human body. Capillary hydrostatic pressure is a filtration force caused when the pressure of the fluid is higher at the arterial end of the capillary than at the venous end. The pressure of the interstitial fluid is negative (−5 mm Hg) because the lymphatic system continuously takes up the excess fluid forced out of the capillaries.

Osmotic pressure is the attraction of water to large molecules such as proteins. Proteins are more abundant in the blood vessels than outside them, so the concentration of proteins in the blood tends to attract water from the interstitial space. Overall, near equilibrium exists between fluid forced out of the capillaries and fluid that is reabsorbed because the lymphatic system collects the excess fluid forced out at the artery ends and eventually drains it back into the two subclavian veins at the base of the neck.

A similar situation exists between the interstitial fluid and the intracellular fluid, although ion pumps and carriers complicate the process. Generally, water movement is substantial in both directions, but ion movement is restricted and depends on active transport via pumps. Nutrients and oxygen, because they are dissolved in water, move passively into cells, whereas waste products and carbon dioxide move out.

TAKE 5

Regulating Fluid Balance

The mechanisms for regulating body fluids are centered in the hypothalamus. The hypothalamus also receives input from the digestive tract that helps control thirst. Antidiuretic hormone (ADH) regulates body fluid volume and extracellular osmosis. ADH influences the body in many ways. One of the major functions of ADH is to increase the permeability of the collecting tubules in the kidneys, which allows more water to be reabsorbed in the kidneys. If the body is lacking fluid intake, as during sleep or during heavy exercise, the result is a concentrated, darker-colored urine of reduced volume. Absence of ADH occurs when the individual is overhydrated. The urine is dilute, pale, or colorless and of high volume.

Primary factors involved in the triggering of ADH production include osmoreceptors and baroreceptors (pressure receptors). Secondary factors include stress, pain, hypoxia, and severe exercise.

Dehydration produced by water loss or lack of fluid intake or relative dehydration in which the body loses no overall water content but rather gains sodium ions stimulates osmoreceptors. The thirst response is connected to the osmoreceptors. How the response actually works is not yet completely understood. Moistening of the mucosal linings of the mouth and pharynx seems to initiate some sort of neurologic response, which sends a message to the thirst center of the hypothalamus. It is perhaps more important that stretch receptors in the gastrointestinal tract appear to transmit nerve messages to the thirst center of the hypothalamus which inhibit the thirst response. Changes in the circulating volume of body fluid also stimulate ADH secretion that results in an increase or decrease in internal pressure monitored by baroreceptors.

A reduction of 8%—10% from the normal body volume of water caused by hemorrhage or excess perspiration results in ADH secretion. Pressure receptors located in the atria of the heart and the pulmonary artery and vein relay their messages to the hypothalamus via the vagus nerve.

Electrolyte Balance

An electrolyte is any chemical that dissociates into ions when dissolved in a solution. Ions can be positively charged (cations) or negatively charged (anions).

The major electrolytes and their charges found in the human body include the following:
- Sodium (Na^+)
- Potassium (K^+)
- Calcium (Ca^{2+})
- Magnesium (Mg^{2+})
- Chloride (Cl^-)
- Phosphate (HPO_4^{2-})
- Sulfate (SO_4^-)
- Bicarbonate (HCO_3^-)

Interstitial fluid and blood plasma are similar in their electrolyte makeup, with sodium and chloride being the major electrolytes. In the intracellular fluid, potassium and phosphate are the major electrolytes. The following information describes the function of electrolytes.

Sodium Balance
Sodium balance plays an important role in the excitability of muscles and neurons and is also crucially important in regulating fluid balance in the body. The kidneys closely regulate sodium levels.

Potassium Balance
Potassium is the major electrolyte of intracellular fluid. Concentration within the cells is 28 times that in the extracellular fluids. As with sodium, potassium is important in the correct functioning of excitable cells such as muscles, neurons, and sensory receptors. Potassium also is involved in the regulation of fluid levels within the cell and in maintaining the correct pH balance within the body. The pH balance of the body also affects potassium levels. In acidosis, potassium excretion decreases, whereas the opposite occurs in alkalosis. Calcium (bicarbonate) increases in alkalosis.

Calcium and Phosphorus Balance
Calcium is found mainly in the extracellular fluids, whereas phosphorus is found mostly in the intracellular fluids. Both are important in the maintenance of healthy bones and teeth. Calcium is also important in the transmission of nerve impulses across synapses, the clotting of blood, and the contraction of muscles. If levels of calcium fall below the normal level, muscles and nerves become more excitable. Phosphorus is required for the synthesis of nucleic acids and high-energy compounds such as adenosine triphosphate. Phosphorus is also important in the maintenance of pH balance. Decreased levels of calcium in the body stimulate the parathyroid gland to secrete parathyroid hormone, causing an increase in the calcium and phosphate levels of the interstitial fluids by releasing them from mineral reservoirs lodged in the bones and the teeth. Parathyroid hormone also decreases calcium excretion by the kidneys. If levels of calcium in the body become too high, the thyroid gland releases a hormone called *calcitonin,* which inhibits the release of calcium and potassium from the bones. Calcitonin also inhibits the absorption of calcium from the gastrointestinal tract and increases calcium excretion by the kidneys.

Magnesium Balance
Most magnesium is found in the intracellular fluid and in bone. Within cells, magnesium functions in the sodium—potassium pump and as an aid to enzyme action. Magnesium plays a role in muscle contraction, action potential conduction, and bone and teeth production. Aldosterone controls magnesium concentrations in the extracellular fluid. Low magnesium levels result in increased aldosterone secretion, and aldosterone increases magnesium reabsorption by the kidneys.

Chloride Balance
Chloride is the most plentiful extracellular electrolyte, with an extracellular concentration 26 times that of its intracellular concentration. Chloride ions diffuse easily across plasma membranes, and their transport is linked closely to sodium movement, which also explains the indirect role of aldosterone in chloride regulation. When sodium is reabsorbed, chloride follows passively. Chloride helps regulate osmotic pressure differences between fluid compartments and is essential in pH balance. The chloride shift within the blood helps move bicarbonate ions out of the red blood cells and into the plasma for transport. In the gastrointestinal system, chlorine and hydrogen combine to form hydrochloric acid.

pH Balance

pH is a measurement of the hydrogen concentration of a solution. Lower pH values indicate a higher hydrogen concentration, or a higher acidity. Higher pH values indicate a lower hydrogen concentration, or a higher alkalinity. Therefore, hydrogen ion balance often is referred to as pH balance, or acid—base balance. Hydrogen ion regulation in the fluid compartments of the body is critically important to health. Even a slight change in hydrogen ion concentration can significantly alter the rate of chemical reactions. Changes in hydrogen ion concentration also can affect the distribution of ions such as sodium, potassium, and calcium, as well as the structure and function of proteins. The normal pH of the arterial blood is 7.4, whereas that of the venous blood is 7.35. The lower pH of the venous blood is caused by the higher concentration of carbon dioxide in the venous blood, which dissolves in water to make a weak acid called *carbonic acid*. When pH changes in the arterial blood, acidosis or alkalosis may result. *Acidosis* is the condition that occurs when the hydrogen ion concentration of the arterial blood increases, and therefore the pH decreases. *Alkalosis* is the condition that occurs when the hydrogen ion concentration in the arterial blood decreases and the pH increases.

Clinical Problems With Fluid Balance

The fluid balance of the body can be upset in many ways, resulting in severe problems and even death.

Dehydration

Dehydration obviously occurs in conditions in which water is unavailable. However, conditions such as diarrhea, severe vomiting, excessive sweating, bleeding, and surgical removal of body fluids also can result in dehydration.

Edema

Edema is an excess of interstitial fluid. This condition often results in tissue swelling and is common whenever lymphatic blockage occurs, or when the lymphatic system, for some other reason, cannot drain the area fast enough. Renal failure, especially the early stages of acute renal failure and the later stages of chronic renal failure, can lead to edema. To test for edema, apply steady pressure with the thumb on the lower leg or other area thought to be affected for 10—20 seconds. If a depression remains after pressure is removed, fluid retention is indicated. This is referred to as *pitting edema*.

Edema is also a symptom of liver and heart failures. Local edema is part of the inflammatory response or can be a protective mechanism, especially in joint dysfunction. A major aspect of massage is support of the body's fluid dynamics. Massage can be targeted to influence the movement of blood, interstitial fluid, and lymph. Important cautions and contraindications may correlate with fluid dysfunction. Cardiac and kidney disease are areas of major concern, as are preeclampsia during pregnancy and side effects from medication.

Massage therapy application can be modified to address simple edema manifesting from logical causes such as sitting or standing for long periods, but severe lymphedema is a pathological condition that requires medical treatment. Lymphedema complications may include:

- Skin infections (cellulitis). The trapped fluid provides fertile ground for germs, and the smallest injury to the arm or leg can be an entry point for infection.
- Sepsis. Untreated cellulitis can spread into the bloodstream and trigger sepsis—a potentially life-threatening condition that occurs when the body's response to an infection damages its own tissues. Sepsis requires emergency medical treatment.
- Leakage through the skin. With severe swelling, the lymph fluid can drain through small breaks in the skin or cause blistering.
- Skin changes. In some people with very severe lymphedema, the skin of the affected limb can thicken and harden so it resembles the skin of an elephant.

TAKE 5

CARDIOVASCULAR SYSTEM

The cardiovascular system is a transport system composed of the heart, blood vessels, and blood. The heart is the pump that sends oxygen and nutrient-rich blood out to the body via the arteries and arterioles. Oxygen and nutrients in the blood leave the capillaries and enter the tissues. Carbon dioxide and metabolic wastes leave the tissues and enter the blood in the capillaries. Venules and veins transport this blood to the lungs, liver, and kidneys. The lungs eliminate carbon dioxide, and the liver and kidneys alter certain substances or eliminate other waste products.

Heart

The heart is the major organ of the cardiovascular system. The heart is a hollow, muscular pump about the size of a fist that is located in the mediastinum—the space between the lungs. The narrow, rounded point of the cone-shaped heart lies just behind the sternum, and the broader, flat base extends slightly to the left of center, near the fifth rib. The *pericardium* is the sac that surrounds and protects the heart and secretes a lubricating fluid that prevents friction caused by the movement of the heart. The pericardium also maintains the location of the heart within the thoracic cavity.

The *myocardium* is cardiac muscle that makes up the thickest part of the heart and generates the contractions. The outer membrane of the heart is called the *epicardium*. The *endocardium* is the smooth, thin, inner lining of the heart. The blood actually slides along the endocardium as it flows through the heart.

The heart is divided into four chambers. The two small, thin-walled upper chambers of the heart are the *atria*, known separately as the *left atrium* and the *right atrium*; these are separated by the interatrial septum. The atria receive blood coming into the heart. The two larger, lower chambers are the left and right ventricles; their thick walls are separated by the interventricular septum. The ventricles pump blood out of the heart. The atria and ventricles are separated by a fibrous structure called the *skeleton of the heart.*

Heart Valves

Created from the folds of the endocardium and maintained within the connective tissue structure of the heart are the heart valves—four sets of valves that regulate the flow of blood through the heart. Atrioventricular valves allow blood to flow into the ventricles from the atria, and they also prevent it from returning into the atria. Strings of connective tissue known as *chordae tendineae cordis* actually connect between the ventricle wall and the valves to help close the valves without letting them collapse backward into the atria. The bicuspid, or mitral (left atrioventricular), valve is located between the left atrium and the left ventricle; the tricuspid (right atrioventricular) valve is located between the right atrium and the right ventricle.

Semilunar valves control the blood flow out of the ventricles into the aorta and pulmonary arteries and prevent any backflow of blood into the ventricles. The aortic valve is between the left ventricle and the aorta, and the pulmonary valve is between the pulmonary artery and the right ventricle. These valves open in response to pressure generated when the blood leaves the ventricle. They close when blood pools in small pockets of the cusps of the valves and pushes the valves closed.

Blood Vessels

The term *blood vessels* refers to the large blood vessels entering or leaving the heart that transport blood to the lungs and the rest of the body. The three great vessels are as follows:

- *Aorta:* The artery that carries oxygen and nutrients away from the heart to the body
- *Pulmonary trunk:* The artery that carries blood to the lungs to release carbon dioxide and take in oxygen
- *Superior vena cava:* The vein that returns poorly oxygenated blood to the right atrium from the upper venous circulation

Other major blood vessels include:

- *Inferior vena cava:* The vein that returns oxygen-poor blood from the lower venous circulation to the right atrium
- *Pulmonary veins:* The four veins, two from each lung, that bring oxygen-rich blood to the left atrium

Blood Supply to the Heart

The two coronary arteries, which originate from the base of the aorta, supply oxygenated blood to the heart muscle.

Coronary veins follow parallel to the arteries and return the blood to the right atrium via the coronary sinus. Both types of coronary vessels run in grooves between the atria and ventricles and between the two ventricles. If either of the coronary arteries is unable to supply sufficient blood to the heart muscle, a heart attack occurs. The most common site of a heart attack is the anterior or inferior part of the left ventricle.

Blood Flow Through the Heart

Blood moves into and out of the heart in a well-coordinated and precisely timed rhythm. For examination purposes, this rhythm can be divided into the following stages:

- *Stage 1:* Deoxygenated blood from the body enters the superior and inferior venae cavae and flows into the right atrium. When the volume of blood in the right atrium reaches a certain volume, it pushes open the tricuspid valve and blood empties into the right ventricle.
- *Stage 2:* The right ventricle contracts and pushes blood through the pulmonary valve into the pulmonary artery. This artery divides into the left and right pulmonary arteries and transports the blood to each lung (these are the only arteries in the body that carry deoxygenated blood). Four pulmonary veins leave the lungs carrying oxygenated blood back to the left atrium (these are the only veins in the body that carry oxygenated blood).
- *Stage 3:* This process takes place at the same time as the process described in stage 1. Blood leaves the left atrium and passes through to the left ventricle via the mitral valve. The left ventricle contracts, and blood pushes through the aortic valve into the aorta. The blood travels through the descending aorta and to all parts of the body except the lungs. The walls of the left ventricle are thicker to provide the extra strength needed to pump blood out to the entire body.

Cardiac Cycle

The heart has its own built-in rhythm. Not only can each cardiac cell contract without nerve stimulus, but the heart can contract even if removed from the body. The ANS does affect the rate of rhythm and force of contraction through sympathetic and parasympathetic activation.

Both atria contract while both ventricles are relaxed, and when the atria relax, the ventricles contract. This synchronization leads to the sequence of events known as the *cardiac cycle.* The cycle consists of one heartbeat, which includes diastole (the relaxation of the ventricles during filling) and systole (the contraction of the ventricles as they empty). Although the heart has an atrial diastole and systole, the stronger ventricular actions are used for identification. Heart rate is identified by the number of cardiac cycles that occur in 1 minute. The average healthy person has 60—70 cycles, or beats, per minute.

The coordinated rhythm of the heart is initiated by the built-in electrical system in the sinoatrial node, which sets the pace of the heart rate. The signal originates in the right atrium and travels to the left atrium, causing the atria to contract. At the precise moment the atria have completed their contraction, the signal travels through the atrioventricular bundle to the right ventricle and into the left ventricle, causing the ventricles to contract. This rhythm can be measured with an electrocardiogram (ECG or EKG), which monitors electrical changes in the heart. A portable electrocardiogram machine, known as a *Holter monitor*, can measure the heart signals over 24 hours. If difficulty with the electrical system develops in the sinoatrial node, physicians can implant a device known as a *pacemaker* to assist with or take over initiation of the signal.

Heart Sounds

Heart sounds can be heard through a stethoscope. Closure of the valves produces two main sounds (valves usually are quiet as they open). The first is a low-pitched "lubb" generated by the swirling of the blood as the mitral and tricuspid valves close. The second is a higher-pitched "dubb" caused by the swirling of the blood as the aortic and pulmonary valves close. **TAKE 5** Extra sounds such as those resulting from faulty valves are referred to as *murmurs*.

Blood Volume and Flow

Cardiac output is the amount of blood pumped by the left ventricle in 1 minute. The average output under normal conditions is 5—6 L of blood. To pump more oxygen and nutrients to the cells during exercise and in times of stress, output may rise to 20 L or more. The speed of the blood flow is fastest in arteries and moderate in veins. The slowest blood movement occurs in the capillaries, to allow for the exchange of nutrients and waste products between tissues and blood.

Vascular System

The *vascular system* is the part of the cardiovascular system consisting of blood vessels that carry blood from the heart to the lungs and body tissues then back to the heart in a continuous cycle. A blood vessel that transports blood from the heart is called an *artery*. Arteries eventually branch off into smaller and smaller arteries, the smallest of which are called *arterioles*. A *capillary* is the smallest type of blood vessel and functions to connect arterioles to *venules* (the smallest of the veins). The veins get larger and larger as they get closer to the heart. The largest veins return blood to the right atrium of the heart.

Arteries

The body has three types of arteries:
- *Elastic arteries* are the large arteries that are capable of undergoing passive stretching. They have thick walls and

recoil when the ventricles relax, which maintains pressure to move the blood. The aorta and pulmonary artery are elastic arteries.
- *Muscular arteries* constitute most of the arteries in the body. These are small- to medium-sized arteries that distribute blood to all tissues by contracting (vasoconstriction), or dilating (vasodilation), to control blood flow. Located between the elastic layers are smooth muscle cells and some collagen. Although the walls of muscular arteries are distensible to a certain extent, as they become smaller and smaller with each successive branching, the amount of elastic tissue decreases, and the muscular component proportionately increases. Arteries are highly contractile, and their degree of contraction or relaxation is controlled by the ANS and by endothelium-derived vasoactive substances. A few fine elastic fibers are scattered among the smooth muscle cells but are not organized into sheets. These are most numerous in the large muscular arteries, which are a direct continuation of the distal end of the elastic arteries. Muscular arteries vary in size from about 1 cm in diameter close to their origin at the elastic arteries to about 0.5 mm in diameter. Muscular arteries are composed almost entirely of smooth muscle. The larger arteries may consist of 30 or more layers of smooth muscle cells, whereas the smallest peripheral arteries have only 2 or 3 layers.
- *Arterioles* are the smallest of the arteries. Any arterial vessel smaller than 0.5 mm in diameter is considered an arteriole. The arterioles offer resistance to blood flow through their small radius, and they are the major site of resistance to blood flow within the vascular network. This area of high resistance to blood flow serves several functions. First, together with the elastic arteries, resistance converts the pulsing ejection of blood from the heart into a steady flow through the capillaries; second, if no resistance were present and a high pressure persisted into the capillaries, considerable loss of blood volume into the tissue would occur by movement of fluid across the capillary wall and around the cells. The arterioles are also important in determining the blood supply to different tissues and regions. They constrict or dilate to control the amount of blood that enters the capillaries.

Massage Application

Massage therapists can increase arterial blood flow by stimulating sympathetic autonomic function to increase the heart rate, providing more push to the blood in the arteries. This action is a reflexive, indirect method that involves the use of homeostatic mechanisms to maintain balance. One can structure massage to be stimulating to the sympathetic ANS. In general, the methods used are brisk and involve active contraction of the muscles coupled with an increased respiratory rate.

Enhancing parasympathetic influences through deep relaxation and encouraging more relaxed diaphragmatic breathing may lead to more balanced pH concentration. Arterial blood flow can be increased mechanically through the pump and tube mechanism of the cardiovascular system, which functions similarly to the fluid dynamics of hydraulics.

Arteries are pliable muscular tubes that carry blood (a fluid) under pressure from the heart pump. Crimping or closing causes pressure to build up between the pump (the heart) and the barrier, like water behind a dam. With removal of the barrier, the buildup of pressure provides an initial extra push to the fluid. Compression over more superficial arteries to temporarily close off the flow of blood results in the same phenomenon. Back pressure builds, and on release of compression, the blood pushes forward with greater force than the heart normally would provide. The massage therapist applies compression against the arteries in the legs and arms to assist peripheral circulation. The rhythm of compression and release occurs at a rate of about 60 beats per minute, to coincide with the heart rhythm. The increase in blood flow is temporary, and in healthy individuals with adequate blood flow, the effect may be negligible.

Veins

The venous system acts as a collecting system, returning blood from the capillary networks to the heart passively down a pressure gradient. The capillaries merge to form venules, which, in turn, unite to form larger but fewer veins, which converge into the venae cavae. The venae cavae empty into the right atrium of the heart. The walls of veins consist of the same three layers as arteries, but the elastic muscle components are much less prominent, and the walls of veins are thinner and more expandable than those of arteries.

The vessels have a large diameter (the inferior vena cava is 2–3 cm in diameter) and thus offer low resistance to blood flow. Some veins, especially those in the arms and legs, include internal folds in the endothelial lining that function as valves and allow blood to flow in one direction only—toward the heart. High venous pressures for long periods can damage these valves by overstretching them, for example, during pregnancy or in persons who stand for extended periods. The valves become weak and lose their function, and varicose veins develop, resulting in edema and varicose ulcers.

A major part of the blood volume, up to 75%, is contained within the venous system, and for this reason, veins sometimes are referred to as *capacity vessels*. Altering the size of the lumen (hollow center) of the venules and veins can modify the capacity of the venous system. These changes are caused by altering the *venomotor tone*, which is the degree of smooth muscle contraction in the vein. Venomotor tone is mainly under the control of the sympathetic nervous system. Changes in venomotor tone can increase or decrease the capacity of the venous circulation and therefore can compensate partially for variations in circulating blood volume.

The veins of the legs contain more valves than the veins of the arms to help fight the effects of gravity and prevent blood from pooling in the feet. Some of the more superficial veins in our hands and arms are visible. All superficial veins empty into the deeper veins which are usually found near arteries.

Venous Return

Venous blood flow occurs along small pressure gradients, and even small variations in resistance and vessel size affect the return flow. The effect of gravity slows venous return. When a person stands upright, the veins are more distended; as the result of hydrostatic pressure produced by a column of blood in the veins below the level of the heart, blood tends to collect or pool in the feet and legs. When the body is vertical, the leg veins take on a circular form that has a greater capacity. When the body is horizontal, the veins take on an elliptical shape with a lower capacity. Increased venomotor tone, which reduces the diameter and hence the capacity of the veins, helps reduce venous pooling. Venous pooling is not blood stagnation but indicates that the veins are accommodating a greater volume of blood.

Maintaining an adequate venous return to the heart at all times is vital because cardiac output depends on venous return (cardiac input). In most instances, the cardiac output equals the venous return. Thus, if the venous return falls, cardiac output and blood pressure also may drop. Several mechanisms are available to help maintain constant venous return. Increasing the venomotor tone is an important mechanism because it decreases the capacity of the venous system and so aids venous return. After a long period of bed rest, when the body is not constantly exposed to the force of gravity and the veins do not have to compensate, venomotor tone is reduced. The therapist should remember this when helping someone up from a massage session. An essential practice is to move the client slowly and steadily while providing support, in case they becomes dizzy and feels faint.

Two systems sometimes referred to as the *skeletal muscle pump* and the *respiratory pump* also assist venous return. Contraction of the skeletal muscles, especially in the limbs, squeezes the veins and pushes blood in the extremities toward the heart; numerous valves prevent backflow. Many communicating channels allow emptying of blood from the superficial limb veins into the deep veins when rhythmic muscular contractions occur. Consequently, every time a person moves the legs or tenses the muscles, these actions push a certain amount of blood toward the heart. The more frequent and powerful such rhythmic contractions are, the more efficient is their action. Sustained continuous muscle contractions, in contrast to rhythmic contractions, impede blood flow through continuous blocking of the veins. The muscle pump mechanism is an efficient system. When an individual stands still for long periods of time, the muscle pump cannot operate, and venous return decreases. The result is that a person may faint because of inadequate cerebral blood flow. Voluntarily contracting and relaxing the muscles of the legs and buttocks aid venous return when one is standing still for long periods.

Respiration produces variations in intrapleural and intrathoracic pressure. Each inspiration lowers the pressure in the thorax and the right atrium of the heart, increases the pressure gradient, and aids blood flow back to the heart; at the same time, movement of the diaphragm into the abdomen raises the intra-abdominal pressure and increases the gradient to the thorax, again favoring venous return. With expiration, the pressure gradients reverse, and blood tends to flow in the opposite direction; fortunately, valves in the medium-sized veins prevent backflow of blood.

Maintaining an adequate circulating blood volume also is necessary. If the blood volume is depleted for some reason, such as dehydration or hemorrhage, the body increases the effective circulating volume over the short term through venoconstriction and vasoconstriction in the blood reservoirs of the body such as the skin, liver, lungs, and spleen. However, restoration of the blood volume eventually requires fluid replacement.

Massage Application

The therapist can incorporate the principles affecting venous return into massage approaches to encourage venous return flow:

- *Muscular pump:* Rhythmic contraction and relaxation of the muscles during movement encourage venous return flow. Restoring normal muscle function and reducing muscle tension supports venous return.
- *Gravity:* Positioning the limbs higher than the heart passively assists venous return flow.
- *Respiratory pump:* Slow, deep diaphragmatic breathing incorporated with or induced by massage modalities enhances venous return flow.
- *Massage application:* Stroking over the veins toward the heart passively moves blood within the veins. This method is particularly effective in the extremities.

The massage therapist can encourage rhythmic contraction of the muscles by having the person move their limbs through a complete range of motion against resistance in a contract-and-relax rhythm of about 60 cycles per minute. The massage therapist then applies short strokes (1 or 2 inches long) over the veins toward the heart at sufficient pressure to push the blood within the superficial veins.

Capillaries (Microvasculature)

Capillaries are composed of small-diameter blood vessels with partly permeable thin walls that permit the transfer of some blood components to the tissues, and vice versa. Capillaries are specialized for diffusion of substances across their walls.

Capillaries, which are the smallest vessels of the blood circulatory system, form a complex interlinking network. Capillaries have the thinnest walls of all blood vessels and are the major sites of gaseous exchange, permitting the transfer of oxygen from blood to tissues, and of carbon dioxide from tissues to blood. Fluids that contain large molecules pass across the capillary walls in both directions. Specialized regions near the junction between the terminal (smallest) arterioles and the capillaries, known as *precapillary sphincters*, consist of a few smooth muscle cells arranged circularly.

Relaxed sphincters allow the capillary beds distal to the sphincters to be open and full of blood. Partially constricted sphincters reduce blood flow to the capillaries, and fully contracted sphincters allow no blood flow.

Some tissues have a much more abundant network of capillaries than others do. For example, dense connective tissue has a poor capillary network compared with cardiac tissue or that of the kidneys and liver.

Another modification in the structure of the microvasculature in tissues is the presence of arteriovenous shunts or arteriovenous anastomoses, which bypass the capillary beds and provide direct connections between the arterial and venous systems. These short, connecting vessels have strongly developed muscular control and are under sympathetic nervous control. They are found in many tissues and organs. In the skin, for example, these connections enable the increase of cutaneous blood flow, which allows dissipation of heat from the body surface during exercise or when exposed to high environmental temperatures.

The capillaries are the most important vessels functionally because they transport essential materials to and from the cells. Efficient exchange between capillary blood and the surrounding tissue fluid occurs because the capillaries are so numerous and so small that blood in the capillaries flows at its slowest rate, which ensures maximum contact time between blood and tissue. This flow of blood through the capillary bed is referred to as *microcirculation*. The capillary network, whatever its form, drains into a series of vessels of increasing diameter to form venules and veins.

Massage Application

The massage therapist can manipulate the network of capillaries with massage, using compression and kneading to encourage movement of blood through the capillaries. **TAKE 5**

Blood Pressure and Pulse

The amount of pressure exerted by the blood on the walls of the blood vessels is called *blood pressure*. Maximal pressure, called *systolic pressure*, occurs when the ventricles contract. *Diastolic pressure* occurs when the ventricles relax. Blood forced into the aorta during systole sets up a pressure wave that travels along the arteries and expands the arterial wall. This expansion can be palpated by pressing the artery against tissue. The number of waves, known as the *pulse*, is a direct reflection of heart rate.

The pulse rate, which is measured when a person is at rest, may be regular or irregular, strong or weak. An irregular pulse occurs commonly with atrial fibrillation and premature contractions. A strong pulse occurs with hyperthyroidism, a weak one with shock and myocardial infarction. A resting heart rate greater than 100 beats per minute is known as *tachycardia*; a heart rate less than 50 or 60 beats per minute is known as *bradycardia*.

The massage therapist can monitor pulses during assessment. In general, pulses should feel bilaterally equal. If the therapist observes differences, he or she should refer the client for diagnosis. The pulse rate ranges from 50 to 70 beats per minute at rest. A rate much slower or faster indicates the need for referral. If the general intent of the massage therapy session is stress management focused toward relaxation with parasympathetic predomination, the pulse rate should slow somewhat over the duration of the session. The opposite is true if the goal is increased arousal of the sympathetic system to energize the client.

Blood pressure is highest during contraction of the heart (systole)—the systolic blood pressure—and is lowest when the heart is relaxed (diastole)—the diastolic pressure. As the vessels become more and more remote from the heart, systolic and diastolic pressures equalize. As the vessels change from arteries to arterioles to capillaries to venules to veins, the pressure decreases, until the pressure may be zero or negative in the large veins. For this reason, when venous blood is drawn, the syringe has to be pulled back.

Blood pressure is measured with a sphygmomanometer. It is recorded as millimeters of mercury (mm Hg), which refers to the number of millimeters of mercury displaced by the changes in pressure. The first number is the systolic pressure, and the second number is the diastolic pressure. When the pressure is recorded, only the numbers are used, and the unit of measure mm Hg usually is dropped.

Sympathetic nerves to the arterioles regulate blood pressure. Normally, arterioles are in a state of partial constriction, called *arteriole tone*. Stimulation of the sympathetic system causes further arteriolar constriction and an increase in blood pressure. Nonstimulation results in a decrease in blood pressure. With hypertension, the sympathetic system is in a state of continuous stimulation, resulting in constant high blood pressure.

Normal Blood Pressure Range

Blood pressure depends on the person's size and age. The average newborn has a blood pressure of 90/60; at 15 years of age, the average blood pressure is about 120/60. An average, healthy young adult has a blood pressure of less than 120/80. Generally, a blood pressure lower than 100/60 is considered hypotension; between 120/80 and 140/90 is considered prehypertension; and a pressure above 140/90 is considered hypertension. Blood pressure changes under various conditions; a single reading should never be used as a final determinant. A systolic increase occurs in temporary conditions such as anxiety and exercise. Hypertension involves an increase in the systolic and diastolic pressures. Hypotension is a decrease in the systolic and diastolic pressures and is an important manifestation of shock, which results from an inadequate blood supply to vital organs.

Massage Application

Stress management programs include methods of movement and moderate aerobic exercise, stretching programs, massage, and other soft tissue methods. Although these approaches initially elevate blood pressure, when continued, they activate parasympathetic responses such as slow deep breathing, and

progressive relaxation; they therefore tend to have a normalizing effect on the blood pressure. These methods are classified as *nonspecific constitutional approaches*; they allow the homeostatic mechanisms to reset to a more effective functional pattern after disruption.

Fluid Flow

The flow of a fluid through a vessel is determined by the pressure difference between the two ends of the vessel, as well as the resistance to flow. For any fluid to flow along within a vessel, a pressure difference must exist; otherwise, the fluid will not move. In the cardiovascular system, the pumping of the heart generates the "pressure head," or force, and a continuous drop in pressure occurs from the left ventricle of the heart to the tissues and from the tissues back to the right atrium of the heart. Without this drop in blood pressure, no blood would flow through the circulatory system. Resistance is the measure of the ease with which a fluid flows through a tube. The easier the flow, the less is the resistance to flow, and vice versa. In the cardiovascular system, resistance usually is described as vascular resistance because it originates primarily in the peripheral blood vessels and is known simply as *peripheral resistance*.

Resistance is essentially a measure of the friction between the molecules of the fluid, and between the tube wall and the fluid. The resistance depends on the viscosity of the fluid and the radius and length of the tube.

Viscosity is a measure of the tendency of a liquid to resist flow. The greater the viscosity (thickness) of a fluid, the greater is the force required to move that liquid. For example, water has less viscosity than a milkshake.

Medulla and Baroreceptors

In the medulla oblongata of the brain, the cells of the reticular formation regulate three vital signs: heart rate, blood pressure, and respiration. They work with signals from various nerve centers in the body. One type of nerve center in the cardiovascular system is the baroreceptor.

Baroreceptors are stretch receptors in the carotid arteries, the aorta, and nearly every large artery of the neck and thorax. When blood pressure increases, arteries stretch. Baroreceptors transmit signals about sudden, brief changes in blood pressure such as when the body changes position. When blood pressure is elevated for a long period, the baroreceptor reflex resets to the new blood pressure level.

When blood pressure suddenly drops, the frequency of signals from the baroreceptors declines. This change sets off a response in the cardioregulatory center of the medulla that increases sympathetic stimulation and decreases parasympathetic stimulation, resulting in an increase in heart rate and blood pressure. Conversely, when blood pressure increases, the signal increases and the medulla oblongata changes its output to slow the heart rate and blood pressure by increasing parasympathetic signals. This is an example of a negative feedback system in the body.

Stimulation of baroreceptors during therapeutic massage could affect blood pressure. The blood pressure could drop, and the client may be light-headed and show other signs of low blood pressure.

Names of Specific Arteries and Veins

The names of most arteries and veins are derived from the anatomic structure they serve. The femoral artery and the femoral vein, for example, are found close to the femur, where these blood vessels serve the tissue of the upper and lower leg. The renal artery is so named because it exits the abdominal aorta and enters the kidney. The renal vein exits the kidney and enters the inferior vena cava. Arteries and veins are found on both sides of the body and are identified as right or left (e.g., the right common carotid artery, the left common carotid artery).

The following is a list of the main arteries and veins:

- The *common carotid artery* is an important pulse-taking artery; damage to this artery may result in a transient ischemic attack.
- The *superficial temporal artery* is a pulse-taking artery located superior and anterior to the ear.
- The *brachial artery* is the main artery for measuring blood pressure and is also a pulse-taking artery. The brachial artery divides at the elbow region into the ulnar and radial arteries, which are also pulse-taking arteries.
- The *ulnar artery* lies deep and medial. The *radial artery* lies more superficial and lateral. Both arteries communicate in the hand via two deep anastomoses and a superficial and deep palmar arch.
- The *dorsalis pedis* is an important pulse-taking artery located on the foot.
- The *great saphenous vein* ascends medially from the foot up the leg to the thigh and drains into the femoral vein. The great saphenous veins may become chronically dilated in some persons and develop into varicose veins. They then may become inflamed and form blood clots, a condition known as *thrombophlebitis*.

The deep veins of the leg may become inflamed, a condition referred to as *deep vein thrombosis*, which is a more serious condition than superficial thrombophlebitis. The clot may break off and travel to the heart and then lodge in the lung as a pulmonary embolism.

Hepatic Portal System

Any portal system is defined by the fact that blood drains from one venous system to another without the presence of arteries between the two. The hepatic portal system begins in the capillaries of the digestive organs and ends in the portal vein. Restriction of outflow through the hepatic portal system can lead to portal hypertension. Portal hypertension is most often associated with cirrhosis. The liver receives approximately 30% of resting cardiac output and is therefore a vascular organ. The hepatic vascular system has a considerable ability to store and release blood and functions as a reservoir within the general circulation.

In the normal situation, 10%—15% of total blood volume is in the liver, with roughly 60% of that in the sinusoids. With loss of blood, the liver dynamically adjusts its blood volume and can eject enough blood to compensate for a moderate amount of hemorrhage. Conversely, when vascular volume increases acutely, as with rapid infusion of fluids, the hepatic blood volume expands, providing a buffer against acute increases in systemic blood volume.

Blood

Blood transports nutrients to the individual cells and removes waste products. Whole blood consists of solid elements (cells and platelets) and the liquid matrix (plasma).

Red blood cells, white blood cells, and platelets are the formed elements of blood which float in the plasma—a thick, straw-colored fluid. Amino acids, carbohydrates, electrolytes, hormones, lipids, proteins, vitamins, and waste materials are the other constituents of blood. A person who weighs 140—150 pounds has about 5 quarts of blood.

In an adult, blood cells form mainly in the red marrow of the bones of the chest, vertebrae, and pelvis. Yellow marrow can convert to red marrow if the body requires increased production of blood cells. The stages of blood cell development in red marrow constitute a process called *hematopoiesis*. Blood cells originate from a common precursor cell called the *stem cell*. Immature blood cells are blast cells. When the cells are mature, they move into the bloodstream. In persons with leukemia, blast cells may be seen in peripheral blood because the body sends them out before they are mature.

Red Blood Cells

Red blood cells, also known as *erythrocytes* or *red blood corpuscles*, make up more than 90% of the formed elements in blood. Because red blood cells cannot divide, they must be produced frequently to replace dead cells. A red blood cell loses its nucleus and most of its organelles during development. Red bone marrow produces enough red blood cells daily to replace dead blood cells. The body needs proper intake and assimilation of iron, vitamin B_{12}, and folic acid to produce new red blood cells.

Erythrocytes contain an iron-protein compound known as *hemoglobin*. Oxygen binds to hemoglobin in the capillaries of the lungs and is transported to all parts of the body. A lack of oxygen, or anemia, can stimulate *erythropoiesis*, the production of red blood cells. Red blood cells also transport a small amount of carbon dioxide from the tissues of the body to the lungs. An abnormal increase in red blood cells is known as *polycythemia*; an abnormal decrease is called *anemia*.

White Blood Cells

White blood cells are also called *leukocytes*, or *white blood corpuscles*. The main function of white blood cells is to protect the body from pathogens and remove dead cells and substances. White blood cells are divided into the following five groups:

- *Neutrophils:* Neutrophils are granular leukocytes; more than 50% of all white blood cells are neutrophils. These cells fight disease by engulfing bacteria in a cell-eating process called *phagocytosis*, which is the ingestion and digestion of particles by a cell. Neutrophils are important in defense of the body against bacterial infection. A buildup of neutrophils and the debris they collect is called *pus*.
- *Lymphocytes:* Lymphocytes account for about 30% of the total number of white blood cells in the body. They produce antibodies and chemicals that are active in regulating disease and allergic reactions and in controlling tumors.
- *Monocytes:* Monocytes are the largest of the white blood cells, yet they account for only about 6% of the total number. They also protect the body through phagocytosis. Monocytes are unique because when they leave the blood and enter the tissues, they can develop into large phagocytic cells called *macrophages*.
- *Eosinophils:* About 3% of the total white blood cell count is made up of eosinophils. However, the number increases greatly with parasitic infections or allergic reactions (e.g., hay fever). Eosinophils are capable of phagocytic activity, and they release chemicals during the inflammatory process.
- *Basophils:* Basophils are also granular white blood cells, and they make up about 1% of the total white blood cell count. Their exact function is not yet understood clearly.

Platelets

- Thrombocytes, also called *platelets*, are the smallest cellular elements of the blood. They are important in the blood clotting process, which prevents blood loss from injury.

Clotting

Damage to a blood vessel causes the release of chemicals. Special proteins, called *clotting factors*, are activated which then form additional clotting factors. A special protein called *fibrin* forms and seals the damaged blood vessels by trapping red blood cells, platelets, and fluid to form a clot. Fibrin then anchors the clot. The clotting process starts the instant the blood vessel is damaged and takes only a few minutes to complete. Calcium and vitamin K are important to the success and speed of the clotting process.

Plasma

Plasma is the straw-colored liquid found in blood and lymph; it is about 90% water, and the rest consists of nutrients, gases, and waste products. Plasma constitutes about 55% of blood and plays a major role in the movement of water between the tissues and the blood.

Pathologic Conditions

Cardiovascular disease is the leading cause of death in Western societies. Cardiac arrest may occur because of several conditions, the most common being a heart attack (myocardial infarction).

Massage Application

In general, cardiovascular disease presents contraindications for therapeutic massage. If the contraindication does not arise from the disease itself, the medication taken to control the disease may pose problems. Anticoagulant medication, for example, increases the possibility of bruising and hemorrhage. Nonetheless, therapeutic massage often is indicated as part of a supervised treatment program. The outcomes of general stress management and homeostatic normalization are desirable for most cardiovascular difficulties. The key is supervision by a qualified healthcare provider. Because the management of cardiovascular diseases can be complex, all treatments should be accounted for as part of a total therapeutic program.

TAKE 5

RESPIRATORY SYSTEM

Of all the basic life support systems in the body, the respiratory system is the only one under voluntary and automatic control. The respiratory system obtains the oxygen necessary to create energy for body functions and to eliminate carbon dioxide produced during cellular metabolism. Considerable voluntary control can be exercised over respiratory movements, most often in connection with speech. Respiration and breath are connected intimately to the expression of emotion, as in laughing or crying, the explosive burst in anger, holding one's breath in fear, and the sigh of relief. This voluntary control of breathing allows regulation of the ANS. Therefore, control of breathing becomes important in many relaxation and meditation practices.

In terms of vital functions, the respiratory system may be considered the most important because the heart and brain require a continuous supply of oxygen to function. Apnea, the lack of spontaneous breathing, can cause irreversible brain damage if it continues for longer than 3 or 4 minutes.

Respiration is the movement of air into and out of the lungs, and the exchange of oxygen and carbon dioxide between the lungs and blood and between blood and body tissues. *Breathing* is a mechanical action of inhalation and exhalation that draws oxygen into the lungs and releases carbon dioxide into the atmosphere. *External respiration* is the exchange of oxygen and carbon dioxide between the lungs and the bloodstream. The exchange of gases between the cells and the blood is called *internal respiration*. The organs of the respiratory system are divided into upper and lower regions. The upper respiratory tract consists of the nasal cavity, all its structures, and the pharynx; the lower respiratory tract consists of the larynx, trachea, and bronchi and alveoli in the lungs.

Lungs

The two lungs are the primary organs of respiration. These soft, spongy, highly vascular structures are separated into left and right lungs by the mediastinum. Each lung is separated into lobes. The right lung has three lobes: an upper, middle, and lower; the left has two lobes: an upper and lower.

The lobar bronchi, which extend from the trachea, each divide into 10 segmental bronchi, which further divide. The amount of cartilage in each tube gradually decreases until the tubes lack cartilage. At this point, the tubes are about 1 mm in diameter and are known as the *bronchioles*, which terminate in the air sacs, or *alveoli*. Capillaries surround the alveoli, and this is where external respiration takes place.

The lungs are enclosed in a pleural cavity lined with two pleural membranes. One connects directly to the lung, and the other attaches to the mediastinum and inside chest wall. This cavity created by the membranes contains approximately 1/2 tsp of lubricating fluid, which reduces friction between the two layers during breathing. Increases in the amount of fluid often occur with diseases such as lung cancer and pulmonary edema and can make breathing difficult. *Pneumothorax* is a condition in which air enters the pleural cavity as a result of trauma or rupture of part of the lung, causing the lung to be no longer able to function. This can be caused by a penetrating injury such as from a bullet or knife or in disease processes such as emphysema. A chest tube called a *thoracostomy tube* inserted between the ribs and connected to a pump removes the air. In hemothorax, physicians can drain blood in the pleural space in a similar manner.

Nerves and Vessels of the Lungs and Respiratory Muscles

The ANS supplies the bronchi and bronchioles. Stimulation of the vagus nerve (parasympathetic) causes contraction of the smooth muscles and narrows the diameter of the tubes (bronchoconstriction). Stimulation of sympathetic nerves initiates smooth muscle relaxation, resulting in widening of the tubes (bronchodilation).

The nerve supply to the intercostal muscles is derived from spinal nerves T1 to T11. The phrenic nerve originates at C3 to C5 and innervates the diaphragm. The reason that the nerve supply originates so distant is that during fetal development, the diaphragm actually begins its growth in the neck and then descends from the neck to the abdomen. A broken neck that injures the spinal cord below C5 still allows the person to breathe because the diaphragm is responsible for the majority of inhalation. Injury to both phrenic nerves or a spinal cord injury above C3 to C5 severely compromises breathing.

The pulmonary arteries and veins participate in the exchange of oxygen and carbon dioxide between the capillaries and alveoli. Branches of the aorta and upper intercostal arteries supply blood to most of the lung tissue. Venous drainage occurs from the azygos vein on the right side of the thorax, and from the first intercostal vein on the left.

Mechanics of Breathing

During the seconds before taking a breath, the pressure inside the lungs and outside the body is equal, whereas the pressure inside the pleural space is slightly lower. When inhalation begins, the external intercostal muscles between the ribs contract, thereby lifting the lower ribs up and out. This creates a vacuum that expands the lungs, causing pressure inside the lungs to decrease. The diaphragm moves down, increasing the volume of the pleural cavities and further decreasing lung pressure. Elastic fibers in the alveolar walls stretch, permitting expansion of the air sacs. The lungs draw air in until the pressure is equal again.

During exhalation, the pressure inside the pleural cavity increases; the external intercostals, diaphragm, and alveolar walls relax; the volume inside the lungs decreases; and the pressure in the lungs increases until it again equals the atmospheric pressure.

In diseases such as asthma, bronchitis, and emphysema, accessory muscles of respiration are often used. Contraction of the sternocleidomastoid and other muscles of the neck aids inspiration, whereas use of the internal intercostals and abdominal muscles aids expiration.

Lung Volumes

Breathing in and out changes the volume of air in the lungs. Four different pulmonary volumes can be measured to use as guidelines in health assessment. The *tidal volume* is the amount of air taken in or exhaled in a single breath during normal breathing, usually while resting. The *inspiratory reserve volume* is the amount of air inhaled forcefully after normal tidal volume inspiration, whereas the *expiratory reserve volume* is the amount of air exhaled forcefully after a normal exhalation. The *reserve volume* is the amount of air that remains in the lungs and passageways after a maximal expiration. The *vital capacity* is the total of the tidal volume, inspiratory reserve volume, and expiratory reserve volume. In the normal, healthy adult lung, vital capacity usually ranges from 3.5 to 5.5 L of air.

In lungs with diseases such as asthma and emphysema, the vital capacity and expiratory reserve volumes are abnormal. A person with asthma, for example, may have a normal tidal volume and vital capacity but decreased expiratory reserve volume, whereas a person with emphysema may have a normal (but often decreased) tidal volume and decreased vital capacity and expiratory reserve volume. Both conditions result in ineffective exhalation.

Transport of Oxygen and Carbon Dioxide

The exchange of oxygen and carbon dioxide takes place by diffusion. In the lungs, carbon dioxide diffuses from the bloodstream through the capillary and alveolar membranes for exhalation by the lungs. Oxygen diffuses in the opposite direction, from the alveoli through both membranes and into the bloodstream.

The pulmonary veins, the only veins to carry oxygenated blood, return it to the left atrium. The oxygenated blood moves from the left atrium into the left ventricle, which pumps it into the aorta. Arteries branch off the aorta and spread to different parts of the body. As the arteries branch, they become smaller and smaller until they enter tissues as arterioles. Arterioles branch into capillaries.

Red blood cells transport oxygen in the blood as oxyhemoglobin. At the arteriole end of the capillary, oxygen leaves the red blood cell and then passes through the capillary membrane into the interstitial fluid. Oxygen then diffuses through the cell membrane to be used for cellular metabolism. Carbon dioxide moves out of the cell in the reverse direction,

The venule end of the capillary joins with venules, which join with small, then large veins. All veins eventually empty the deoxygenated blood into the superior and inferior venae cavae, which empty into the right atrium. Blood moves from the right atrium into the right ventricle, which pumps it into the pulmonary trunk. The pulmonary trunk branches into pulmonary arteries, the only arteries to carry deoxygenated blood, which transport the blood to the lungs. The bicarbonate ion releases carbon dioxide, which diffuses from the bloodstream into the alveoli so it can be exhaled from the lungs.

TAKE 5

Control of Breathing

The *respiratory center* is a group of nerve cells in the medulla oblongata and pons. A variety of stimuli affect the respiratory center. Impulses from the cerebral cortex under voluntary control modify respiration, as do changes in the carbon dioxide content and acidity of blood and cerebrospinal fluid. Chemoreceptors, nerve cells found near the baroreceptors, are sensitive to the oxygen level and to a lesser extent to carbon dioxide and pH levels in the bloodstream. Two chemoreceptors are located near the arch of the aorta (aortic bodies), and one is in each carotid artery (carotid bodies). The aortic bodies transmit impulses to the respiratory center in the medulla through the vagus nerve; the carotid bodies transmit by way of the glossopharyngeal nerve. A low concentration of oxygen in the body stimulates the chemoreceptors, and the respiratory rate increases.

Respiratory Rate

The respiratory rate in adults is about 12–16 breaths per minute, and in the newborn it is about 35, gradually decreasing to adult values at about age 20. Emotions are a powerful stimulus for respiratory change. Fear, grief, and shock slow the rate, whereas excitement, anger, and sexual arousal increase the respiratory rate.

Besides the effects of emotions, changes in breathing rates can occur as a result of increased oxygen requirement from exercise, due to obesity as a result of increased vessel resistance, during infection and fever because of increased energy requirements, in heart failure from decreased oxygen flow, during pain because of increased nervous stimulation, with anemia because of decreased oxygen transport, in

hyperthyroidism from an increase in metabolic rate, and during emphysema as a result of blockage of oxygen.

Hyperpnea is fast breathing, and *tachypnea* is rapid, shallow breathing. This type of breathing can lead to acute hyperventilation or chronic overbreathing called *breathing pattern disorder*, which causes a variety of signs and symptoms, as discussed later in this section.

Bradypnea, or slow breathing, occurs in alcohol and other depressant drug intoxication states because of the depressant action on the brain. Bradypnea also occurs as the result of increased intracranial pressure from pressure on the respiratory center and during a diabetic coma.

Periods of hyperpnea alternating with periods of apnea (no breathing) sometimes occur during the sleep of infants, particularly premature ones. These patterns also appear in brain injury and in the terminally ill.

Reflexes That Affect Breathing

Foreign matter or irritants in the trachea or bronchi stimulate the cough reflex. The epiglottis and glottis reflexively close, and contraction of the expiratory muscles causes air pressure in the lungs to increase. The epiglottis and glottis open suddenly, resulting in an upward force of air in a cough that removes the offending contaminants in the throat.

The sneeze reflex is similar to the cough reflex, except contaminants or irritants in the nasal cavity provide the stimulus. A burst of air moves through the nose and mouth, forcing contaminants out of the respiratory tract.

A *hiccup* is an involuntary, spasmodic contraction of the diaphragm that causes the glottis to close suddenly, producing a characteristic sound.

A *yawn* is a slow, deep inspiration through the open mouth. Scientists still have not found the actual physiologic mechanism for yawning.

Pathologic Conditions

Respiratory disease is a major healthcare concern. The respiratory system is vulnerable to infection. Chronic disease is also common. Massage application for respiratory disease typically is involved with supporting the mechanisms of breathing.

Any of the listed disorders of the respiratory system of viral or bacterial origin are usually contraindicated for massage until the disease runs its course. Whenever the body is under stress, as with respiratory infection, further stress in the system can worsen the condition. Simple palliative measures to provide comfort and encourage sleep are appropriate. The practitioner should follow all sanitary procedures and standard precautions.

In chronic conditions such as asthma or emphysema, general stress management and maintenance of normal respiratory muscle function is beneficial. Always gauge that the added stress of massage stimulation is appropriate. In cystic fibrosis, percussion helps loosen the phlegm but should not be attempted without medical supervision and training.

Disordered breathing occurs when the inhale is longer than the exhale, oxygen intake exceeds physical demand, and accessory muscles are used excessively. Almost every meditation or relaxation system uses breathing patterns because they are a direct link to altering ANS patterns, which, in turn, alters mood, feelings, and behavior. Therapeutic massage approaches and moderate application of movement therapies such as tai chi, yoga, or aerobic exercise often help breathing pattern disorder.

The shoulders should not move during normal breathing. Activation of the accessory muscles of respiration located in the neck area should only occur when increased oxygen is required for fight or flight. This is the pattern for sympathetic breathing. If the person does not use the additional oxygen through increased activity levels, blood gas levels change and symptoms appear. Constant activation of the accessory muscles of respiration such as the scalenes, sternocleidomastoid, serratus posterior superior, levator scapulae, rhomboids, abdominals, and quadratus lumborum will result in dysfunctional muscle patterns related to forced inhalation and expiration. Therapeutic massage and general stress management techniques can reduce anxiety and bring balance into these areas to encourage a more effective breathing pattern—specifically diaphragmatic "belly" breathing.

Although detailed discussion of the many meditations, breathing modulators, or retraining measures is beyond the scope of this text, two basic types of systems exist: one leading to physiologic hyperarousal and one to hypoarousal. Both processes facilitate the reestablishment of homeostasis, just as a muscle can be encouraged to relax by tensing it first and then releasing it, or by using the antagonist pattern to initiate reciprocal inhibition to allow the muscle to relax. Hyperarousal systems increase sympathetic activity with a secondary parasympathetic balance. Aerobic exercise is an example. Hypoarousal systems directly activate parasympathetic responses. Examples include quiet reflection and meditative methods combined with slow exhalation during breathing.

 TAKE 5

MUSCLE SKELETAL SYSTEM AND CONNECTIVE TISSUE

Mechanical characteristics of contractile and noncontractile tissue, as well as the neurophysiologic properties of contractile tissue, determine how soft tissue functions.

When soft tissue is stretched, elastic or plastic changes occur. *Elasticity* is the ability of soft tissue to return to its resting length after passive stretch. *Plasticity* is the tendency of soft tissue to assume a new and greater length after the stretch force has been removed. Both contractile and noncontractile tissues have elastic and plastic qualities.

The soft tissues that can restrict joint motion are muscles, connective tissue, and skin. When stretching procedures are applied to these soft tissues, the speed, intensity, and duration of the force creating tension stress, as well as the temperature of the soft tissues, all affect how these tissues respond. Other qualities of touch applied during massage—depth of pressure, direction, duration, rhythm, speed, frequency, and drag—also affect how soft tissues respond.

Muscle is composed primarily of contractile tissue but is attached to and interwoven with the noncontractile tissues of tendon and fascia. The connective tissue framework in muscle, not its contractile components, is the primary source of resistance to passive elongation of muscle.

Adhesions can develop after an impact injury, wounds, or surgery. Because the superficial fascia in the dermis is connected to the underlying deep fascia coverings of the muscles, these adhesions decrease soft tissue mobility. Adhesions in the superficial fascia can also entrap the cutaneous nerves, leading to pain, numbness, and tingling. Accumulative change to the tissue pliability is problematic.

How massage and stretching increase tissue pliability and length is still not fully understood. The response of tissue to excessive mechanical force can result in injury. However, if these same mechanical forces are applied in a purposeful and controlled manner during massage, the client benefits.

Connective Tissue

Connective tissue consists of hard and soft tissues. It forms the structures of the organs and blood vessels and binds joints together through ligaments and joint capsules. It forms tendons, which transmit muscle fiber contractions to produce movement. Strains of muscles or tendons, and sprains of ligaments are common injuries that damage the connective tissue.

Connective tissue, which forms tensegritic tension lines that traverse the body in many directions, is made up of ground substance and fibers. Ground substance is a transparent, viscous fluid (like raw egg whites) that surrounds all the cells in the body. It is formed from glycosaminoglycans (GAGs) and water. GAGs draw water into the tissue and bind it. Water makes up approximately 70% of ground substance. Think of ground substance as Silly Putty, wallpaper paste, or Jell-O. Ground substance is a source of nutrition and a carrier for waste products resulting from cellular function. It is a lubricant and a spacer between collagen fibers that prevents the fibers from adhering to each other. Ground substance has a thixotropic quality. Thixotropy pertains to a substance that becomes more fluid when agitated and more solid when still. Heat and agitation create a change in the ground substance from thick and stiff to a more fluid or pliable state.

With disuse and immobilization, the tissues become cool, and the ground substance becomes thicker and more gel-like. Stiffness and aching, decreased circulation and nutrition, and decreased lubrication result. Theoretically massage therapy can change the viscosity of the ground substance from a gel to a more fluid state through the introduction of mechanical forces.

Active and passive movement of tissues during massage stimulates the synthesis of ground substance and GAGs, promotes the circulation of blood and lymph, and supports ground substance pliability, creating increased lubrication to the tissue. Tissue movement also transports nutrients and promotes the exchange of waste products.

Chondrocytes, a type of cartilage cell, are found in the collagen matrix of cartilage. Chondrocytes synthesize new cartilage in the normal turnover of cells and in the repair of damaged cartilage. Chondrocytes are involved with joint illness, injury, and repair.

Osteocytes, or the bone cells, transport materials to maintain the structure of the bones and are active in the repair of bone. Piezoelectric effects support bone repair and guide the tensegritic nature of bone formation. *Piezoelectricity* is the ability of a tissue to generate electrical potentials in response to the pressure of mechanical deformation. Piezoelectricity is a property of most, if not all, living tissues.

Reticular fibers form a mesh network that supports organs and glands. Elastin fibers are more elastic than collagen and are found in ligaments and the linings of arteries. Collagen forms approximately 80% of tendons, ligaments, and joint capsules, and a large percentage of cartilage and bone, providing shape to the soft tissue. It forms the structural support for the skin, muscles, blood vessels, and nerve fibers. Normal stresses in the form of exercise and activities of daily living increase collagen synthesis and strengthen connective tissue. This is an important aspect of fitness, especially for the elderly.

Collagen stabilizes the joints through the ligaments, joint capsules, and periosteum by resisting the tension or pulling force transmitted through the joints by movement or gravity. Collagen transmits the pulling force of muscle contraction through the fascia within the muscle as well as the tendon attachment. Collagen fibers tend to orient to parallel and longitudinal alignment along the lines of mechanical stress imposed by loading of the tissue during activity. Normal gliding/sliding of collagen fibers is maintained by movement and lubrication from connective tissue ground substance.

Immobilization or lack of use decreases collagen production, leading to atrophy in the connective tissue and to osteoporosis in the bone. Without movement, collagen is laid down in a random orientation, with the fibers packed close together, forming microadhesions. *Adhesions* are abnormal deposits of connective tissue between gliding surfaces. This atrophy and random orientation of the fibers create weakness in the tissue and instability of the associated joint. This condition is more common in those who are just beginning a fitness regimen and increases injury potential. The aging process decreases the amount and quality of the collagen structure; therefore, exercise helps to prevent age-related soft tissue dysfunction.

Too much mechanical and repetitive stress results in excessive deposits of collagen, causing abnormal cross-fiber links and adhesions. The fibers pack closer together, lubrication decreases, and the water content of ground substance is reduced. This, in turn, decreases the ability of the fibers and fascicles to slide relative to each other. This condition is often called *fibrosis.*

Massage may mechanically deform the collagen fibers by introducing bind, shear, torsion, compression, and tension loading.

Tendons

Tendons are a continuation of the connective tissue within the muscle. They attach muscle to bone by weaving into the connective tissue covering of the bone called the *periosteum.* Tendons transmit the force of muscle contraction to the bone, thereby producing motion of the joint. They also help stabilize the joint and act as a sensory receptor through Golgi tendon organs. Tendons consist of long spiraling bundles of parallel collagen fibers, oriented in a longitudinal pattern along the line of force stress, and are embedded in ground substance with a small number of fibroblasts. Tendons have a microscopic "crimp" or wavelike structure that acts like a spring, enabling them to withstand large internal forces. The musculotendinous junction is where the muscle fibers end and the connective tissue that forms the tendon begins. This area is vulnerable to injury. Tendons may be cordlike, such as the Achilles tendon; a flattened band of tissue, such as the rotator cuff; or a broad sheet of tissue called an *aponeurosis*, such as the attachment of the latissimus dorsi. They are surrounded by a loose connective tissue sheath. In areas of high pressure or fiction, such as where tendons rub over the bones of the wrist and ankle, the tendon sheath is lined with a synovial layer to facilitate gliding.

A *strain* is an injury to muscle and/or tendon. Tendon strains are tears of the collagen fibers occurring at the musculotendinous junction, the tenoperiosteal junction, or within the body of the tendon. Loss of normal motion in a tendon through illness and injury or immobilization creates loss of collagen fibers and adhesions between the tendon and surrounding structures, including the tendon sheath.

Ligaments

Ligaments attach bones at joints, help stabilize joints, and help guide joint motion, prevent excessive motion, and act as sensory receptors. Ligaments are composed of dense, white, short bands of nearly parallel bundles of collagen fibers embedded in a matrix of ground substance and a small number of fibroblasts. They contain some elastic fibers and a "crimp" structure, giving them greater elasticity, and are pliable and flexible. All ligaments surrounding the joints contain proprioceptors, mechanoreceptors, and pain receptors, which provide information about posture and movement that plays an important role in joint function.

Under normal conditions, when the joint moves, the ligament is stretched and the crimp in the tissue straightens out. The ligament returns to its normal length when the joint returns to a neutral position. If sustained mechanical tension or force is slowly applied to a ligament consistently and is sustained, the tissue assumes the new length because of its viscous nature. This condition can lead to overstretched or lax ligaments that compromise stability of the joint. Because ligaments stabilize joints and act as neurosensory structures, injuries to ligaments can create dysfunction of the joint and surrounding soft tissue. There is a reflex connection between

TAKE 5

the ligaments of a joint and the surrounding muscles, which affects muscle tone. In the case of lax ligaments, tone in muscles reflexively increases to provide joint stability.

A *sprain* is an injury to ligaments resulting in overstretched or torn collagen fibers. Repeated sprains may result in permanent joint instability. This is a common issue associated with ankle dysfunction.

The joint capsule and the ligaments typically respond to injury by becoming stretched, with resulting joint instability. However, these structures can also shorten, resulting in loss of a joint's normal range of motion and joint stiffness. Immobilization causes ligaments to atrophy and weaken, which changes the normal gliding motion of the joint. Ligaments can twist into abnormal positions. Irritation or injury of the ligaments usually causes a reflexive contraction or inhibition in the surrounding muscles. Muscle energy methods that address gait and muscle activation sequence firing patterns can help restore normal function temporarily because the muscle is connected to the ligaments with a neurologic reflex. However, the condition will continue to occur because the instability of the joint is the underlying causal factor.

Injured ligaments can become thick and fibrous from increased collagen formation, abnormal cross-fiber links, and adhesions. This is especially common if inflammatory responses are slow to resolve or have remained chronic.

Massage applied to ligaments that have developed adhesions is performed across the fiber direction to increase pliability and realign fiber structure. If ligaments are too lax, exercise and rehabilitation can stimulate the production of new collagen and help restore normal joint integrity. External stabilization such as braces and other types of supports can be used if necessary. Friction massage can be used to create small, controlled inflammation in the ligament structure to stimulate collagen production as well.

Periosteum

Periosteum is a dense, fibrous connective tissue sheath that covers the bones. The outer layer consists of collagen fibers parallel to the bone and contains arteries, veins, lymphatics, and sensory nerves. The inner layer contains osteoblasts (cells that generate new bone formation). Repetitive stress can stimulate the inner layer of the periosteum to create bone outgrowths, called *spurs*. This often occurs at the heel when the plantar fascia is short.

The periosteum weaves into ligaments and the joint capsule. Stretching of the periosteum provides mechanoreceptor information regarding joint function at these junctions. The periosteum also blends with the tendons, forming the tenoperiosteal junction, where the muscle pulls on the bone during joint movement. Sensory nerves in the periosteum are sensitive to tension forces.

A common site of soft tissue injury is the *tenoperiosteal junction*. An acute tear or cumulative microtearing of the periosteum can cause the orientation of the collagen in the area to become random, leading to the development of

abnormal cross-fiber links and adhesions. Massage can address this abnormal fibrotic developed at the tenoperiosteal junction. Friction is used to introduce small amounts of controlled inflammation, resulting in an active acute healing process. When coupled with appropriate healing and rehabilitation, massage leads to a more functional outcome.

Fascia

The term *fascia* is defined in multiple ways, including the following:

- Soft tissue component of the connective tissue system
- Fibrous collagenous tissues that are part of a body-wide tensional force transmission system

Fascia is a fibrous connective tissue that is arranged as sheets or tubes. Fascia can be thick and dense (like duct tape) or can consist of thin, filmy membranes (like plastic wrap) or be fluffy (like a cotton ball) as found in loose connective tissue.

Fascia is connected throughout the body, creating a unified form. Superficial fascia lies under the dermis of the skin and is composed of loose, fatty connective tissue.

Deep fascia is dense connective tissue that surrounds muscles and forms fascial compartments called *septa*, which contain muscles with similar functions. These compartments are well lubricated in the healthy state, allowing the muscles inside to move freely. Fascia can tear, adhere, torque, shorten, or become lax, just as other connective tissue structures can, and responds well to connective tissue massage methods, which are described later in this section.

A common source of musculoskeletal pain is the deep somatic tissues. These include the periosteum, joint capsule, ligaments, tendons, muscles, and fascia. The most pain-sensitive tissue is found in the periosteum and the joint capsule. Tendons and ligaments are moderately sensitive, and muscle is less sensitive. This is an important matter of awareness for massage therapists, who sometimes are overly focused on muscle function as opposed to the total soft tissue system. Hyaluronan (HA) is a slippery gel-like substance found in fascia that allows slipping between adjacent fibrous fascial layers. The deep fascia has a layer of HA between fascia and the muscle and within the loose connective tissue that divides different fibrous sublayers and compartments of the deep fascia. If the loose connective tissue inside the fascia alters its density because of changes in hyaluronan, the normal sliding behavior of the deep fascia and underlying muscle will become compromised.

Massage Application

In general, it is theorized that mechanical forces applied during massage stimulate cellular activity and create heat within the tissues. This heat stimulates cellular activity and improves lubrication of the fibers by making the ground substance more fluid. Fascia is embedded with mechanoreceptors and smooth muscle bundles that respond to the mechanical forces applied during massage to decrease fascial tone and increase pliability.

Effectively focused massage may support the following results:

- Stimulate the fibroblasts to repair the injured collagen
- Introduce mechanical forces to realign the collagen fibers to their normal parallel alignment
- Lengthen shortened tissue and increase ground substance pliability
- Separate adhered tissue layers
- Stimulate fluid distribution and tissue layering to promote normal tissue gliding

Concepts such as acupressure and trigger point therapy may alter fascial tone through mechanical stimulation of embedded nerves.

Friction methods may be used to create controlled focused inflammation to increase collagen proliferation, especially in lax structures. Proper healing and rehabilitation must be combined with this approach for a beneficial outcome. Otherwise, the result can be increased adherence and scar tissue formation.

TAKE 5

Joint Structure and Function

Joints are innervated by the articular nerves, which are branches of the peripheral nervous system. Branches of these nerves also supply the muscles that control the joint. This innervation is one of the reasons why muscles can cause joint dysfunction, and joint dysfunction can cause muscle problems. Many sensory receptors surround the joint. The four types of joint receptors are located in joint capsules, ligaments, periosteum, and articular fat pads.

- Type 1: Located in the superficial layers of the superficial joint capsule. They are mechanoreceptors that provide information concerning the static and dynamic position of the joint.
- Type 2: Located in the deep layers of the fibrous joint capsule. They are dynamic mechanoreceptors that provide information on acceleration and deceleration of movement.
- Type 3: Located in the intrinsic and extrinsic joint ligaments. They are dynamic mechanoreceptors that monitor the direction of movement and have a reflex effect on muscle tone to provide deceleration.
- Type 4: Located in joint capsules, ligaments, and periosteum. They are pain receptors.

These receptors send information to the CNS regarding the functional status of the joint and its surrounding soft tissue. The reflex control of the muscles surrounding the joint is called the *arthrokinematic reflex.* The CNS produces contraction or relaxation of the muscles to protect the joint. The arthrokinematic reflex coordinates agonists, antagonists, and synergists around the joint, as well as other jointed areas, for large movements and fine muscular control.

Proper function of these reflex mechanisms is extremely important in posture, coordination, and balance; direction and speed of movement; position of the joint and body; and pain in the joint.

Irritation of pain receptors and mechanoreceptors typically causes the flexors of the joint to be facilitated and to become short/tight and hypertonic, whereas the extensors of the joint become inhibited or weak, long, and taunt.

Irritation of the joint receptors also can lead to abnormalities in posture, muscle coordination, control of movement, balance, and awareness of body position. These are major issues for clients. Assessment and treatment of gait patterns and firing patterns, with the use of massage and muscle energy methods, can support normal reflex functions. Joints are classified as follows:

- *Fibrous joint:* United by fibrous tissue that has little movement
- *Cartilaginous joint:* United by fibrocartilage and has slight movement
- *Synovial joint:* Bones are not united directly; instead the joint has a joint cavity filled with synovial fluid and is surrounded by a joint capsule; this structure allows the joint to move freely

The joint capsule is composed of two layers. The outer layer is fibrous connective tissue and the inner layer is synovial tissue. The outer layer contains intrinsic ligaments that thicken within the body of the capsule and extrinsic ligaments that lie superficial to the capsule. Many of the tendinous insertions of muscles weave into the joint capsule.

The outer layer of the joint capsule helps stabilize the joint, guide joint motion, and prevent excessive motion. It is innervated by mechanoreceptors and pain fibers. The mechanoreceptors sense the rate and speed of motion and the joint position, and they have reflex connections to the muscles that affect the joint. Irritation and injury to the joint capsule can create muscle contractions designed to protect the joint. This response of the muscle is called *guarding/splinting.*

The inner synovial layer of the joint capsule secretes synovial fluid when it is stimulated by joint motion. Synovial fluid is thick, clear, and viscous, to provide lubrication and nutrition for the joint.

Fibrosis or thickening of the outer layer of the joint capsule is caused by acute inflammation, immobilization, or irritation/inflammation caused by imbalanced stresses on the joint. A tight, fibrotic joint capsule results in compression of certain areas of the cartilage and degeneration of joint surfaces. The capsule and supporting ligaments may be overly lengthened due to injury or excessive stretching during activities such as dance and gymnastics. If immobilization causes a loss of adequate motion, the fibrous layer of the joint capsule atrophies, creating joint instability.

The synovial membrane also can become injured or dysfunctional as the result of acute trauma to the joint, immobilization, and cumulative stresses from chronic irritation caused by imbalanced forces on the joint. Joint swelling occurs during inflammation. The swelling typically causes abnormal function of the muscles controlling the joint. During immobilization, the synovial fluid thickens with disuse, and the amount of synovial fluid secreted decreases. This leads to adhesions between the capsule and the articular cartilage, tendon sheaths, and bursae, contributing to stiffness and joint degeneration.

Massage Application

A fibrotic joint capsule is addressed by using massage to introduce mechanical forces into the tissue to increase pliability. The fibrotic capsule is treated with manual pressures on the capsule itself. The massage strokes are applied in all directions, addressing the irregular alignment of the collagen. Active and passive movement and stretching are used to reduce intraarticular adhesions.

A capsule that is too loose needs exercise rehabilitation to help lay down new collagen fibers, as well as proprioception exercises to help restore neurologic function. Appropriate friction massage might stimulate an acute inflammatory response that stimulates collagen formation.

An acute, swollen joint capsule is treated with gentle rhythmic compression and decompression of the joint. Pain-free, passive joint movement also is used to act as a mechanical pump. If there is too little fluid in the joint, passive and active movement helps stimulate the synovial membrane, increasing synovial fluid production, and thereby supporting lubrication and nutrition.

Cartilage

Cartilage is a dense, fibrous connective tissue that is composed of collagen, ground substance, and cartilage cells called chondrocytes. Hyaline or articular cartilage covers the ends of bones and provides a smooth gliding surface for opposing joint surfaces. Articular cartilage creates new cells with use and deteriorates with disuse. It has no nerve or blood supply and is composed mostly of water. It is elastic and porous, and it has the capacity to absorb and bind synovial fluid. Intermittent compression and decompression create a pumping action, thereby causing the movement of synovial fluid into and out of the cartilage, which is self-lubricating as long as the joint moves. Normal joint movements open and close the joint surfaces, compress and decompress the cartilage, and tighten and loosen the joint capsule and ligaments, all of which support joint lubrication and nutrition.

Synovial joints generate compression and decompression through movement, intermittent contraction of the muscles, and twisting and untwisting of the joint capsule. Massage application that includes passive joint movement introduces compression and decompression and supports joint health.

Cartilage damage is common. An arthritic joint is a joint with degeneration of the cartilage. Damage to articular cartilage may be caused by an acute trauma or by cumulative stresses. These stresses are often the result of imbalances in the muscles surrounding the joint, a tight joint capsule, or a loose joint capsule. A tight capsule creates high-contact areas to cartilage and decreased lubrication. A loose capsule allows inappropriate joint laxity, creating potential for misalignment and rubbing of the articulating bones. Dysfunctions of the muscles that move the joint create excessive pressure on the cartilage. The cartilage degenerates, beginning with damage to the collagen fibers and depletion of the ground substance.

Studies have shown that cartilage cells can create new cartilage. The joint must be moved to stimulate the synthesis of chondrocytes and the secretion of synovial fluid. Compressing and decompressing the joint capsule pumps synovial fluid into and out of the cartilage, rehydrating the cartilage. In addition to appropriate exercise, massage and muscle energy methods support joint health through the following methods: contract/relax, reciprocal inhibition, pulsed muscle, or a combination of these methods; active/passive movement and compression/decompression of the joint of the joint to promote fluid exchange.

Fibrocartilage consists of dense, white fibrous connective tissue arranged in dense bundles or layered sheets. The fibrocartilage has great tensile strength combined with considerable elasticity. Fibrocartilage will deepen a joint space, such as the labrum of the hip and shoulder, the menisci of the knee, and the intervertebral disks of the spine. It also lines bone grooves for tendons, such as the bicipital groove for the long head of the biceps brachii. Common joint injuries include various types of fibrocartilage damage.

Bursa

Bursae are synovial filled sacs lined with a synovial membrane that are found in areas of increased friction. A bursa secretes synovial fluid, which decreases friction in the area. Bursitis typically is caused by excessive friction of the muscles and connective tissue (tendons and fascia) that overlie the bursa. Massage can lengthen structures that are rubbing and may support drainage of excessive fluid from the area through lymphatic drain methods.

TAKE 5

Joint Stability

For a joint to perform a full and painless range of motion, it must be stable. A rule for joint health is stability before mobility, mobility before agility. Otherwise, abnormal forces move through the joint, leading to excessive wear and tear on the articular surfaces. Joint stability is determined by the following:
- The shape of the bones that make up the joint. This is called *form stability*.
- Passive stability provided by the ligaments and the joint capsule. This is called *form stability*.
- Dynamic stability provided by the muscles. This is called *force stability*.

If instability of the joint is caused by the form (e.g., bones, ligaments), soft tissue massage methods are palliative and targeted to condition management. However, if force instability is present, joint function can be improved with exercise and massage.

It is important for the tone of the muscles that cross a joint to be balanced, or the forces on the joint will create uneven stresses, leading to dysfunction and eventual degeneration of the cartilage.

When a joint is in the close-packed position, the capsule and the ligaments are tightest. In the loose-packed position, the joint is most open, and the capsule and ligaments are somewhat lax. Generally, extension closes and flexion opens the joint surfaces. Midrange of the joint is typically the loosest packed position and the point at which the joint is most vulnerable to injury. For performance of most traction methods, the joint should be positioned in the midrange.

Dr. John Mennell introduced the concept of "joint play," which describes movements in a joint that can be produced passively but not voluntarily. In most joint positions, a joint has some "play" in it that is essential for normal joint function.

Joint Degeneration

One common cause of joint degeneration is loss of normal function of the joint. This altered function can occur as the result of a prior trauma or cumulative stress on the joint and is common in athletic performance. Most conditions called *arthritis* no longer involve an active inflammatory response and should be referred to as *arthrosis*, meaning "joint degeneration." *Osteoarthritis* and *degenerative joint disease* typically are used interchangeably to describe chronic degeneration of a joint, although *osteoarthritis* may be used to describe a true inflammatory joint condition. Many people will develop arthritis and arthrosis. Technical advances have increased the success of joint replacement surgery and rehabilitation.

Massage Application

Appropriate massage addresses adhesions and tightening of the joint capsule or ligaments, sustained contraction of the muscles surrounding the joint, muscle and motor tone imbalances, and irregular muscle activation sequences (firing patterns). Short and tight muscles are lengthened and relaxed, and muscles that are weak and inhibited need to be reeducated and exercised to regain their normal strength.

Joint mobilization is any active or passive attempt to increase movement at a joint. Joint mobilization within the normal range of motion is within the scope of practice for the massage therapist. The movement must not be forcefully abrupt or painful.

The goals of joint mobilization are as follows:
- To restore the normal joint play
- To promote joint repair and regeneration
- To stimulate normal lubrication by stimulating the synovial membrane to promote rehydration of articular cartilage
- To normalize neurologic function
- To decrease swelling
- To reduce pain

Joint manipulation can be valuable but should only be performed by qualified healthcare providers such as osteopathic physicians, chiropractors, and physical therapists.

TAKE 5

Muscle

What we think of as a muscle is more appropriately called the muscle organ, because it consists of tissues that combine to work together to perform a function. The structural unit of skeletal muscle is the muscle fiber. The fibers are arranged in parallel bundles called *fascicles*. Each fascicle is composed of many myofibrils. The myofibril is composed of thousands of strands of proteins, also arranged in parallel bundles called *myofilaments*, and these are further divided into actin and myosin, the basic proteins of contraction. Muscles contain satellite cells that can regenerate muscle fibers to a certain extent.

The muscle fibers are so interwoven with connective tissue that it is hard to separate the two. A more appropriate term may be *myofascial*, for the combination of muscle and fascia.

The connective tissue of muscle transmits the pulling forces of contracting muscle cells to the bones and gives the muscle fibers organization and support. Collagen fibers found in the epimysium, perimysium, endomysium, and other connective tissue components of muscle converge to form the tendon. Tendon fibers weave into the connective tissue of the periosteum, joint capsule, and ligaments. All these connective tissue layers are lubricated in the healthy state, so that muscles can slide over each other during movement. When this does not happen, function is altered. This commonly occurs as part of the aging process, or when adhesions form during the injury repair process.

Muscles are also dynamic stabilizers of the joints because they actively hold the joints in a stable position for posture and movement. Proprioceptors in muscle tissue sense joint movement and body position. Muscles are connected to the nerves in the skin, and to the nerves in the neighboring joint capsule and ligaments, through neurologic reflexes. If the skin or the joint is irritated or injured, the associated muscles may go into a reflexive spasm, be inhibited, or do whatever bests protect the area. Muscles have pain receptors that fire with chemical or mechanical irritation. Muscles act as a musculovenous pump because contracting skeletal muscle compresses the veins and moves blood toward the heart. A similar process assists lymphatic movement.

Muscle Function Types

Muscles exert a pulling force when the muscle fibers are stimulated to contract. There are three types of muscle function.
- *Isometric:* In an isometric contraction, the muscle contracts, but its constant length is maintained. The main outcome is stabilization.
- *Concentric:* Concentric contraction occurs when a muscle shortens while it contracts. The main outcome is movement/acceleration.
- *Eccentric:* Eccentric contraction occurs when a muscle lengthens while it contracts. The main outcome is control of movement/deceleration.

All movements in the body are accomplished by more than one muscle. The muscles that contract concentrically to perform a certain movement are called the *agonists.* This action is called *acceleration,* and the muscle is also called the *prime mover.* For example, the biceps brachii is an agonist for elbow flexion. The muscles that perform the opposite movement to that of the agonists are called the *antagonists;* they provide control through deceleration during eccentric function. Triceps brachii is the antagonist for biceps brachii because it extends the elbow and controls flexion of the elbow. The muscle that works with another muscle to accomplish a certain motion is a *synergist.* The term *synergist* refers to stabilizers and neutralizers.

Typically, when the agonist is working concentrically, the antagonist is functioning eccentrically. Sherrington's law of reciprocal inhibition states that neurologic inhibition of the antagonist occurs when the agonist is working. When the biceps brachii contracts to flex the elbow, the triceps brachii is being inhibited neurologically, which allows it to lengthen during elbow flexion. Co-contraction is an exception to this rule. Co-contraction occurs when the agonist and the antagonist are working together. For example, when you make a fist, the flexors and extensors of the wrist are co-contracting to keep the wrist in a position that ensures the greatest strength of the fingers.

Human movement seldom involves pure forms of isolated concentric, eccentric, or isometric actions. This is because body segments are periodically subjected to impact forces, as in running or jumping, or because some external force such as gravity causes the muscle to lengthen. In many situations, the muscles first act eccentrically, with a concentric action following immediately, mixed in with isometric stability function.

Two types of motor nerves supply each muscle. Alpha nerves fire during voluntary contraction of a muscle. Gamma nerves have voluntary and involuntary functions and unconsciously help to set the motor tone of the muscle, its resting length, and function during voluntary activities for fine muscular control.

As discussed previously, five types of sensory nerve receptors supply each muscle. The sensory nerves are sensitive to pain, chemical stimuli, temperature, deep pressure, and mechanoreceptor stimuli. There are two specialized receptors: the muscle spindle, which detects changes in length of the muscle, and the Golgi tendon organ, which detects changes in tension in the muscle.

TAKE 5

Muscle Length–Tension Relationship

A muscle develops its maximum strength or tension at its resting length or just short of its resting length because the actin and myosin are positioned to form the maximum number of cross bridges. When a muscle is excessively shortened or lengthened, the amount of tension that the muscle is able to generate decreases. This is called the *length-tension relationship.* A muscle can develop only moderate tension in the lengthened position and minimum tension in the shortened position. Massage can effectively normalize this situation by changing the length (making longer or shorter) of the muscle and restoring the normal resting length.

Reflexive Muscle Action

Protective coordinated muscle reflex action is an important consideration when providing massage. The following are reflex actions:

- Withdrawal reflexes, such as pulling away from a hot stove, involve instantaneous muscle contraction.
- Righting reflexes and oculopelvic reflexes from the eyes, ears, ligaments, and joint capsules communicate with the muscle and stimulate instantaneous contraction for protection of the joint and associated soft tissue; they also support upright posture.
- Arthrokinematic reflexes describe unconscious contraction of muscles surrounding a joint, caused by irritation in the joint.

Splinting, guarding, or involuntary muscle contraction can be caused by various types of muscle pathology. Emotional or psychological stress creates excessive and sustained muscle tension.

Viscerosomatic reflexes occur when irritation or inflammation in a visceral organ causes muscle spasm. Efficient motor function is an effectively integrated, multiplanar (frontal, sagittal, transverse) movement process that involves acceleration, deceleration, and stabilization of muscle and fascial tissue and joint structures.

Physical fitness protocols need to follow a sequence. Stability must develop before effective mobility can be attained. The core is considered the lumbo-pelvic-hip complex, thoracic spine, and cervical spine. The core operates as an integrated functional unit to dynamically stabilize the body during functional movements. Systems of stabilization must function optimally if prime movers are to produce efficient and powerful mobility. Many low back pain conditions are directly related to problems with core stability.

Functional movement patterns occur at every joint and involve acceleration, stabilization, and deceleration. Frontal plane movement includes adduction and abduction. Sagittal plane movement includes flexion and extension. Transverse plane rotational movements include internal and external rotation.

Functional Movement

During functional movement patterns, almost every muscle has the same synergistic function: to eccentrically decelerate protonation or to concentrically accelerate supination. The central nervous system recruits the appropriate muscles in an optimal firing pattern during specific movement patterns.

When in a closed kinematic chain (standing upright), full body protonation is multiplanar (frontal, sagittal, and transverse), synchronized joint motion that occurs with eccentric muscle function. Supination is multiplanar (frontal, sagittal, and transverse) synchronized joint motion that occurs with concentric muscle function. This means that for one joint pattern to move effectively, all the involved joints have to move. Movement can be initiated at any joint in the pattern, and restriction of any joint in the pattern will restrict motion or increase motion in interconnected joints.

To briefly describe functional biomechanics, we will review the gait cycle. During walking or other locomotor activities such as running, motion at the subtalar joint is linked to transverse plane rotations of the bone segments of the entire lower extremity. During the initial contact phase of gait, the subtalar joint pronates, which creates internal rotation of the tibia, femur, and pelvis. At midstance, the subtalar joint supinates, which creates external rotation of the tibia, femur, and pelvis. Poor control of protonation decreases the ability to eccentrically decelerate multisegmental motion and can lead to muscle imbalances, joint dysfunction, and injury. Poor production of supination decreases the ability of the kinetic chain to concentrically produce appropriate force during functional activities and can lead to synergistic dominance.

Joint arthrokinematics refers to roll, slide, glide, and translation that occur between two articular partners. *Joint play* is defined as the involuntary movement that occurs between articular surfaces that is separate from the range of motion of a joint produced by muscles. It is an essential component of joint motion and must occur for normal functioning of the joint. Predictable patterns of joint arthrokinematics occur during normal movement patterns. Optimal length-tension and force-couple relationships ensure maintenance of normal joint kinematics.

Optimal muscle posture supports the development of high levels of functional strength and neuromuscular efficiency. *Functional strength* is the ability of the neuromuscular system to perform dynamic eccentric, isometric, and concentric actions efficiently in a multiplanar environment. This process allows the appropriate muscle activation sequence to be chosen to perform an activity and ensures that the right muscle contracts at the right joint, with the right amount of force, and at the right time. If the kinetic chain is nonoptimal, the individual will have decreased structural efficiency, functional efficiency, and performance. For example, if one muscle is short and tight (altered length-tension relationships), the force couples around that particular joint are altered. If the force couples are altered, the normal arthrokinematics is altered, and joint pain can occur.

Arthrokinematic inhibition is the neuromuscular phenomenon that occurs when a joint dysfunction inhibits the muscles that surround the joint. For example, a sacroiliac joint dysfunction causes arthrokinematic inhibition to the deep stabilization mechanism of the lumbo-pelvic-hip complex (transversus abdominis, internal oblique, multifidus, and lumbar transversospinalis). All these neuromuscular phenomena occur as the result of postural dysfunction. Various movement systems such as Feldenkrais and Alexander technique may interact with this mechanism.

TAKE 5

Development of Muscle Imbalances

Muscle imbalances are caused by postural stress, pattern overload, repetitive movement, lack of core stability, and lack of neuromuscular efficiency. Tonic/postural/stabilizing muscles play a primary role in maintenance of posture and joint stability. The primary role of phasic (moving) muscles is quick movement. It has been found that tonic/postural stabilizing muscles react to stress by becoming short and tight, and that phasic/mover muscles react to stress by becoming inhibited and weak.

An important difference between the two muscle groups is that a small reduction in the strength of an inhibition-prone muscle initiates a disproportionately larger contraction of the antagonist tightness-prone muscle. This is because work and recreational activities favor tightness-prone muscles getting stronger, tighter, and shorter as the inhibition-prone muscle becomes weaker and more inhibited (long). If daily movement is not balanced, dysfunctional patterns become exacerbated. This is one of the reasons why the length-tension relationship becomes important. Some muscles, such as quadratus lumborum and the scalenes, can react with either tightness or weakness.

Muscle dysfunction from illness or injury, job or exercise activity, reduced recovery time, chronic pain, and inflammation can create disturbances in normal muscle function and may stimulate neurologically based tightness (shortening) or weakness (lengthened inhibition) of a muscle.

Muscles that curl you toward your belly button (flexors, adductors, internal rotators) get short and pull the posture forward (make a cave). In response, the opposite muscles, which would uncurl you (extensors, abductors, external rotators), are pulled long and become stretched (taut) over the "hills." These muscles feel taut and tight and often hurt, but only because the muscle groups are fighting the ones that curl you forward, trying to maintain some aspect of upright posture. A simple massage approach is to massage and increase pliability of the fascia and muscle structure in the "cave" and use exercise to strengthen the muscles on the "hills."

A short tight muscle is held in a sustained contraction. The muscle is constantly working and consumes more oxygen and energy, and generates more waste products, than a muscle at rest. Circulation is decreased because the muscle is not performing its normal function as a pump, leading to ischemia that causes pain receptors to fire. Sustained tension in the muscle pulls on its attachments to the periosteum, joint capsule, and ligaments, creating increased pressure, uneven forces, and excessive wear in the joint.

Short tight muscles often compress nerves between the muscles or through a muscle, which is a form of impingement syndrome. Weak long muscles (feel tight but are taut) are unable to support joint stability and contribute to poor posture, excessive tension and compression of adjunct structures, and abnormal joint movements. Muscle activation sequences and gait reflexes are disturbed. Inhibited muscles interfere with vascular and lymphatic movements.

Reciprocal inhibition is the process whereby a tight muscle (psoas major, for example) causes decreased neural impulse transmission to its functional antagonist (gluteus maximus). This process decreases contraction by the prime mover and leads to compensations by the synergists, called *synergistic dominance.* Synergistic dominance occurs when synergists compensate for weak or inhibited prime mover patterns. Synergistic dominance is the process whereby a synergist compensates for a prime mover to maintain force production. For example, if a client has a weak gluteus medius, synergists (tensor fasciae latae, and quadratus lumborum) become dominant to compensate for the weakness. This alters normal joint alignment, which further alters the normal length-tension relationships around the joint where the muscles attach. This process leads to altered movement. It often occurs from activity performed while fatigued. People complain of heavy or labored movement if synergistic dominance is occurring.

Poor posture and muscle imbalance that produce reciprocal inhibition and synergistic dominance further cause altered joint alignment. Altered joint alignment is created by muscle shortening and muscle weakness. Altered arthrokinematics is further changed as the result of altered force-couple relationships. If synergists are dominant, then normal joint movements are altered, because muscles are activating out of sequence. This is a continuous and cyclic process. Muscle shortening, muscle weakness, joint dysfunction, and decreased neuromuscular efficiency all can initiate this dysfunctional pattern.

Massage Application

Massage application is particularly effective in dealing with these conditions and supports other professional treatments. Mainly, massage lengthens short tight muscles and increases tissue pliability. These benefits support therapeutic exercise to treat long (taut) weak inhibited muscles. In other words, treatment involves massage and elongation of short and tight tissues and exercise for long and weak muscles. Massage and stretch the "caves"—strengthen the "hills."

Massage appears to do the following:

- Create a mechanical force on the soft tissues to encourage relaxation and pliability
- Normalize fluid movement using rhythmic cycles of compression and decompression, rocking, and specific methods such as lymphatic drain to restore the natural rhythmic movement of the body's fluids
- Normalize ANS, neurotransmitter, and endocrine function; deliberate use of stimulation or inhibition and optimal pressure levels encourage appropriate neurochemical function

Massage targets both the connective tissue and neuromuscular aspects of muscle tissue function because tension within a muscle and its fascia is created by active and passive elements. The passive elements include collagen fibers and ground substance, which are influenced by massage with the introduction of various mechanical forces. Because muscle contains ground substance, it demonstrates viscous behavior. It becomes thicker and stiff when it is stretched quickly, is cold, or is immobilized. It becomes more fluid-like if it is stretched slowly or is warmed up. Active components include the contractile proteins (actin and myosin), and the nerves. Massage influences length-tension relationships and neurochemical stimuli.

TAKE 5

Massage-Related Research Findings

The findings discussed in this section provide evidence supporting the following benefits of massage therapy:

- May play a role in reducing detrimental stress-related symptoms
- Is pleasurable
- Appears to manage some muscle/fascia type pain
- Supports social bonding
- Likely improves the perception of quality of life in individuals who enjoy massage
- Typically is safe when provided in a conservative and general manner with sufficient pain-free pressure

The benefits of massage may occur when normalizing tissues that are tense, tight, deformed, twisted, or compressed by introducing mechanical forces (e.g., pulling, pressing, bending, and twisting) into body tissues using massage, stretching, mobilization, etc.

Fascia is everywhere, connecting everything so that the body functions as a single, integrated unit instead of individual parts. The specific massage applications that best influence fascia are still unknown. Focused tension (stretching) of the tissues currently appears to be the most effective mechanical force for influencing the fascia.

Current understanding indicates that the effects of massage are derived through interrelationships of the peripheral and central nervous systems (and their reflex patterns and multiple pathways) and the ANS, neuroendocrine control, and response of the fascial network to mechanical forces applied during massage.

Based on research, it is difficult to state confidently that massage influences the movement of body fluids, even though research seems to support the theory that massage affects the water content of fascia. It is logical to apply massage in a way that mimics normal function.

The main component of body fluid is water. It seems reasonable to expect that the mechanical forces applied during massage at least affect the fluid in a particular area while the tissue is massaged. Squeezing and compressing fluid in tissue, which occurs during massage, should help the body move and process the various body fluids. However, more research is needed before a specific massage effect on blood, interstitial, and lymphatic movement can be stated with confidence.

The use of methods thought to influence blood, interstitial fluid, and lymph movement is appropriate. However, massage professionals must explain to clients that although the methods appear to be clinically effective, research as yet is unable to prove the outcomes.

Research supports massage as a means of managing anxiety related to pain and a means of altering mood, the pain threshold, and the perception of pain. General full body massage appears to directly and indirectly influence many structures, and can help individuals adapt and cope while assisting restoration of function.

Research has not yet been able to specifically identify the results of individual, specific applications, because massage encompasses many different elements. Benefits can be derived from the quiet, nurturing presence of the massage therapist, the duration of the massage, the massage environment, and the unlimited variations in methods, pressure, speed, and so forth. A well-performed, full body massage is somewhat like a tasty cookie—ingredients are all mixed together in the right proportions, baked at the correct temperature for the right amount of time, and served in a relaxing environment.

COMPREHENSION CHECK FOR REVIEW PART THREE CHAPTERS 5 AND 6

Using a Scenario to Stimulate Comprehension

Following are short real-world examples of entry-level professional practice and how the various MBLEx categories could be reflected in multiple choice question form. There are four scenarios each with 20–30 questions. The answer key is found in appendix C.

This exercise has two parts:

• Answering the question
• Writing a rationale for why the correct answer is the best response and why the other answers are not the best response to the question posed.

A rationale is when you give the reasoning or justification for the choice you made when answering the question. This activity solidifies comprehension of Chapter 5 and 6 content and prepares you for the next review phase targeting review by individual content areas. While the sample test questions in this review guide have rationales written as part of the answer key, this activity challenges your ability to use critical thinking as you choose the best answer and understand why you made that decision.

Use the information in this review guide, your textbooks used while in school and the internet. The internet is very helpful when writing rationales. You can search keywords from the question to help you with the critical thinking process.

Three examples are provided.

➤ Targeting massage/bodywork application to the shoulder would involve understanding
   a. regional anatomy.

b. developmental anatomy.
c. gross anatomy.
d. comparative anatomy.

Correct answer and rationale **a**.

Regional anatomy: The study of all the structures of a particular area would be the answer that best fits the intent of the question-massage/bodywork of an area.

Incorrect answers rationales.

Developmental anatomy is how anatomy changes over the life cycle. Gross anatomy is the study of body structures large enough to be visible to the naked eye. Comparative anatomy is the study of structures and the functions of these structures of other animals corresponding to the human body.

➤ The hip joint is abducted. The massage practitioner asks the client to move the hip toward the midline. How would the muscle group that returns the hip to the anatomical position be functioning?
   a. Lengthening
   b. Shortening
   c. Stabilizing
   d. Flexing

Correct answer and rational **b**.

The adductors of the hip would need to be shortening producing a concentric contraction to return to the anatomical position.

Incorrect answers rationales.

The adductor group would be lengthened when the hip is in the abductor position. The muscle group would need to be contracting pulling into adduction, not flexion, to move back to anatomical position. There would be stabilizing involved but the question is asking for what is happening during a movement.

➤ What is an ethical issue related to legislated draping regulations in the massage practice?
   a. Veracity
   b. Autonomy
   c. Respect
   d. Beneficence

Correct answer and rational **c**.

Respect is esteem and regard for clients, other professionals, and oneself.

Incorrect answer and rationales.

Client autonomy and self-determination is the freedom to decide and the right to sufficient information to make the decision. Veracity is the right to the objective truth. Beneficence means to act for the benefit of others.

Scenario 1

A 24-year-old student was referred to you by their parents, who are regular clients. The individual is experiencing school stress, especially since finals are coming up. The history intake form reveals that in addition to considerable stress from a full load of college classes. This individual also is working approximately 15 hours a week as a server at local restaurant. The medical history reveals seasonal allergies and ongoing neck pain from carrying trays of food at the restaurant. The only medications are birth control pills, and they take a multivitamin. The client describes the neck pain as a dull ache that comes and goes combined with at a level of 5—6 (on a 0—10 Visual Analog scale, with 0 being no pain and 10 being unbearable pain). Your assessment shows mildly restricted range of motion in the neck during left lateral flexion, with moderately palpable muscle tenderness in the right trapezius with increased muscle tone in the right cervical muscles.

Anatomy and Physiology

1. Which of the following hormones would be most affected by birth control pills?
   a. Progesterone
   b. Testosterone
   c. Aldosterone
   d. Thyroxine
2. When a client is stressed, increased activity in sympathetic autonomic nervous system often occurs interfering with which restorative function supported by massage therapy?
   a. Exercise
   b. Hygiene
   c. Eating
   d. Sleep
3. C fibers are
   a. small myelinated fibers which carry sharp pain
   b. large unmyelinated fibers which carry burning pain
   c. small unmyelinated fibers which carry burning pain
   d. large myelinated fibers which carry sharp pain
4. Nociceptors are
   a. bipolar cells
   b. free nerve endings
   c. epithelial receptors
   d. Pacinian corpuscles

Kinesiology

5. Which of the following is involved in lateral flexion in the cervical region and may function as a breathing muscle?
   a. Anterior scalene
   b. Splenius capitis
   c. Middle trapezius
   d. Pectoralis minor
6. If a client's work activities involve lifting and holding a moderate weight at shoulder level, which joint type would be most difficult to stabilize?
   a. Ball and socket
   b. Pivot
   c. Saddle
   d. Hinge

Pathology, Contraindications, Areas of Caution, Special Populations

7. What headache type involves soft tissue changes as the primary cause?
   a. Tension

b. Sinus
   c. Vascular
   d. Cervicogenic
8. Nasal congestion and irritated eyes would be major symptoms for _____
   a. sepsis
   b. contact dermatitis
   c. seasonal allergies
   d. anaphylaxis

Benefits and Physiological Effects of Techniques That Manipulate Soft Tissue

9. A client describes work-related stress, tension-type headache, and neck and shoulder stiffness. Which of the following best justifies a general massage approach for this client?
   a. Stress with breathing changes can be the underlying cause of the more specific symptoms.
   b. Tissue changes related to stress are only affected with general massage.
   c. Targeted mechanical force application would not affect the sensation of tissue stiffness.
   d. The client is too fragile to adapt to a targeted and localized massage application.
10. A client indicates they have sinus congestion. Which massage therapy positioning would most likely increase the symptom?
    a. Seated
    b. Prone
    c. Supine
    d. Sidelying

Client Assessment, Reassessment, and Treatment Planning

11. During review of the health history coupled with postural assessment it is noted that the work-related activities may be a perpetuating aspect of the shoulder and neck stiffness the client describes. Which of the following assessment procedures could confirm this suspicion?
    a. Have client demonstrate positions that both aggravate and alleviate symptoms.
    b. Palpate the affected area screening for tissue changes and trigger point activity.
    c. Perform joint movement assessment having client indicate if movement aggravates symptoms
    d. Instruct the client to demonstrate common work postures and activities.
12. During intake a practitioner notices that the client places their hand on serratus posterior inferior. What would be the most logical question to ask related to this behavior?
    a. Have you tripped and almost fallen?
    b. Have you been coughing?
    c. Have you been constipated?
    d. Are you experiencing any discomfort around your scapula?

Ethics, Boundaries, Laws, Regulations

13. When increasing stress responses are unable to be managed with methods such as massage therapy, what ethical principle would most influence the massage practitioner when providing a referral for the client?
    a. Respect (esteem and regard for clients, other professionals, and oneself)
    b. Client autonomy and self-determination (the freedom to decide and the right to sufficient information to make the decision)
    c. Veracity (the right to the objective truth)
    d. Proportionality (the principle that benefit must outweigh the burden of treatment)

14. The practitioner is licensed as a massage therapist and trained as a Yoga teacher. The client indicates they are stiff especially in the morning. What could create an ethical dilemma?
    a. Dual role
    b. Scope of practice
    c. Transference
    d. Confidentiality

15. A client is displaying long-term stress-related symptoms. Why would it be advisable for the practitioner and the client to wear a mask during the massage session?
    a. Long-term stress can reduce immune function
    b. Stress changes the breathing rate increasing droplet transmission of pathogens
    c. Masks are an effective way to decrease the transmission of skin-related conditions
    d. The stressed client can more easily transmit infections

Guidelines for Professional Practice

16. A massage therapist is seeking an employment position. What should they expect?
    a. a 1099
    b. Employer withholding income tax
    c. a rental agreement
    d. required to provide supplies

17. A client is requesting an appointment schedule outside of normal business operations when the practitioner typically has a full day scheduled. The client's parents are regular clients. The dilemma involves
    a. business structure
    b. financial concerns
    c. practitioner self-care
    d. facility access

18. The massage practitioner is developing an efficient 30-minute session. How can the time be best used?
    a. Using the seated position instead of prone or supine
    b. Eliminating the postural assessment
    c. Adapting session to be applied over clothing
    d. Providing sessions in a nonprivate setting

19. The practitioner is employed by a chiropractor. A client is asking for a fee discount. Who has the ability to make this decision?

a. Practitioner
b. Receptionist
c. Employer
d. Insurance provider

Scenario 2

Mrs. Ellen Fitch, age 32, was in a serious car accident 16 months ago. She experienced multiple injuries, many of which have affected her CNS functions. She had a skull fracture. She also developed an abscess from a secondary bacterial infection, which has resolved with antibiotic treatment. As a result of the trauma, Mrs. Fitch has a closed head injury that affects her linear reasoning. She has difficulty processing any sort of sequence, such as following the steps of a recipe or the instructions for using an appliance. She experiences a lot of pain, including headache. Concern has arisen that she is developing a dependency on pain medication. She also suffered a contusion injury of the spinal cord in the lumbar area. She is not fully paralyzed but has weakness in both legs, more so on the left. She is able to walk using a walker for support, and she is receiving physical therapy, making slow progress. There is mild swelling in ankles and feet related to reduced mobility. She also is depressed and experiencing posttraumatic stress symptoms that interfere with her sleep. Mrs. Fitch is angry about the accident and obviously stressed. She is unable to work as a retail manager and wonders if she will ever be able to go back to work. Her family and the healthcare team believe that massage can help manage some of the symptoms and aid in her recovery.

Anatomy and Physiology

1. What part of the central nervous system might be damaged if an individual has difficulty planning, organizing, and implementing daily life activities?
    a. Cauda equina
    b. Cerebellum
    c. Brain frontal lobe
    d. Brainstem

2. What dermatome is located in the lumbar area?
    a. L3
    b. T2
    c. C6
    d. S4

3. The fluid causing interstitial edema originates from the
    a. urinary system.
    b. lymphatic system.
    c. immune system.
    d. circulatory system.

4. Excess fluid in the interstitium is collected by the
    a. lymph nodes.
    b. lymph capillaries.
    c. lymph duct.
    d. lymph trunk.

Kinesiology

5. When a client uses a walker which of the following muscles are used to hold the handles?
   a. Flexor digitorum profundis
   b. Flexor hallucis longus
   c. Fibularis longus
   d. Flexor carpi ulnaris

6. Which of the following muscles is involved in walking and acting both at the hip and knee?
   a. Psoas
   b. Quadriceps femoris
   c. Gastrocnemius
   d. Vastus lateralis

7. What muscle can cause flexion at both the wrist and elbow?
   a. Flexor carpi radialis
   b. Brachialis
   c. Flexor hallucis longus
   d. Flexor pollicis longus

8. Which of the following joint types would be considered polyaxial joints?
   a. Fibrous
   b. Synovial
   c. Ball and socket
   d. Cartilaginous

Pathology, Contraindications, Areas of Caution, Special Populations

9. Which of the following is a brain injury?
   a. Concussion
   b. Fracture
   c. Infection
   d. Strain

10. A client taking an opiate-based pain medication may commonly experience which of the following conditions that may be helped by massage therapy?
    a. Itching
    b. Coughing
    c. Constipation
    d. Dizziness

11. An antibiotic medication would be used to treat
    a. flu
    b. athlete's foot
    c. scabies
    d. staph

12. A client is experiencing simple edema in their ankles and feet which has been improved by massage therapy. What best describes this condition?
    a. Congestion in the veins
    b. Increased fluid in the interstitial space
    c. Densification of connective tissue
    d. Swollen lymph nodes

Benefits and Physiological Effects of Techniques That Manipulate Soft Tissue

13. A client reports that the pain level decreased after the massage. Which is the most biologically plausible reason for this result?
    a. Sensory stimulation creating hyperstimulation analgesia
    b. Decrease in fascial adhesions entrapping nerves
    c. Increased blood flow reducing ischemia
    d. Therapeutic inflammatory provocation

14. A client prefers moderate pressure and requests that light pressure be avoided. Which is the most logical reason?
    a. Feverish
    b. Depressed
    c. Ticklish
    d. Diabetic

15. A client experiencing simple edema in ankles and feet would benefit by
    a. Legs bolstered so feet are raised
    b. Seated with a pillow at the chest
    c. Prone with bolster under abdomen
    d. Supine with legs flat

16. A massage client indicates simple edema in ankles and feet improved after a bodywork session. What method was likely used to address this issue?
    a. Myofascial release
    b. Neuromuscular technique
    c. Ischemic compression
    d. Rhythmic gliding

Client Assessment, Reassessment, and Treatment Planning

17. The client history indicates residual muscle weakness in the legs related to impact trauma. When asked to lift the legs to position the bolster the practitioner observes that the client is able respond but did not lift the right leg high enough to place bolster under the knees. Using this information what grade for a manual muscle test is most accurate?
    a. 5—Normal strength
    b. 4—Movement against gravity and resistance
    c. 3—Movement against gravity (resistance eliminated)
    d. 2—Movement with gravity eliminated

18. Which of the following conditions is most easily objectively assessed?
    a. Chronic pain
    b. Anxiety
    c. Muscle weakness
    d. Fatigue

Ethics, Boundaries, Laws, Regulations

19. Treatment for which of the following conditions would be most likely outside the scope of practice for massage therapy?
    a. Headache

b. Depression

c. Pain

d. Simple edema

20. What is required to for the practitioner to legally work with an orthopedic focus?
    a. Certificate of achievement
    b. Board Certification
    c. License
    d. Professional assessment

21. An occupational therapist is providing massage in a rehabilitation clinic. A massage practitioner working in the same environment is concerned if this is ethical. A factor to consider would be
    a. Transference
    b. Certification
    c. Jurisprudence
    d. Scope of practice

Guidelines for Professional Practice

22. What equipment will be most beneficial when working with a client experiencing mobility issues?
    a. Percussion tool
    b. Electronic table
    c. Hot towel cabinet
    d. Aromatherapy diffuser

23. A practitioner has agreed to provide in home services for an individual unable to drive. Which of the following is appropriate?
    a. Practitioner bringing pet dog to the session
    b. Practitioner asking to bring their young child with them to the client's home
    c. Removal of the client's service dog from the premises while practitioner onsite
    d. Adding a travel and setup fee to the price for service

24. A complex client is seeking massage therapy to manage a variety of symptoms related to a car accident. In which situation would a newly licensed practitioner be most apt to help this client's complicated health issues?
    a. A rehabilitation center
    b. A solo practice
    c. A fitness center
    d. Mobile practice

Scenario 3

Client played little league, high school, and currently college softball. The only major physical problem is recurring bursitis in the right shoulder. This is problematic because it is the pitching arm. The trainer has used ice and various other treatments, and the pain is reduced, although the pain returns if the client plays consecutive games. The client had one cortisone injection 12 months ago which was helpful, but additional injections are not advised at this time. They are taking celecoxib (CELEBREX). This client has also modified the pitching style somewhat which reduced shoulder discomfort but has noticed increased tension in the forearm. Massage has not been used specifically to address the underlying factors causing the bursitis. Goals for massage intervention will be targeted toward reducing the irritation causing the bursitis and providing general athletic performance support.

Anatomy and Physiology

1. Which body system experiences the most adverse side effects from nonsteroidal antiinflammatory medication?
    a. Endocrine
    b. Digestive
    c. Respiratory
    d. Skeletal

2. Cortisone based medication mimics and replaces a hormone most related to the
    a. liver
    b. pancreas
    c. adrenals
    d. interstitium

3. Systemic and local inflammation is most related to the
    a. immune system
    b. cerebral spinal fluid
    c. sleep–wake cycle
    d. skeletal system

4. Productive acute inflammation promotes
    a. sepsis
    b. fascial dysfunction
    c. injury healing
    d. muscle atrophy

Kinesiology

5. The subacromial bursae would be prone to bursitis with overuse involving which movement?
    a. Knee flexion
    b. Cervical rotation
    c. Glenohumeral circumduction
    d. Supination

6. In order to kick a ball, which muscle functions in the frontal plane for leg stability?
    a. Plantaris
    b. Gluteus medius
    c. Gastrocnemius
    d. Illiacus

7. Increased tone would occur in what muscle during an exercise involving squeezing a ball in the hand?
    a. Brachioradialis
    b. Supinator
    c. Flexor hallucis longus
    d. Flexor digitorum profundus

8. A client is experiencing discomfort near the lessor trochanter during hip flexion. What muscle is most likely involved?
    a. Tensor Facia Lata
    b. Sartorius
    c. Illiacus
    d. Adductor longus

9. The boney landmark that is the attachment of structures involving hip extension is the
   a. iliac crest
   b. acromion process
   c. glenoid fossa
   d. trochlear notch

Pathology, Contraindications, Areas of Caution, Special Populations

10. What inflammatory condition would be most commonly experienced by a college softball athlete?
    a. Stress fracture
    b. Plantar fasciitis
    c. Pancreatitis
    d. Gout
11. A grade 2 sprain of the medial collateral ligament is considered in the subacute healing phase when there is
    a. repair of the injured tissues.
    b. tissue remodeling.
    c. heat, swelling, and pain.
    d. organization of the collagen fibers.
12. A client is experiencing a sensation of stiffness in their upper body. What best describes this condition?
    a. Congestion in the veins
    b. Increased fluid in the interstitial space
    c. Densification of connective tissue
    d. Swollen lymph nodes

Benefits and Physiological Effects of Techniques That Manipulate Soft Tissue

13. A client reports that the discomfort level increased after the massage. Which is the most biologically plausible reason for this result?
    a. Sensory stimulation was too aggressive
    b. Methods created fascial adhesions entrapping nerves
    c. Increased blood flow caused edema
    d. Improved distribution of pain-modulating neurotransmitters
14. A regular client prefers moderate to firm pressure. Which is the most biologically plausible reason?
    a. Athletes require more pressure for results.
    b. Younger clients believe more pressure increases benefits
    c. Clients with soft tissue stiffness may require more pressure
    d. The client has been told that therapeutic massage involves heavy pressure

Client Assessment, Reassessment, and Treatment Planning

15. Which of the following conditions is most easily objectively assessed?
    a. Chronic pain
    b. Anxiety
    c. Inflammation

d. Fatigue

16. A common assessment for bursitis is
    a. palpation for tenderness near the joint
    b. observation of gait
    c. muscle testing of adjacent joint
    d. postural assessment
17. An assessment used to identify location of inflammation is
    a. muscle strength testing
    b. palpation for heat
    c. interview about medication
    d. joint movement

Ethics, Boundaries, Laws, Regulations

18. Treatment for which of the following conditions would be most likely outside the scope of practice of massage?
    a. Tendinosis
    b. Gout
    c. Pain
    d. Simple edema
19. What is required to for the practitioner to legally work with a physical therapist?
    a. Sports massage certificate
    b. Board Certification
    c. Associates degree
    d. License
20. A massage practitioner regularly observes a coworker using hot packs with a specific client who is not charged extra for the service. An ethical factor to consider would be
    a. countertransference
    b. certification
    c. jurisprudence
    d. scope of practice

Guidelines for Professional Practice

21. A client has limited finances and the practitioner's fee structure does not support the client receiving massage on a regular basis. The practitioner is considering options for this client since they have a strong social media following that could support increased exposure for new clients. This would be considered
    a. management
    b. strategic planning
    c. advertising
    d. financial planning
22. An athletic client is seeking massage therapy to support recovery posttraining and competition. What would the practitioner need to consider related to their self-care?
    a. Scheduling availability for the client during regular business hours
    b. What type of personal protective equipment would be required
    c. Does the client have sufficient income to cover the cost of frequent sessions
    d. Regular updates from the training team on client status

Scenario 4

A 20-year-old college soccer player has been referred to the team massage therapist for management of delayed-onset muscle soreness. The client also reports being constipated, and sleep is interrupted by frequent need to urinate. Gluteus maximus is short and tight bilaterally. Goals for massage are to reduce the aching and stiff feeling and to enhance athletic performance. The trainer's goal is management of delayed-onset muscle soreness.

Anatomy and Physiology

1. Lymph moving from the legs into the thorax filter through
   a. inguinal lymph nodes.
   b. axillary lymph nodes.
   c. mesenteric lymph nodes.
   d. mediastinal lymph nodes.
2. The main function of the colon is to
   a. mechanically break down food.
   b. absorb nutrients.
   c. reabsorb water.
   d. release bile.
3. Which of the following is involved in the regulation of digestion?
   a. Trigeminal nerve
   b. Accessory nerve
   c. Vagus nerve
   d. Saphenous nerve
4. Which of the following hormone's primary function relates to fluid balance?
   a. Aldosterone
   b. Androgen
   c. Prolactin
   d. Progesterone
5. The sympathetic autonomic nervous system affects the bladder in what way?
   a. Stimulates the detrusor muscle to contract, causing the person to urinate
   b. Stimulates the internal urinary sphincter to remain tightly closed so urine collects in the bladder
   c. Increases the potential for stress incontinence and inability to stop urinating
   d. Decreases the stress response therefore decreasing stress incontinence

Kinesiology

6. Which category of muscles contracts to apply a force when kicking a ball?
   a. Agonists
   b. Hip extensors
   c. Lateral rotators
   d. Antagonists
7. Which synovial joint type moves only in the sagittal plane?
   a. Saddle
   b. Fibrous
   c. Hinge

   d. Syndesmoses
8. The main function of the gluteus maximus is
   a. hip flexion
   b. hip extension
   c. hip abduction
   d. hip medial rotation

Pathology, Contraindications, Areas of Caution, Special Populations

9. When there is an increase or change in exercise that involves eccentric movement which of the following is most likely to occur?
   a. Plantar Fasciitis
   b. Delayed-onset muscle soreness
   c. Exertional Rhabdomyolysis
   d. Compartment syndrome
10. When there is a significant increase in exercise intensity which of the following might occur and is considered a medical emergency?
    a. Plantar Fasciitis
    b. Delayed-onset muscle soreness
    c. Exertional Rhabdomyolysis
    d. Grade two muscle strain
11. A client indicates they are significantly constipated. Which of the following would indicate the need for referral?
    a. Bowel obstruction
    b. Bladder infection
    c. Opioid pain medication
    d. Inguinal hernia
12. What is a common injury experienced by an athlete?
    a. Hamstring strain
    b. Hip dislocation
    c. Femur fracture
    d. Hiatal hernia

Benefits and Physiological Effects of Techniques That Manipulate Soft Tissue

13. What massage application would be common to address both lymphatic and venous return?
    a. Percussion
    b. Gliding
    c. Friction
    d. Vibration
14. The outcome for the massage session is relaxation and sleep support. Which approach is the best choice?
    a. Focused regional compression, active movement, kneading, and shaking
    b. General short session using slow gliding, fast petrissage, and shaking
    c. Focused regional rhythmic shaking with targeted kneading and friction
    d. Generalized rhythmic gliding, kneading, and rocking
15. The most biologically plausible explanation for why massage therapy alters pain perception is

a. biofeedback

b. hyperstimulation analgesia

c. reduction of superficial facia gliding

d. increased sympathetic ANS arousal

16. Alternating applications of hot and cold is called

   a. contrast hydrotherapy

   b. decompression or cupping therapy

   c. instrument assisted soft tissue manipulation

   d. reflexology

17. A client scheduled a 30-minute massage session with concentration on the shoulders and hips but cannot comfortably lay on their stomach. Which positioning would provide the best access to both these areas in the time allotted?

   a. Seated

   b. Supine

   c. Prone

   d. Slide-lying

18. Which of the following massage methods is most easily used over clothing?

   a. Kneading

   b. Gliding

   c. Compression

   d. Friction

19. A term used in classical massage that indicates gliding/stroking would be

   a. gymnastics

   b. tapotement

   c. petrissage

   d. effleurage

Client Assessment, Reassessment, and Treatment Planning

20. An athletic trainer refers an athlete to a massage therapist indicating general nonspecific massage to support recovery. What would be the main reason for assessment for this client?

   a. To develop a self-help program to support performance

   b. To identify areas of caution and possible contraindications

   c. To develop a treatment plan of care for the athletic trainer to approve

   d. To identify specific applications to improve performance

21. A client outcome for massage is for stress management. Which would be the appropriate question to ask during the verbal intake related to this goal?

   a. Do you have pain in your joints?

   b. Are you taking any antiinflammatory medication?

   c. What is the quality of your sleep?

   d. Have you had any abdominal surgeries?

22. Which of the following assessment methods specifically targets tissue texture?

   a. Joint movement

   b. Palpation

   c. Strength assessment

   d. Observation

23. A client has been evaluated by a physician with the recommendation of knee joint replacement. The client asks if massage therapy can help support this procedure's recovery. They ask how the massage applications would be determined. This is an example of

   a. Client treatment goal setting

   b. Formulation of treatment strategy

   c. Ability to rule out contraindications

   d. Informed consent and therapeutic relationship

24. During history taking the client indicated they are using four different medications related to depression, hypertension, and gastroesophageal reflux disease. The massage practitioner gathers information about the medications and determines adaptations of massage application needed for this client. This is an example of

   a. Client consultation and evaluation

   b. Verbal intake using a health history form

   c. Clinical reasoning

   d. Research literacy

25. Postural and joint movement assessment would be most relevant for

   a. mobility

   b. pain

   c. stress

   d. well-being

Ethics, Boundaries, Laws, Regulations

26. A practitioner with less than 1 year of experience identifies during palpation assessment that the client has moderate edema in the legs, most pronounced at the ankles. What is the best course of action?

   a. Inform client of the finding, ask clarifying questions, and potentially refer to client's physician

   b. Complete session incorporating passive joint movement and refer to a more experienced practitioner

   c. Inform client of the finding, ask clarifying questions, and continue with session

   d. Modify application to target fluid movement and recommend increased fluid intake

Guidelines for Professional Practice

27. Client has been seeing practitioner for 6 months. They inform the practitioner they are beginning gender-affirming hormone therapy. The practitioner is unfamiliar with the process and has become uncomfortable communicating with the client. Which is the most appropriate course of action for the practitioner?

   a. Seek guidance from a peer with more experience in this area

   b. Question the client about motivation for making this decision

   c. Ignore uncomfortable feelings and continue to work with the client

   d. Refer the client to a practitioner who is curious about gender fluidity

28. A practitioner recently began working with a college athletic department with the assistant athletic trainer being the direct supervisor. Multiple professionals in the department are sending athletes for sessions without notifying the supervisor. Which of the following best describes this situation?
    a. Scope of practice issue
    b. Standard of care
    c. Needs assessment
    d. Communication dilemma

29. In which practice setting would it be common for the practitioner to be provided with treatment orders?
    a. Wellness center
    b. Destination spa
    c. Chiropractic office
    d. Fitness center

30. A practitioner is advertising that a package of 12 sessions will prevent post exercise soreness. Which of the follow describes why this is a concern?
    a. Lack of specialized training
    b. Misleading claims about benefits
    c. Scope of practice infringement
    d. Power differential dual role

TAKE 5

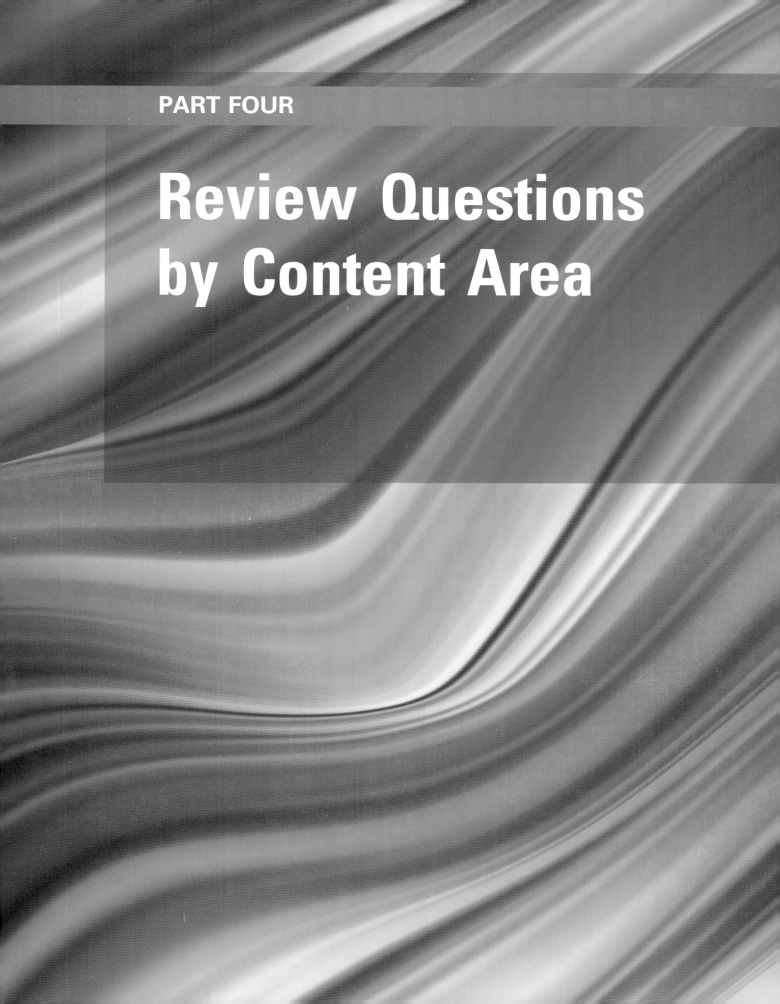

PART FOUR

Review Questions by Content Area

REPETITION, REPETITION, REPETITION: THEN MORE REPETITION

Study Tips and Test-Taking Habits

This part of the review guide is set up by content area, which means that a specific topic, such as the skeletal system, massage application, or ethics, is addressed. This part consists of a specific content area and various types of questions that represent how the content can appear on exams. A brief review of each content area is provided. Recommendations for review and study target the specific content area.

In this section, each question is a mini lesson. By approaching each practice question in this way, you can learn to do the following:

- Understand what the question is trying to measure.
- Determine what the question is trying to teach.
- Identify the problem the question poses.
- Use clinical reasoning skills to solve the problem in the question.

Remember, the goal is not to get the right answer to the question while you are studying. When studying, the goal is to do these things:

- Understand the type of question: factual recall/knowledge, concept identification/comprehension, or clinical reasoning synthesis/application.
- Determine whether you understand the terminology, and if not, review Part 2, and use the glossary or dictionary to define words.
- Identify the various ways that information can be presented in a question.
- Practice using clinical reasoning to solve the problem presented by the question.

The goal is to be able to demonstrate competency as a massage professional. Massage professionals use clinical reasoning!

The questions are arranged in two groups: (1) factual recall/knowledge and (2) application and concept identification/comprehension—clinical reasoning and synthesis/application.

Factual recall questions are first. Remember, these are primarily vocabulary questions. The study strategy is to define each relevant word in the question and possible answers. Although these questions are not common on exams, they are excellent for reinforcing the meaning of terminology. Terminology study involves repetition and memorization. Review Part 2 if you struggle with these questions.

Next, the concept identification and clinical reasoning and synthesis questions are grouped. Concept identification questions use the terminology to measure an understanding of relationships. These question types are common on exams because they move beyond memorization into a basic level of understanding. Because they are based on definitions of terms, these questions can be validated readily with the use of

textbooks and reference material. The focus of the question remains objective, which is important for the legal defensibility of the exam. This group of questions presents the content in a format in which a connection is made between concepts. It is necessary first to know the definition of all words in the question and potential answers and then to understand how the concepts relate to each other. Most questions on licensing exams are of this type; thus, most of the questions in this guide are application and concept applications. If you struggle with these questions, review Parts 2 and 3 of this review guide.

Clinical reasoning and synthesis questions are the most advanced question type, and they truly assess your understanding of the material. To answer these questions, you must know the meanings of all the words and how the concepts relate to each other. Then, based on that information, you decide which is the best, most logical answer. The goal is to solve the problem the question presents. Many may recognize these as story problems. These are the most difficult questions to write and answer, and no matter how hard you look, *the answers will not be in the textbooks*; the only thing in textbooks and references is information—not decisions. These questions are complex, and the reader's ability to figure out the best answers demonstrates his or her ability to use the clinical reasoning model. They do not appear on exams as often as they should, which is unfortunate because they measure competency best. If you struggle with these types of questions, review Part 3.

Not all content areas include all types of questions because some content lends itself more easily to vocabulary assessment, and other content is applied better to application and problem solving.

If you have a good grasp of the content in the review of Parts 2 and 3, then read the summaries provided at the beginning of each content area, and you should progress through each type of question with increasing levels of understanding.

Correct Answers and Rationales

Correct answers and rationales are provided in Appendix C. Rationales of questions for factual recall refer to definitions. If you do not know what the individual words mean, you cannot decipher the meaning of the question. The rationale may not provide the definitions because these can be looked up easily in the glossary, Part 2 of this text, or a dictionary. If you experience difficulty with this question type, study the terminology, review Part 2, and read the glossary.

Rationales for the concept identification questions describe the relationships of the concepts. Rationales for the clinical reasoning questions reflect the decision-making process and justify the correct answer.

Remember, the questions in this part are not meant to mimic various licensing exams—they have been developed to help you *study* for the exams. Some are easy, some are hard, and some are really long and complex. All questions are designed to help you understand the material.

The practice exams provided in Part 5 and on the Evolve site are more like typical licensing exams. When you have worked your way through the content area questions in this part, you will be ready to do the practice exams in Part 5, which mixes up the questions. Once you complete the Part 5 practice tests, then you are ready to challenge the 10 additional practice exams on the Evolve site that are presented in a computer-based format similar to how actual licensing exams appear.

CHAPTER 7

Therapeutic Massage

FOUNDATIONS OF THERAPEUTIC APPLICATIONS OF TOUCH

Review Tips

The information in this content area provides a foundation for professional behavior. Test questions written on the foundations of therapeutic applications of touch include vocabulary, professional behavior, and historical influence on current trends in the professional evolution of therapeutic massage. This content is often found in case study questions, especially in combination with content on ethical behavior and communication skills.

The vocabulary targets terms used to describe interactions of persons in social and professional settings. When studying the vocabulary, pay particular attention to words used in each of the example questions. Use textbooks and the glossary in this book to look up terms that are unclear.

Culture, gender, age, life events, spirituality, and diversity all influence the experiences of touching and being touched. There are inappropriate forms of touch and appropriate forms of professional touch. Therefore, an understanding of the subjective experience of touch is important.

Typically, licensing exams do not have questions about historical dates. Questions about historical figures may appear on some exams, but usually not many. Therefore, do not memorize this content. An understanding of massage history from ancient times to the present is important. However, focus more on information regarding the progression of massage therapy and understanding the professional aspects of therapeutic touch.

Quick Content Review

- Professional touch is a skilled touch that is delivered to achieve a specific outcome, with the recipient in some

way reimbursing the professional for services rendered. Personal interpretations of touch and their influence on professional interactions include personal space, culture and subculture (such as social structure and spiritual discipline), gender, age, and life events.

- Therapeutic massage has a rich heritage and history. Massage or touch as a method of healing has many cultural origins. This means that no one culture owns massage, and that some sort of underlying, instinctive mechanism spurred the development of a type of massage in most, if not all, cultures on the planet.

- Scientific research is the key to validation. Massage has been validated by the science of the day. Many of the ideas that past scientists had were incorrect. The important thing to remember is that even though the "scientific rationale" from the past for massage was incorrect, the benefits of massage are real. It is important to remember the value of objective research for validation. Pain research has uncovered many physiologic explanations for the benefits of massage. History does repeat itself, and massage has reemerged in every age. The best results have occurred when science is advanced enough to figure out why massage works. It will be exciting to move into the future, keeping in mind the lessons of the past.

- The skin is the largest sensory organ of the body. Many subcutaneous soft tissue structures (e.g., muscles, connective tissue), as well as visceral structures (e.g., the lungs, heart, digestive organs), project sensation to the skin. The autonomic nervous system (ANS), which regulates the visceral and chemical homeostasis of the body, is highly responsive to skin stimulation in support of well-being. Mood (the way a person feels) often is reflected in the skin. We blush with embarrassment, flush with excitement, and pale with fear.

- Personal space, culture and subculture, including social structure and spiritual discipline, gender, age, and life events can influence an individual's experience of touch. Forms of inappropriate professional touch include the following:

- Hostile touch
- Aggressive touch
- Sexual touch
- The development of a common terminology is important as modern massage moves toward standardization.

Factual Recall Questions

1. Professionalism is defined as _____.
   a. An occupation that helps people
   b. A service provided for others
   c. An intricate system that is structured and systematic
   d. Adherence to qualified status, methods, standards, and character
2. Which of the following defines culture?
   a. Race as defined by color and where you live
   b. Arts, beliefs, customs, institutions, and all products of human work and thought created by a specific group of people at a particular time
   c. What you study, the profession you choose, the family you grew up in, and whom you marry
   d. The workplace, including the people, environment, physical location, and financial management
3. A form of touch technique is touch that is _____.
   a. Socially stereotyped
   b. Mechanical
   c. Inadvertent
   d. Ritualized
4. The approach to care that acknowledges the whole person is
   a. biopsychosocial
   b. based on fixed outcomes
   c. population specialization
5. As important to the client outcome as the methods used is the
   a. therapeutic alliance
   b. practitioner's education
   c. practice setting
6. A bodywork form using compression over loose clothing is
   a. Manual lymph drain
   b. Swedish
   c. Shiatsu
7. An approach that targets connective tissue by modifying application to move superficial tissue is
   a. Myofascial release
   b. Polarity therapy
   c. Lymphatic drainage
8. Passive treatment in this system includes terms like effleurage, petrissage, and tapotement:
   a. Neuromuscular therapy
   b. Swedish massage
   c. Myofascial release
9. A bodywork form considered modern and western is
   a. neuromuscular therapy
   b. classical massage
   c. Thai massage
10. Which touch modality is based on the premise that change can be affected in different parts of the body by working the corresponding reflex areas in the feet, hands, or ears?
    a. Polarity therapy
    b. Reflexology
    c. Shiatsu

Application and Concept Identification Question

1. A characteristic of an individual response to professional therapeutic touch is that it _____.
   a. Is consistent with cultural influences
   b. Cannot be predetermined
   c. Is gender specific
   d. Depends on outcomes
2. A middle-aged client is reluctant to work with a 22-year-old massage therapist. The most likely reason why is because of _____.
   a. Gender issues
   b. Genetic predisposition
   c. Age issues
   d. Body sensitivity

Using the previous questions as examples, write at least three more questions. Develop plausible wrong answers and be sure the correct answer is truly the best answer. Then write a rationale for each question. The more questions you write, the better you will understand the material.

PROFESSIONALISM AND LEGAL ISSUES

Review Tips

Professionalism and legal issues are considered important on most exams because they influence ethical professional behavior. One of the purposes of exams is to determine whether persons will behave in an appropriate manner so that clients are not harmed. The reason for legislation is to protect the public, and questions on this content attempt to determine safe and professional practice. Some states require a jurisprudence exam. Jurisprudence is the study of the law. When a massage therapist seeks licensing from a particular state, the jurisprudence exam would cover content related to the massage legislation for that state.

Specific terms are used to describe this content and concepts. Use the vocabulary in the questions as a guide for study. Use textbooks and the glossary in this book to look up terms that are unclear.

This content often is tested in the case study/example type of format. The clinical reasoning process is necessary to determine the correct answer. The facts are presented in the question, and the possibilities are given in the four potential answers. Analyze each potential answer against the facts in the question to determine the best response.

Quick Content Review

- Professionalism is the skill, competence, or character expected of a member of a highly trained profession. Therapeutic massage is the application of systematic touching for health purposes. The variety of massage methods makes it difficult to encompass all approaches in a concise definition for the massage and bodywork profession.
- A scope of practice defines the knowledge base and practice parameters of a profession as determined by each state in the regulatory legislation.
- Ethics is the system of rules, based on morals, values, and standards of accepted conduct, that guide correct behavior. The following 10 principles guide professional ethical behavior:
    1. Respect—Esteem and regard for clients, other professionals, and oneself
    2. Client autonomy and self-determination—The freedom to decide, and the right to sufficient information to make the decision
    3. Veracity—The right to the objective truth
    4. Proportionality—The principle that benefit must outweigh the burden of treatment
    5. Nonmaleficence—The principle that the profession shall do no harm and shall prevent harm from happening
    6. Beneficence—The principle that treatment should contribute to the client's well-being
    7. Confidentiality—Respect for privacy of information
    8. Justice—Equality
    9. Fidelity—The building of trusting relationships and keeping of promises
    10. Fiduciary duty—The obligation to maintain trust and the legal responsibility to act solely in the best interest of another party
- These ethical principles direct the development of standards of practice. Standards of practice provide specific guidelines and rules that form a concrete professional structure. Standards of practice guidelines direct quality care and provide a means of measuring the quality of care. They usually are more concrete than ethical principles.
- The relationship between the massage professional and the client is based on professional trust and safety. If the client is unable to make an informed choice, the trust is broken and the touch is not safe. In professional relationships where expectations and rules are understood clearly, clients can make informed choices about their behavior. If the situation is vague and the rules change from week to week, the expectations between client and practitioner become unclear. Completing an informed consent process with clients allows for informed choice.
- Take ethics into consideration in maintaining professional boundaries and the therapeutic relationship. The massage

therapist's touch needs to be safe and nonjudgmental. How could we ethically say that we are providing this service for a client for whom we feel dislike, disapproval, or fear? All boundary concerns should be resolved with the intent that the therapeutic relationship be equitable and balanced. We invade a person's boundaries when our needs are put above their needs. If a massage professional wishes to maintain a nondiscriminatory approach but cannot best serve a particular client, clear, honest, and respectful disclosure to the client of the massage practitioner's problem allows the massage professional to best serve the needs of the client without discrimination.
- Effective listening involves the development of focusing skills. Reflective listening involves restating the information to indicate that you have received and understood the message. Active listening may clarify a feeling attached to the message but does not add to or change the message. Listening does not involve giving advice, resolving the problem presented, or in any other way interjecting information about what was said. Effective listening occurs when we listen to understand, instead of to respond. I-messages share feelings and concerns. You-messages put a person down, blame, or criticize and provoke anger, hurt, embarrassment, and feelings of worthlessness.
- It is important to understand the nature of implicit bias. Bias consists of attitudes, behaviors, and actions that are prejudiced in favor of or against one person or group compared to another. Implicit bias is a form of bias that occurs automatically and unintentionally, that nevertheless affects judgments, decisions, and behaviors. Thoughts and feelings are "implicit" if we are unaware of them or mistaken about their nature. We have a bias when, rather than being neutral, we have a preference for (or aversion to) a person or group of people. Thus, we use the term "implicit bias" to describe when we have attitudes toward people or associate stereotypes with them without our conscious knowledge.
- The massage professional must refer the client to other healthcare professionals when appropriate. Often, it may be tempting to answer a client's questions related to a diagnosis, but it is better to refer the client to their physician to avoid problems.
- Short-lived feelings of sexual arousal that occur when a person relaxes have a physiologic basis. If the client has experienced essential touch only in a sexual situation, the client logically connects the two experiences. Education and explanation help clients understand the difference. Acting sexual in the context of the therapeutic relationship is always inappropriate.
- Harassment of all types including sexual harassment is always inappropriate. Maintain a "zero tolerance" policy for this type of behavior.
- Use a problem-solving approach to enhance ethical decision-making. If each massage professional establishes professional boundaries, and if these are respected through equal consideration of each person's needs in a situation, the massage professional's respect for the client and the

client's understanding of professional ethics will support decision-making in most vague situations.

- Massage practitioners must know what credentialing is required by law to practice massage therapy, and what types of credentialing are voluntary. Credentials must be issued by verifiable sources.
- The main purpose of a law is to protect the public's health, safety, and welfare.
- The massage professional needs to understand legislative issues, local ordinances, and zoning regulations. Depending on where the massage therapist wants to practice, these legal issues to a large extent determine the requirements for starting a business.
- Identify and report the unethical conduct of colleagues. Depending on the seriousness of the infraction and the colleague's response, it may be necessary to file a formal complaint through the professional organization or the legal system in your area. It is unprofessional to ignore unethical behavior in colleagues. A willingness to be involved with profession-wide ethical concerns supports professional integrity as a whole. Carefully document the concerns and the process of intervention. Follow all ethical principles in these types of situations.
- The Health Insurance Portability and Accountability Act (HIPAA) of 1996 was signed into law by President Bill Clinton on August 21, 1996. Conclusive regulations were issued on August 17, 2000, to be instated by October 16, 2002. HIPAA requires that transactions regarding all patient healthcare information must be formatted in a standardized electronic style. In addition to protecting the privacy and security of patient information, HIPAA includes legislation on the formation of medical savings accounts, the authorization of a fraud and abuse control program, the easy transport of health insurance coverage, and the simplification of administrative terms and conditions. HIPAA encompasses three primary areas, and its privacy requirements can be broken down into three types: privacy standards, patients' rights, and administrative requirements.
- Ethical behavior is professional behavior. It revolves around a high regard and respect for our clients; for other health, training, and service professionals; and for ourselves. Being a professional is a compassionate and caring responsibility that requires a commitment to continued learning, self-reflection, and the highest good for all concerned. Ethics is the system of rules, based on morals, values, and standards of accepted conduct, that guide correct behavior.
- Ethical behavior needs to be considered with the use of social media. Information available to the public affects the massage profession as a whole. If an individual presents themselves as a massage therapist, their behavior publicly impacts the massage profession as a whole through multiple venues such as advertising and social media (Facebook, Twitter, Instagram, etc.,).
- The massage professional needs to understand the scope of practice for other professionals. With additional training beyond entry-level education, massage therapists can become important team players and can work within the scope of practice of other healthcare professionals to assist them in providing the best care for their clients.
- Massage practitioners must avoid falling into a situation that could allow them to be accused of practicing medicine. To avoid such situations, massage professionals must not focus on specific treatment for specific problems; rather, they must provide a service that helps the client maintain or enhance good health. The massage professional also must refer the client to other healthcare professionals when appropriate.

Factual Recall Questions

1. The knowledge base and the practice parameters of an occupation determined by law is called _____.
   a. Scope of practice
   b. Informed consent
   c. Dual role
   d. Therapeutic relationship
2. A client, a professional dancer, is basically healthy but is seeking massage to manage minor injury and support recovery. Which approach to care description best describes these outcomes?
   a. Wellness/normal function
   b. Healthcare services
   c. Dysfunction and athletic performance
   d. Illness/trauma
3. A massage professional is careful to provide an informed consent process for each client and updates informed consent regularly. Which of the following ethical principles is being followed?
   a. Confidentiality of client information
   b. Justice
   c. Proportionality
   d. Client autonomy and self-determination
4. Taking a client's history and providing a physical assessment to develop a massage care plan is called a _____.
   a. Initial assessment
   b. Brochure and policy statement
   c. Jurisprudence
   d. Chart
5. A massage professional has worked hard to develop a policy statement and has included types of services offered, information on training and experience, appointment policies, client and practitioner expectations, sexual appropriateness, and recourse policy. What did the professional forget to include?
   a. Number of appointments needed to meet therapeutic goals
   b. Fee structure
   c. Objective progress measurements
   d. Methods of clinical reasoning
6. A massage practitioner made a practice of careful and modest draping during the massage, used low lighting and soft music to help clients relax, always locked the

door to maintain privacy, provided informed consent, and maintained charting. Which of these activities has the greatest potential for ethical concerns?
a. Locked door
b. Low lighting
c. Soft music
d. Confidential charting

7. A client seems to interrupt often when the massage practitioner is attempting to gather information about the client's condition before the massage. The client often provides inaccurate information when asked questions. Where might the client need assistance in the communication process?
a. Formulating I-messages
b. Listening
c. Open-ended question
d. Word choice

8. A client informs a massage professional that another massage practitioner in the practice is soliciting clients to move to a new private practice the therapist is starting. Everyone in the current practice signed a contract agreeing to avoid soliciting clients in this manner. After careful consideration of the situation and discussion with a peer in a similar situation in another state, what is the next step the massage professional would take?
a. Formal reporting
b. Contacting a lawyer
c. Talking with those involved
d. Speaking to fellow workers

9. Local legislation that controls the location of a business is called _____.
a. Licensing
b. Building codes
c. DBA—Doing Business As
d. Zoning

10. What is the struggle between interdependent people called?
a. Communication skills
b. Reflective listening
c. Conflict
d. Brainstorming

11. A massage therapist is frustrated with the supervisor over charting each massage using new forms. When voicing concerns, the supervisor told the massage therapist to stop arguing, and they could leave. Which of the following describes the conflict resolution method the supervisor was using?
a. Power/dominance
b. Denial
c. Collaboration
d. Negotiation

12. Which of the following best describes HIPAA?
a. Credentials
b. Clinical reasoning
c. Reciprocity
d. Privacy standards

Application/Concept Identification and Clinical Reasoning/Synthesis Questions

1. A massage professional becomes angry with a client who complains about personal problems during the massage. The massage practitioner is displaying _____.
a. Transference
b. Therapeutic relationship
c. Ethical behavior
d. Countertransference

2. A massage professional fails to regularly drape clients in a modest and professional manner. Which of the following best describes this conduct?
a. Engaging in a dual role
b. Breach of a standard of practice
c. Misuse of scope of practice
d. Need for additional training in boundary setting

3. A massage professional uses a variety of methods for athletes, those with chronic pain, and clients who require teaching on stress management. Which of the following is most likely the massage application style the massage therapist uses?
a. Structural and postural approaches
b. Deep tissue massage
c. Integrated approaches

4. A massage professional has been working with a particular client for 12 months. Recently, the client has been experiencing increasing difficulty with family communications. Discussions during massage are centered on solving this problem. Which of the following best describes this situation?
a. The massage professional is having difficulty maintaining informed consent.
b. Scope of practice violations, particularly involving psychology, are occurring.
c. The client should be referred for acupuncture or chiropractic treatment.
d. The client is engaged in countertransference.

5. A massage professional with entry-level training has been seeing a client who was recently given a diagnosis of diabetes. The massage professional is becoming more uncomfortable providing massage as the client displays more symptoms. What is the most likely reason for the massage professional's discomfort?
a. Being in a dual role with the client now that the client is ill
b. Having more demands from the client
c. Failing to abide by the definition of massage
d. Functioning outside the personal scope of practice

6. Which of the following is a violation of confidentiality?
a. Maintaining client records in a secure location
b. Asking the client questions about the work environment
c. Approaching and speaking to a client in a restaurant
d. Speaking to a client's chiropractor with appropriate releases

7. Which of the following would be an appropriate disclosure to a client?
   a. The fact that the practitioner has a cold
   b. Business financial concerns
   c. Discussion about a mutual acquaintance
   d. Marital difficulties

8. A practitioner has been asked to work with a support group for persons with cerebral palsy. The therapist is well trained and has 7 years of experience but is uncomfortable with persons with disabilities, especially those for whom communication is problematic. Which of the following can serve as grounds for refusal on the part of the practitioner?
   a. Lack of skills
   b. Lack of peer support
   c. Inability to serve without bias

9. A massage professional with 15 years of experience but minimal continuing education is in charge of a massage clinic. A recent massage graduate on staff at the clinic notices that their current skills, particularly in charting and critical thinking, are more sophisticated than those of the supervisor, but is hesitant to discuss the issue. What is the best description for this situation?
   a. Power differential
   b. Dual role
   c. Professionalism

10. The best example of transference is a practitioner who _____.
    a. has bias toward a client because of political beliefs
    b. receives small gifts from a client to express affection
    c. asks a client to attend a meeting about a nutritional product
    d. angers a client by being late for the last three appointments

11. Which of the following is the most likely reason a client became confused by becoming mildly sexually aroused during the massage?
    a. The massage practitioner was sexualizing the massage.
    b. The client was sexualizing the massage.
    c. The client was experiencing parasympathetic sensations.
    d. The massage practitioner was massaging erotic zones.

12. A massage therapist is angry with a coworker about the scheduling of the massage room. The massage therapist is busier than the coworker and wants to schedule more time on Saturdays. What type of conflict is this?
    a. Relationship
    b. Data
    c. Interest

13. A massage professional is troubled over a client's responses during the last four massage sessions. There is nothing specific about the client's behavior, but something has changed in the client's response to the massage. Which activity would most help the massage professional?
    a. Credentialing review with certification
    b. Managing intimacy issues

c. Changing body language
d. Decision-making with peer support

Exercise

Using the previous questions as examples, write at least three more questions—one of each type: factual and recall and comprehension, application and concept identification, and clinical reasoning and synthesis. Develop plausible wrong answers and be sure that the correct answer is clearly correct. Then write a rationale for each question. The more questions you write, the better you will understand the material.

BUSINESS CONSIDERATIONS FOR A CAREER IN THERAPEUTIC MASSAGE

Review Tips

The content on standard business practices is what most commonly appears on exams. Legally defensible exams cannot present questions based on opinion. Therefore, questions typically take the factual recall and comprehension format presented in the case study style. Business terminology must be learned so one can decipher the meaning of the question and possible answers. Make sure that you know why the wrong answers are incorrect.

Quick Content Review

- Motivation provides the inner strength to stay with a project long enough to succeed. If we understand all aspects of ourselves, then it is easier to determine where difficulties may arise, where we will need help from others, or what other skills we may need to learn to support our weak areas. A successful business depends on maximum utilization of strengths and compensation for and understanding of weaknesses.
- Burnout occurs when we expend more energy than we restore. It also could be described as taking care of others better than we take of ourselves. To prevent burnout, we can keep our lives balanced by participating in a wellness program, taking continuing education classes, and taking a vacation.
- A résumé helps us present the professional experience, qualifications, and attributes that we bring to a business relationship.
- A business plan is a map of a business's future. It provides direction, clarity of purpose, and a mechanism for setting smaller goals to achieve along the way.
- Start-up costs reflect the amount of money it takes to begin a business. One start-up cost that often is forgotten is a reserve of money for subsidizing living expenses during the first year of business.

- Web-based advertising, as well as the use of social media, has become a primary mode of marketing and advertising. It is important to maintain ethical and professional behavior when communicating through electronic platforms such as Twitter, Facebook, and web-based advertising.
- Massage therapy practice includes the time it takes to do a massage, as well as the time between massages and the time needed to complete the client's records. In addition, self-employed massage professionals must realize that the time spent on business record-keeping and paperwork requirements will equal approximately the time spent performing the actual massage.
- The two main types of business opportunities available for the massage professional are (1) self-employment and (2) employee status (earning an hourly wage or salary). An independent contractor is self-employed. The legal classification of an independent contractor in massage therapy rarely occurs. Most often if this classification is used the actual status should be employee.
- Professional liability or malpractice insurance and premise liability insurance ("trip and fall" insurance) are crucial for the protection of the massage professional. Other types of insurance are available, depending on the complexity of the business.
- A record-keeping system accurately reports business income, keeps track of client progress, and allows the massage professional to evaluate past successes and mistakes to achieve better business operation in the future.
- The client-practitioner agreement and policy statement is useful if it is presented in a format that the client can easily understand, enables the client and the therapist to set realistic expectations about what is required, and determines the boundaries of the professional relationship.

Factual Recall Questions

1. A massage professional is considering a position at a local day spa. Which would be an advantage of being an employee?
   a. Variable income
   b. Stable income
   c. Subject to employer's regulations
   d. Independent ability to set work hours
2. Expenses used to begin new business operations are called _____.
   a. Business plan
   b. Reimbursement
   c. Investments
   d. Start-up costs
3. A massage therapist is involved in developing a web-based promotional campaign to increase massage business since taking on a part-time massage employee. What is this called?
   a. Marketing
   b. Business plan
   c. Résumé

4. A massage practitioner has just redesigned the brochure and has included the types of massage provided, what the massage is like, information about the practitioner's qualifications, and client responsibilities. What did they forget?
   a. Tax structures
   b. Type of premise liability insurance
   c. Fees
   d. Client-practitioner agreement
5. A client notices that the massage office is clean, neat, and efficient, and that licenses and certificates are posted on the wall. These demonstrate the massage practitioner's abilities in _____.
   a. Applications of massage
   b. Communication skills
   c. Marketing
   d. Management
6. A massage professional wants to check to see whether the location for an office being considered for rental is in an appropriate business distinct. Where is this information found?
   a. Local zoning office
   b. Facility rental agreement
   c. State licensing bureau
   d. County clerk's office
7. Gross income minus expenses equals _____.
   a. Deductions
   b. Deposits
   c. Net income
8. What type of insurance will protect the massage professional in case a client falls while at the business location?
   a. Malpractice
   b. Premise liability
   c. Product liability
   d. Disability
9. A massage practitioner's business model is sole proprietorship with a DBA. They obtained required licenses and permits for the business location and have had an attorney develop the business checking account and tax plan. They contacted a local insurance agent for appropriate business insurance and are a member of a professional organization that supplies professional liability insurance. They have developed a marketing plan and client-practitioner agreements. What business plan component is missing?
   a. Retirement investment
   b. Zoning approval
   c. Salary structure
   d. Accounting plan
10. Who is eligible for federal and state unemployment?
    a. Employees
    b. Self-employed
    c. Independent contractors
11. For the self-employed, what is similar to the social security and Medicare taxes withheld from the pay of most employees?
    a. Self-employment tax

b. Income tax

c. Workers' compensation.

12. What covers employees if injured on the job?

a. Social security

b. Medicare

c. Workers' compensation

13. A business conducted from a residence may be eligible for some tax deductions if it

a. Has barrier-free access and adjacent restroom.

b. Is used regularly and exclusively as a principal place of business.

c. Meets zoning requirements.

14. The healthcare provider identification system adopted by the U.S. Department of Health and Human Services as part of the implementation of the Health Insurance Portability and Accountability Act (HIPAA) uses a/n

a. National Provider Identification (NPI) number

b. Employer Identification number

c. Taxpayer Identification Numbers

Application and Concept Identification Question

1. A self-employed massage professional has been working 2 years, 8–10 hour/day, 5 days a week seeing 30 clients per week. Lately, the practitioner is tired and out of sorts and fails to rebook clients who cancel. What is the most logical explanation for their behavior?

a. Motivation

b. Coping

c. Burnout

d. Infection

Exercise

Using the previous questions as examples, now write at least three additional questions. Develop plausible wrong answers and be sure that the correct answer is clearly correct. Then write a rationale for each question. The more questions you write, the better you will understand the material.

MEDICAL TERMINOLOGY

Review Tips

Medical terminology for professional record-keeping lends itself to definition-type factual recall questions. The most effective study strategy for this type of content is memorization. Use flashcards and similar study aids to prepare for testing on this content.

Various types of record-keeping procedures are acceptable. The massage community tends to follow the SOAP style (subjective data, objective data, analysis/assessment, and plan). Intake procedures are relatively standardized—history-taking, assessment, and treatment plan development.

Quick Content Review

- The three word elements used in medical terms are *prefix*, *root*, and *suffix*. Prefixes are placed at the beginning of the root word to change the meaning of the word. Root words contain the basic meaning of the word. A suffix is placed at the end of a word to change the meaning of the word. A good plan when translating medical terms is to begin with the suffix.

- Abbreviations are shortened forms of words or phrases. When using abbreviations in any record-keeping, including charting, provide an abbreviation key on the forms or in a conspicuous place on the file. Excessive use of abbreviations is discouraged. To maintain the integrity of client charts, make sure that any abbreviations used are universally understood, or write out the word.

- Steps for effective professional record-keeping are based on clinical reasoning. The four steps for a common clinical reasoning approach are as follows: (1) review the facts and the information collected, (2) brainstorm the possibilities in terms of solutions, (3) consider the logical outcome of each possibility, and (4) consider the ways in which people are affected by each possibility. Decisions made through this process are reflected and recorded in the care/treatment plan.

- A care/treatment plan typically involves clinical reasoning to develop a comprehensive plan involving a series of sessions to attain outcome goals for a client. Session planning involves clinical reasoning to develop a specific session within the context of the treatment plan.

- The written account of the clinical reasoning process is called *documentation*. Charting or recording individual sessions requires an organized system. A common approach is SOAP notes, which include the following:

  S: Subjective data recorded from the client's point of view.

  O: Objective data acquired from inspection and palpation, and a list of assessment procedures and interventions used during the session.

  A: Analysis or assessment of subjective and objective data and an analysis of the effectiveness of interventions/actions taken, along with a summary of the most pertinent data.

  P: A plan, including the method used for intervention and the progress noted in the sessions, is developed and recorded.

- Record-keeping/documentation skills and the ability to use necessary language/terminology are important parts of professional development. Clear communication through writing and when speaking fosters understanding and accurate exchange of information.

- Outcome goals for the massage must be quantified. This means that they are measured in terms of objective criteria. Measurement of joint range of motion is an example of a quantified goal. Some goals may be qualified. Qualified goals are measured in terms of subjective criteria. The question to be answered is "How will we know when the goal is achieved?" or "What will the client be able to do after the goal has been reached that he or she is not able to do now?"

- Documentation involves multiple procedures. Intake procedures are done once and updated periodically. Charting is ongoing after each session. To maintain the integrity of client charts, make sure that any abbreviations used are universally understood, or write out the word. Comply with electronic record-keeping when required. If writing by hand, use black pens. Make sure handwritten notes are readable. Never erase or white-out a correction. Draw a single line through any error and make the correction above or next to the error. It is important to share the charting notes with and explain them to the client regularly. If electronic charting is used, it is important to follow software program processes.

Factual Recall Questions

1. The process for client record-keeping/documentation involves _____.
   a. Charting each session of the ongoing process
   b. Having the client fill out a general information packet
   c. Creating a written record of intake procedures, informed consent, assessments, recording of each session, and release of information
   d. Filing each piece of information received from physicians and insurance companies and payments received from clients

2. Charting can be defined as the _____.
   a. Record of each payment made by the client
   b. Record of the time spent with each client
   c. Written record of the intake procedure
   d. Ongoing process of recording each session

3. Massage treatment goals must be quantified, meaning _____.
   a. That they are achievable
   b. That they are measured in terms of objective criteria
   c. How they will be done

4. Which term means a cavity that contains pus?
   a. Abscess
   b. Cellulitis
   c. Cyanosis

5. Which of the following suffixes indicate a sensitivity to pain?
   a. -algesia
   b. -itis
   c. -asthenia

6. The purpose of assessment is to _____.
   a. Provide methods to correct deviations from the norm
   b. Identify effective functioning to eliminate massage to that area
   c. Do a visual and functional assessment but not a palpation assessment
   d. Identify effective functioning and deviations from the norm

7. To analyze the data gathered during the assessment, the massage professional must _____.
   a. Increase mechanical application of skills for application of the treatment plan
   b. Generate quantifiable goals and methods that can be used to achieve client goals
   c. Consider the information based on examination, investigation, and analysis in relation to outcomes
   d. Compare information versus generalized norms and protocols for treatment

8. The treatment plan is characterized as _____.
   a. An exact protocol developed by client and practitioner
   b. A fluid guideline developed by client and practitioner
   c. Being completed at the end of the first session and is without revision
   d. Being completed before the massage begins, avoiding use of information gathered during the massage

9. The P (plan) part of SOAP should include which information?
   a. Client medication history
   b. Client self-care
   c. Key symptoms
   d. Relation of outcomes to goals

10. The suffix in angioplasty means _____.
    a. Tumor
    b. Enlargement
    c. Surgical repair
    d. Disease

11. While reading the history, the massage professional sees that the client has myalgia. Which of the following defines *myalgia*?
    a. Muscle condition
    b. Spine pain
    c. Muscle pain
    d. Muscle paralysis

12. While reviewing a file on a client referred from another massage therapist, the massage professional finds information in the SOAP charting that indicates that applications of effleurage/gliding to the legs resulted in vasodilation. Which body system was affected directly?
    a. Cardiovascular
    b. Urinary
    c. Immune
    d. Digestive

13. Where would a massage professional record this statement on a SOAP note: "Palpation identified mild scoliosis"?
    a. S
    b. O
    c. A
    d. P

Application/Concept Identification and Clinical Reasoning/Synthesis Questions

1. An example of a quantified outcome goal is that the client will be _____.
   a. Able to increase range of motion of the lateral flexion of the cervical area by 15 degrees
   b. Able to resume normal work activities
   c. Reassessed in 12 sessions
   d. Recovering the skills to play golf

2. The objective data part of a SOAP note would include that the client _____.
   a. States that they have interrupted sleep
   b. Is currently taking melatonin
   c. Has upper chest breathing from observation and palpation
   d. Wishes to have weekly appointments for the next 2 months
3. In the SOAP note, the most important area in terms of determining future intervention procedures based on results is _____.
   a. Subjective
   b. Objective
   c. Analysis
   d. Plan
4. The purpose of using a clinical reasoning model is to _____.
   a. Think through an intervention process and justify the effectiveness of a therapeutic interaction
   b. Provide to other healthcare professionals a primary means of effectively supporting diagnosis
   c. Integrate all modalities and techniques into a user-friendly charting process for all to understand
   d. Provide a framework to use for charting protocols and collecting data on the client
5. Which of the following is necessary to develop a valid analysis of massage benefits in a SOAP chart?
   a. Completion of a treatment plan
   b. Preassessment and postassessment procedures
   c. Prior development of a problem-oriented medical record
   d. Dates of reassessment
6. A massage professional lists "reducing neuritis" as a long-term client goal in the treatment plan. The desired outcome would be to _____.
   a. Relieve intestinal spasm
   b. Decrease joint mobility
   c. Stimulate nerve conduction
   d. Decrease nerve inflammation

Exercise

Using the previous questions as examples, write at least three more questions. Develop plausible wrong answers and be sure that the correct answer is clearly correct. Then write a rationale for each question. The more questions you write, the better you will understand the material.

RESEARCH LITERACY AND EVIDENCE-BASED PRACTICE

Review Tips

- Research is important to the massage profession, but this content is difficult to write text questions about because the information changes often in response to research findings. Test questions must have clearly right and wrong answers, and if the knowledge base shifts, the questions may become obsolete.
- More consistent content includes terminology and the generally accepted effects of massage. The questions in this chapter rely heavily on the correct use of terminology. When using these questions for study, make sure to define all terms in the questions and possible answers. Use the textbooks, references, and the glossary in this book to look up any terms you do not understand.

Quick Content Review

- **Research literacy** (or *scientific literacy*) is the knowledge and understanding of scientific concepts and processes required for personal and professional decision-making. When we are research literate, we can find, read, and understand the research and use critical thinking to determine the validity of the information presented by the paper. Critical thinking and the scientific method are very similar.
- Developing an inquiry-based approach to life also is important. This means that we learn to ask relevant questions. Relevant questions evolve from mindfulness and intuition. For example, "Why and how does massage reduce uncomfortable stress responses?" Only when we have relevant questions can we begin the research process. Scientifically based research methods are a way to seek answers to those questions.
- A research-literature search discovers information from researchers who designed and conducted a study to look for answers to some of the same questions we might have. Part of reading research articles involves making sure the research was conducted properly and that the information is scientifically valid and not just opinion.
- Effective outcomes from massage applications are achieved when massage methods interact with physiologic processes. Because massage has demonstrable physiologic effects, those effects can be studied through the scientific method. Because people behave, feel, and function differently before and after massage, these outcomes can be studied with valid research. Massage therapy research generally falls into two types: what works and why it works. What works—based research involves outcomes such as reduced pain perception, improved sleep patterns, and decreased anxiety. What works—type research can be targeted to a specific condition such as degenerative joint disease or fibromyalgia. Why it works—based massage research attempts to identify the physiological changes as a result of massage, such as alteration in neurochemicals, changes in inflammatory markers, and shifts in neuro-responses.
- Research also can be categorized by determining efficacy and effectiveness. Efficacy means that something can produce an effect, especially in very controlled situations such as a research experiment. Effectiveness is more about how

valuable an intervention, such as massage, is when used in less-controlled situations.

- The **scientific method** is a means of objectively researching a concept to determine whether it is valid. Research begins with a **hypothesis** (i.e., "If this happens, then that will happen"). The hypothesis must then be tested; this usually is accomplished through an **experiment.** Interpretation of the data collected during the experiment is expressed in statistical form; therefore, the reader must be able to interpret terms used in statistical reporting. This requirement sometimes makes reading research papers difficult for the general public. However, you do not have to be an expert in statistics; you simply must understand what the statistical terms mean. Usually, the statistical results are presented in a chart or graph, which is helpful.
- The experiment must follow accepted design measures so that others can replicate it to see whether they get the same result to make sure the original researcher did not have any biases that influenced the outcome of the research. The results of the experiment should either prove or disprove the hypothesis. Often the results of the research generate more questions, leading to more research.

Different types of experiments are performed in research:

- *Randomized controlled trials* involve a randomization procedure in which each subject has an equal chance of being assigned to an intervention group that actually receives the treatment or a control group that receives a fake treatment. Randomization helps prevent researchers from knowingly or unknowingly creating bias in the outcomes. Randomized controlled trials are the gold standard for establishing the effects of a treatment.
- *Cohort studies*, also called *prospective* or *longitudinal studies*, use observation as the research method. The interventions are not manipulated; rather, the researchers select and follow a large population of people who have the same condition or are receiving a specific intervention over a period of time. The progression and results of treatment are compared with a group not affected by the condition.
- *Outcomes research* involves a larger group of individuals who receive the same intervention. They are evaluated for outcomes after the intervention is complete.
- A *case series* is a collection of comprehensive reports that follow the research method on a series of clients with the same condition who are receiving the same intervention.
- A *case report* involves a report on the intervention and outcome for a single client. These cannot be taken as evidence based, as the sample size is too small to have a definite cause and effect relationship. However, case reports can be good to determine specific means to handle a certain patient type.
- *Systematic reviews* and *meta-analyses* combine multiple research studies that are similar in design. A systematic review usually is restricted to random controlled studies, which are considered valid evidence if they are well done. A group of reviewers searches the available literature databases by entering common terminologies into the

databases and retrieving copies of all the articles written on a specific topic. After all the research has been collected, the reviewers use critical thinking methods to evaluate the validity of each study and then synthesize the results. The final product reports on properly completed, meaningful research that is relevant to practitioners and clinicians.

- A meta-analysis is a type of systematic review that uses statistical methods to combine and analyze multiple investigations. Two important sources of systematic reviews that involve massage are the Cochrane Database of Systematic Reviews (commonly called the Cochrane Reviews) and the Database of Abstracts of Reviews of Effects.
- **Evidence-based practice** comprises interventions for which consistent scientific and clinical evidence shows improved client outcomes. **Evidence-informed practice** uses the best available information to guide professional practice. The best evidence to determine whether an intervention, such as massage, actually causes the outcome is the double-blind, randomized controlled clinical trial. It consists of the randomized assignment of subjects or participants in a double-blind design, in which neither the investigators nor the study subjects know the actual treatment group in which the subjects are placed. This type of trial also uses a control group, in which no intervention is used, and a sham group, in which a fictional treatment is provided. This type of trial is difficult to design for massage therapy research. One of the biggest challenges is devising fake or fictional massage. However, progress is being made, and more quality research should be forthcoming in the future.
- The quality of research for massage remains less than satisfactory; however, there appears to be enough research for therapeutic massage to be an evidence-informed practice. Evidence-informed practice allows expanded types of evidence.
- Systematic reviews (including meta-analyses), randomized controlled trials, and other types of experimental research are considered in evidence-based practice. In evidence-informed practice, the following are also considered: nonexperimental research (e.g., surveys), qualitative research, conference and seminar reports, examples of good practice, and expert opinion.
- Research studies currently provide evidence that massage therapy:
  - May play a role in reducing detrimental stress-related symptoms
  - Is pleasurable
  - Appears to manage some types of soft tissue pain
  - Supports social bonding
  - Likely improves the perception of quality of life in individuals who enjoy massage
  - Typically is safe when provided in a conservative and general manner with sufficient pain-free pressure
- The benefits of massage appear to be related to the application of mechanical forces to soft tissue. The manual techniques of massage are physiologically specific and well defined by the following:

- Mode of application (i.e., rubbing, pulling, pressing, touching)
- Speed (sustained or slow, rhythmic, staccato, or fast)
- Intensity and depth of pressure of touch (light touch, moderate/medium touch or firm/heavy touch, or a combination)
- Part of the therapist's body used to apply the techniques (fingers, hands, forearms, knees, or foot)
- Massage methods involve the application of mechanical forces. Possible results of these methods include the following:
  - Altered pliability of connective tissue
  - Stimulation of nerve endings in the fasciae
  - Changes in local circulation
  - Changes in the tone of muscles
- The benefits of massage may occur when methods normalize tissues that are tense, tight, deformed, twisted, or compressed by introducing mechanical forces (e.g., pulling, pressing, bending, and twisting) into body tissues using massage, stretching, mobilization, etc. The fascia is found throughout the body, connecting everything so that the body functions as a single, integrated unit instead of individual parts. The specific massage applications that best influence the fascia are still unknown.
- How often and how long a massage should be received has not yet been determined definitively. This would be determined by dosing research. A few dosing studies indicate that the weekly 60-minute massage session is most effective.
- Research supports massage as a means of managing anxiety related to pain and a means of altering mood, the pain threshold, and the perception of pain. Expanding on what we learned about massage earlier, we can say that massage therapy:
  - Appears to reduce stress
  - Is pleasurable
  - Improves the perceived quality of life
  - May help move fluids around
  - Is safe when provided in a conservative and general manner with sufficient pain-free pressure
- Some applications of massage can mimic normal physiological function for benefit. An example is abdominal massage supporting large intestine function.
- Overall, it appears that a general full-body massage can directly and indirectly influence many structures and functions to help the person adapt and cope and to help restore function. The results of individual, specific applications may not be able to be identified because massage encompasses many different elements.
- Benefits can be derived from the quiet, nurturing presence of the massage therapist, the duration of the massage, the massage environment, and the unlimited variations in methods, pressure, speed, and so forth.

Factual Recall Questions

1. Science is defined as _____.
   a. Knowing something without going through a conscious process of thinking
   b. The ability to pay attention to a specific area and maintain an unconscious focus and intent
   c. The process of using all mental and physical resources available to better understand, explain, and predict normal and unusual natural phenomena
   d. Craft, skill, and technique that enable a person to monitor and adjust involuntary or subconscious responses

2. Centering/mindfulness is defined as _____.
   a. A craft, skill, technique, and talent
   b. The ability to pay attention and maintain specific focus
   c. Knowing something without going through a conscious process of thinking
   d. The objective researching of a concept to see whether it is valid

3. The purpose of valid research in bodywork is to _____.
   a. Generate more questions
   b. Objectively research the physiologic process
   c. Subjectively research the bodywork process
   d. Justify bodywork as an art

4. Which of the following is an example of a method that provides manual external sensory stimulation?
   a. Music
   b. Kneading
   c. Centering
   d. Breathing

5. Most agree that the effects of massage can be explained by which two categories?
   a. Sensory stimulation and mechanical methods
   b. Centering and intuition
   c. Art and experimentation
   d. Art and intuition

6. Which type of method specifically targets the nervous system?
   a. Mechanical
   b. Circulatory
   c. Sensory stimulation
   d. Energetic

7. Which of the following is an example of biochemicals being responsible for problems in behavior, mood, or perception of stress and pain?
   a. Anxiety
   b. Obstructive sleep apnea
   c. Eczema
   d. Farsightedness

8. If massage can increase fine motor movements such as handwriting, then which neurotransmitter is influenced?
   a. Serotonin
   b. Oxytocin
   c. Dopamine
   d. Growth hormone

9. If massage can be shown through research to reduce cravings for food or to reduce hunger, then which neurotransmitter is responsible?
   a. Epinephrine
   b. Serotonin
   c. Dopamine
   d. Norepinephrine

10. Hans Selye described body responses to stress in three stages. The middle stage is called which reaction?
    a. Alarm
    b. Exhaustion
    c. Resistance

11. What general term is used to describe the initial activation of the sympathetic nervous system?
    a. Alarm
    b. Stress
    c. Entrapment
    d. Randomization

12. Parasympathetic patterns are described as _____.
    a. Restorative; adrenaline is secreted, mobility is decreased, and the bronchioles are constricted
    b. Occurring as physical activity is curtailed, digestion and elimination are increased, and bronchioles are constricted
    c. Involving increased physical activity, dilated pupils, halted saliva secretion, and increased stomach secretion
    d. Restorative; heartbeat speeds up, bladder emptying is delayed, and saliva secretion is increased

13. Three main types of proprioceptors are muscle spindles, tendon organs, and _____.
    a. Cervical/lumbar plexus
    b. Spinal nerves
    c. Joint kinesthetic receptors
    d. Sphincter muscles

14. A client gets a cramp in the hamstrings when elongating the muscles too quickly. Which reflex prompted the action?
    a. Stretch
    b. Hooke's
    c. Flexor
    d. Tendon

15. What reflex is involved in maintaining balance?
    a. Flexor
    b. Withdrawal
    c. Tendon
    d. Crossed extensor

16. Gate control theory refers to _____.
    a. Reduction in perception of sensation of a sensory receptor by adaptation
    b. Control of homeostasis by alteration of tissue or function
    c. A method of teaching the body to deal with stress through meditation and entrainment
    d. Painful stimuli being prevented from reaching the spinal cord by stimulation of other sensory nerves

17. When a research experiment is performed more than once to make sure that the results were unbiased, it is called _____.
    a. Double blind
    b. Control
    c. Hypothesis
    d. Replication

18. What is the first aspect of research?
    a. Conclusions
    b. Question
    c. Hypothesis
    d. Experiment

19. What is it called when the researcher is exploring existing information about a research question?
    a. Discovery
    b. Discussion
    c. Scientific method
    d. Framework

20. What is the broad explanation that synthesizes many different, unrelated facts and findings to explain a process or phenomenon?
    a. Experiment
    b. Introduction
    c. Variable
    d. Theory

21. In which group is the variable present?
    a. Control
    b. Experimental
    c. Replication
    d. Discussion

22. Which of the following defines the experiment?
    a. Testing the conclusions
    b. Discovering the variables
    c. Testing the hypothesis
    d. Comparing the results

23. In a typical research paper, where is the actual experiment described?
    a. Introduction
    b. Results
    c. Conclusions
    d. Methods

24. When a researcher's opinions influence the outcome of the research, the research is considered _____.
    a. Valid

b. Biased
c. Abstract
d. Replicated

Application/Concept Identification and Clinical Reasoning/Synthesis Questions

1. A client states a goal of wanting to relax and complains of having headaches, gastrointestinal problems, and high blood pressure. The client is likely to be experiencing _____.
   a. Excessive parasympathetic output
   b. Excessive sympathetic output
   c. Normal entrainment
   d. Sleep deprivation

2. A person experiencing fluid retention, muscle weakness, vertigo, hypersensitivity, fatigue, weight gain, and break-down in connective tissue most likely has _____.
   a. An infection disease
   b. Long-term high blood levels of cortisol
   c. First-stage/alarm reaction

3. Massage to support arterial circulation based on mimicking normal physiological function would be performed in which way?
   a. A 50-minute massage using gliding but avoiding heavy pressure
   b. A 45-minute compressive massage against the vessels proximal to the heart and moving in a distal direction
   c. A 50-minute massage using short pumping techniques and gliding toward the heart
   d. A 30-minute massage emphasizing gliding strokes distal to proximal and active joint movement

4. A researcher is conducting an experiment in which massage is introduced to determine whether endorphin levels change. What part of the experiment is the massage?
   a. Hypothesis
   b. Controlled variable
   c. Independent variable
   d. Abstract

5. What type of massage would be most helpful for a client who has reached the exhaustive reaction phase of the general adaptive response to stress and has been there for longer than 6 months?
   a. Weekly appointments over 1 month using 15 minutes of tapotement and shaking
   b. Weekly sessions over 3 months with light pressure, pulling and pressing
   c. Weekly appointments over 6 months with slow strokes, broad-based compression, and rocking
   d. Weekly sessions for 6 months with staccato, fast deep pressure

Exercise

Using the previous questions as examples, write at least three more questions. Develop plausible wrong answers and be sure that the correct answer is clearly correct. Then write a rationale for each question. The more questions you write, the better you will understand the material.

INDICATIONS AND CONTRAINDICATIONS FOR THERAPEUTIC MASSAGE

Review Tips

The indications and contraindications for therapeutic massage serve as the foundation for safe practice. Massage provides benefits that are justified by research and clinical experience. It is important for massage to benefit clients and not harm them. The major reason for massage licensing is to protect the public from harm. It would be prudent to test this content extensively on exams. Questions typically are written in all three question forms. The best study strategy for factual recall and concept identification questions is memorization of the terminology, using the clinical reasoning process, and identifying wrong answers as well as figuring out why they are wrong. Use these questions to help determine whether you comprehend the vocabulary used. Look up any terms you do not understand.

This content can be tested in the case study type of question, which assesses the ability to synthesize information and requires clinical reasoning to identify the best answer based on facts supplied in the question.

Quick Content Review

- Indications for massage are based on physiologic effects that provide the benefits of massage. Massage is beneficial for most people, yet contraindications do exist and harm to clients can occur. This is called an adverse effect. The responsible massage professional always refers a client for diagnosis and treatment by a qualified health professional without delay—as soon as any condition is noticed that may suggest an underlying physical or mental health problem. Massage may prove beneficial and supportive to the interventions of the healthcare professional and may enhance the healing process by temporarily reducing pain, relaxing the client, reducing stress responses, and much more. In addition, the client's subjective experience with the one-on-one contact and compassionate touch given by the massage professional may provide support during a difficult time, thereby reducing feelings of frustration, isolation, anxiety, and depression which often accompany illness or periods of stress.
- An indication is a condition for which an approach would be beneficial for health enhancement, treatment of a particular disorder, or support of a treatment modality other than massage.
- A contraindication is a condition for which an approach could be harmful. The following contraindications occur:
  - General avoidance of application—Do not massage.

- Regional avoidance of application—Do massage, but avoid a particular area.
  - Application with caution—Do perform massage, but carefully select the types of methods to be used, the duration of the massage, the depth and intensity of pressure, and the frequency of application.
- Most contraindications are best described as cautions. This means that massage will need to be adapted to ensure that the client is not harmed.
- Approaches to care are: therapeutic change, condition management, restorative care, and palliative care.
- Therapeutic change is a beneficial alteration produced by massage that is targeted to return the individual to a state of improved function.
- Condition management involves the use of massage methods to support clients who are not able to undergo a therapeutic change process but wish to be treated as effectively as possible within an existing set of circumstances.
- Restorative care approach to massage supports normal rest and restorative function. It helps restore the body to a state of calm and allows it to relax and repair. The massage approach supports parasympathetic and enteric ANS function. With a restorative approach, the client is generally healthy and has adaptive capacity. This care approach can be considered preventive and part of health maintenance.
- Palliative care is provided when the condition most likely is going to become worse and degenerative processes will continue (e.g., terminal illness, dementia). It often relates to approaches that reduce suffering. Palliative care is also considered general relaxation massage for pleasure and well-being.
- Health is more than the absence of disease. Health is the optimal functioning of the body and mind. Dysfunction is the in-between state of "not healthy" but "not sick" (experiencing disease). Massage professionals serve many people at the beginning of dysfunctional patterns—when the client does not feel his or her best but is not yet sick. It is important to monitor the client to make sure that they do not progress further into dysfunctional patterns. The benefits of massage are most effectively focused on assisting people to stay within the healthy range of functioning.
- Homeostasis is a state of balance. In acute conditions, homeostatic balance is recovered quickly. In chronic diseases, the body is stressed, and a fully normal state of balance may never be restored.
- Risk factors may put a client at risk for developing a disease or injury. Sometimes signs and symptoms may be contraindications with cautions requiring a cautious and informed approach to massage or may show the need for referral to a physician. A massage therapist may be the first to recognize the early warning signs of disease and will need to determine whether a massage will benefit or interfere with the process and whether a client needs to be referred to another healthcare professional.
- Inflammation is the body's method of healing; however, if inflammation does not resolve, the condition may become chronic.

- Pain is a complex, private, abstract experience. For acute pain, massage can activate the parasympathetic nervous system, thereby relaxing the client. For chronic pain, a massage therapist needs to work as part of a multidisciplinary healthcare team to provide symptomatic relief of pain and to initiate hardiness. With intractable pain, massage may provide short, temporary, symptomatic relief.
- Localized pain is confined to a specific area at the site of origin. Projected pain is a nerve pain that is continued along the nerve tract. Radiating pain is diffused around the site of origin and is not well localized. Referred pain is felt in an area distant from the site of the painful stimulus. Somatic pain arises from stimulation of receptors in the skin or the fascia and deeper soft tissues and can be called *deep somatic pain*. Visceral pain results from stimulation of receptors in the viscera (internal organs). Neurogenic pain is defined as pain due to dysfunction of the peripheral or central nervous system, in the absence of nociceptor (nerve terminal) stimulation by trauma or disease. Other terms used to describe some (but not all) forms of neurogenic pain include neuropathic pain.
- If the client has a recurring pain pattern that resembles referred pain patterns, they should be referred to a physician for a more specific diagnosis. When pain is referred, it is usually to a structure that developed from the same embryonic segment or dermatome as the structure in which the pain originates.
- Phantom pain is a type of pain frequently experienced by clients who have had a limb amputated. These clients experience pain or other sensations in the area of the amputated extremity, as though the limb were still there.
- The difference between entrapment and compressed nerve impingement indicates when massage is most effective. Entrapment is pressure on a nerve from soft tissue. Compression is pressure on a nerve from bony structures. Massage applied to soft tissues is most beneficial for entrapment.
- Endangerment sites are areas in which nerves and blood vessels surface close to the skin and are not well protected by muscle or connective tissue. Areas with fragile bony projections are also considered endangerment sites. Areas that are pressure sensitive such as the eyes are considered endangerment sites.
- Important warning signs that indicate that the client should be referred to a physician for specific diagnosis include persistent unexplained fatigue; inflammation; lumps and tissue changes; rashes and changes in skin; edema; mood alterations (e.g., depression, anxiety); infection (local and general); changes in appetite, elimination, or sleep; bleeding and bruising; nausea, vomiting, or diarrhea; and changes in temperature (hot [fever] or cold).
- The massage therapist should be able to assess the effects of the medications and should discover the ways that massage may interface with these effects. When researching the action of medications, pay extra attention to the side effects as an indication for potential referral.

- Clients must always be referred to their personal healthcare professionals. The massage therapist should make no attempt to direct clients to different healthcare professionals. If the client does not have a doctor, chiropractor, or counselor, a list of professionals who have been contacted and educated about therapeutic massage should be provided.
- Use clinical reasoning methods and the best available information to function in an evidence-informed approach.

Factual Recall Questions

1. Which of the following is *not* a type of contraindication?
   a. Application of a modality other than massage
   b. General avoidance of an application
   c. Regional avoidance of an application
   d. Application with caution

2. Which of the following is *not* a general benefit of massage?
   a. Decrease in perceived stress
   b. Enhanced elimination
   c. Inhibition of homeostasis
   d. Increased pain tolerance

3. The generally accepted definition of chronic pain is that it _____.
   a. Is a symptom of a disease or a temporary aspect of medical treatment
   b. Is frequently experienced by clients who have had a limb removed
   c. Persists or recurs for indefinite periods, usually longer than 6 months
   d. Often subsides with or without therapy

4. Which of the following is a description of burning pain?
   a. Short-lived but intense and easily localized
   b. Constant but vague in location
   c. Slow to develop; lasts longer and is less accurately localized
   d. Blocks blood supply to the muscle, and contraction causes pain

5. Somatic pain is defined as pain _____.
   a. Resulting only from stimulation of receptors in the skin
   b. Resulting only from stimulation of receptors in the skeletal muscles, joints, or tendons
   c. Resulting only from stimulation of receptors in the internal organs
   d. Arising from stimulation of receptors in the skin, skeletal muscles, joints, tendons, and fascia

6. What type of pain is experienced in a surface area away from the stimulated organ?
   a. Muscle
   b. Referred
   c. Deep
   d. Acute

7. Neck pain on the right side can be indicative of referred pain from what organs?
   a. Appendix and kidney
   b. Colon and bladder
   c. Heart and lungs
   d. Liver and gallbladder

8. Lung and diaphragm pain may be referred to which cutaneous area?
   a. Left side of the neck
   b. Right side of the chest
   c. Right side of the neck
   d. Left side of the hip

9. A person who is experiencing an impingement of the cervical plexus would have which symptoms?
   a. Shoulder pain, chest pain, arm pain, wrist pain, and hand pain
   b. Low back discomfort with a belt distribution of pain, as well as pain in the lower abdomen, genitals, and thigh
   c. Gluteal pain, leg pain, genital pain, and foot pain
   d. Headaches, neck pain, and breathing difficulties

10. Sacral plexus nerve impingement is indicated by _____.
    a. Gluteal pain, leg pain, genital pain, and foot pain
    b. Headaches, neck pain, and breathing difficulties
    c. Shoulder pain, chest pain, arm pain, wrist pain, and hand pain
    d. Low back discomfort with a belt distribution of pain and with pain in the lower abdomen, genitals, thigh, and medial lower leg

11. What is the definition of *health*?
    a. Prepathologic state
    b. Homeostatic and restorative body mechanisms are unable to adapt
    c. Anatomic and physiologic functioning limits
    d. Optimal functioning with freedom from disease or abnormal processes

12. *Pathology* can be defined best as _____.
    a. The in-between state of "not healthy" but "not sick"
    b. Anatomic and physiologic functioning limits
    c. The study of disease
    d. The processes of inflammatory tissue repair

13. A sign of disease is _____.
    a. Subjective abnormalities felt only by the patient
    b. Objective abnormalities seen or measured by someone other than the patient
    c. A dysfunctional process noted by the patient

14. *Homeostasis* can be defined as _____.
    a. The process of counterbalancing a defect in body structure or function
    b. A group of signs and symptoms
    c. The relative constancy of the internal environment of the body
    d. Subjective abnormalities felt by the patient

15. The general adaptation syndrome is characterized as _____.
    a. Being always a preexisting condition
    b. Involving three stages: alarm, resistance, and exhaustion
    c. Involving three stages: inflammatory response, swelling, and pain

16. The inflammatory response has five signs: loss of function, redness, swelling, pain, and _____.
    a. Stickiness
    b. Liquid
    c. Heat
    d. Mucus

17. What term describes the process of new cells replacing similar cells?
    a. Egestion
    b. Fibrosis
    c. Inflammation
    d. Regeneration

18. Regional contraindications are characterized as _____.
    a. Those that require a physician's evaluation to rule out serious underlying conditions before any massage
    b. Being present when health is the optimal functioning goal
    c. In effect when a client is in the in-between state of "not healthy" but "not sick"
    d. Those that relate to a specific area of the body

19. The difference between benign tumors and malignant tumors is that _____.
    a. Early detection is easier for benign than for malignant tumors
    b. Malignant tumors are bigger than benign tumors
    c. Benign tumors remain localized; malignant tumors tend to spread
    d. Benign tumors grow slowly; malignant tumors grow rapidly

20. Massage and medication stimulate a body process, replace a chemical in the body, and _____.
    a. Work on a cure for the problem
    b. Work from a pathologic base
    c. Inhibit a body process
    d. Remove cellular debris

21. What occurs when medication and massage stimulate the same process?
    a. Antagonism
    b. Synergism
    c. Metastasis
    d. Impingement

22. Intractable pain is described as a(n) _____.
    a. Cutaneous distribution of spinal nerve sensations
    b. Diffuse, localized discomfort that persists for indefinite periods
    c. Chronic pain that persists even when treatment is provided
    d. Abnormality in a body function that threatens well-being

23. Predisposing conditions that may make the development of disease more likely are called _____.
    a. Metastasis
    b. Pathology
    c. Signs and symptoms
    d. Risk factors

24. Objective abnormalities that can be seen or measured by someone other than the client are referred to as _____.
    a. Stress
    b. Memory
    c. Signs
    d. Pain

25. What type of tissue supports, provides structure, spaces, stabilizes, and forms scars?
    a. Connective
    b. Membranous
    c. Epithelial
    d. Fibrotic

Application/Concept Identification and Clinical Reasoning/Synthesis Questions

1. What is the major reason massage practitioners need to be aware of endangerment sites?
    a. These are soft areas that are unable to tolerate any pressure or movement.
    b. They may signal a life-threatening disorder.
    c. The remaining proximal portions of sensory nerves are exposed here.
    d. These areas could be damaged by deep sustained pressure.

2. Which of the following is an example of condition management?
    a. Managing the existing physical compensation patterns
    b. Assisting the client through learning to walk again
    c. Restoring a client's range of motion to preinjury state
    d. Using massage to help a client feel better about self and to change jobs

3. A client enters the massage room complaining of a bad back from working at the computer. This is a stage 1 dysfunction, and the client wants to reverse the condition. Which approach would be the most effective?
    a. Referral to a back specialist
    b. Therapeutic change
    c. Condition management
    d. Palliative care

4. Which of the following clients may require only palliative care from a massage therapist?
    a. Athlete with a sprained ankle
    b. Person with a broken arm
    c. Individual with terminal cancer
    d. Pregnant client in the first trimester

5. Therapeutic inflammation is best used in situations in which _____.
    a. There is compromised immune function
    b. Fibrotic connective tissue causes dysfunction
    c. Active inflammation is already present
    d. A condition such as fibromyalgia exists

6. Which is the most effective massage method for working on impingement syndromes?
    a. Tapotement and shaking

b. Gentle stretching

c. Rapid deep compression

d. Friction

7. Acute pain is most effectively managed with which intervention?

a. An inhibitory method

b. An aggressive rehabilitation approach

c. One that is less invasive and supports the current healing process

d. One that involves compression on a nerve in a bony structure

8. Which technique would be contraindicated for a client taking an anticoagulant?

a. Holding stroke

b. Friction

c. Superficial gliding

d. Rocking

9. Which of the following is contraindicated for application of deep sustained compression?

a. Lymph nodes

b. Trigger points

c. Dermatomes

d. Ground substance

10. A doctor referral is indicated if the client _____.

a. Has mild edema in the lower legs after a plane flight

b. Complains about care at the local outpatient clinic

c. Bruises and fatigues easily

d. Is beginning a new medication

Exercise

Using the previous questions as examples, write at least three more questions. Develop plausible wrong answers and be sure that the correct answer is clearly the best answer. Then write a rationale for each question. The more questions you write, the better you will understand the material.

HYGIENE, SANITATION, AND SAFETY

Review Tips

Hygiene, sanitation, and safety continue the theme of maintaining a safe massage experience for the client. This content typically is assessed with factual recall questions. Effective study strategy involves a review of the terminology. The content covers pathogenic organisms and how to control the spread of these disease-causing agents through hygiene and sanitation. Standard precautions have been developed to maintain a safe environment not only for the client but also for the massage therapist. Fire safety, environmental safety, and premise safety are main topics. It is also important to identify various types of harassment behavior and to understand strategies to deal with these situations.

Quick Content Review

- This information supports a safe, professional practice. It is a good idea to review procedures regularly. Always prioritize a safe, sanitary massage environment for clients. As massage professionals, we must understand the use of standard precautions and fire and premise safety measures to serve our clients in a health-promoting and hazard-free manner. Standard precautions are an expansion of the previous universal precautions developed by the Centers for Disease Control (CDC). Transmission-based precautions are used when people have diseases that can spread through contact, droplet, or airborne routes and are always used in addition to standard precautions.

- Respiratory protection protects the wearer. Respiratory protection refers to respirators, which are protective devices that cover a person's nose and mouth or the entire face or head to help reduce the wearer's exposure from breathing in air that contains contaminants, such as small respiratory droplets from a person who has COVID-19. This type of protection can include filtering facepiece respirators (FFRs), like N95 respirators.

- Source control protects others. Source control refers to the use of masks to cover a person's mouth and nose and to help reduce the spread of large respiratory droplets to others when the person talks, sneezes, or coughs. This can help reduce the spread of SARS-CoV-2, the virus that causes COVID-19, and other respiratory conditions.

- It is our responsibility to act reliably in emergencies, which includes basic first aid and CPR taught by the American Red Cross.

- The massage professional's hygiene and appearance are important because the massage professional represents all massage practitioners and therefore reflects the sanitary and safety practices of the massage business. If the professional's appearance does not reflect attention to hygiene and sanitation, concern may develop about the sanitation measures practiced by all massage professionals. Also, if massage professionals are not careful, they can transmit disease between clients. Careful hygiene limits this possibility.

- Tobacco smoke, breath odor, body odor, essential oils, incense, and perfume are some of the odors that may be offensive or may pose a health risk to clients.

- Alcohol and drug abuse, along with use of some prescription medications, affect a person's ability to function. The sensitivity and perception of the massage professional are altered. This definitely interferes with the ability to give the best massage possible and could even put the client in danger.

- The massage professional's awareness of pathogenic organisms is necessary because pathogenic organisms can cause disease in a client who is stressed, fatigued, injured, or weakened. Bacteria usually can be controlled with various prescription antibiotics. Today, many resistant strains of bacteria make antibiotics less effective. Viruses are not controlled easily. The few available antiviral agents only slow the reproduction of the virus. The best resistance to a virus is provided by the body's own immune system. Fungi, protozoa, and pathogenic animals can thrive only on or in a weakened host.

- The massage practitioner's main focus is wellness. If a disease is present, the body will be weak. Precautions must be taken to prevent the spread of disease and to avoid putting a weakened body at further risk. The massage professional must understand the mechanisms of disease to practice massage safely.

- The skin provides the main defense against invasion of pathogens and infection. Many serious diseases first manifest as skin symptoms. Because the massage practitioner observes and touches so much of the client's skin, it is important that he or she be able to recognize the major types of skin lesions. It also is important that the massage professional prevents the spread of infection by not massaging over breaks in the skin.

- Diseases caused by pathogenic organisms are spread by (1) environmental contact (e.g., food, water, soil, contaminated surfaces), (2) opportunistic invasion (when a person is weakened and the conditions are right for invasion), and (3) person-to-person contact through droplet transmission from direct contact or from airborne particles and body fluids.

- Aseptic methods include sterilization that kills everything; disinfection kills almost everything, antisepsis slows or stops the growth of most pathogens, and isolation separates or puts up a barrier against pathogens. Disinfection procedures using hot, soapy water and a 10% chlorine bleach solution (freshly made each day) or a commercial disinfectant are adequate for most massage situations. Alcohol and hydrogen peroxide are also considered disinfectants. Quaternary ammonium products can be used for disinfection on surfaces but are not considered effective for body fluid contamination. Although quaternary ammonium products are less cohesive than chlorine bleach, they also are less effective in the general sanitation process because they lose potency when exposed to hard water, cotton, or any other organic material. Chlorine bleach remains the most effective and least costly broad-spectrum disinfecting agent.

- Disinfection procedures are used for all laundry and cleaning, and the disinfectant should be allowed to air-dry on surfaces.

- The main concepts that support sanitation are keeping everything clean and disinfected. Keep areas or items that are contaminated separate from clean items. The massage environment must be constructed and maintained in such a way as to prevent the spread of disease by insects or other vermin.

- The main goal of standard precautions is to prevent the spread of infection through person-to-person contact or through contact with body fluids. Methods of isolation, including the use of a mask, gloves, and a gown, along with disinfection and sterilization procedures, prevent the spread of communicable disease.

- The massage professional needs to remain current about various contagious diseases, including hepatitis, human immunodeficiency virus (HIV), acquired immunodeficiency syndrome (AIDS), tuberculosis, bacterial infection, staphylococcal infection, severe acute respiratory infection (SARS), COVID-19, methicillin-resistant *Staphylococcal aureus* (MRSA) infection, as well as any other contagious disease.

- Microbes can be spread from one source to another. This is known as cross-contamination.

- It is the responsibility of the massage professional to stay current with new information, especially through the Centers for Disease Control and Prevention (CDC). Massage professionals need to understand the contamination routes. They need to know when their own germs may pose a threat to those who are immune suppressed, including those with HIV infection or AIDS. Massage professionals need to understand that casual contact is not a transmission route for hepatitis or HIV. Tuberculosis can be transmitted through droplets of mucus spread by coughing and sneezing.

- A vector is a means of infection transmission usually by an insect or animal that is not directly affected but acts as a passive carrier to the next host. Routes of infection transmission include person-to-person, contaminated blood or other bodily fluids, environmental contact, airborne, food, water, insects and other animals, and fomites (nonliving objects such as bedding, towels, or toys).

- Remember, the sanitation method that is most effective in controlling the spread of disease is careful hand washing and, for massage therapists, washing of any part of the body (e.g., the forearms) that is used in massage delivery.

- The main precautions necessary for preventing falls and accidents include the following:
  - Do not leave anyone who is at risk of falling alone in the massage therapy room
  - Keep all traffic areas hazard free
  - Provide good lighting
  - Regularly check all equipment for safety and make any repairs immediately

- The main way to prevent a fire is to make sure that all electrical equipment and wiring are in proper working order. Avoid any type of open flame in the area, including candles. Do not allow any smoking in the facility.

- Everyone should be skilled in first aid, cardiopulmonary resuscitation (CPR), and emergency care. The American Red Cross and similar organizations in other countries are best equipped to provide this training.

- The most common form of the crime of solicitation is prostitution, which is offering money to someone to have sex. But solicitation can be committed in the commission of any crime, such as murder or arson. The actual crime does not have to take place for someone to be charged with solicitation. Any form of solicitation should be reported to the police.

- Harassment is unwelcome conduct that is based on race, color, religion, sex (including sexual orientation, gender identity, or pregnancy), national origin, older age (beginning at age 40), disability, or genetic information (including family medical history). Harassment can include a range of verbal or physical behavior, including:

- Offensive jokes
- Demeaning remarks
- Name-calling, offensive nicknames, or slurs
- Offensive pictures or objects, including pornographic images
- Bullying
- Physical assaults
- Threats
- Intimidation

Factual Recall Questions

1. Pathogenic disease-causing organisms include _____.
   a. Dirt, sweat, and grime
   b. Paint, tar, and dust
   c. Viruses, bacteria, and fungi
2. A group of simple parasitic organisms that are similar to plants but are without chlorophyll and live on skin or mucous membranes are _____.
   a. Viruses
   b. Fungi
   c. Bacteria
   d. Protozoa
3. Which of the following is a route by which pathogens are spread?
   a. Opportunistic invasion
   b. Clean uniform
   c. Intact skin
4. The three primary ways that pathogens are spread include person-to-person contact, opportunistic invasion, and _____.
   a. Hand washing
   b. Standard precautions
   c. Shoes
   d. Environmental contact
5. A pressurized steam bath would be an example of what common aseptic technique?
   a. Isolation
   b. Sterilization
   c. Disinfection
6. The simplest, most effective deterrent to the spread of disease is _____.
   a. Hand washing
   b. Sterilization technique
   c. Using a towel barrier
7. An example of disinfection is _____.
   a. Using chemicals such as alcohol or soap
   b. Using extreme temperature
   c. Sanitary disposal of tissues
   d. A pressurized steam bath
8. The definition of acquired immunodeficiency syndrome is _____.

   a. An inflammatory process caused by a virus
   b. An irritation in the immune system
   c. A group of clinical symptoms caused by a dysfunction in the immune system
   d. A disease contracted by casual contact such as shaking hands or sharing bathroom facilities
9. Which of the following is an unsafe professional practice?
   a. Assisting the elderly onto and off the massage table
   b. Burning candles for atmosphere in the massage room
   c. Maintaining good lighting in massage areas
   d. Checking cables regularly on portable massage tables
10. Standard precautions are defined as _____.
    a. Emergency care given to all ill or injured persons before medical help arrives
    b. Procedures developed by the Centers for Disease Control and Prevention to prevent the spread of contagious disease
    c. The process by which all microorganisms are destroyed
    d. The process by which all pathogens are destroyed
11. Severe acute respiratory syndrome and COVID-19 are _____.
    a. Noncontagious
    b. Spread by person-to-person contact
    c. Harmless
    d. Controlled with nutrition

Clinical Reasoning and Synthesis Question

1. The massage professional is running behind today, and the next client has been waiting for 15 minutes. It is most important that the massage professional _____.
   a. Maintains scheduled appointments on time
   b. Has materials and activities available for clients to entertain themselves
   c. Makes sure sheets and linens are changed and equipment is disinfected between massages
   d. Apologizes to the client for being late
2. Thirty minutes into the session a client asks if sexual release is available for an additional fee. The next best action of the practitioner is
   a. leave the session and report solicitation to the police.
   b. explain sexual harassment to the client.
   c. leave the session and make note on client record.
   d. leave session after explaining no tolerance policy.

Exercise

Using the previous questions as examples, write at least three more questions. Develop plausible wrong answers and be sure that the correct answer is clearly correct. Then write a rationale for each question. The more questions you write, the better you will understand the material.

BODY MECHANICS

Review Tips

The information on body mechanics varies among textbooks; therefore, writing exam questions on this content is difficult if the exam must be legally defensible. The content is important and describes ergonomics. Because textbooks do not agree, questions typically are general and avoid controversial areas.

One of the best study strategies is to identify why all the wrong answers in the sample question are incorrect. Terminology is not standardized, so studying vocabulary is important but is not as effective as in other content areas.

Quick Content Review

- To maintain effective body mechanics and weight transfer, massage professionals need to be attentive to posture and balance, use the larger muscles to do the work, rely on leverage to apply pressure, and maintain a stable and relaxed body. Massage professionals must avoid using upper body strength to exert pressure for massage. Instead, they should use leverage and leaning to shift the center of gravity using body weight to provide pressure during massage. It is also important to maintain relaxed hands and wrists while giving massage.
- Avoid the use of the thumb when applying massage. When the thumb must be used, a stabilized joint position protects it. Massage professionals should use the hand as a unit and should rely on the forearm for many massage strokes, including most forms of gliding and compression.
- Massage professionals must learn to keep their lower backs straight and to avoid bending or curling at the waist and hips while giving a massage. Trunk flexion at the hip should not exceed 20 degrees. Frequent posture shifting also helps protect the massage professional's lower back.
- Knee problems can be avoided by respecting the basic design of the knee and frequently shifting the weight from foot to foot. Avoid hyperextension of the knee. Maintain an asymmetrical stance with one leg ahead of the other and move the position of the legs often.
- The ankle and the foot are protected by an asymmetrical stance, frequent position changes, and sitting when possible to do massage. Asymmetrical standing is the most efficient standing position.
- The massage professional needs to be comfortable and dressed in loose, nonrestrictive clothing that does not interfere with movement.
- Before your massage day begins, warm up your body with some general aerobic activity and gentle stretching. During the day, take breaks between massages, and move all the muscles you use while giving a massage. Massage your own arms, hands, and shoulders after each massage. The massage professional benefits from receiving regular massage.
- The massage table must be set at a comfortable height. Use a higher table for moderate to light pressure. A lower table can

be used if applying heavy pressure. Measure table height related to not exceeding 20 degrees of trunk flexion at the hip with a client on the table. This generally falls about where the hip joint is located. The size of the client will modify table settings. A higher table supports using the forearm for method application.

- If the massage professional carries a portable table, they must pay attention to the body mechanics used to lift and move the table. Lift the table with the knees and the hips—not the waist. Do not reach for the table when moving it from the car. Avoid habitually carrying the table on only one side.
- Massage professionals can protect their wrists by avoiding excessive compressive forces. Use a proper wrist angle, maintaining a relaxed wrist and fingers.
- Core strength is important to keep the trunk stable and in a neutral position.
- The basic principles of body mechanics are leaning and using the body weight focused from the foot to create ground reaction forces.
- The general rules for body mechanics are as follows:
  - Make sure your body is in good alignment and that your feet provide a wide base of support. The arm that is generating downward pressure should be opposite the back weight-bearing leg that creates the ground reaction force.
  - Weight is kept on the back leg and full foot (not toes), and the client's body is in front. The front non—weight-bearing leg is used to modulate pressure levels and to provide some stability.
  - Keep your head up.
  - Make sure that the wrists and the hands are always relaxed.
  - Avoid using your fingers and thumbs. Keep kneading strokes to a minimum. Grasping is stressful on the hands and forearms. Do not use the thumb for direct pressure.
  - Do not use the triceps portion of your arm. You can damage your ulnar nerve. Use the forearm just below the elbow.
  - Do not reach for the stroke. Keep the client close to you. The length (excursion) of the stroke on the client's body is no more than 24 inches.
  - Never hyperextend the wrist or knees. The weight-bearing knee will move into the normal knee-lock position; this is not hyperextension, which damages the knee. Make sure the angle of the wrist is no greater than 45—50 degrees of extension or flexion. This voids compression of the nerves in the wrist. Keep the elbows straight most of the time but do not allow elbows to hyperextend.
  - Change your position and method often.
  - Face the area you are working to avoid twisting.
  - Turn your whole body when you change the direction of your movements and shift the body weight to the back foot.
  - Kneading combines pushing and pulling. Pushing mechanics include shifting forward while flexing the front

knee with the rear knee extended. Pulling mechanics include rocking backward while flexing the rear knee and extending the front knee.

- If heavy pressure is required, do not push harder. Instead, use counterpressure, which is a force or pressure that acts in a contrary direction to pressure being applied.
- Work with smooth and even movements.
- Allowing your body to rock and sway with the movements is important. Slow rocking keeps your strokes slow. The resulting rhythmic movement keeps your body relaxed and is comforting to the client.

Factual Recall Questions

1. When a practitioner is in a relaxed standing posture supporting the gravitational line with the normal knee-locked position, which muscles are used for balance?
   a. Psoas major and psoas minor
   b. Gastrocnemius and soleus
   c. Hamstrings group
   d. Quadriceps group
2. What is the most efficient standing position (stance) for applying massage?
   a. Symmetrical
   b. Feet placed wide
   c. Asymmetrical
3. Most massage applications use a force generated in which direction?
   a. Downward
   b. Forward
   c. Downward and forward
   d. Forward and across
4. When compression is applied down and forward, weight transfer is most efficient when the massage therapist puts weight on the _____.
   a. Back leg and foot
   b. Front leg and knee
   c. Back foot and toes
   d. Front foot and toes
5. Increasing levels of pressure are achieved by _____.
   a. Moving closer to the massage table
   b. Increasing force into the back weight-bearing foot
   c. Standing on the toes

Application/Concept Identification and Clinical Reasoning/Synthesis Questions

1. A client keeps complaining of discomfort at the end of the massage stroke. The most likely reason is because the _____.
   a. Practitioner is pushing with the legs
   b. Practitioner is off balance and is using counterpressure
   c. Skin is being pulled from lack of lubricant
   d. Force is distributed over a narrow base at the end of the stroke
2. Observation of a fellow massage practitioner indicates that the shoulder girdle is aligned with the pelvic girdle, with the pressure-bearing arm opposite the weight-bearing leg, the fingers relaxed, the head up, the back straight, truck flexion is at 40 degrees, and the stance asymmetrical. Which of these areas needs correction?
   a. Back position
   b. Elbows
   c. Stance
   d. Shoulder position
3. When stretching the legs of a client by applying a pull against the ankle, the massage practitioner should _____.
   a. Fix the feet and pull with the shoulders
   b. Move to a symmetrical stance and lean back
   c. Maintain an asymmetrical stance and lean back, keeping the back straight
   d. Bend the knees and push back
4. The massage therapist needs to have _____ to be effective with body mechanics.
   a. Core stability
   b. Hyperflexibility
   c. Hypoflexibility
   d. Forearm strength
5. A massage professional is feeling strain in the shoulders and arms after completing four massage sessions. Which of the following is the most logical reason?
   a. Muscle strength in the arms is being used to exert force.
   b. An asymmetrical stance is being used.
   c. The client is positioned for best mechanical advantage.
6. A massage practitioner has been experiencing increasingly severe low back pain. What could the massage practitioner do to reduce back strain?
   a. Bend the knees past 15 degrees of flexion while performing massage
   b. Raise the table height to prevent torso bending
   c. Keep the head forward and down to change the center of gravity
   d. Externally rotate the back foot away from the line of force
7. A massage professional is complaining of pain in the wrist and near the elbow. Which of the following is an appropriate corrective action?
   a. Maintain the hands in a clenched fist to promote stability
   b. Increase the movement of the stroke at the shoulder joint
   c. Relax the hand and fingers during massage
   d. Shift the force application to the fingers and thumb
8. A massage professional is feeling strain in the knees. Which of the following is the most logical cause?
   a. Doing massage on hard floors
   b. Working with clients in the side-lying position

c. Keeping the knees flexed and static

d. Moving whenever the arm reach is beyond 45 degrees

Exercise

Using the previous questions as examples, write at least three more questions. Develop plausible wrong answers and be sure that the correct answer is clearly correct. Then write a rationale for each question. The more questions you write, the better you will understand the material.

PREPARATION FOR MASSAGE: EQUIPMENT, SUPPLIES, PROFESSIONAL ENVIRONMENT, POSITIONING, AND DRAPING

Review Tips

The content for the preparation for massage section includes massage equipment, draping, sanitation, hygiene, lubricant types, the massage environment, and how to communicate and give and receive feedback in the professional setting. The difficulty with this content is that it is more opinion based than fact based, so writing legally defensible questions is difficult. The case study format is common, and the key to finding the best answer is to eliminate the wrong answers. When reading the content in your textbook, identify the content areas that are not as opinion based. For example, draping clients and using massage lubricant generally are expected. Specifically, how the drape is used or how the lubricant is applied is more a matter of opinion. As with all content areas, there is unique terminology to be studied.

Quick Content Review

- The different locations and environments for massage set the mood and reflect the personality of the massage practitioner. Careful consideration of equipment (e.g., massage tables, body supports), supplies (e.g., oils, linens), music, and other amenities results in a professional yet personalized approach.

- Taking time to explain massage procedures to a client, taking a health history, and learning and understanding the expectations and outcomes for each massage help create an approach that meets the client's needs.

- Providing safe, respectful touch by using careful, modest draping and positioning is essential to massage therapy practice.

- Therapeutic massage is provided in many different environments. To maintain the integrity of the professional relationship, the environment created for the massage setting, including decorations and the reading material provided for clients, should reflect the scope of practice of massage. Whatever the physical location of the massage environment, the most important aspect is to present and deliver the highest standard of professional care to the public.

- Whether the massage takes place in a private office or clinical setting, in a public setting, onsite at a client's business or home, or outdoors, the general conditions for massage areas that must be considered include temperature, the fresh air supply, privacy, and accessibility. It is important to consider designated areas for business operations and the massage session and to provide privacy if any clothing needs to be removed. The massage practitioner must be attentive to cigarette or other smoke odors, cold hands, keeping pets out of the massage area, and other such considerations.

- The equipment, supplies, and setup procedures required for beginning a massage practice include portable and free-standing and hydraulic adjustable height massage tables, massage mats, massage chairs, and body supports. The setup of the massage area consists of supplies, table supports for positioning, modest draping materials, lubricant, music, and appropriate temperature of the massage area. The massage practitioner and the client must enjoy the music and want to listen to it. The rhythm and the beat of the music should match the desired effect for the massage session.

- The lighting is indirect so it does not cast a glare into the client's eyes. The practitioner must be able to dim or reduce the intensity of the light and to increase it for visibility when it is time to clean the room. Practitioners never work in a dark or candle-lit room.

- The massage practitioner completes preparations before beginning the massage. The room has to be set up and all necessary supplies gathered. The type of lubricant used and how it is dispensed, the temperature of the massage room, and the warmth of the practitioner's hands are all considerations. Massage professionals benefit from developing a method, referred to as *centering*, to help them focus on the client and the session to come.

- Client positioning and modest, appropriate draping procedures also must be considered. The practitioner then uses history-taking and assessment procedures to identify client outcomes and to formulate the approach for the massage. The plan is discussed with the client, and informed consent is obtained. All of this is done before the massage begins.

- Massage therapists must explain massage procedures to the client. Clients respond better and are less anxious if they understand procedural details such as sanitation methods, draping, where to hang their clothes, and what types of lubricant will be used.

- It is necessary to effectively drape and position a client. Two basic methods of draping are contour and flat draping. Pillows, rolled towels, and specially cut pieces of foam are used to contour the flat surface of the massage table and provide stability and comfort. Sheets, towels, or other large pieces of fabric are used to cover the client during the massage to provide privacy, modesty, and warmth. All draping materials are laundered with hot soapy water and bleach or another approved disinfecting solution. A fresh set of drapes is used for each client.

- When a client is lying prone, supports under the ankles, the lower abdomen and possibly around the chest are used. When supine, supports are placed under the knees and the neck. Side-lying with supports at the legs and under the arms and head is beneficial.

- Opaque draping materials must be used, and only the area that is being massaged is undraped. A chest towel or pillowcase is used to drape the breast area while the larger drape is pulled back to expose the abdomen. The towel is placed over the flat sheet and stabilized, and then the larger flat sheet is pulled out. The genital area is never undraped. A woman's breasts are not undraped or massaged as part of the general full-body approach. During a typical full-body massage, the client has to remove most clothing. The drape provides separation from the massage practitioner and defines the client's personal space.

- A portable and/or freestanding massage table, massage mat, and chair for seated massage can all be used when providing massage. The table should be simple and sturdy with adequate width and length and should be portable if the table is to be moved often. The massage table should have a face cradle, a covering that can be disinfected, and adequate padding for comfort and firm support. A height adjustable table or a hydraulic lift table best supports body mechanics. The massage table, including all connectors, bolts, cables, and hinges, must be checked for structural stability, to ensure the client's safety.

- Body supports that are used for massage clients include pillows, rolled towels, and specially cut pieces of foam, to contour the flat surface of the massage table and provide stability and comfort.

- Lubricants are used only to reduce friction on the skin caused by massage methods. Massage practitioners do not use lubricants for medicinal or cosmetic purposes. Types of lubricants include oils, creams, and gels. Lubricants must be dispensed in a contamination-free manner, and they should be as natural as possible. Scents should be avoided.

Factual Recall Questions

1. The most important stability feature of a portable massage table is the _____.
   a. Frame
   b. Cable support
   c. Adjustable legs
   d. Center hinge
2. Regardless of the type of draping material used, which characteristic is required?
   a. Disposable
   b. Large
   c. Opaque
   d. Cotton fabric

3. To maintain sanitary practice, draping material must be _____.
   a. Laundered in hot soapy water with a disinfectant such as bleach
   b. Sterilized and heat pressed
   c. Professionally laundered
4. To prevent allergic reactions, all lubricants should be _____.
   a. Oil based
   b. Water based
   c. Dispensed in sanitary fashion
   d. Scent free
5. The purpose of lubricant is to _____.
   a. Moisturize the skin
   b. Reduce drag on the skin
   c. Transport nutrients
   d. Provide counterirritation
6. Which environment is the most difficult for maintaining professional boundaries?
   a. Public events
   b. Private office in a commercial building
   c. Onsite at a residence
   d. Home office

Application/Concept Identification and Clinical Reasoning/Synthesis Questions

1. A client is particularly concerned with safety and is afraid of falling. Which piece of massage equipment would make the client most comfortable?
   a. Mat
   b. Stationary table
   c. Portable table
   d. Chair
2. A massage professional has just rented office space and fully decorated the area. The room has a window as well as overhead and indirect lighting. The central thermostat is in another area, but the massage room has a fan and an electric heater to adjust temperature. The small waiting area is bright and comfortable, with many flowering plants. A private restroom is just off the waiting room. The massage room is without a closet but does have hooks for clients' clothing. A closed cabinet holds supplies. The business area is small but includes a locked file cabinet and a small desk. What suggestion would improve the massage environment?
   a. Add an aromatherapy atomizer
   b. Put a lock on the massage room door
   c. Move the file cabinet into the massage room
   d. Remove the flowering plants
3. A massage practitioner has been seeing the same client weekly for 3 months. The client often discusses personal issues with the massage practitioner. During the previous session, the massage professional provided some reading material to help the client and talked with the client about how the practitioner had dealt with a similar issue. The

client has canceled the last two appointments. What is the most logical reason?

a. Feedback about the massage broke down.

b. Conversation with the client overshadowed the massage.

c. Gender issues are influencing the session.

d. The orientation process needs to be repeated.

4. A massage professional is preparing an orientation process for a new client. The professional has developed the following checklist: Show client the massage area, where to change and hang clothes, massage table draping and positioning, how to get on and off the massage table, music choices, and location of restrooms. Explain charts and equipment, lubricant types, sanitary procedures, and privacy methods. What is missing?

a. Explaining the general idea of massage flow

b. Providing a centering meditation with the client

c. Providing education on self-help

d. Introducing the client to products for sale

5. A client complains of mild general low back pain. Which approach is appropriate?

a. Use a side-lying position with leg and knee support

b. Work with the client prone, without support under the ankles

c. Work with the client supine, using support only under the neck

d. Position the client in a seated position and avoid supports

6. A client is shy and modest. Which of the following draping methods would be the best choice?

a. Contoured draping with towels

b. Partial body towel draping

c. Full-body sheet and towel draping

d. Sheet draping without towels

7. For which client should the massage therapist stay in the treatment room and assist the client onto and off the massage table?

a. A client in the first trimester of pregnancy

b. A 65-year-old man with diabetes

c. An elderly woman with high blood pressure

d. An adolescent with a wrist cast

8. An adolescent is coming in with a parent for a massage. The massage therapist has been informed that the client is uncomfortable with disrobing. Which of the following is the most logical alternative?

a. An educational session about the benefits of treatment

b. A draping demonstration

c. Working only with the client's feet

d. Having the client wear loose shorts and T-shirt

9. A client regularly lingers after the massage session to talk, causing the massage professional to get behind schedule. What is the most likely cause of this problem?

a. Boundaries regarding leaving promptly after treatment are unenforced.

b. Longer appointments are required.

c. More frequent appointments are required.

d. Transference and countertransference issues are being acted out.

Exercise

Using the foregoing questions as examples, write at least three more questions—one of each type: factual recall and comprehension, application and concept identification, and clinical reasoning and synthesis. Develop plausible wrong answers and be sure that the correct answer is clearly correct. Then write a rationale for each question. The more questions you write, the better you will understand the material.

MASSAGE MANIPULATIONS AND TECHNIQUES

Review Tips

Content about massage manipulations and techniques introduces many new terms. By this time, you should know to look up all terms you do not understand, and you should be able to use the terminology correctly. This content often is found in the factual recall question style.

Massage methods should be used in a safe and appropriate way. This content usually is assessed in a concept identification or clinical reasoning/synthesis type of question. Case studies are common. Anatomy and physiology terminology is common in these questions. You must be able to interpret the language in the question and possible answers and to use the clinical reasoning process to find the correct answer.

Effective study strategies include explaining a concept in different words than the text, to give examples of what the text is talking about, and to develop metaphors about the content.

Quick Content Review

Physiologic Effects of Massage

- All massage methods use some form of external sensory information from applied mechanical forces that can stimulate or inhibit body processes, depending on their use. In general, a fast, specific application of methods tends to stimulate, whereas a slow, general application tends to inhibit.

- Methods that move through the skin to the underlying tissue tend to be more mechanical and stimulate localized chemical responses.

- Painless, deep, broad-based compression encourages parasympathetic dominance.

- Massage manipulations and techniques that stay within the skin and superficial fascial layer tend to have a direct reflexive effect on the nervous system because many sensory nerves are located in the skin. These methods also tend to stimulate the release of hormonal and other body chemicals that provide a general systemic (whole-body) effect.

- Lighter methods may stimulate sympathetic dominance.

- Methods that move the body, cause muscles to contract and relax, and change joint position deliver sensory input to the proprioceptors and are more neurological in nature.

- Most massage methods that exert force on soft tissue result in neurological, mechanical, and chemical changes.

Massage Methods

- Basic massage methods include gliding (effleurage), kneading (pétrissage), compression, vibration, shaking, rocking, tapotement, percussion, and friction.
- The holding position is used for initial contact, stillness, calling attention to an area of the body, and adding body heat; reestablishing contact allows stillness when intermixed with the other movements of massage. The body needs time to process all the sensory information it receives during massage. Stopping the motions and simply resting the hands on the body provides this moment of stillness.
- Gliding (effleurage; French word meaning "to skim" or "to touch lightly on") refers to gliding methods applied horizontally in relation to the tissues. It is used for applying lubricant, warming the area with increasing pressure, connecting one area to another, evaluating, and providing abdominal massage. It results in tension stress in soft tissue when lubrication use is minimal, which creates drag and provides local tissue stretch.
- Kneading (pétrissage, from the French verb petrir, meaning "to knead") requires that the soft tissue be grasped, rolled, and squeezed. The main purpose of this manipulation is to twist tissue, thus applying bend, shear, and torsion stress into the tissue.
- Compression moves down into the tissues with varying depths of pressure, adding bending and compressive stress into the tissue. Very specific pinpoint compression, called *direct pressure* or *ischemic compression*, can be used on acupressure points and trigger points. The superficial application resembles the resting position but uses more pressure. The manipulations of compression usually penetrate the subcutaneous layer, whereas in the holding position, they stay on the skin surface. Much of the effect of compression results from pressing tissue against underlying structures including bone, causing it to spread and be squeezed from two sides.
- Vibration is a powerful method if it can be done long enough and at an intensity sufficient to produce physiologic effects. All vibration begins with compression. After the depth of pressure has been achieved, the hand needs to tremble and transmit the action to surrounding tissues.
- Shaking is a massage method that is effective for relaxing muscle groups or an entire limb. Shaking methods may confuse the positional proprioceptors because the sensory input is too disorganized for the integrating systems of the brain to interpret; muscle relaxation is the natural response in such situations. Shaking warms and prepares the body for deeper bodywork and addresses the joints in a nonspecific manner. Shaking is effective when the muscles seem extremely tight. This technique is primarily neurological in effect, but a small mechanical influence may be exerted on the connective tissue as well because of the lift-and-pull component of the method. Rhythmic shaking can also support fluid movement.
- Rocking is a soothing, rhythmic method that is used to calm people. Rocking is both neurological and chemical in its effects. Rocking also works through the vestibular system of the inner ear and feeds sensory input directly into the cerebellum. Other reflex mechanisms probably are affected as well.
- Tapotement (percussion) comes from the French verb *tapoter*, which means "to rap, drum, or pat." Tapotement techniques require that the hands or parts of the hand administer springy blows to the body at a fast rate. These blows are directed downward to create a rhythmic compression of the tissue. Percussion is divided into two classifications: light and heavy. The difference between light and heavy tapotement lies in whether the force of the blows penetrates only to the superficial tissue of the skin and subcutaneous layers (light), or more deeply into the muscles, tendons, and visceral (organ) structures, such as the pleura in the chest cavity (heavy). Heavy percussion should not be done over the kidney area or anywhere there is pain or discomfort. The various types of tapotement include hacking, cupping, beating, pounding, slapping, and tapping.
- Vibration, rocking, shaking, and tapotement can be called oscillation methods.
- Friction moves superficial tissue over deeper underlying tissue. Movement of the hands briskly on the skin is a form of friction. To prevent sliding on the skin, during deeper tissue layer massage, no lubricant is used. Movements are applied to a specific location and are transverse to the grain of the tissue or are circular.
- Two methods are used to apply friction:
  - No lubricant is used. Braced fingers, hand, or forearm or tool compresses the tissue to the depth required to access the tissue in which friction is to be used. The massage practitioner does not slide but rather moves the tissues back and forth or around.
  - The practitioner applies compression over the area in which friction is to be used. Instead of moving the application hand, the practitioner moves the adjacent joint of the client while sustaining compression. The friction results from the action of the underlying bone against the tissue.
- The five types of tissue stress (compression, tension, bending, shear, and torsion) occur when mechanical force (push/pull) is applied to the body.
- Compression occurs when two structures are pressed together.
- Tension (also called *tensile*) occurs when two ends of a structure are pulled apart from one another.
- Bending represents a combination of compression and tension. One side of a structure is compressed, while the other side is exposed to tensile stress.
- Shear is a sliding stress, often resulting in significant friction between the structures that are sliding against each other.
- Torsion stress is best thought of as twisting force. Massage methods that use kneading introduce torsion stress into the tissue.

- The seven aspects of quality of touch are depth of pressure, drag, direction, speed, rhythm, frequency, and duration.
- Depth of pressure can be light, moderate, heavy, or variable.
- *Drag* is the amount of pull (stretch) on the tissue.
- The direction can move from the center of the body out (centrifugal) or in from the extremities toward the center of the body (centripetal). It can proceed from origin to insertion (or vice versa) of the muscle, following the muscle fibers, transverse to the tissue fibers, or in circular motions.
- The speed of application can be fast, slow, or variable.
- *Rhythm* refers to the regularity with which the technique is applied. If the method is applied at regular intervals, it is considered even, or rhythmic. If the method is disjointed or irregular, it is considered uneven, or nonrhythmic.
- *Frequency* is the rate at which the method repeats itself within a given time frame. In general, the massage practitioner repeats each method about three times before moving or switching to a different approach.
- *Duration* is the length of time that the method lasts or that the manipulation stays in the same location.
- It is important to be able to organize a systematic approach to the massage so that all soft tissue is addressed and all joints are moved in a rhythmic, pleasurable manner. The body will adapt to repetitive sensory stimulation and will stop responding to the sensory input. Varying the touch quality prevents adaptation and continues to stimulate the body.
- A basic flow pattern is important so that all soft tissue is addressed and all joints are moved. The pattern for abdominal massage is always the same to facilitate the natural flow and elimination pattern of the large intestine.
- The use of joint movement techniques can make massage methods more effective. These techniques warm the tissues, relax the nervous system, and relax and lengthen the muscles, thus reducing the need for repetitive massage in an area.
- Three types of proprioceptors are affected by movement techniques:
  - Joint kinesthetic receptors detect position and rate of movement.
  - Muscle spindles detect stretch of muscle.
  - Golgi tendon organs detect muscle tension at the tendon.
- Two different types of joint movement are known: active (produced by the client) and passive (produced by the massage professional).
- The pathologic range-of-motion barrier is the point at which motion causes a bind, a catch, or pain.
- Hand placement for joint movement is as follows. One hand should be placed close to the joint to be moved. This hand acts as a stabilizer and is used for evaluation. The other hand is placed at the distal end of the bone and provides the movement.
- Methods can be used both as assessment to determine the status of the body and as an intervention to change

the status of the body. Some approaches are primarily intervention such as ischemic compression and friction.
- Muscle energy methods are an intervention. The methods involve the controlled used of muscle contraction to support tolerance to the sensation of tissue stretching. Positioning is very important. Muscle energy methods are focused on specific muscles and associated connective tissues and resultant joint function. For the muscles to be accessed for proper contraction, they must be positioned (actively or passively) in such a way that the tissue is shortened (attachments close together), then lengthened (attachments separate).
- Various types of muscle actions are used for muscle energy techniques:
  - Isometric, which involves no movement, only effort.
  - Isotonic, which involves movement against resistance. There are three types:
    1. Concentric isotonic: Attachments (origin and insertion) come together against resistance.
    2. Eccentric isotonic: Attachments (origin and insertion) separate against resistance.
    3. Multiple isotonic: Concentric and eccentric actions combine against resistance for a full range of movement for a joint.
- Postisometric relaxation (PIR) or contract relax (CR) is relaxation after a contraction.
- Contract-relax-antagonist-contract (CRAC) involves both the agonist and antagonist to support stretching.
- Pulsed muscle energy methods differ from all other methods. Instead of one strong contraction, small, light, rapid contractions of the muscles are used to activate the receptors.
- The target muscle is the muscle or muscle group on which the massage practitioner is specifically focusing a particular response.
- The amount of strength required during the contraction for the muscle energy method to work is usually no greater than 25% of muscle strength. The exception to this is strengthening of weak muscles. In this case, a stronger contraction or repeated contraction may be required.
- Positional release/strain-counterstrain is used when specific tender points are found, or when the client is in pain and positioned so that the painful sensation is reduced. It is a good method for gentle, painless release of all specific sore spots regardless of pathology (what is wrong). The tender point is the guide to proper positioning of the client. Use a full-body approach in positioning, and do not focus solely on the area around the tender point.
- Stretching is not always an appropriate method to use. Stretching is not used in acute situations. Do not stretch beyond normal range of motion.
- Two basic types of stretching may be used: longitudinal stretching, which pulls tissue in the fiber direction, and cross-directional stretching, which pulls tissue against the fiber direction, often with a twisting component.

- Massage consists of a mixture of techniques. A base of general, broad application methods is needed to form the structure of the massage. The methods most commonly used are gliding, compression, and rocking.
- General massage has a goal—to stimulate all sensory receptors, touch all layers and types of tissue, and move all major joints of the body. There are a million ways to do a massage. Subtle shifts and changes in pressure and intensity, methods used, positioning, sequence, and focus allow each massage to be different. Each client is different, and therefore each massage is different.

Factual Recall Questions

1. Massage methods are characterized as _____.
   a. Skillful use of the hands and forearms to affect the soft tissue directly
   b. Skillful use of the hands to affect the joints directly
   c. Application of methods using heat and equipment to affect soft tissue
   d. Application of compressive forces to affect meridians
2. Which of the following is produced voluntarily?
   a. Joint play
   b. Arthrokinematic movement
   c. Osteokinematic movement
   d. Joint end feel
3. Lifting the tissue away from underlying structures is the primary effect of which of the following methods?
   a. Compression
   b. Kneading
   c. Gliding
   d. Vibration
4. A client requests massage without lubricant. Which method would be inappropriate?
   a. Shaking
   b. Compression
   c. Kneading
   d. Gliding
5. A client is ticklish, particularly on the chest. Which method would be the best choice for this area?
   a. Compression over the client's own hand
   b. Friction with a tool
   c. Gentle gliding
   d. Fingertip compression
6. A client is feeling fatigued and wishes to be passive and quiet during the massage. Which of the following methods would be appropriate?
   a. Positional release
   b. Pulsed muscle energy
   c. Integrated approach
   d. Rocking
7. Isolate the target tissue in passive contraction, have the client contract the target group, have the client relax, and then lengthen the target muscles. Which method does this procedure describe?
   a. Positional release
   b. Postisometric relaxation
   c. Contract-relax-antagonist-contract
   d. Pulsed muscle energy
8. A major contraindication to massage of the legs is _____.
   a. Acne
   b. Brachial nerve compression
   c. Disk compression
   d. Thrombophlebitis
9. Which of the following Swedish methods is best for general broad applications when lubricant is requested?
   a. Pétrissage
   b. Compression
   c. Effleurage
   d. Vibration
10. Which of the following is of most concern when massaging the face?
    a. Proximity to mucous membranes and the transmission of pathogens.
    b. The skin of the face is thin.
    c. Facial muscles are weak.
    d. Compression damages underlying cranial sutures.
11. Which of the following body areas requires special attention to draping?
    a. Hand
    b. Leg
    c. Chest
    d. Shoulder
12. Which of the following body areas often is massaged longer than is effective?
    a. Hands
    b. Abdomen
    c. Legs
    d. Back
13. *Gliding* most effectively creates which tissue deformation?
    a. Shear
    b. Tension
    c. Torsion
    d. Resting
14. A massage application that twists tissue creates which of the following?
    a. Bend
    b. Torsion
    c. Gliding
15. Which of the following creates shear stress?
    a. Gliding
    b. Compression
    c. Tapotement
    d. Friction
16. Kneading is effective when creating _____.

a. Resting stroke
b. Tapotement
c. Bend and torsion stress

Application/Concept Identification and Clinical Reasoning/Synthesis Questions

1. A massage practitioner uses massage methods in a brisk and specific way. Which of the following client goals is best served by this approach?
   a. Decreased alertness
   b. Increased parasympathetic response
   c. Decreased sensory awareness
   d. Increased alertness

2. A massage client is unhappy with the massage. The main complaint is a feeling of choppiness and lack of continuity. Which of the following qualities of touch is most responsible?
   a. Pressure
   b. Drag
   c. Rhythm

3. Which of the following methods of abdominal massage is most beneficial for mechanically encouraging fecal movement in the large intestine?
   a. Gliding
   b. Holding position
   c. Tapotement/percussion
   d. Compression

4. A client requests that percussion be used at the end of the massage to stimulate the nervous system. Which is the best choice for the face?
   a. Hacking
   b. Cupping
   c. Tapping
   d. Slapping

5. Which of the following methods would be most effective for assessing for the physiologic and pathologic motion barrier?
   a. Passive joint movement
   b. Active-resistive movement
   c. Postisometric relaxation
   d. Concentric isotonic contraction

6. Which component is essential for the effective application of joint movement?
   a. Stabilization to isolate movement to the targeted joint
   b. Tapotement to stimulate joint kinesthetic receptors
   c. High-velocity manipulative movement

7. A client's muscles cramp when the massage professional attempts to contract/relax to lengthen a shortened group of muscles. Which of the following methods would be a better choice for lengthening the muscle group?
   a. Skin rolling
   b. Active-resistive joint movement
   c. Contract antagonist
   d. Stretching

8. When the outcome for the massage is to produce parasympathetic dominance, which combination of methods would be the best choice?
   a. Gliding, rocking, and passive joint movement
   b. Compression, shaking, and friction
   c. Active joint movement, contract antagonist, and rocking
   d. Tapotement, compression, and vibration

9. A client is requesting extensive massage to the neck and upper shoulders. Which is the most efficient client position for massaging these areas easily?
   a. Prone
   b. Supine
   c. Seated
   d. Side-lying

10. Which method is beneficial to use on the hands and feet to stimulate lymphatic movement?
    a. Deep gliding
    b. Skin rolling
    c. Shaking
    d. Pumping compression

11. A client complains of a stiff and stuck feeling in the lumbar area. Assessment indicates that the fascia in that area is thick and dense. Which method would best restore pliability to this tissue?
    a. Skin rolling
    b. Shaking
    c. Holding position
    d. Vibration

12. A client has a lot of body hair on the back. During the first massage, lubricant was used. At the return visit, the client requests that lubricant not be used on places on the body where there are large amounts of hair. Which method could be used?
    a. Gliding
    b. Kneading
    c. Compression
    d. Pétrissage

13. A client has an outcome goal for the massage of increased range of motion for the knee. Which of the following is the best approach?
    a. Neurologic methods focused on chemical changes
    b. Mechanical methods focused on the area
    c. Mechanical methods to influence neuroactivity reflexively
    d. Reflexive methods to increase compressive force to the viscera

14. The primary outcome for the massage is to increase shoulder mobility. Which method would be the best choice?
    a. Friction
    b. Focused stretching
    c. Hydrotherapy

15. The client has stiffness and reduced mobility since a fall and has been receiving massage weekly for 2 months. The main goal is to increase mobility in the lumbar and hip region. General massage and muscle energy

methods with stretching have produced mild improvement. Which of the following methods has the potential to enhance results?
a. Lymphatic drainage
b. Connective tissue methods
c. Contract/relax
d. Strain-counterstrain

16. A client with a hyperkyphosis likes to have the back massaged and asks that most of the massage time be focused there. However, each week the client complains that the massage is ineffective in reducing back pain the day after the massage. What is the best explanation that can be given to the client?
a. The soft tissue of the back often is tight because of extensive pulling and shortening of tissues in the chest; massage of the chest may help.
b. Massage to the back limits blood flow, so the soft tissues remain in contracture.
c. Massage on the extremities would be better to reduce the pain in this area because the mechanical effect is more concentrated.

17. A client complains about stiffness in the neck but is particularly sensitive to pressure applied in the neck area, flinching and stiffening in a protective manner whenever the neck is massaged. The current approach consists of primarily using kneading with the client in the prone position. What would be the most effective alternative?
a. Change position to supine and use gliding
b. Use the side-lying position and broad-based compression
c. Combine passive joint movement and friction with the client seated
d. Use the seated position and deep kneading

18. A client arrives late for a massage appointment and only 30 minutes remains. The goal for the session is general relaxation. Massage on which areas would best achieve desired outcomes in the allotted time?
a. Back, gluteals, and hips
b. Face, hands, and feet
c. Hands, arms, and back

Exercise

Using the previous questions as examples, write at least three more questions. Develop plausible wrong answers and be sure that the correct answer is clearly correct. Then write a rationale for each question. The more questions you write, the better you will understand the material.

ASSESSMENT PROCEDURES FOR DEVELOPING A CARE PLAN

Review Tips

The content related to assessment procedures for developing a care plan includes unique terms but is more concerned with

integration of information into the actual application of massage. The clinical reasoning and synthesis case study question is the most effective way to assess proficiency in knowledge.

The best study strategy for factual recall and concept identification questions is memorization of the terminology, use of the clinical reasoning process, and identification of wrong answers. Use the sample questions to help you determine whether you comprehend the vocabulary. Look up any terminology you do not understand.

This content can be tested by the case study type of question to assess for the ability to synthesize information and use clinical reasoning to identify the best answer based on the facts supplied in the question.

Quick Content Review

- Massage is a whole-body discipline. Assessment skills serve as the basis for developing critical thinking and clinical reasoning because they encourage one to pay closer attention and become more skilled in interpreting assessment information. With practice and experience, these skills become almost second nature.
- An assessment is the collection and interpretation of information provided by the client, the massage practitioner, and referring medical professionals. An assessment is performed to decide whether the client should be referred to a medical professional and to gather information to be used in designing a massage that meets the individual's specific needs. The most important source of information during the assessment process is the client.
- A massage professional modifies methods to best address the client's needs.
- The more reliable the assessment information, the more likely it is that interpretation of it will be accurate. The more accurate the interpretation, the more specific is the application of massage methods. Massage techniques are relatively basic. Soft tissue can be pushed, pulled, shaken, stretched, and pounded, regardless of the bodywork system. Forces applied change the shape of the soft tissue resulting in tension, bend, shear, compression, and torsion stresses. The only variables are the location of the application; the intensity, including drag, depth of pressure, and rhythm; the direction; the frequency; and the duration.
- The therapist should not hesitate to ask for help and should refer a client when the problem is beyond the individual professional skills as specified by the scope of practice for massage therapy. By joining in the team approach with other health professionals, the massage practitioner can adapt the massage to become an important part of the client's treatment.
- It is important to have rapport with clients. Rapport is the development of a relationship that is based on mutual trust and harmony. It is the responsibility of the massage professional to create an environment that supports rapport.
- When observing the general presence of the client, look for efficiency of movement, breathing patterns, and the general state of sympathetic or parasympathetic activation.

By watching a person's gestures, such as the way a person points and touches the body during conversation, you can obtain information and clues as to whether the problem is muscular, joint related, or visceral.

- Three factors influence posture: heredity, disease, and habit. Habit is the easiest to adjust. Habitual patterns are occupational, recreational, and sleep related.
- Mechanical balance has a fundamental nature. The gravitational line falls through the axis of the weight-bearing joint. If it does not, extra effort is required of the muscles to maintain the upright position. To stand up, the person's body must cooperate and use various segments. Passive tension of ligaments, fascia, and the connective tissue elements of the muscles support the skeleton. Muscle plays a small part through activity of the postural muscles, by continually repositioning the body over the mechanical balance point. If mechanical balance is disrupted, postural muscles struggle with this function.
- The position of the client during assessment of the standing position is a symmetrical stance, with eyes focused forward.
- The importance of bony landmarks in the assessment process is to provide markers for checking levelness and symmetry.
- Assessment for efficient gait patterns is important because walking is something that is done every day. Walking is a full-body experience that demands many coordinated activities of the arms and legs, neck and trunk, and eyes and ears. Almost every joint, muscle, and bone is involved in every step taken. Walking is one of the most important survival activities. The body expends a lot of energy to walk. If this pattern is inefficient, more energy is used than is necessary for the activity. This can translate into fatigue and possibly pain during walking.
- The sacroiliac joint is important during walking because it moves in an alternating-side figure-eight pattern. If the joint is limited in this function, the entire gait pattern is disrupted.
- Look for two main factors when assessing gait: identify areas that move too much as well as those that do not move enough during walking. It is important to consider the entire body when looking for these patterns because the activity of the arms provides a counterbalance to the legs.
- The most common reasons for dysfunctional walking patterns are pain, muscle weakness, muscle shortening, limitation of joint movement, and changes in bone or soft tissue. Full-body massage is beneficial for efficient gait patterns.
- Palpation is involved in touch assessment that differentiates between tissue textures within the same tissue types. Palpation is a way to compare tissue to other tissue and check for heat and cold. A good time to observe skin color and the state of the hair and nails is during palpation.
- The hand is an effective assessment tool. Proprioceptors and mechanoreceptors of the hand receive stimulation from palpated tissue. The brain devotes a large sensory area for the hand. The refined discriminatory sense of the hand can perceive subtle sensory shifts.
- Palpation skills are not limited to the hand. The whole body can be used to pick up sensory information. The areas most sensitive to posture shift and movement changes are the massage therapist's joints because of the large concentration of positional receptors found in and around joint capsules. Therefore, when the therapist's hip, elbow, knee, and foot are placed against the client, sensory data about client movement can be detected.
- It is important to trust first impressions during palpation. Sensory receptors in the massage practitioner's hand adapt quickly and do not respond as well to prolonged stimulation; you simply do not feel it the second time you try. Thinking about what you are feeling also interferes with the perception of sensory data. Do not think until after you have felt.
- We can feel things that do not touch us. Skin sensory receptors are designed to detect subtle changes in heat, air pressure, and air movement. This survival mechanism becomes most sensitive at a distance of about an arm's length from the person or object. The following information is gathered with near-touch or palpation that does not actually touch the body: heat and cold, and areas of not enough or too much sensitivity to air pressure changes.
- Intuition is the subconscious awareness of all sensory stimulation that we have receptor mechanisms to detect. Sensitivity, or intuition, is the ability to work with this information on a conscious level. It does not depend on extrasensory skills but rather on conscious awareness of everything.
- Certain things are noticed when the skin is palpated, such as whether the skin is damp or dry; whether there are goose bumps, moles, or surface growths; the elasticity of the skin; the surface texture; and the mobility of the skin against superficial connective tissue.
- The superficial connective tissue layer is a gelatinous layer. The superficial blood and lymph vessels are located in the superficial connective tissue; these vessels feel like soft tubes. Any changes in the superficial connective tissue affect circulation. You can feel pulses in the arteries, but if you press too hard, you lose the pulse. This may give some idea of how to locate the superficial connective tissue layer.
- Clients with enlarged lymph nodes should be referred to a physician because the lymph nodes can be indicators of many different conditions, from a minor local infection to a life-threatening condition. Only a physician is equipped to make that determination.
- Skeletal muscle has a distinct, ribbed feeling created by the fiber direction. It should feel firm and resilient without feeling stringy. Skeletal muscle within a specific area usually consists of three and sometimes more layers, and these layers crisscross and slide over one another. It is important to systematically palpate through all the layers and assess the ability of individual muscles to slide on top of one another.

- The importance of the musculotendinous junction is that it serves as the transition area between muscle and tendons. For this reason, this area is the site of greatest strain and therefore most frequent injury. In addition, this is the area where the nerves often enter, and it is the location of the motor points that activate the muscle. Most muscle dysfunction arises at the musculotendinous junction.

- Tendons do not attach only to bone. Tendons are just as likely to adhere to all surrounding connective tissue. The fascial sheaths, ligaments, and other tendons, as well as bone, serve as attachment points. During palpation, it is important to be able to trace the tendon, rather than rely on the bony attachment sites shown in diagrams.

- Fascial sheaths separate individual muscles, wrap and organize muscles into functional units, expand the skeleton, and provide stability. They include grooves in which the nerves, blood, and lymph vessels lie. Fascial sheaths run primarily horizontally and vertically through the body. They must be pliable and distinct to serve these important functions.

- It is important for the massage therapist to be able to palpate and recognize a ligament. Ligaments support and connect joints. Connection and separation of the joint are very important for posture because of positional receptors in the joint. If the function of the ligaments is disrupted, postural distortion develops. Because of their limited blood supply, ligaments do not heal well if injured.

- A joint should feel stable, supported, resilient, and unrestricted within a normal and functional movement range. Joint end feel is the perception of the joint at the limit of its range of motion. It is either hard or soft. Normal end feel is perceived as soft but resilient at the physiologic barrier. If the area is dysfunctional, the end feel will be hard, restricted, protective, and painful. The anatomic barrier may be reached if the ligament structure at the joint is too loose or lax and the joint is hypermobile.

- The basic configuration of muscles around a joint is a short lever; a one-jointed muscle initiates and stabilizes joint movement. With a long lever, a one-jointed muscle provides for full range of movement and power in the movement. A two-jointed muscle coordinates movement with the joint above or the joint below and assists the long-lever muscle.

- Hypertonic muscles and shortened connective tissue can pull the alignment of a joint out of its optimal anatomic position. Usually, the flexor and adductor muscles are the muscles that pull the joint out of alignment because they are approximately 30% stronger than the extensor and abductor muscles. Trauma also may push or pull a joint out of alignment.

- It is important to differentiate between joint and soft tissue dysfunction. Joint dysfunction is out of the scope of practice for massage. The two ways to determine this are as follows: (1) pain on traction usually is soft tissue dysfunction, and (2) pain on compression usually is joint dysfunction. If active range of motion produces pain and passive range of motion does not, the problem usually involves the soft tissue. If both cause pain, the problem usually involves a joint. Always refer clients with suspected joint problems to a physician.

- Palpate bones to locate bony landmarks for comparison of symmetry and muscle attachments.

- There are important things to look for when palpating the abdomen, such as hard and spongy areas, referred pain patterns, and the location of the liver and large intestine. If any unusual areas are noted, refer for diagnosis.

- The primary body rhythms are respiration and blood and lymph circulation. Rhythms ebb and flow in an undulating fashion. The breath is particularly important. The rhythm of normal relaxed breathing is an inhalation as the abdomen expands and the diaphragm flattens and a longer exhalation as the diaphragm muscle returns to it domed shape. The inhalation phase of breathing is shorter than the exhalation phase. The normal exhalation takes at least twice as long as the inhalation. This pattern is reversed as physical activity increases. Massage tends to stabilize and even out these rhythms.

- There are two basic types of muscle testing. Strength muscle testing seeks to discover whether the muscle being tested is responding with sufficient strength. Neurologic muscle testing evaluates the ability of the nerves to respond appropriately to a signal. With strength testing, the muscle to be isolated is placed in contraction and the client holds it in place with a stabilizing force, while the massage practitioner attempts to pull or push the muscle from its contracted position without recruiting other muscles. Strength patterns must be compared against a similar area, such as the same muscle on the other side, or against antagonist patterns. Neurologic muscle testing uses the same isolation of muscles, and the client holds the stabilizing force. The massage therapist provides light pressure to evaluate the response of the muscle. A normal response would be the ability to respond to the stimulus without using full strength and without recruiting other muscle action.

- There are two basic types of muscle functions. Postural muscles are made up of slow-twitch red fibers that can maintain a sustained contraction; these muscles are used to keep the body balanced against gravity. When stressed, they tend to shorten. Phasic muscles are used primarily for movement and are made up of fast-twitch white fibers that contract quickly but fatigue easily. They tend to weaken in response to postural muscle shortening. A muscle can serve a dual role and can have a mixed fiber configuration.

- Muscle imbalances set up patterns because the body moves in segments. These areas counterbalance each other against gravity and during movement. A typical muscle imbalance pattern bounces front to back and side to side at the segments.

- Remember that muscle function is integrated with the structural integrity of the fascial system and connective tissue structures.

- Interpretation of assessment data is done after the assessment. With experience, the two are not separated. When a student is learning the process, it is easy to jump to conclusions if all the information is not gathered first. Interpretation is the process of piecing together all the information and then designing the best massage for the client.

- Some key elements are required for designing a massage to meet the client's requested outcomes. Note the client's general presence and the sequence that the client uses in gesturing and explaining. Also, consider the symmetry of posture, efficiency of movement, tissue texture and condition, and areas that are hot or cold and overactive or underactive.

- The purpose for designing a massage is to provide balance by respecting current patterns and providing stimulation to encourage more efficient function. Put simply, the purpose is to cool down the hot spots, warm up the cold spots, lengthen the short areas, strengthen the weak areas, "unstick the stuck spots," and so forth.

- Reassessment is important because it allows the massage practitioner and the client to determine what was successful during the massage process. Information given before and after the massage reinforces the benefits of massage for the client.

- Most conditions with which the massage professional deals are chronic or self-limiting problems. Symptomatic relief, combined with activity to pass the time while the body heals itself, goes a long way toward assisting clients with this type of difficulty.

Factual Recall Questions

1. A client seems nervous and unwilling to provide information during the history-taking process. The massage therapist is becoming impatient. What is lacking?
   a. Rapport between client and practitioner
   b. Prior information from the physician
   c. State-dependent memory status

2. When is the data collected during the assessment process interpreted for patterns of dysfunction and methods of massage application?
   a. As the history-taking progresses
   b. During the physical assessment
   c. When the information is charted in the subjective part
   d. After the data have been collected and analyzed

3. During the initial greeting, a client seems generally healthy and in good spirits; however, when the client is speaking, the breathing pattern seems strained. What assessment process is being used?
   a. Palpation
   b. Physical
   c. Interviewing
   d. Observation

4. A massage practitioner asks a client the following question, "Please explain to me how you would like to feel after the massage." This communication is appropriate because the massage practitioner _____.

   a. Used an open-ended question
   b. Directed the response to reduce rapport
   c. Formulated a response while listening to the answer
   d. Used a closed-ended question to use time effectively

5. A massage practitioner carefully listens to a client during the interview portion of the assessment process and then proceeds to the physical assessment. What communication step was missed?
   a. Using open-ended questions and analysis
   b. Charting and developing a treatment plan
   c. Summarizing and restating information
   d. Using understandable language

6. A vacationing client will have only one massage from the massage practitioner. Which is the appropriate assessment process?
   a. Physical assessment for symmetry and gait assessment for movement patterns
   b. Palpation assessment of soft tissues to identify treatment areas
   c. Subjective and objective assessment for contraindications

7. During postural assessment, symmetry involves the _____.
   a. Shoulders rolling forward evenly, leveling the clavicles
   b. Circumference of the muscle mass in the legs being similar
   c. Ribs being more fixed on the left and springy on the right

8. Which of the following is part of a normal gait pattern?
   a. Arms are swinging freely opposite the leg swing.
   b. Knee is maintained in the "screw-home" mechanism.
   c. Toes contact the floor first and then roll to the heel.

9. During the massage, the massage professional notices a temperature difference in the tissue of the lumbar area. Which type of assessment is being used?
   a. Postural
   b. Gait
   c. Palpation
   d. Observation

10. Which method is most effective for assessing potential areas of muscle hyperactivity when the focus of the palpation is on the surface of the skin?
    a. Compressing until the striations of the underlying muscles are felt
    b. Light fingertip stroking to assess for areas of dampness or drag
    c. Skin rolling to assess for any adherence of superficial fascia to the skin
    d. Moving the skin on top of the superficial fascia to locate areas of bind

11. Passive joint movement as an assessment method identifies which of the following?
    a. End feel
    b. Viscosity
    c. Vessels

12. Bilateral assessment of the dorsalis pedis pulse would provide information about _____.

a. Respiration
b. Abdominal viscera
c. Lymph nodes
d. Arterial circulation

13. Where would the massage practitioner focus palpation assessment for the status of nerve gliding?
   a. Tendons at the proximal attachment
   b. Ligaments of synovial joints
   c. Grooves in fascial sheaths
   d. Myotomes

14. During muscle strength testing, the flexors and the extensors of the elbow seem equally strong. Why is this a dysfunctional pattern?
   a. Gait patterns should inhibit the flexors.
   b. Flexors should be about 25% stronger than extensors.
   c. Extensors should be 30% stronger than adductors.
   d. Postural muscles are inhibited by gait reflexes.

15. An objective measurement of connective tissue shortening in the lumbar area would be _____.
   a. Measuring a skinfold by lifting the tissue
   b. Have the client lift the chest into extension while prone
   c. Measuring hot and cold skin temperature
   d. Palpating adjacent pulse points for evenness

Application/Concept Identification and Clinical Reasoning/Synthesis Questions

1. A massage practitioner identifies an area of restricted tissue and immediately uses skin rolling to increase connective tissue pliability. How did this interfere with assessment?
   a. Localized treatment proved ineffective.
   b. Pattern was changed before it was understood.
   c. Therapist performed treatment before charting the affected area.
   d. Method was inappropriate to the condition.

2. Which of the following is incorrect when using muscle strength testing?
   a. Isolate muscles and position attachments as close together as is comfortable.
   b. Use a force sufficient to recruit a full response of the tested muscles and the surrounding muscles.
   c. Use a slow and even counterpressure to pull or push the muscle out of the isolated position.
   d. Compare muscle tests bilaterally for symmetry.

3. During the interview process, a client continues to grab the tissue at the back of the neck and pull it. What is the most logical explanation for this gesture?
   a. Nerve entrapment
   b. Joint compression
   c. Trigger point
   d. Connective tissue shortening

4. A physician refers a client for massage for circulation enhancement to the limbs. The client complains of cold hands and feet. Assessment indicates decreased pliability of the tissues around the elbows and knees. Work-related activities require repetitive movement in these areas. The massage professional presents three main approaches for the physician to consider:

Option 1. General massage and rest
Option 2. General massage with connective tissue stretching in restricted areas
Option 3. Compression focused specifically on the arteries to encourage circulation

After considering all three options, the physician eliminates option 1 as too time-consuming. Option 2 seems viable, but the client responds poorly to methods that may be painful. Option 3 seems too limited an approach to the massage professional. The decision is to begin with option 3 and expand to connective tissue methods when the client is able to tolerate them. Which part of this process best reflects brainstorming possibilities?
   a. Data collection
   b. Analysis of outcomes based on pros and cons
   c. Generating the options
   d. Assessment for additional facts

5. A client experienced an episode of severe low back pain 3 years ago. The diagnosis was a stenosis at L4. The condition has stabilized, and pain is experienced only occasionally. Assessment indicates shortened lumbar fascia, increased lateral flexion to the right, and a high shoulder on the right. The massage professional specifically addressed these areas and noted improvement following the massage. The next day, the client called to complain that the low back was in spasm. What is the most logical reason?
   a. The phasic muscles were too weak to maintain posture.
   b. The gait shifted so there was a more normal heel strike.
   c. Facilitated segments in the skeletal muscles went into spasm.
   d. Resourceful compensation patterns were disturbed.

6. When evaluating a treatment plan for successful client compliance, which of the following would provide the most helpful information?
   a. Any referral information from the healthcare provider
   b. Completing a comprehensive physical assessment
   c. Generating multiple treatment options
   d. Indications of enthusiasm for the plan by the client and any support system

7. If, during walking and running, shoulder flexion on the right is activated and hip flexors on the left are assessed, the most logical result is that the muscles should be _____.
   a. Inhibited
   b. Facilitated
   c. Functioning eccentrically
   d. Fibrotic and adhered

8. During postural assessment, the massage professional observes that the client's shoulder girdle is rotated to the left. The most likely cause is that the client _____.
   a. Regularly reaches to the left when answering the phone
   b. Often wears boots when riding horses
   c. Does weight-bearing exercise with machines three times a week

9. A regular client has a grade 2 left ankle sprain and is using a crutch to maintain balance when walking. During assessment of posture, the massage therapist notices an elevated right shoulder. The most likely cause is that the _____.
   a. Client is closing an open kinetic chain pattern
   b. Muscles of the right lower leg are inhibited
   c. Symmetrical stance is enhanced
   d. Body is displaying compensation patterns
10. If the area between C7 and T12 is pulled forward, making the chest concave, with a right rotation pattern making the right shoulder more forward than the left, where are the shortened soft tissues?
    a. Anterior thorax on the right
    b. Right lumbar posterior
    c. Left thorax posterior
    d. Lower abdominal on the right
11. A client has increased internal rotation of the right shoulder. Which of the following is the best massage approach to reverse the condition?
    a. Frictioning and traction to the external rotators
    b. Muscle energy with lengthening and then stretching of the internal rotators
    c. Compression and tapotement to the internal rotators
    d. Stretching of the flexors and extensors with lengthening to the external rotators
12. During range-of-motion assessment, if full extension of the shoulder has a hard end feel, a logical conclusion would be that the shoulder _____.
    a. Assesses as normal.
    b. Has a firing pattern dysfunction.
    c. Has an anatomic range of movement that is dysfunctional.
    d. Has joint dysfunction.

Exercise

Using the previous questions as examples, write at least three more questions. Develop plausible wrong answers and be sure that the correct answer is clearly correct. Then write a rationale for each question. The more questions you write, the better you will understand the material.

COMPLEMENTARY BODYWORK SYSTEMS

Review Tips

Complementary bodywork systems are generally not considered in therapeutic massage but are often included as an adjunct (add-on) to the massage. This distinction is becoming less apparent as massage methods targeting fluids, connective tissue, and trigger points are commonly included in the general type of massage. Again, there is new terminology to understand, so the factual recall and comprehension question is common.

Questions often cover safe and appropriate inclusion of the methods into the general massage. It is appropriate for the massage therapist to have a general understanding of the application and concepts of adjunct methods.

Quick Content Review

Continuing education is required to use adjunct methods and complementary bodywork systems effectively because each method has so much to offer and can stand alone as a therapeutic approach. It is impossible to provide a thorough study in the few pages devoted here because a book could be written on each topic. A higher skill level is attained with concentrated study. However, a massage therapist needs to understand the general approach and value of adjunct and complementary methods for referral purposes and to consider during the massage application. Some complementary systems have aspects that are easily and safely incorporated into massage.

Hydrotherapy and Thermotherapy

- Thermotherapy uses temperature to affect the body. The most common forms of thermotherapy involve the use of water and are part of hydrotherapy.
- The primary effects of hydrotherapy are mainly neurological and focus on the ANS. The addition of heat energy or dissipation of heat from the tissue may be classified as mechanical in effect. In general, cold stimulates sympathetic responses, and heat activates parasympathetic responses. Short and long applications of hot or cold produce different results. Most short cold applications stimulate and increase circulation. Long cold applications depress and decrease circulation. A short application of heat depresses and depletes tone, whereas a long hot application results in a combined depressant and stimulant reaction. Hot and cold compresses can be used. Some simple hydrotherapy methods that do not require special equipment are as follows:
  - A footbath is easy to incorporate.
  - A bag of frozen peas makes a great ice pack.
  - Hot water bottles are safer to use than heating pads.
  - Water frozen in a paper cup with a stick in it makes an effective ice massage tool.
- The following are important conditions that contraindicate the use of ice: vasospastic disease, cold hypersensitivity, cardiac disorder, compromised local circulation, rheumatoid conditions, an area of paralysis, and coronary artery disease. When using ice, it is important to consider the following precautions:
  - Do not use frozen gel packs directly on the skin.
  - Do not use cryotherapy applications for extended periods; 15-minute therapy sessions are recommended.
  - Do not do exercises that cause pain after cold applications.

- The use of methods that apply hot and cold to the body can create risk for the client. Be especially careful when using heat applications, including hot stones and seed bags. Ice applications can cause "freezer burn" damage to the tissues.

Aromatherapy

- The physiologic effect of essential oils is primarily chemical. The chemistry of essential oils is complex. Hundreds of components, such as terpenes, aldehydes, and esters, make up the oils. Lavender, for example, has antiseptic, antibacterial, antibiotic, antidepressant, analgesic, decongestant, and sedative properties. Essential oils are thought to reach the bloodstream through inhalation. When inhaled, they pass through the tiny air sacs to the surrounding blood capillaries by the process of diffusion. Once in the bloodstream, the aromatic molecules may interact with the body's chemistry.
- In addition to their medicinal properties, essential oils have the ability to uplift the client's spirits through inhalation. The sense of smell is interrelated with the limbic system, an area of the brain primarily concerned with emotion and memory. This influence of aromas on the psyche has led many aromatherapists to practice a form of aromatherapy called psychoaromatherapy, in which essential oils are used to enhance the client's mood and emotions. The massage therapist needs to be cautious of the scope of practice and ethical boundaries when oils are used for specific treatment of physical or mental disorders.
- An aromatherapy massage can help a person deeply relax and let go of worries, even if only for a short time, which may help activate the body's self-healing abilities. Combining the physical and emotional effects of massage with the medicinal and therapeutic properties of essential oils can alleviate stress and improve a person's mood.

Safety Guidelines for the Use of Essential Oils

As mentioned previously, essential oils are highly concentrated, volatile substances that, if used correctly, can have therapeutic benefit. Although many oils are useful, some are not safe to use at all, and proper safety guidelines must always be followed when using essential oils. Practitioners should receive advanced training in the use of essential oils before offering aromatherapy massage.

Note: The following cautions and information do not in any way replace medical and professional advice and may not include all cautionary information available.

- Always dilute essential oils in a carrier oil to prevent skin irritation and burning. Never use undiluted essential oils directly on the skin. Experienced aromatherapists may break this rule, but without extensive training it is important to use these substances with caution. Some clients can tolerate some oils, such as tea tree and lavender, in an undiluted form. However, caution is always advised because severe reactions and sensitivity are possible.
- When using a new oil on your client, it is important to patch test for sensitization and irritation. To patch test, apply a small amount of the diluted oil to the client's skin and leave it there for 24—48 hours to determine whether a reaction occurs. Even if working with an oil that does not commonly cause irritation, the patch test is an important measure of safety.
- Be familiar with essential oils that are contraindicated during pregnancy or for clients with diseases and illnesses such as asthma and epilepsy.
- Only small amounts of essential oils are needed, and you should use the smallest amount possible for effective treatment. If an additional drop is not necessary, do not use it.
- Many essential oils are not appropriate for use in aromatherapy. Do not assume that every essential oil can be used safely. Some oils, such as wormwood, onion, bitter almond, pennyroyal, camphor, horseradish, wintergreen, rue, and sassafras, should only be used by a qualified aromatherapist. Some oils should not be used at all.
- Keep essential oils out of children's reach. These oils can be tempting because the scents are appealing and children may think they are lotions or even candy or sweet drinks (e.g., citrus oil). Treat these oils as medicines or poisons when considering storage.
- Keep essential oils away from animals.
- Do not eat, drink, or otherwise ingest essential oils. With extreme caution, a qualified aromatherapy practitioner may prescribe internal use of an essential oil, but only after detailed consultation with the client.
- Essential oils are flammable. Store them properly and keep them away from fire hazards.
- Keep oils away from the eyes. If a drop or so of oil accidently gets in the eye, put some vegetable oil (e.g., almond oil) in the eye; the vegetable oil will absorb the essential oil, and a tissue then can be used to remove the oil. Do not use water, which will spread the oil. If burning or itching occurs, seek medical treatment.
- Do not use the same oils for a prolonged period.
- Use photosensitizing oils cautiously (i.e., bergamot, verbena, lime, angelica root, bitter orange, lemon, and grapefruit). Advise the client to avoid sun exposure and the use of tanning beds for 12 hours after application of these oils. Photosensitization occurs when oils containing furanocoumarin compounds are applied to the skin and the skin is immediately exposed to sunlight or ultraviolet (UV) light. Furanocoumarin compounds allow the UV rays to penetrate the skin more readily, resulting in abnormal skin pigmentation or mild to severe burns. Remember, UV rays are present even on cloudy days.
- Store essential oils away from light and heat and keep the cap tightly closed. Essential oils are volatile and evaporate readily.
- Some aromatherapy experts believe that certain essential oils should not be used unless administered by qualified

aromatherapists, and some oils should not be used even by qualified practitioners.

Aromatherapy Applications

Essential oils can be used in various ways in combination with hydrotherapy and massage.

- Aromatic bath, hot tub, or sauna: Put 4—10 drops of essential oil in the water just before the person gets into it. Gently stir the water to disperse the oil. For a sauna, dilute the oil with 70%—90% water and spray it on the rocks and into the air. The bottle must be shaken continually to keep the oil in suspension in the water.
- Aromatic compress: Put three to five drops of oil into one to two cups of hot or cold water, depending on the need for a compress. Fold a clean cloth and submerge it in the water, then squeeze the excess water from the compress into the basin. Apply immediately to the treatment area.
- Aromatic facial steam: Use one to two drops of oil per one cup of boiling water. Place the oil in the bowl or basin after the water has boiled. Stir the water to disperse the oil. Immediately place a towel over the head and place the face as close as possible to the aromatic steam without causing any discomfort.
- Environmental and room fragrance: Electronic diffusers offer an easy, effective way to fragrance a room for aesthetic and therapeutic purposes. Use only pure essential oils or synergies of pure essential oils. Never use essential oils cut with carrier oils in diffusers because this clogs the diffuser.
- Aroma lamps: Aroma lamps are great for adding environmental fragrance. Add 10 drops of essential oils to one teaspoon of water and place in the designated receptacle on the lamp. The heat of the light disperses the fragrance.

Systemic Massage Methods

Systemic massage methods focus on massage on a specific body system; two forms of systemic massage are lymphatic massage and circulation massage. The intent is to mimic and support normal physiologic function.

- Lymphatic massage consists of a combination of short, pumping, and active gliding strokes, followed by long surface gliding strokes that influence the movement of interstitial fluid, as well as deep breathing and passive range of motion, which support lymph movement more specifically. The direction of action is toward the drainage points with application generally beginning proximal and sequentially moving distally. The focus of the pressure and drag is on the dermis just below the surface layer of skin and the layer of fascial tissue just beneath the skin and above the muscles; it then may gradually increase. Rhythmic kneading, compression, and rocking of the thorax and abdomen support lymphatic movement.

- Circulation massage consists of compression applied over the main arteries, beginning near the heart or proximally to it, and systematically moving distally, ending at the tips of the fingers or toes. The strokes are applied over the arteries and pump at a rhythm of approximately 60 beats per minute or at the client's resting heart rate. The next step is to assist venous return flow. A combination of short gliding strokes, long gliding strokes, and joint movement is used. With venous return flow, the strokes move distal to proximal, or from the finger and toes to the heart, over the major veins. Short strokes are about 3 inches long and move the blood from valve to valve. Long strokes carry the blood through the entire vein. Passive and active joint movements promote venous circulation. Placing the limb or area above the heart allows for gravity assistance.

Reflexology

- The foot has many joint and reflex patterns. Sensory information about position and posture from the joint kinesthetic receptors is extensive. Sensory and motor centers of the brain devote a large area to the feet and hands. Nerve distribution to the feet and hands is extensive. The position of the foot sends a great deal of postural information through the central nervous system.
- Stimulation of the feet seems to activate the responses of the gate control mechanism, or hyperstimulation analgesia, as well as parasympathetic dominance. Body-wide effects are achieved by this technique. Many nerve endings in the feet and hands correlate with acupressure points, which in turn may release endorphins and other endogenous chemicals when stimulated. In addition, major plexuses for the lymph system are located in the hands and feet. Compressive forces in this area stimulate lymphatic movement.
- An excellent way to massage a foot is to apply pressure and movement systematically to the entire foot and ankle complex. This pressure stimulates circulation, nerves, and reflexes. Moving the joints stimulates large-diameter nerve fibers, initiating hyperstimulation analgesia and joint kinesthetic receptors. The result is a shift in proprioceptive and postural reflexes. This same approach can be used to massage the hands.

Connective Tissue and Trigger Point Approaches

Techniques that specifically target connective tissue are classified as connective tissue or myofascial approaches.

- Connective tissue methods stretch, pull, drag, elongate, and move the tissue. The intent of connective tissue massage is to soften the ground substance of connective tissue to support tissue pliability or to introduce tissue layer gliding.

- Most connective tissue methods move soft tissues into bind and hold at that point until change is perceived. This approach is considered a direct method.
- Implement-assisted methods include scraping and suction. Tissue scraping methods that drag an instrument over the skin are adjunct approaches to introducing tissue inflammation. Because tissue damage is occurring, it is necessary to use the method cautiously. Suction or cupping methods lift tissue, creating localized stretch of connective tissues. Caution is required since prolonged suction can affect surface circulation and result in blood from the capillaries pooling in the interstitial spaces. Fragile skin and anticoagulant medication also present cautions and contraindications.
- A trigger point is thought to be an area of local nerve facilitation of a muscle that when aggravated by stressors affects the individual. Trigger points are small areas of hypertonicity within muscles. If these tight areas of muscle fibers are located near motor nerve points, referred pain may result from nerve stimulation. Often the area of the trigger point is the point at which nerve stimulation initiates a contraction in a small sensitive bundle of muscle fibers (motor point) that in turn activates the entire muscle. A variety of tender points exist, which can be difficult to differentiate. Any clustering of nerve endings as part of normal anatomy in the skin and superficial fascia, as well as other body tissues, can become hypersensitive and display pain symptoms.
- Using light palpation, the massage practitioner needs to notice whether the skin feels tense and whether there is resistance to gliding strokes. The skin may be slightly damp with perspiration from sympathetic facilitation. The temperature in a local area increases in acute trigger/tender points but decreases in chronic trigger points as a result of ischemia, which is an indication of fibrotic changes within the tissues around the trigger point.
- Edema produces an impression of fullness and congestion within the tissues. In instances of chronic dysfunction, edema is replaced gradually with fibrotic (connective tissue) changes, and the tissue texture feels cemented.
- During deep palpation, the massage therapist establishes contact with the deeper fibers of the soft tissues and explores them for immobility, tenderness, edema, muscle tension, and fibrotic changes.
- With both light and deep palpation, gliding strokes cover a region of 2–3 inches at a time. The trigger point is painful to pressure and refers pain to other areas.
- The trigger point is hyperstimulated by using various methods such as compression, pushing together or apart on the spindle cells, or active contraction of the muscle. Hyperstimulation is followed by stretching of the muscle fibers that contain the trigger point.
- After treatment of a trigger point, the target (referred) area should be searched to uncover satellite or embryonic trigger points that need to be treated. Immediately afterward, the area should be massaged to increase local circulation. Placing a damp warm or hot towel over the region is soothing and useful. The area requires rest for a few days, with all stressful activity avoided.

Traditional Methods

A person is body, mind, and spirit. These are not separate pieces but parts of a whole. Health is achieved when harmony exists in all areas. Most cultures have historic forms of bodywork methods that have evolved into health systems. Examples include traditional Chinese medicine and Ayurveda. Dr. Stone trained in various systems and incorporated these methods with a Western knowledge base to create an eclectic, multifaceted system called polarity. Although the theoretical, assessment, and intervention process may vary, the commonality is the shared human anatomy and physiology.

- Most acupuncture points correspond with motor points or nerve endings; meridians lie over or close to main nerve tracts; yin is parasympathetic; and yang is sympathetic. Acupuncture points usually lie in fascial divisions between muscles, near the origin, and insertion. The point feels like a small hole, and pressure elicits a "nervy" feeling.
- Unlike a trigger point, which may be present on only one side of the body, acupuncture points are bilateral (located on both sides of the body). To confirm the location of an acupuncture point, locate the point in the same place on the other side of the body.
- To stimulate a hypoactive or "not enough energy" acupuncture point, use a short vibrating or tapping action. This method is used if the area is sluggish or if a specific body function needs stimulation.
- To sedate a hyperactive "too much energy" point for pain reduction, elicit the pain response within the point itself. Use sustained holding pressure until the painful energy dissipates and the body's own painkillers are released into the bloodstream. The pressure techniques are similar to those used for trigger points, although it is not necessary to lengthen an acupuncture point after treatment.

Implement-Assisted Methods

An implement is some sort of device that is used to augment the massage application. The device can roll, press, scrape, or suction. The two main reasons for using an implement are as follows:

1. The device reduces the effort required to apply massage, making massage application easier for the massage therapist.
2. The device can apply mechanical force to the soft tissue more effectively than the massage therapist's hands, forearms, or other part of the body used to apply massage methods.

Remember that massage methods apply mechanical forces to deform soft tissue and that mechanical forces are a push or a pull. Any devices incorporated into massage should assist this process. There are many implements that can be used to push into tissue. In general, these devices are used to create compression stress. Rollers, balls, knobs, and so forth in a variety of designs are made from different types of material including plastic and wood. The stones used in hot and cold stone massage are implements.

- The main safety concerns are compression injury to soft tissue and sanitation. The various tools must be disinfected after every use. Compression injury is called a contusion. A contusion (bruise) is an injury to the soft tissue often produced by a blunt force resulting in pain, swelling, and discoloration. Nerves are especially susceptible to compression injury.
- Implements can also be used for percussion and vibration. Bundled sticks, usually bamboo or rattan, and soft head mallets are examples of tools that can be used to replace the hands when performing percussion methods.
- The main safety concern is the tissue damage that could occur with aggressive percussion. The tissue can be bruised, and depending on the implement (e.g., bundled sticks), the skin could be cut.
- Electric devices can create percussion and vibration to augment massage application. A percussion device moves in-out and up-down like hammers or pistons. A vibration device moves back and forth.
- The main safety concern for electrical devices is the prolonged exposure of hand-arm vibration to the massage therapist, which causes damage to hands and fingers. The resulting condition is known as white finger disease, Raynaud phenomenon, or hand-arm vibration syndrome (HAVS). One of the symptoms is that affected fingers may turn white, especially when exposed to cold. Caution is required.
- Traction devices pull. Traction is the act of applying a mild stretch at constant pressure to the body tissues, especially muscles and ligaments, around jointed areas. Most often implements that assist the massage therapist in performing traction are straps and bands.
- The main safety concern from straps is skin damage. There is also a potential for traction application to be too aggressive when a strap is used to assist the method.
- Vacuum manual therapy/cupping is a suction method that is an ancient traditional and complementary medicine practice. Vacuum manual therapy is performed by applying a suction device to selected skin points and creating a subatmospheric pressure by suction.
- Suction is contraindicated directly on surface veins, arteries, nerves, skin inflammation, any skin lesion, body orifices, eyes, lymph nodes, or varicose veins. Suction is also contraindicated on open wounds, bone fractures, and sites of deep vein thrombosis.
- Because of the capillary breakage caused by the suction, the skin can become marked with dark red or purplish areas in the shape of the suction device. These areas are not bruising which is tissue damage caused by compression. The discoloration can be significantly reduced or avoided by moving the suction device or only leaving it stationary for short periods such as 15 seconds.

Factual Recall Questions

1. Bodywork methods that focus on meridians and points fall into which category?
   a. Eastern and Asian
   b. Reflex
   c. Energetic
   d. Structural
2. Cold applications of hydrotherapy to reduce swelling are called _____.
   a. Analgesic
   b. Antipyretic
   c. Antispasmodic
   d. Antiedemic
3. The secondary effect of a local cold application is _____.
   a. Sedative
   b. Increased localized circulation
   c. Diaphoretic
   d. Decreased systemic circulation
4. What is the water temperature for a neutral bath?
   a. 65–92°F
   b. 98–104°F
   c. 92–98°F
   d. 56–65°F
5. A folded towel soaked in water of the desired temperature and placed on a large area of skin is called _____.
   a. Tonic friction
   b. Cupping
   c. Gua Sha
   d. Pack
6. Because of a skin condition, general massage is contraindicated for a client, but they are allowed to have feet and hands worked on. The client complains of neck stiffness. If using foot reflexology theory, where would the massage practitioner focus massage on the foot to affect the neck?
   a. Heel
   b. Tips of the toes
   c. Base of the large toe
   d. Sole of the foot
7. Reflexology can be beneficial because _____.
   a. The complex structure of the foot is highly innervated and sensitive to changes in pressure and position, making it highly responsive to massage manipulation.
   b. The flexor withdrawal mechanism of the foot is inhibited by pressure to the foot, and this inhibits neural activity in the dorsal horn of the spinal cord.
   c. Specific mapped areas of reflex activity in the foot to organs have a direct relationship to visceral/cutaneous responses.
   d. Stimulation of zone therapy points on the bottom of the foot activates meridian energy movement in the chakra system.
8. Myofascial methods are focused most specifically on change in the _____.
   a. Motor point
   b. Lymph nodes

c. Gait control mechanism

d. Ground substance

9. Deep transverse friction applied correctly will ____.

   a. Inhibit circulation

   b. Create controlled inflammation

   c. Provide broad-based application

10. Which of the following is correct application of trigger point therapy?

    a. 15-minute application in combination with focused stretching

    b. 45-minute application with hydrotherapy cold applications

    c. Limiting application to latent trigger points only

    d. Using pressure methods first and limiting stretching

11. A characteristic of trigger points is that they _____.

    a. Require surgery

    b. Occur only in the feet

    c. Cause inflammation

    d. Refer pain

12. Which of the following essential oils would be used often in the spa environment?

    a. Clove

    b. Lavender

    c. Spirulina

    d. Paraffin

13. A spa treatment that is said to stimulate circulation is _____.

    a. Body polish

    b. Dry brush

    c. Mud mask

    d. Mylar wrap

Application/Concept Identification and Clinical Reasoning/Synthesis Questions

1. A client has been receiving massage for a mild peripheral arterial circulation problem. Which of the following would be an appropriate self-help method to teach the client?

   a. Lymphatic drainage

   b. Skin rolling

   c. Alternating applications of hot and cold

2. A client injured their right shoulder 3 years ago. Assessment indicates decreased mobility of the superficial tissue surrounding the shoulder coupled with a painful but normal range of motion. Which is the best treatment option for this client?

   a. Deep transverse friction

   b. Superficial myofascial release

   c. Compression

   d. Lymphatic drainage

3. An active trigger point that is left untreated for 6 months often will _____.

   a. Become an ashi point

   b. Become hot to the touch

   c. Undergo fibrotic changes

   d. Elicit only referred pain

4. Which of the following characterizes trigger point treatment?

   a. Direct pressure methods and squeeze methods should be used first.

   b. Positional release with lengthening is the first application method.

   c. Connective tissue stretching needs to accompany muscle energy application.

   d. Lengthening of the tissue housing the trigger point is effective only with a local tissue stretch.

5. Which is most correct about the application of lymphatic drainage methods?

   a. Pressure levels are only sufficient to drag the skin.

   b. The direction is toward the heart.

   c. The rhythm is variable and moderate to fast.

   d. Pressure is variable, slow and rhythmic toward drain patterns.

6. Which type of spa is likely to involve medical intervention?

   a. Luxury

   b. Resort

   c. Day

   d. Weight loss

7. Which of the following typically is found in some form in the spa environment?

   a. Shiatsu

   b. Stone ritual

   c. Hydrotherapy

8. A client has mild edema in their lower legs from a long plane fight the previous day. Which of the following is an appropriate treatment plan?

   a. Short, light gliding strokes focused on the legs. Compression to the soles of the feet. Active and passive joint movement for the ankle, knee, and hip. Placing the legs above the heart.

   b. Compression to the legs focused on the medial side from proximal to distal. Muscle energy and lengthening combined with stretching in the area of greatest accumulation of fluid.

   c. Deep gliding strokes from proximal to distal on the legs. Placing the legs above the heart. Limiting movement to encourage drainage.

   d. Superficial and deep compression along the vessels in the lateral leg. Active-resistive joint movement combined with shaking.

9. A client is getting ready to play a tournament tennis game in 60 minutes and wants to increase circulation and prepare their muscles for the game. Which of the following treatment plans is the best option?

a. 45-minute massage using long gliding strokes from distal to proximal focused toward the heart combined with rocking.

b. 20-minute massage using broad-based compression to the soft tissue of the limbs generally focused from proximal to distal combined with shaking and tapotement.

c. 45-minute full-body massage with muscle energy methods and lengthening.

d. 15-minute massage with compression, superficial myofascial release, and trigger point work focused on the limbs combined with passive joint movement and shaking.

10. An indication for using lymphatic drainage during the massage would be a client who has _____.

a. Edema in the lower extremities but no logical reason for the fluid retention

b. Premenstrual bloat and edema

c. Kidney disease, although dialysis is unnecessary

d. Fever and general lethargy and achiness

Exercise

Using the previous questions as examples, write at least three more questions. Develop plausible wrong answers and be sure that the correct answer is clearly correct. Then write a rationale for each question. The more questions you write, the better you will understand the material.

ADAPTIVE MASSAGE

Review Tips

The content on serving special populations is more about unique circumstances involving individuals. The relevance is how the massage therapist needs to adapt to the specific needs of individuals who have unique challenges. Again, there is terminology to study, but by this time you should know various study strategies for learning vocabulary. This content usually is assessed by the case study type of question, to identify whether the massage practitioner knows how to make appropriate accommodations in the environment and alterations in massage delivery to benefit and not harm the client.

Quick Content Review

- The three main career tracks for massage can be categorized as follows:
  1. Health and wellness (spa/franchise)
  2. Medical care (clinical/medical)
  3. Sports performance and fitness

  These career tracks are typically defined by the location where the massage is provided, common outcomes requested for the massage, and parameters that define a specific population.

- Massage therapists who want to focus their professional skills to best meet the specific needs of each client must seek out training and information pertinent to the therapeutic needs of the client. Often the knowledge required to provide massage to many populations becomes extensive, and it becomes necessary to specialize. When this is the situation, such as when a massage professional obtains additional training in oncology massage, geriatric massage, or sports massage, the information is built on the fundamentals of massage with additional training focused toward application in specific environments or unique circumstances.

- Communication skills are important for working with a client with special needs. Always remember to interact with the person who has a special need. Do not allow yourself to become over focused on the situation. Consider the person first. The client is the best source of information. Even if the client lacks technical knowledge about a particular illness, sport, pregnancy, disability, or emotional pattern, he or she still is the only one who really understands the effects of any situation.

- Athletes can be given three forms of restorative massage: *recovery massage*, which primarily focuses on the athlete who wants to recover from a strenuous workout or competition when no injury is present; *remedial massage*, which is used for minor to moderate injuries; and *rehabilitation massage*, which is used for severe injury or as part of intervention after surgery. Compensation patterns that may develop from any sport respond well to maintenance massage methods. In addition, recovery occurs more quickly and performance is enhanced by regular massage. Organizing a sports massage team to provide general postevent massage is a great public education and promotional concept. It is important to develop a simple, 15- to 30-minute routine that all massage practitioners can use.

- Children's attention spans are shorter; therefore, the massage may need to take less than an hour; 15—30 minutes is typical. Touch is important during the growing years. Massage is an organized approach to touch, and the nervous system likes to learn from it. Wrestling and horsing around—both activities that many children engage in—may provide massage-like responses. Massage provides temporary relief from growing pains. Massage is a great, organized, and safe way to touch. This may help families stay in touch during both difficult and good times. The parent or guardian provides informed consent and must supervise the massage session.

- Chronic illness presents a variety of problems in living. For many, "healing" is the act of taking back self-control—not getting rid of the illness, but learning to live with it in a resourceful manner. It is important for the massage professional to focus on helping the client feel better for a while, rather than trying to eliminate the chronic illness. Massage can help the process by providing temporary symptomatic relief in cases of chronic illness. Hardiness, or toughening, is the ability to physically and mentally withstand external stressors. Because of a decrease in physical activity and isolation, those with a chronic illness become less hardy and resilient. Massage is a gentle, organized, and controlled way to provide physical and mental opportunities to change. It gives the client the opportunity to begin to assimilate and adjust to sensory input in a way that increases hardiness and resilience.

- Many individuals with a chronic illness are taking medication or undergoing other medical interventions. It is important for the medical professional to be able to monitor the effects of different therapies. Because massage interacts with the nervous and endocrine systems, it is important that massage effects be monitored as part of the entire therapeutic outcome. A reduction in medication dosage and thereby in side effects may be possible through a multidisciplinary approach to deal with chronic illness.

- Individuals who are in their 50s or older can benefit from massage as the aging process becomes more evident. Because of reduced joint space and changes in soft tissue, it is common to find nerve compression and resulting pain. It is important to understand the physiology of aging and the physical changes that take place. An older client may take medication to control various physiologic processes, but in general, the only requirements of the therapist are basic massage skills and an attentive, caring approach.

- Posttraumatic stress response is a normal response to traumatic events. Examples include accidents, soldiers returning from combat, abusive relationships, rape, national disasters, and many other short-term or long-term events that require more than normal coping mechanisms. When the stress response is no longer beneficial over a reasonable period of time, it should be resolved. If this does not occur, posttraumatic stress disorders develop, which can include symptoms such as flashback memory. Occasionally a client will dissociate or become emotional. The massage therapist needs to be aware that these responses can occur but are rare and to simply become quiet and calm while maintaining gentle contact with the client. Trauma-informed care shifts the focus from "What's wrong with you?" to "What happened to you?" Trauma-informed care seeks to realize the widespread impact of trauma; recognize the signs and symptoms of trauma; integrate knowledge about trauma into policies, procedures, and practices; and actively avoid re-traumatization.

- If a client experiences an emotional response during the massage, it is important to stay connected with the client but distanced from the experience, which belongs to the client. Maintain gentle contact with the client and ask whether they would like you to continue the massage. Continue the massage methods that triggered the response only if the client agrees. Slow the methods and allow the body time to integrate and resolve the body memory. Refer the client if additional coping and counseling skills are indicated.

- When a client self-abuses, they may discount the injury, provide a cover story, feel guilty or ashamed, or be surprised that the injury is there. It is important for the massage therapist to not press the issue and to realize that self-abuse is a coping mechanism that may calm the person. The massage therapist should not perpetuate an abuse pattern by providing invasive massage. Refer the client if additional coping and counseling skills are indicated.

- Fundamental massage skills are sufficient for working with those who are pregnant. As in the aging process, pregnancy is a normal event, not a sickness. General wellness massage is indicated. Consideration must be given to positioning, and emotional swings linked to hormonal changes need to be taken into account. The abdomen is never massaged deeply, and changes such as swelling should be referred to the physician or midwife. Massage is beneficial both as the pregnancy progresses and during labor. Watch for fever, edema, varicose veins, and severe mood swings. Pregnancy is typically considered a hypercoagulable state—meaning that most pregnant women clot blood more readily than normal and are predisposed to deep vein thrombosis or other clot-related conditions. Keep in mind that blood clots during pregnancy are rare, but they are serious conditions that may become life-threatening when the blood clot is dislodged from the site of formation.

- Massage for infants provides an organized sensory stimulation that helps the nervous system to grow and begin to integrate information. It also provides a bonding method for parent and infant. Primary caregivers gain the most from massaging the baby. The massage professional serves both the infant and caregivers by teaching infant massage. Infants instinctively know when a touch is not safe. They will not respond well to a nervous touch but depend instead on a confident touch. It is important to honor an infant's physiologic state and give him or her time to respond to the touch.

- Those who are dying are undergoing a meaningful and serious process which can be supported by the compassionate presence and touch of the massage therapist. Being privileged to share in the process can teach us how to die with dignity. A hospice is one of the best resources, and the massage practitioner is encouraged to support and learn from the dedicated individuals who work in hospices. Massage supports other comfort measures within palliative care. Physical touch can be an important link to this world. Just listening to the person and maintaining regular massage sessions for as long as they desire throughout the process is important. Gentle touch and a spirit willing to connect and to mourn an inevitable loss are all that is necessary.

- Medical care environments present unique adaptations. Supervision provided within a healthcare team requires tempering of independent treatment and clearance of all interventions to ensure they coordinate with the total treatment plan. Charting is essential, as is attention to effective communication. The environment may be noisy, with interruptions and lack of privacy. The client may be taking medications or using special equipment, such as intravenous lines.

- Many clients with a variety of conditions will require adaptation. Some of these individuals will function with disabilities. Ask the client to explain the disability to you, as well as any limitations and the type of assistance needed. Then pay attention to the person, not the disability. In all situations, remember to see and address the person first, and then to accommodate the individual's special needs by offering assistance and following the client's directions. Special care must be taken to ensure that the client is able to provide informed consent. Massage can be beneficial in reducing general stress levels.

- Many adaptations necessary during massage are related to the size and comfort of the client as well as any assistive equipment. The massage professional serving clients who are large, especially tall or short in stature, will require equipment adaptation such as stools; additional draping material; and alteration to the width, length, and weight capacity of massage tables. Barrier-free access to the massage location and restrooms is necessary.

- In providing wellness massage, as opposed to rehabilitative massage, the skills are no different. What is different is the situation presented by the client. An athlete has certain needs based on the sport, adaptation based on the pregnancy is individualized, and those with a chronic illness adaptation is based on the illness pattern. The massage practitioner needs additional training in the various situations and conditions to use the fundamental massage skills purposefully and confidently.

Factual Recall Questions

1. Which area requires additional study for the massage professional who works with any population needing treatment adaptation?
   a. Massage methods
   b. Special situations
   c. Psychology
   d. Relaxation methods

2. A massage professional has been working with an 86-year-old client who lives independently with some outside support. How does this client most likely benefit from weekly massage?
   a. Physical and emotional stimulation
   b. Increased circulation
   c. Friendship

3. Which of the following is encouraged for a parent who is massaging their infant?
   a. Hardiness
   b. Dissociation
   c. Development
   d. Bonding

4. A massage therapist has just started a job at a family practice medical center. The center deals with many clients who exhibit stress-related symptoms. Which of the following professional skills will the massage therapist need to perfect?
   a. Muscle energy methods
   b. Restorative massage
   c. Charting and record-keeping

   d. Lymphatic drainage

5. A client just began to work with a massage professional who specializes in massage for those with physical disabilities. Which of the following would be a likely accommodation that the client would notice?
   a. The building is barrier free.
   b. Special massage methods are used.
   c. All clients have guardians.
   d. All clients set quantifiable and qualifiable goals.

6. A massage therapist has developed a referral network with a group of physicians and physiologists to deal with anxiety and panic disorders. Which of the following will the therapist need to effectively manage with massage?
   a. Exercise protocols
   b. Nutrition
   c. Support group interactions
   d. Breathing pattern dysfunction

7. A massage client is in the first trimester of their third pregnancy. Which of the following is contraindicated?
   a. Prone position
   b. Massage of the feet
   c. Deep abdominal massage
   d. Lymphatic drainage

8. A long-term client has just notified the massage professional that they have a terminal illness. Which of the following approaches will be used as the client approaches death?
   a. Therapeutic change
   b. Palliative care
   c. Remedial massage

9. Which of the following is a medical emergency?
   a. Nausea
   b. Heatstroke
   c. Capsulitis
   d. Heat cramp

Application/Concept Identification and Clinical Reasoning/Synthesis Questions

1. An adult client has many surgical scars on the chest and abdomen. History indicates that the client had surgical intervention as a child to repair congenital malformations. The client enjoys massage on the limbs and back in the prone position but appears distant and unsettled when turned to the supine position. What is the most logical explanation for this response?
   a. Abuse
   b. Reenactment
   c. Dissociation
   d. Integration

2. A college football player is seeking massage as part of a healing program for an injured knee that required surgical intervention. The athletic trainer is supervising the massage. The massage consists of general full-body massage that addresses any developing compensation caused by gait change while the knee is healing. Specific applications of kneading and myofascial release are being used to

maintain pliability in the soft tissue of the upper and lower leg. What type of massage is being performed?
   a. Post-event
   b. Recovery
   c. Rehabilitation
3. In which of the following circumstances would breast massage with specific informed consent be most appropriate?
   a. General body treatment
   b. Adjunct to cancer treatment
   c. Scar tissue management
   d. Examination for lumps
4. What is the most challenging countertransference situation that a massage professional faces when working with clients with chronic illness?
   a. Understanding the combined effects of massage and medications
   b. Decreasing frustration with a client whose condition fails to improve
   c. Maintaining boundaries with a client who sees bodywork as the answer to all physical problems
   d. Managing acute episodes of chronic illness
5. A massage practitioner has been asked by a group of mental health professionals to begin work at a residential facility. Which of the following should be their highest priority?
   a. Types of mental health issues
   b. Obtaining informed consent
   c. Learning specific massage protocols for each condition
6. In which of the following circumstances would massage without supervision by a healthcare professional best benefit children?
   a. Growing pains
   b. Anxiety disorder
   c. Touch sensitivity
7. Which of the following complaints by athletes can be addressed by lymphatic drainage?
   a. Muscle guarding
   b. Laceration
   c. Delayed-onset muscle soreness
   d. Cramp
8. Which of the following conditions in the second trimester of pregnancy requires referral to the client's physician?
   a. Breast changes
   b. Constipation
   c. Preeclampsia
9. Which of the following athletic injuries is addressed most effectively through massage?
   a. Grade 3 acute strain
   b. Dislocation
   c. Stress fracture
   d. Chronic tendinopathy

Exercise

Using the previous questions as examples, write at least three additional questions—one of each type: factual recall and

comprehension, application and concept identification, and clinical reasoning and synthesis. Develop plausible wrong answers and be sure that the correct answer is clearly correct. Then write a rationale for each question. The more questions you write, the better you will understand the material.

WELLNESS EDUCATION

Review Tips

The content concerning wellness education is important for ensuring that the massage professional has a broad-based understanding of the different factors that support wellness and health. Content of this type is also important when developing self-care strategies for the massage therapist. Massage is an important part of health maintenance, illness and injury prevention, and well-being. This content is interesting, but exams typically contain only a few questions involving this information and how massage is part of the health practice. Therefore, do not overemphasize this content.

All three question types are used to assess this content. Study all the terminology. Develop examples and metaphors and explain the content in words different from those used in your textbooks.

Quick Content Review

- Massage is an important part of any wellness program because it restores body balance and provides a connection with other human beings. It is necessary for the massage professional to understand how massage fits into the overall wellness picture.
- It is not possible to define a step-by-step process that provides for wellness because each person responds in an individual manner. Wellness programs can be built around the body; these include nutrition, light and dark exposure, sleep, breathing, physical fitness, and sensory stimulation; the mind, including relationships with self and others, communications, beliefs, and intellectual stimulation; and the spirit, which includes purpose, connection, faith, hope, and love. We are considered well when body, mind, and spirit are in ideal balance. We are not well when imbalance exists and balance cannot be restored.
- The basic components of a wellness program are as follows:
  - Body—nutrition, sleep, breathing, and physical fitness
  - Mind—relationship, communication belief, and intellectual stimulation
  - Spirit—purpose, connection, faith, hope, and love
- Stress is our response to any demand on the body or mind to respond, adapt, or alter. It is a state of readiness to survive, requiring hypervigilance from the body and mind. Stressors are any internal perceptions or external stimuli that demand a change in the body. It is our emotional reaction to stress that may be the difference between positive

action and destructive breakdown, especially if many of the stressors seem beyond our control. Defensive measures are the ways our bodies defend against stressors, as through production of antibodies and white blood cells or behavioral and emotional defenses. Sometimes defending is not the best way to deal with stress. It is important and resourceful to know when to quit or surrender.

- Signs of stress result from fluctuations in the ANS and resulting endogenous chemical shifts. Common stress responses include the following:
  - General irritability, hyperexcitation, or depression
  - Pounding of the heart
  - Dryness of the throat and mouth
  - Impulsive behavior and emotional instability
  - Overpowering urge to cry, run, or hide
  - Inability to concentrate
  - Weakness or dizziness
  - Fatigue
  - Tension and extreme alertness
  - Trembling and nervous tics
  - Intermittent anxiety
  - Tendency to be easily startled
  - High-pitched, nervous laughter
  - Stuttering and other speech difficulties
  - Grinding teeth
  - Insomnia
  - Inability to sit still or physically relax
  - Sweating
  - Frequent need to urinate
  - Diarrhea, indigestion, queasiness, and vomiting
  - Migraine and other tension headaches
  - Premenstrual tension or missed menstrual cycles
  - Pain in the neck or lower back
  - Reduced or excessive appetite
  - Increased use of chemicals, including tobacco, caffeine, and alcohol
  - Nightmares
  - Neurotic behavior
  - Psychosis
  - Proneness to accidents
- Wellness training requires an extensive amount of information about diet, exercise, lifestyle, and behavior patterns most of which are out of scope of practice for massage therapy.
- Remember, only a few symptoms combine to create a huge array of illness and disease patterns. Fortunately, a combination of only a few lifestyle changes is required to redirect a disease pattern toward a more resourceful and healing pattern. Taking care of ourselves is what wellness and massage are all about.
- Communication is one of the biggest problems for humans because it is so subjective. It is difficult to be truly objective; knowing this is an important part of wellness. Wellness requires assuming responsibility for our communication.
- Wellness often revolves around simplification of lifestyle. Simplification requires choices, boundaries, discipline, and "letting go" in many dimensions. Sometimes an event

in life removes some part of us. It could be a body part, a body function, a relationship, a member of our family, or a job. Loss heals through grieving. To heal, we need to reconstruct that part or learn to live resourcefully without it. Many professionals can help us with specific therapeutic interventions as the wellness program is developed. Doctors, counselors, other healthcare providers, educators, and religious and spiritual advisors can all play an important part in helping us become well again or maintain our wellness.

- A wellness program needs to change as we change. When a good wellness program is carried out, a person looks forward to getting back to living life to the fullest and, at the appropriate time, dying with dignity.
- The care of our bodies is an important part of any wellness program. Areas that require attention in a wellness program designed to support the body include nutrition, breathing, exercise and stretching, relaxation, and sleep.
- Nutritional experts have varying opinions on the ideal diet. All agree that a balanced diet that uses natural ingredients with low quantities of fats and sugars is healthy for the body. Adequate hydration and fiber maintain bladder and bowel habits that support wellness. A balanced diet is low in saturated fats and refined foods—no trans fats—and high in vegetables, fruits, grains, and beans; moderate consumption of lean protein, including fish and dairy, is required, as is an adequate intake of fiber and water.
- Breathing provides us with air, an essential nutrient, and can alter ANS patterns, which, in turn, affect mood, feelings, and behavior. Most individuals do not breathe efficiently. Almost every meditation or relaxation system uses breathing patterns.
- Normal breathing consists of a shorter inhale in relation to a longer exhale. Inhalation is produced by contraction of the diaphragm and expansion of the abdominal wall, as well as activation of the external intercostals to expand the thorax. Breathing pattern disorder tends to correlate with excessive activation of neck and shoulder muscles during inhalation, resulting in upper chest breathing. Quiet exhalation most often is a passive action. It occurs through relaxation of the external intercostals and elastic recoil of the thoracic wall and tissue of the lungs and bronchi, with gravity pulling the rib cage down from its elevated position. Essentially, no muscle action is occurring. Forced exhalation brings in muscles that can pull down the ribs and muscles that compress the abdomen, forcing the diaphragm upward. Forced exhalation such as coughing activates additional muscular action. Therapeutic massage can support more effective breathing. The steps for efficient, relaxed breathing are as follows:
  - Inhale while the abdomen expands.
  - Exhale as the abdomen contracts.
  - Intake of air is shorter than exhale.
  - Auxiliary breathing muscles are relaxed.
- The main components of a physical fitness exercise program are intensity, duration, and frequency. The main components of an exercise program include the following:

- Warm-up
- Aerobic exercises
- Cooldown
- Changes that occur with exercise are an increase in cardiac function and a decrease in sympathetic ANS stress response. Respiratory changes include more efficient breathing and an increase in uptake of oxygen and elimination of metabolic waste. Mitochondria in cells increase. Body fat decreases and bone density increases.
- Flexibility is the ability to move joints through a normal unrestricted, pain-free range of motion. Stretching is a therapeutic modality that lengthens and softens short soft tissues and supports flexibility. It is possible to be too flexible called hypermobility, which can be a source of soft tissue dysfunction as the muscles and connective tissue compensate to maintain stability.
- Exercise and stretching programs are important parts of any wellness program because they provide the activity our body was designed to have. Any exercise and stretching program must begin slowly. Activity levels can be increased gradually each week. It takes about 7—8 weeks for those who are new to movement to reach a level of comfort. Activities may be added slowly once the body has adapted.
- *Fitness* is a general term that is used to describe the ability to perform physical work. Performing physical work requires cardiorespiratory functioning, muscular strength and endurance, and musculoskeletal flexibility. To become physically fit, individuals must participate regularly in some form of physical activity that challenges all large muscle groups and the cardiorespiratory system and promotes postural balance.
- Relaxation methods initiate a parasympathetic response. Because muscle tension patterns are habitual, most successful relaxation methods combine moving, stretching, tensing, and then releasing muscles (progressive relaxation). The focus of relaxation is to quiet the physical body—not to create a spiritual experience; however, many prayer systems use similar patterns, which are beneficial for relaxation as well.
- Restorative sleep is necessary for wellness. Lack of quality sleep is becoming a major health concern. Many individuals do not get enough sleep. An absolute minimum of 6 hours of uninterrupted sleep is required, with 8—9 hours necessary for most people. During sleep, the body renews, repairs, and generally restores itself. Growth hormone is an important factor in this process, with more than half of its daily secretions taking place during sleep.
- Feelings represent the body's interpretation of emotions. They occur as a response to the effects of hormones, neurotransmitters, and other endogenous chemicals. Often if a person's physiology can be changed, his or her feelings also can be changed. The easiest way to change physiology is to move, as in exercising or breathing.
- The mind is the part of us that reasons, understands, remembers, thinks, and adapts. It coordinates the conscious and subconscious parts of us that influence and direct mental and physical behavior. This interaction between mind and body forms the basis for current approaches to mind/body medicine. The mind involves emotions, behavior, self-concept, and coping.
- Emotions are feelings driven by thoughts. They lead to actions that represent the consequences of how we think and what we do. What we think and feel and how we live are all inextricably linked. Emotions can be powerful. If used resourcefully, they can provide us with the empowerment to reach our goals. Many good things have come from an emotion turned into resourceful behavior. Wellness comes from using the emotion instead of the emotion using us. Used resourcefully, emotions can provide the motivation to achieve wellness; if not, they can make us ill and may be destructive to those who share our lives.
- Behavior is what we do in response to feelings, to trigger thoughts and feelings, and occasionally to avoid feelings. Addictive behavior can take many forms. A person who is addicted to food, drugs, alcohol, exercise, pain, crisis, or loss will develop a lifestyle that both protects and supports the substance or behavior of choice. Addiction requires a great deal of time and energy. Addictive behavior throws the balance of wellness off course. It takes hard work and lots of support to change an addictive behavior.
- Self-concept is what we think about ourselves and how we talk to ourselves; it is an important contributor to wellness. Most of us want a purpose and a sense of achievement, success, and self-confidence. This is achievable when we stop comparing ourselves with one another. Instead, wellness involves reaching out to others for support and information. When we have developed a healthy relationship with ourselves, we can develop and sustain healthy relationships with others.
- Resourceful coping consists of commitment, control, and challenge. *Commitment* is the ability and willingness to be involved in what is happening around us and to have a purpose for being. *Control* is characterized by the belief that we can influence events by the way we feel, think, and act. Healthy control is considered internal control supporting resourceful adaption to the circumstances around us. Living each day as a challenge—filled with things to learn, skills to practice, tasks to be accomplished, and obstacles to overcome—supports wellness.
- Our spirit is the part of us that transcends. Our spiritual selves "know our truth." Spiritual wellness consists of faith, hope, and love. *Faith* is the ability to believe, trust, and know certain things that science cannot prove. Faith is the strength of wellness and involves the expression of that connecting strength each day through faith in ourselves, our partners, our families, and humanity as a whole. Faith is essential to wellness. *Hope* is the belief, assurance, conviction, and confidence that our future somehow will be okay. It is the belief that the choices we make now will be resourceful as we create our future. Without hope, no sense of continuity exists. *Love* has no concrete explanation. Love is a prerequisite for wholeness, and wholeness is necessary for wellness. This is not

romantic love; it is bigger, stronger, more empowering, and mightier. It is quiet, gentle, forgiving, and nonjudgmental.

- Spiritual fitness supports resourceful coping because of the balance in faith, hope, and love, which provides meaning to life and motivates one to commitment, internal control, and energy to meet life's challenges.

Factual Recall Questions

1. During the massage, a client often speaks of problems with children respecting house rules. This is a _____ issue.
   a. Body
   b. Mind
   c. Spiritual

2. A massage practitioner notices that they become a bit aloof if they get behind and are running late for scheduled massage sessions. What type of issue is this?
   a. Denial measure
   b. Defensive measure
   c. Exhaustion phase response
   d. Lack of purpose

3. Wellness usually involves simplification of lifestyle to reduce demands. A stressful outcome of this process is often _____.
   a. Hyperventilation syndrome
   b. Financial stability
   c. Dealing with loss and letting go

4. Which of the following describes breathing in the normal relaxed pattern?
   a. The inhale is longer than the exhale.
   b. Deep inspiration is accentuated.
   c. Accessory muscles work only on exhalation.
   d. The exhale is longer than the inhale.

5. Which of the following may improve sleep?
   a. An afternoon cup of coffee
   b. Taking a long nap in the afternoon
   c. Going to bed and watching television
   d. Spending at least 30 minutes outdoors

6. Feeling confident with commitment, control, and challenge in life describes _____.
   a. Coping well
   b. Using behavior modification
   c. Functioning from an external locus of control

d. Relying on defense mechanisms

Application/Concept Identification and Clinical Reasoning/Synthesis Questions

1. Which of the following best explains why communication is more difficult to improve than diet?
   a. Diet and nutrition are more concrete and objective than subjective communication.
   b. Diet is much more dependent on others, whereas communication is independent of others.
   c. Stress focuses change toward a diet of healthy food choices and improves communication.
   d. Communication skills are highly genetically influenced, but diet has little to do with genetics.

2. In which of the following intervention areas is massage most effective for wellness?
   a. Promoting exercise
   b. Restoring an appropriate eating and sleep cycle
   c. Normalizing breathing mechanisms
   d. Promoting belief system changes

3. A client has been relatively inactive. Recently, the client has been diagnosed with diabetes and needs to begin an exercise program. Which of the following best describes the client's level of fitness?
   a. Deconditioned
   b. Endurance
   c. Flexibility
   d. Aerobic

4. A client has begun an exercise program by walking an hour per day. Which of the following best describes the program?
   a. Stretching and flexibility
   b. Aerobic continuous training
   c. Circuit-interval training
   d. Metabolic anaerobic

Exercise

Using the previous questions as examples, write at least three more questions. Develop plausible wrong answers and be sure that the correct answer is clearly correct. Then write a rationale for each question. The more questions you write, the better you will understand the material.

CHAPTER 8

Anatomy, Physiology, and Pathology

THE BODY AS A WHOLE

Review Tips

The content concerning the body as a whole typically creates a platform for understanding the design of the body and how the body functions. The sciences are described in essentially a foreign language. To be able to understand this content, it is necessary to learn the language. Science studies in general, not only in this chapter, place a heavy emphasis on terminology.

This content usually is tested in the factual recall type of question, which relies on correct use of terminology. The best study skill is rote memorization of the terminology. In the answer key at the end of this chapter, many of the rationales indicate that the correct answer is the definition of the term.

Know the definition of each term and be able to use the term correctly. More complex questions use the terminology in the question and possible answers, and unless the language is deciphered, it is difficult to know what the question or the provided answers mean. There is no easy way to study terminology. Using flashcards, reading glossaries, and doing labeling exercises reinforce the definitions of the various terms. Use the study resources in this guide and the Evolve site, and make sure that when reading the textbooks, you understand what the words mean. Also, make sure to understand the meaning of the general language used to write the questions. If the meaning of a word is unclear, look it up in the dictionary.

Quick Content Review

- Define characteristics of life.
  - Maintenance of boundaries: Keeping the internal environment distinct from the external environment
  - Movement: The ability to transport the entire being, as well as internal components

- Responsiveness: The ability to sense, monitor, and respond to changes in the external environment
- Conductivity: The movement of energy from one point to another
- Growth: A normal increase in the size or number (or both) of cells
- Respiration: The absorption, transport, and use or exchange of respiratory gases (oxygen and carbon dioxide)
- Digestion: The process by which food products are broken down into simple substances to be used by individual cells
- Absorption: The transport and use of nutrients
- Secretion: The production and delivery of specialized substances for diverse functions
- Excretion: The removal of waste products
- Circulation: The movement of fluids, nutrients, secretions, and waste products from one area of the body to another
- Reproduction: The formation of a new being; also, the formation of new cells in the body to permit growth, repair, and replacement
- Metabolism: A chemical reaction that occurs in cells to effect transformation, production, or consumption of energy
- Understand the levels of organization.
  - Chemical level (atoms and molecules): The chemical properties of a substance have to do with the way it reacts with other substances or responds to a change in the environment. Molecules are the smallest part of a substance that can exist independently without loss of the physical and chemical properties of the substance. Atoms combine to form molecules. The atoms most commonly found in living things are hydrogen, carbon, nitrogen, and oxygen. An atom can achieve a state of maximal stability by gaining or losing electrons to fill or empty its outer shell. A chemical reaction or

chemical change results in the breakdown of substances and the formation of new ones.

- Organelle level: Molecules combine in specific ways to form organelles, the basic structures found in cells. Organelles perform specific functions within the cell; the sum property of these structures allows each cell to live. More than two dozen organelles have been identified.
- Cellular level: A cell is the basic structural and functional unit of a living organism. Cells are self-regulating, which allows them to adjust to change by attempting to remain constant and maintain homeostasis.
- Tissue level: A tissue is a group of similar cells that usually have a similar embryologic origin and are specialized for a particular function.
- Organ level: Organs are more complex than tissue. An organ is a group of two or more types of tissue, arranged so they can perform a special function.
- System level: Organs that work together to perform more complex bodily functions are called systems. The 11 systems of the human body are the integumentary, skeletal, muscular, nervous, endocrine, cardiovascular, lymphatic and immune, respiratory, digestive, urinary, and reproductive systems.
- Organism level: The body as a whole is an organism. Each part of the body works with the other parts to support the whole. The mutually dependent nature of the cells and the organization of complex systems allow us the endless possibilities of diversity that we experience.
- Epithelial tissue covers and protects the surfaces of the body; lines cavities; specializes in moving substances into and out of the blood during secretion, excretion, and absorption; and forms many glands.
- Connective tissue is specialized to support and hold together the body and its parts, to transport substances through the body, and to protect the body from foreign substances.
- Muscle tissue has the ability to effect movement by shortening through contraction. Muscle tissue enables the body to move, maintain posture, and produce heat.
- Nervous tissue regulates and coordinates body activity quickly. Nervous tissue has developed greater excitability and conductivity than other types of tissues.
- Anatomy is the scientific study of the structures of the body and the relationships of its parts. Physiology is the scientific study of the processes and functions of the body that support life.
- Gross anatomy is the study of body structures large enough to be visible to the naked eye. Regional anatomy is the study of all of the structures of a particular area. Systemic anatomy is the study of the body divided into its systems. Surface anatomy is the study of internal body structures as they can be recognized and related to the overlying skin surface.
- An atom is the smallest particle of an element that retains the properties of that element. Molecules are the smallest

parts of a substance that can exist independently without losing the physical and chemical properties of that substance.

- Metabolism refers to the chemical reactions in the body. A chemical reaction that releases energy as it breaks down complex compounds into simpler ones is catabolism. Anabolism is a chemical reaction that uses energy as it joins simple molecules together to form more complex molecules. Anabolism requires energy supplied from the molecule adenosine triphosphate (ATP). Enzymes are proteins that speed up chemical reactions but are not consumed or altered in the process. The acidity/alkalinity of a solution is measured in terms of pH.
- A cell is the basic structural and functional unit of a living organism. Interphase is the period when the cell grows and carries on most of its activities. Mitosis occurs when the cell divides; it is the process by which the cell reproduces itself. Meiosis is a special form of mitosis that halves the number of chromosomes in reproductive cells. Hypertrophy is an increase in the size of a cell; atrophy is a decrease in cell size.
- Organelles are the basic structures inside the cells, and they perform specific functions. Diffusion is the movement of ions and molecules from an area of higher concentration to an area of lower concentration. Bringing substances into the cell by forming vesicles is endocytosis, and transporting substances out of the cell is exocytosis.
- A tissue is a group of similar cells that usually have a similar embryologic origin and that are specialized for a particular function. The tissue surface that faces the inside of the body is known as the basal surface.
- Epithelial tissue covers and protects the surfaces of the body; lines body cavities; specializes in moving substances into and out of the blood during secretion, excretion, and absorption; and forms many glands. A membrane is a thin, sheetlike layer of tissue that covers a cell, an organ, or a structure; lines tubes or cavities; or divides and separates one part from another. The four types of membranes are cutaneous, serous, mucous, and synovial.
- Connective tissue is specialized to support and hold together the body and its parts, to transport substances through the body, and to protect it from foreign substances. Within the matrix of connective tissue is a shapeless or amorphous ground substance containing molecules that expand when bound with electrolytes and water molecules. Of all the hundreds of different protein compounds in the body, collagen is the most abundant, accounting for more than one-fourth of the protein in the body.
- Collagenous fibers are strong fibers with minimal stretch capacity. They have a high degree of tensile strength, which allows them to withstand longitudinal stress. Reticular fibers are delicate connective tissue fibers that occur in networks, which support small structures such as capillaries, nerve fibers, and the basement membrane. Elastic fibers are extensible and elastic. They are made from a protein called elastin, which returns to its original length after it is stretched.

- Muscle tissue provides movement, maintains posture, and produces heat. Skeletal muscle fibers are made up of large, cross-striated cells connected to the skeleton, and under voluntary control of the nervous system. Cardiac muscle fibers are small, striated, involuntary fibers that enable the heart to pump blood. Smooth muscle fibers are neither striated nor voluntary. They help regulate blood flow through the cardiovascular system, propel food through the gut, and squeeze secretions from glands.
- Nervous tissue is able to regulate and coordinate body activity quickly. Nervous tissue has developed more excitability and conductivity than other types of tissues.

Factual Recall Questions

1. Adenosine triphosphate releases energy in muscles through what process?
   a. Mitosis
   b. Interphase
   c. Catabolism
   d. Anabolism
2. The substance between cell tissues made up of ground substance and fibers is called _____.
   a. Matrix
   b. Nucleic acids
   c. Basement membrane
3. The chemical reaction that occurs in cells to effect transformation, production, or consumption of energy is _____.
   a. Absorption
   b. Digestion
   c. Responsiveness
   d. Metabolism
4. Atomic bonding to form molecules occurs because of the action among _____.
   a. Nuclei
   b. Protons
   c. Electrons
   d. Neutrons
5. When chemical bonds are broken and new ones are formed, what has occurred?
   a. Mitochondrial reactivity
   b. Hydrolysis response
   c. Conductivity interaction
   d. Chemical reaction
6. The physiologic process that converts food and air into energy is called _____.
   a. Metabolism
   b. Homeostasis
   c. Responsiveness
7. In which of the following chemical reactions are complex compounds formed?
   a. Anabolism
   b. Meiosis

   c. Catabolism
   d. Mitosis
8. Which of the following organelles is involved in the manufacture of proteins?
   a. Muscle spindle
   b. Mitochondria
   c. Lysosomes
   d. Ribosomes
9. The most abundant component in cells is _____.
   a. Water
   b. Protein
   c. Lipids
   d. Carbohydrates
10. Cell division is the reproductive process of cells called _____.
    a. Interphase
    b. Mitosis
    c. Cytosol
11. When a cell is able to perform a specialized function, the structure of the cell is modified. This is called _____.
    a. Hypertrophy
    b. Atrophy
    c. Differentiation
12. Basement membrane connects epithelial tissue to what type of tissue?
    a. Muscle
    b. Nervous
    c. Cardiac
    d. Connective
13. Which of the following is considered a cutaneous membrane?
    a. Skin
    b. Mucous membrane
    c. Serous membrane
    d. Collagen
14. Which of the following membranes lines cavities not open to the external environment and many organs?
    a. Basement
    b. Mucous
    c. Serous
    d. Cutaneous
15. Which of the following type of tissue is the most abundant in the body?
    a. Epithelial
    b. Connective
    c. Muscle
16. Specialization of connective tissue is focused toward _____.
    a. Support
    b. Contractility
    c. Excitability
    d. Differentiation
17. The connective tissue type with the greatest blood flow is _____.
    a. Cartilage

b. Dense irregular
c. Areolar
d. Dense regular

18. The type of connective tissue most often found in ligaments and tendons is _____.
    a. Dense regular
    b. Dense irregular
    c. Areolar

19. Which of the following cell types is found in the connective tissue matrix that secretes bone?
    a. Fibroblast
    b. Chondroblast
    c. Osteoblast

20. What property of collagen may make it viable in the generation of electrical potentials?
    a. Resistance to deformation
    b. Piezoelectric aspects
    c. Colloid formation
    d. Macrophagic activity

21. If a bruise is charted as located on the client's thigh, which of the following correctly describes where the bruise is located?
    a. Systems anatomy
    b. Regional anatomy
    c. Pathophysiology
    d. Collagenous fibers

22. The terms *basement membrane* and *reticular fibers* relate to which of the following?
    a. Epithelial and connective tissue
    b. Nervous tissue and neural tissue
    c. Cardiac and smooth muscle
    d. Cytoplasm and filtration

Application/Concept Identification and Clinical Reasoning/Synthesis Questions

1. How is physiology used in the application of massage?
   a. Location of structures to be manipulated
   b. Specific positioning of the client for assessment
   c. Decision-making related to projected outcomes
   d. Directional communication in charting

2. Characteristics of life involve which of the following concepts?
   a. Physiology
   b. Yin
   c. Anatomy

3. Homeostasis often begins at what level of body organization?
   a. Chemical
   b. Cellular
   c. Tissue
   d. Organ

4. How does massage affect chemical reactions?
   a. Generates a stimulus
   b. Encourages interphase

c. Supports hypertrophy
d. Disrupts differentiation

5. Why is the study of chemical actions in the body important to the massage professional?
   a. Charting depends on these interactions.
   b. Many treatment benefits are derived from chemical reactions.
   c. Validation of subtle energy is atomic.
   d. Chemical reactions are responsible for all pathologic conditions.

6. The diverse forms of connective tissue are attributed to _____.
   a. Properties of cells and composition of matrix
   b. Extensive distribution of blood vessels
   c. Distribution of chondroblasts in the matrix

7. Which of the following tissues is most likely to be damaged from wear and tear of the hip or knee joint?
   a. Hyaline cartilage
   b. Fibrocartilage
   c. Elastic cartilage
   d. Reticular cartilage

8. Massage methods applied to connective tissue affect its thixotropic properties by _____.
   a. Stimulating mast cells to release histamine to reduce inflammation
   b. Separating the desmosomes and gap junctions to allow flexibility
   c. Increasing the secretion of synovial fluid to increase joint mobility
   d. Agitating ground substance and encouraging a softer, more pliable texture

9. A massage therapist notices that a client's heart rate has decreased and the client's breathing has become slower and deeper. Which of the following best describes this outcome from the massage?
   a. Characteristics of life
   b. Organizational physiology
   c. Change in physiology
   d. Change in anatomy

10. A client reports that they have a hormonal imbalance related to a diet low in lipids, which means that the diet is _____.
    a. Acidic and high in fat
    b. Low in amino acids
    c. Excessively low in fat
    d. Low in carbohydrates

Exercise

Using the previous questions as examples, write at least three more questions. Develop plausible wrong answers and be sure that the correct answer is clearly correct. Then write a rationale for each question. The more questions you write, the better you will understand the material.

MECHANISMS OF HEALTH AND DISEASE

Review Tips

The content regarding mechanisms of health and disease is targeted to physiology and anatomy. This content can be tested with all three question types, although the factual recall question is most commonly used because language is still the main focus. Information in this content area is often used in case study types of questions, which combine massage application with physiologic outcomes. These questions are based on the clinical reasoning and synthesis model. Be aware of this factor in future chapters when the content becomes more complex.

As explained previously, you must know the definitions of the terms and you must be able to use the terms correctly. More complex questions use the terminology in the question and possible answers, and unless you can decipher the language, you will not know what the question or the provided answers mean. There is no easy way to study terminology. Using flashcards, reading glossaries, and doing labeling exercises reinforce the definitions of the various terms. Use the study tools in this guide and on the Evolve site, and make sure that when you read your textbooks, you know what the words mean. Also, make sure that you understand the meaning of the general language used to write the questions. If you are not sure of the meaning of a word, look it up in a glossary or dictionary. One of the challenges of any entry-level study is learning the ABCs of the system. It does not matter what you are studying—massage, computers, cooking, carpentry—you have to learn the names and meanings of the materials and equipment. For massage, this means you must learn anatomy and physiology medical terminology.

Quick Content Review

- Health is the capacity to maintain homeostasis in response to stress.
- Stress is anything that causes the body to respond or change so as to maintain homeostasis.
- The sympathetic nervous system triggers the fight-or-flight response (accelerator pedal).
- The parasympathetic nervous system reverses the fight-or-flight response (brake pedal).
- Various effects of excessive stress include overbreathing, muscle stiffness, anxiety, depression, fatigue, heightened blood pressure, digestive problems, sleep disorders, and inhibited immune system function.
- Humans adapt to and manage stress.
- Mental and physical health influence adaptive capacity and resilience. A balanced lifestyle contributes to mental and physical health. Stress management techniques include massage, meditation, mindful breathing, and exercise.
- Homeostasis is the relatively constant state maintained by the physiology of the body.
- Afferent signals move toward a particular center or point of reference, whereas efferent signals move away from a particular center or point of reference.
- Biologic rhythms represent the internal, periodic timing of an organism generated within the body. Entrainment is the synchronization of rhythms.
- Pathology is the study of disease.
- Congenital disease is something present at birth, not something accrued during life, whereas inherited disease is acquired naturally, not as a result of circumstance.
- Etiology is the study of all the factors involved in causing a disease.
- Uncontrolled cell division, or hyperplasia, can result in a neoplasm or an abnormal growth of new tissue called a tumor.
- A benign tumor is a contained and encapsulated neoplasm. Anaplasia is the reproduction of abnormal and undifferentiated cells that fail to mature into specialized cell types.
- Cancer is a nonencapsulated malignant cell mass that invades surrounding tissue. These cells have the devastating ability to break away from the primary tumor and form secondary cancer masses in a process called metastases.
- Inflammation is a protective response of the tissues to irritation or injury. The inflammatory response has four primary signs: heat, redness, swelling, and pain. A fifth sign is loss of mobility.
- Pain is an unpleasant complex, private, abstract experience. Acute pain can be a symptom of a disease condition or a temporary aspect of medical treatment. The pain acts as a warning signal, activating the sympathetic nervous system, and is usually temporary, of sudden onset, and easily localized. Chronic pain persists or recurs for indefinite periods, usually for longer than 6 months. The pain frequently has an obscure onset, and the character and quality of the pain may change over time. The pain is usually diffuse and poorly localized.
- Somatic pain arises from stimulation of receptors in the skin, in which case it is called superficial somatic pain, or from stimulation of receptors in skeletal muscles, joints, tendons, and fasciae, in which case it is deep somatic pain.
- Visceral pain results from stimulation of receptors in the viscera or internal organs.
- Phantom pain frequently is experienced by persons who have had a limb amputated and experience pain or other sensations in the extremity, as if the limb were still there. Pain may be brought on by mechanical, electrical, thermal, or chemical stimuli.
- Nociceptive pain occurs when actual or threatened tissue damage occurs as a result of the activation of nociceptors. Nociceptive pain typically starts as acute pain that lessens with time and tissue healing. This protective and productive response is a normal and appropriate function of the nervous system.
- Neuropathic pain refers to pain that is generated or sustained by the nervous system. It is the result of nerve damage or a malfunctioning nervous system and involves problems with signals from the nerves. Neuropathic pain

commonly is associated with a variety of neurodegenerative, metabolic, and autoimmune diseases. By definition, neuropathic pain is chronic and may escalate over time. There are two categories of neuropathic pain:

1. Central neuropathic pain results directly from CNS injury (e.g., a stroke).
2. Peripheral neuropathic pain is related to injury or disease of the peripheral somatosensory nervous system.

These conditions often begin with productive, normal nociceptive pain. However, in chronic neuropathic pain, the nervous system responds inappropriately to the damage through multiple mechanisms, misreading sensory inputs and generating nonproductive painful sensations. Secondary symptoms that commonly accompany neuropathic pain include depression, sleep disturbance, fatigue, and decreased physical and mental functioning.

- Neuroplastic changes commonly occur with neuropathic pain. After a peripheral nerve injury, anatomical and neurochemical changes can occur within the CNS that can persist long after the injury has healed. When the problem begins in the peripheral nerves, it is called peripheral sensitization. The increased responsiveness in the CNS is called central sensitization. Central sensitization is a factor in chronic pain in which peripheral stimuli are interpreted as more painful than in a normal function. Central sensitization results in amplification of peripheral signals. It is not an independent pain generator in peripheral neuropathic pain conditions. There are three main dysfunctions:

1. Allodynia is pain, generally on the skin, caused by something that wouldn't normally cause pain. Allodynia is believed to be a hypersensitive reaction that may result from central sensitization.
2. Hyperalgesia is an increased pain response—basically, pain that is more painful than it should be.
3. Paresthesia is the experience of unpleasant or painful feelings even when there is nothing touching you, and no stimulus.

- The neuromatrix theory of pain addresses the complex nature of pain in these ways:
  - Pain is an output of the brain that is produced whenever the brain concludes that the body is in danger and action is required. Each person's brain has developed an individual neural network, referred to as the body-self neuromatrix. Pain is a multisystem output that is produced when an individual's pain neuromatrix is activated.
  - An individual's neuromatrix consists of genetic neural programs, individual experience, and behavior. The intensity and location of sensory inputs from the skin, organs, and other somatic receptors influence the perception of a situation as dangerous, triggering activity of the body's stress-regulation systems.
  - Pain becomes chronic as the pain neuromatrix is strengthened by nociceptive and non-nociceptive mechanisms; this means that less input, both nociceptive and non-nociceptive, is required to produce pain. This is called sensitization.

- Pain research has helped explain that acute pain and chronic pain are very different, and actual tissue damage does not always correspond to the intensity of the pain experience. The conscious awareness of pain is a subjective experience that is brain/CNS based. What has emerged is the importance of pain neuroscience education. Educating ourselves and our clients reduces fear and stress. Pain management must be person centered, multidimensional, and comprehensive, taking into consideration the biopsychosocial, spiritual, and cultural factors affecting the person. Pain management should be an interprofessional team effort.

- Guide to Acute Injury Care: ICE/RICE/PRICE/POLICE/MEAT/MCE/MICE/CRIME.
  - ICE, RICE, PRICE, POLICE/MEAT/MCE, MICE, and CRIME are all acronyms for methods to manage an acute soft tissue injury, such as a sprain or strain. The process began with ICE and since has evolved, adding methods and letters to the acronym. Ice is no long recommended to reduce inflammation in the acute healing phase, since the inflammatory response is productive for tissue repair. Ice remains appropriate for pain management.

  I—Ice. Ice, or cryotherapy, is the application of cold, typically by applying an ice pack to the injured area. Ice lowers the skin and tissue temperature, which reduces nociceptive signaling and can lead to a reduction in pain sensation. The use of ice has stirred some controversy because it can reduce the productive acute inflammatory response. However, ice is a much better pain management strategy than pain medication. When applying ice to a local area, do not apply it directly to the skin, to prevent frostbite. The ice application should not exceed 20 minutes.

  C—Compression. Compression after an injury helps prevent further swelling. Compression usually is applied to a local area with an elastic bandage wrap. The bandage should not be so tight that it causes discomfort or interferes with blood flow.

  E—Elevation. Elevating the injured area reduces hydrostatic pressure, which in turn reduces the accumulation of interstitial fluid and manages edema.

  - Next, R and P were added, giving us RICE and PRICE.

  R—Rest. The intention of rest is to support the healing process. The person should not rest excessively, but taking it easy for 24 hours may be prudent.

  P—Protection. Protection prevents further injury. It involves some type of immobilization, such as the compression bandage or reduced weight bearing or demand (e.g., crutches or a sling).

  - Over time, best practices showed that PRICE needed updating, and POLICE came into being. The R was removed, and OL was added:

  OL—Optimal loading. Optimal loading uses movement, weight bearing, and resistance to stimulate the healing process in bones, tendons, ligaments, and muscles. The intensity of the loading increases as the healing progresses. The right amount of activity can help manage swelling.

- Recently a new protocol has been advocated—MEAT (movement, exercise, analgesics, and therapy). This protocol incorporates elements of optimal loading by recommending movement, exercise, and therapy (e.g., physical therapy). Analgesics are used to reduce pain enough to support movement, exercise, and therapy. The use of ice is discouraged in the acute healing phase.
  - AND THE VARIATIONS CONTINUE: MCE: (Move safely, Compression, Elevation) AND ICE IS AGAIN PART OF THE PROTICAL….MAYBE. MICE: (Motion, Ice, Compression, Elevation) CRIME: (Compression, Rest, Ice, Motion and Elevation).

Factual Recall Questions

1. Any stimulus that disrupts internal homeostasis is called _____.
   a. Allodynia
   b. Negative feedback
   c. Stress
   d. Pathology
2. A sensor mechanism, an integration/control center, and an effector mechanism are parts of a _____.
   a. Stress response
   b. Postisometric relaxation
   c. Stimulus response
   d. Feedback loop
3. Feedback that reverses the original stimulus, thereby stabilizing physiologic function, is _____.
   a. Positive
   b. Negative
   c. Stimulus response
   d. Reflex mediated
4. Biologic rhythms are related to _____.
   a. Circadian patterns
   b. Pathogenesis
   c. Negative feedback
   d. Positive feedback
5. Evidence of a healthy state includes _____.
   a. Adaptive capacity to stress
   b. Strain in response to stress
   c. Susceptibility to bacterial infection
   d. Stress exceeding adaptive capacity
6. The study of disease processes is called _____.
   a. Physiology
   b. Pathology
   c. Epidemiology
   d. Pharmacology
7. A group of signs and symptoms that identify a pathologic condition linked to a common cause is called a _____.
   a. Disease
   b. Diagnosis
   c. Pathogenesis
   d. Syndrome
8. A disease with a vague onset that develops slowly and remains active for a long time is considered _____.
   a. Acute
   b. Communicable
   c. Chronic
   d. Idiopathic
9. Which of the following is considered to be a pathogenic organism?
   a. Parasite
   b. Chemical
   c. Allergen
10. A neoplasm resulting from hyperplasia that is contained and encapsulated is considered _____.
    a. Acute
    b. Chronic
    c. Benign
    d. Malignant
11. Reproduction of abnormal and undifferentiated cells that fail to mature into specialized cell types is called _____.
    a. Replacement
    b. Carcinogens
    c. Metastasis
    d. Anaplasia
12. Heat, redness, swelling, and pain are signs of _____.
    a. Cancer
    b. Degeneration
    c. Counterirritation
    d. Inflammation
13. Inflammatory exudate that accumulates during an inflammatory process _____.
    a. Reduces swelling
    b. Dilutes irritants
    c. Inhibits tissue repair
14. Which of the following is an inflammatory mediator that dilates blood vessels?
    a. Histamine
    b. Prostaglandin
    c. Inflammatory exudate
15. The purpose of increased tissue fluid volume during inflammation is to _____.
    a. Allow parenchymal cells to regenerate the area of injury
    b. Allow immune cells to travel quickly to destroy pathogens
    c. Support the activity of labile cells during tissue repair
    d. Increase the activity of histamine and kinins during tissue repair
16. Tissue repair that results in a scar is called _____.
    a. Stroma
    b. Replacement
    c. Regeneration
    d. Idiopathic
17. A major component of scar tissue is _____.
    a. Epidermis
    b. Epithelium
    c. Fibroblasts
    d. Collagen
18. Genetics, age, lifestyle, stress, environment, and preexisting conditions are considered _____.
    a. Determinants of immune hypersensitivity
    b. Predisposing risk factors for development of disease

c. Potential distribution routes for pathogens

d. Warning signs of cancer

19. What do people complain about most to their healthcare professionals?
    a. Decreased circulation
    b. Joint stiffness
    c. Breathing difficulty
    d. Pain

20. Potential tissue damage is signaled by _____.
    a. Pain
    b. Inflammation
    c. Steroids
    d. Stress

21. The term for pain that is poorly localized, nauseating, and associated with sweating and blood pressure changes is _____.
    a. Superficial somatic
    b. Superficial visceral
    c. Aching
    d. Deep

22. Which of the following terms describes pain that may be a symptom of an organ disorder?
    a. Superficial somatic
    b. Deep somatic
    c. Aching

23. Pain that arises from stimulation of receptors in the skin or from stimulation of receptors in skeletal muscles, joints, tendons, and fasciae is called _____.
    a. Visceral
    b. Phantom
    c. Somatic
    d. Referred

24. A massage application that creates superficial somatic pain that blocks transmission of deep somatic or visceral pain is called _____.
    a. Counterirritation
    b. Pain-spasm-pain cycle
    c. Reflex contraction

25. When pain is felt in a surface area away from the stimulated receptors, particularly in organs, it is called _____.
    a. Visceral
    b. Phantom
    c. Somatic
    d. Referred

26. Aspirin is used in pain management because its effects include _____.
    a. Stimulating inflammation
    b. Inhibiting enkephalins
    c. Inhibiting prostaglandins
    d. Stimulating A delta nerve fibers

27. According to Hans Selye, the overall response of the body to stress is called the _____.
    a. Fight-or-flight response
    b. Resistance reaction
    c. Exhaustion phase
    d. General adaptation syndrome

28. A common breathing disturbance in excessive or long-term stress is _____.
    a. Hyperventilation syndrome
    b. Immune suppression
    c. Gastritis
    d. Tetany

29. At which life stage is homeostasis most effectively maintained?
    a. Birth to 3 years old
    b. 4 years old to 12 years old
    c. Adolescence to midlife
    d. 65 years old and older

Application/Concept Identification and Clinical Reasoning/Synthesis Questions

1. A reduction in blood pressure as a massage outcome is characterized as a _____.
   a. Positive feedback response
   b. Virulent response
   c. Feedback loop
   d. Reduction of a fistula

2. Massage that stimulates sensory receptors to encourage homeostatic mechanisms is best described as which of the following?
   a. Allodynia
   b. Feedback loop
   c. General adaptation syndrome
   d. Threshold and tolerance

3. What do biofeedback, massage, aromatherapy, medication, and hypnosis all have in common?
   a. Strategies for pain management
   b. Methods of massage
   c. Risk factors for pain
   d. Methods of controlling inflammation

4. A client has noticed hair loss, mouth ulcers, and bladder urgency. These symptoms are related because they are _____.
   a. Examples of inflammatory responses
   b. Stress and pain modulators
   c. Genetic disease risk factors
   d. Stress-related disease symptoms

5. Feedback is an essential aspect of homeostasis because of _____.
   a. Afferent discharge
   b. Reflex arcs
   c. Information exchange
   d. Efferent signaling

6. The effects of massage are processed by the body as a _____.
   a. Controlled condition
   b. Control center
   c. Response
   d. Stress stimulus

7. Many benefits of massage are a result of _____.
   a. Nonspecific stress stimulus that encourages feedback response to more optimum function
   b. Precise application of selected stimulus-creating positive feedback
   c. Positive feedback response to return function to homeostasis
8. People experience relaxed mood states when _____.
   a. Sympathetic ANS dominates
   b. Breathing is rapid
   c. Heart rate is rapid and irregular
   d. Parasympathetic ANS patterns dominate
9. The chronic form of inflammation may be helped with what form of massage?
   a. Extensive application of deep transverse friction
   b. Light surface stroking
   c. Controlled use of friction, stretching, and pulling
   d. Brisk beating and pounding
10. A client's low back pain returns within 3 hours of receiving massage. What organ may be the cause for referred back pain?
    a. Bladder
    b. Kidney
    c. Stomach
    d. Gallbladder
11. Massage used as a pain management strategy is a form of _____.
    a. Stimulus-induced analgesia
    b. Acupuncture
    c. Dermatomal inhibition
12. The first response of the alarm reaction is the _____.
    a. Sympathetic centers are activated
    b. Hypothalamus is stimulated
    c. Adrenal cortex releases glucocorticoid
    d. Adrenal medulla releases epinephrine
13. A client complains of an aching pain just under the ribs to the right of the midline, under the right scapula, and in the right neck and shoulder area. This pain has been occurring more frequently and is now almost constant. The referred pain pattern might indicate problems with what organ?
    a. Bladder
    b. Kidney
    c. Stomach
    d. Gallbladder
14. The client asks for very deep pressure. The massage professional keeps asking whether the pressure is causing discomfort, and the client says no. It seems that any deeper pressure may cause bruising and other tissue damage. This client may be exhibiting _____.
    a. Counterirritation
    b. Reduced influence of beta-endorphins
    c. High pain tolerance
    d. Hyperstimulation analgesia

15. A client has had to deal with multiple stressors, including a death in the family and having a car stolen. The client is 69 years old, is sleeping poorly, and tells the massage therapist about feeling unable to deal with it all. The most logical explanation is the client's _____.
    a. Reduced stress threshold is straining the cortisol enhancement of the immune system
    b. Ability to adapt to multiple stressors is challenged by increasing age
    c. Adaptive capacity is adequate, but the family death is enough to increase mental strain
    d. Stress response is increasing adaptive capacity that is challenged by age-related immune suppression

Exercise

Using the previous questions as examples, write at least three more questions. Develop plausible wrong answers and be sure that the correct answer is clearly correct. Then write a rationale for each question. The more questions you write, the better you will understand the material.

MEDICAL TERMINOLOGY

Review Tips

The content about medical terminology is all about language. When studying, memorize all of the lists of prefixes, root words, and suffixes that combine to make medical terms—just like sounding out words using phonics. If you know what the parts mean, you can decipher what the word means.

This is another area for which you have to memorize the language. Again, use the study aids in this text, read glossaries, and look up words you do not understand. It may be helpful to obtain a medical terminology textbook and use it as a self-teaching tool. Elsevier has many medical terminology books and dictionaries from which to choose.

Quick Content Review

- A word element is part of a word. A prefix is placed at the beginning of a word to alter the meaning of the word. A vowel added between two roots or a root and a suffix to make pronunciation easier is a combining vowel. The root word element contains the basic meaning of the word, and the suffix is placed at the end of a root to change the meaning of the word. A shortened form of a word or phrase is an abbreviation.
- Combine word elements into medical terms. Examples of word elements combined into medical terms are shown in Table 8.1.

TABLE 8.1 Word Elements Combined Into Medical Terms

Term	Word elements	Definition
Antiseptic	Anti: against; septic: germs	Effective against germs
Contralateral	Contra: opposing; lateral: side	The opposite side
Subaxilla	Sub: under; axilla: armpit	Under the armpit
Neurogenic	Neur: nerve; genic: origin	Originating in the nerves
Bradycardia	Brady: slow; card: heart (i.e., a state or condition)	Slow heartbeat
Neuralgia	Neur: nerve; algia: pain	Nerve pain
Contraindication	Contra: opposing; indication: desired result	Opposite of the desired result
Periosteum	Peri: around; oste: bone	Around the bone (the periosteum is a specialized membrane that surrounds bone)
Intracephal	Intra: within; cephal: head	Within the head
Arthroplasty	Arthro: joint; plasty: surgical repair	Reconstruction of a joint

- Identify abbreviations used in healthcare and provide their meanings. Table 8.2 provides examples of abbreviations used in healthcare, along with their meanings.
- A chart is a written record of professional interactions representing a clinical reasoning method that emphasizes a problem-solving approach. The POMR is a problem-oriented medical record, and SOAP is the acronym (subjective, objective, assessment/analysis, and plan) for the four parts of the written account of the health assessment.
- In a problem-solving model of charting, the practitioner collects a database before beginning the process of identifying the client's problems. The database contains all available subjective and objective information that contributes to therapeutic intervention. Next, the information is analyzed. Each identified problem represents a conclusion or a decision that arises from examination, investigation, and analysis of the data collected. A decision then is made about a plan of intervention. The plan needs to be implemented, reevaluated, and adjusted as necessary. The action taken, its effectiveness, and the outcome are recorded progressively from session to session.
- Western science is a young discipline that uses scientific methods of observation; it involves measuring concrete entities, accumulating data, and analyzing findings. Ancient approaches also require observation, measurement, and accumulation and analysis of data, but in addition, they have validated the importance of intuition. Ancient or indigenous healing practices do not separate the body, mind, and spirit as Western science does, but this is changing. Most ancient healing systems are grounded in concepts similar to those presented in the Asian model, mainly the idea of bringing the body into balance to promote health, rather than simply eliminating symptoms, as has been the method of the young Western scientific approach. Western mind/body medicine is developing according to similar theories.

- Common to these ancient and indigenous healing traditions is the use of soft tissue methods, movement, meditation and inner reflection, exercise, dietary influences and naturally occurring herbs for medicinal purposes, and emotional influences and spiritual connections to help make human beings one with their environment and the universe. Metaphors based on naturally occurring phenomena that can be observed often are correlated with physical and psychological function. Western scientific theories are not in opposition to these practices; they actually are complementary.
- Define terms used to describe the positions of the body in relation to other body parts:
  - Anterior or ventral: Front of the body
  - Posterior or dorsal: Back of the body
  - Distal: Farthest from the torso
  - Lateral: To the side
  - Medial: Toward the middle
  - Proximal: Closest to the torso
  - Ipsilateral: Same side
  - Contralateral: Opposite side
  - Cephalad: Toward the head
  - Caudal: Toward the tail
  - Superior: Above
  - Inferior: Below
  - Peripheral: Outside
  - Volar: Palm of the hand
  - Plantar: Bottom of the foot
  - Varus: Bow-legged
  - Valgus: Knock-kneed
  - Dextral: Right hand
  - Sinistral: Left hand
  - Internal: Inside
  - External: Outside
  - Deep: Away from the surface
  - Superficial: Toward the surface

TABLE 8.2 Abbreviations Used in Healthcare

Abbreviation	Meaning
ADLs	Activities of daily living
ad lib	As desired
a.m.a.	Against medical advice
ANS	Autonomic nervous system
as tol	As tolerated
BP	Blood pressure
CC	Chief complaint
c/o	Complains of
Dx	Diagnosis
h (hr)	Hour
H_2O	Water
Hx	History
IBW	Ideal body weight
ICT	Inflammation of connective tissue
id	The same
L	Left; length; lumbar
lig	Ligament
M	Muscle; meter; myopia
meds	Medications
ML	Midline
n	Normal
NA	Nonapplicable
OTC	Over the counter
P	Pulse
PT	Physical therapy
Px	Prognosis
R	Respiration; right
R/O	Rule out
ROM	Range of motion
Rx	Prescription
SOB	Shortness of breath
SP, spir	Spirit
Sym	Symmetrical
T	Temperature
TLC	Tender loving care
Tx	Treatment
WD	Well developed

Factual Recall Questions

1. A prefix, root, or suffix is based on Latin or Greek _____.
   a. Grammar
   b. Basic word meaning
   c. Word elements
2. The prefix *auto-* means _____.
   a. Self
   b. Hear
   c. Against
   d. Both sides

3. The prefix meaning "against" or "opposite" is _____.
   a. Circum-
   b. Caud-
   c. Contra-
   d. Brach-
4. The prefix *mal-* means _____.
   a. Large
   b. One or single
   c. Form or shape
   d. Illness or disease
5. The prefix for hard is _____.
   a. Schist(o)-
   b. Sepsi-
   c. Scler(o)-
6. The root word *pneum(o)-* means _____.
   a. Vein
   b. Lung or gas
   c. Chest
   d. Breathing
7. The root word for kidney is _____.
   a. Nephr(o)-
   b. Neur(o)-
   c. Uro-
   d. Phleb(o)-
8. The suffix for pain is _____.
   a. -asis
   b. -ase
   c. -algia
   d. -emia
9. The suffix *-pnea* means _____.
   a. To breathe
   b. Paralysis
   c. Putrefaction
10. The ability to think through and justify an intervention process is called _____.
    a. History taking
    b. Assessment
    c. Database collection
    d. Clinical reasoning
11. The history-taking interview provides data for which part of the SOAP note charting process?
    a. Subjective data
    b. Objective data
    c. Analysis
    d. Plan
12. The aspect of the physical assessment that identifies altered movement patterns is considered _____.
    a. Visual
    b. Functional
    c. Palpation
13. Physical assessment provides information for which SOAP charting area?
    a. Subjective data
    b. Objective data
    c. Analysis

14. For the data collected during the interview process and physical assessment to be focused on a particular outcome for the client, the information must be _____.
    a. Recorded in a SOAP note
    b. Communicated to the client
    c. Analyzed through a logical process
    d. Written in medical terminology

15. Referral to another healthcare professional is based on which part of the clinical reasoning process?
    a. Assessment of data
    b. Data collection
    c. Plan development
    d. History interview

16. The head, neck, trunk, and spinal cord are considered to be which region of the body?
    a. Appendicular
    b. Thoracic
    c. Axial
    d. Ventral

17. The bladder is located in which region of the abdomen?
    a. Epigastric
    b. Umbilical
    c. Left iliac
    d. Hypogastric

18. The liver is located in which quadrant?
    a. Right upper
    b. Left upper
    c. Right lower
    d. Left lower

19. Which movement decreases the angle of a joint?
    a. Flexion
    b. Extension
    c. Retraction
    d. Adduction

20. The term meaning "on the same side" is _____.
    a. Lateral
    b. Contralateral
    c. Ipsilateral
    d. Dextral

21. The term meaning "closer to the trunk or point of origin" is _____.
    a. Anterior
    b. Posterior
    c. Distal
    d. Proximal

22. A commonality of the point phenomena is that they _____.
    a. are often located over motor points
    b. refer pain patterns
    c. are located over A delta and C afferent nerve fibers
    d. are located in meridian pathways

23. What do the following have in common: *circum-*, *andro-*, and *steno-?*
    a. Root words
    b. Prefixes
    c. Suffixes
    d. Abbreviations

24. A massage therapist identified a short muscle in the occipital area. Where is this located?
    a. Leg
    b. Ankle
    c. Neck
    d. Arm

Application/Concept Identification and Clinical Reasoning/Synthesis Questions

1. During assessment, the client appears twisted, which means the client _____.
    a. Has frontal plane distortion
    b. Is rotated in the transverse plane
    c. Is unable to abduct in the sagittal plane
    d. Has limited flexion and extension in the transverse plane

2. The use of abbreviations in charting is characterized as _____.
    a. Being universally understood
    b. Being time consuming
    c. Requiring a deciphering key
    d. Communicating information clearly

3. Many ancient healing practices were developed on the basis of _____.
    a. Measurement of concrete functions
    b. Experiential observation
    c. Scientific methods
    d. Meridian system

Exercise

Using the previous questions as examples, write at least three more questions. Develop plausible wrong answers and be sure that the correct answer is clearly correct. Then write a rationale for each question. The more questions you write, the better you will understand the material.

NERVOUS SYSTEM BASICS AND THE CENTRAL NERVOUS SYSTEM

Review Tips

Researchers are identifying many interactions between massage and the nervous system. To understand the physiologic mechanisms of massage that benefit the client, it is important to understand both the terminology and the physiology. This is a different sort of study. Comprehension is necessary to appreciate how various aspects of the nervous system work together and how these functions affect massage. Studying for terminology/word definitions is like the ABCs. Comprehension is about how you recognize how the ABCs go together or form words that are symbols for meaning.

An effective study strategy is to explain a concept in words different from those in the text or to give an example of what the text is talking about or to develop a metaphor about the content. A metaphor is different from an example. A metaphor is more of a comparison. Here is an example of a metaphor: Myelin is like the insulation around an electrical cord. As for the previous parts, look up any terminology you do not understand, and make sure you know why the wrong answers are wrong.

Review the content that lists pathologic conditions related to the body system and related indications and contraindications for massage. Massage examinations tend to target safe practice content. As a result, the appropriateness of massage for various pathologic conditions is emphasized. Review Appendix A at the back of this book.

Quick Content Review

Nervous System and Endocrine System

- The nervous system, the most complex of the body systems, is composed of more than 110 billion nerve cells. The nervous system is divided into the central nervous system (CNS), which is composed of the brain, spinal cord, and coverings, and the peripheral nervous system (PNS), which includes the cranial nerves, spinal nerves, and ganglia.
- The peripheral nervous system is divided further into autonomic and somatic divisions. These subdivisions combine and communicate to innervate the somatic and visceral parts of the body.
- The somatic division is associated with the bones, muscles, and skin.
- The visceral or autonomic division is associated with the internal glands, organs, blood vessels, and mucous membranes.
- The autonomic nervous system (ANS) is divided further into two subdivisions:
  1. The sympathetic nervous system activates arousal responses and expends body resources to respond to emergency situations or any activity of excitement or acceleration.
  2. The parasympathetic nervous system reverses the response of the sympathetic nervous system by returning the body to a nonalarm state and restoring body resources. The sympathetic division is considered the "flight, fight, fear" system. However, any highly emotional state of joy, excitement, and elation is also sympathetic. The parasympathetic nervous system is associated with the relaxation response. Much of the interaction between body and mind takes place through ANS activity.
- The ANS can also be divided into three divisions: sympathetic, parasympathetic, and enteric, which focuses on the gastrointestinal system in vertebrates (the gut).
- The basic structure of the nervous system is the neuron, or nerve cell. The nerve cell is an impulse-transmitting fiber that connects the CNS with all parts of the body. Three basic types of neurons exist:
  1. Afferent or sensory neurons, which carry impulses to the CNS
  2. Connecting or associative interneurons, which transmit nerve impulses between neurons
  3. Efferent or motor neurons, which transmit impulses away from the CNS to the muscles, organs, and glands
- The parts of the neuron include the neuroglia, dendrites, axon, and neurilemma.
- A nerve impulse is a self-perpetuating wave of electrical energy that travels along the surface of the plasma membrane of the neuron. Nerve impulses have to be initiated by a stimulus that changes the environment of the neuron. A neuron is said to be excited when a stimulus triggers the opening of additional Na^+ (sodium ions) channels, allowing the membrane potential to move toward zero. Inhibition occurs when the stimulus triggers the opening of additional K^+ (potassium ions) channels, thereby increasing the membrane potential. The electrical disturbance stimulates a similar change in the next part of the membrane, resulting in a nerve impulse that travels in one direction along the surface of the neuron. After a local area of a neuron membrane has been stimulated and a nerve impulse has been generated, the neuron resists restimulation and will not respond to a stimulus, no matter how strong. This is called the refractory period.
- In myelinated fibers, action potentials in the membrane occur only at the nodes of Ranvier. If the traveling impulse encounters a part of the membrane that is covered with insulating myelin, it jumps over the myelin, resulting in faster transmission than is possible in nonmyelinated parts.
- Neurotransmitters are chemical compounds that regulate many body activities and states. Neurotransmitter effects may be excitatory—increasing activity—or inhibitory—decreasing activity.
- Chemical synapses occur at presynaptic cells that release chemical transmitters called neurotransmitters across a tiny gap to the postsynaptic cell. The plasma membrane of a postsynaptic neuron consists of protein molecules that serve as receptors for the neurotransmitters. When a nerve impulse reaches a synaptic knob, thousands of neurotransmitter molecules flow into the synaptic cleft and bind to specific receptors, generating an action potential. The action of the neurotransmitter is terminated quickly by neurotransmitter molecules that are transported back into the synaptic knob or that are metabolized into inactive compounds. Many drugs act by disturbing the termination phase.
- The major neurotransmitters include acetylcholine, serotonin, histamine, epinephrine, norepinephrine, dopamine, glutamate (or glutamic acid), gamma aminobutyric acid, substance P, somatostatin, cholecystokinin, and vasoactive intestinal peptide.
- Change in neurotransmitter concentrations at various synapses causes change in behavior. Mental illness behaviors

and much of daily behavior, especially pain, pleasure, and survival behavior, are determined by brain chemistry. An ongoing dynamic balance in this chemical soup allows for resourceful behavior for each situation encountered. In addition, people behave in certain ways to increase or decrease levels of neurotransmitters or hormones.

- When medication is used to manage neurotransmitters, mood and behavior are affected.
- A pain-inhibiting system exists in the body. Internal, or endogenous, opiates (endorphins and enkephalins) produced by the body block pain impulses in various portions of the pathway, probably as a protective device. The neurotransmitter substance P is blocked by enkephalins. Endorphins and enkephalins also affect mood.
- The brain, which is the center for interpreting, regulating, integrating, and coordinating physiologic functions, is divided into the following major segments:
  1. Major functions of the cerebrum involve interpretation of sensory information received from the eyes, ears, and nose, and from taste, tactile, and other sensory structures of the body. The cerebrum also transmits motor impulses that initiate voluntary movements and some involuntary movements in response to sensory data, and it performs functions that allow learning, reasoning, recall, language, and consciousness.
  2. The frontal lobe of the cerebral cortex is the anterior area positioned behind the frontal bone. Its major function is to control the voluntary skeletal muscles in an area called the precentral gyrus. The frontal lobe is active in functions of problem-solving that involve concentration and planning. The parietal lobe is located next to the parietal bones of the skull; it contains the postcentral gyrus, which is the sensory area of the brain that assists with sensory data reporting of temperature, pressure, touch, and pain. The temporal lobe, which is positioned next to the temporal bones, is responsible for the sensory functions of hearing and smell. The occipital lobe is located just anterior to the occipital bone of the skull and is responsible for control of eyesight.
  3. The brainstem contains centers for vital functions connected with survival; vomiting, coughing, and sneezing; posture; and basic movement patterns; it houses the cranial nerves. Located in the brainstem are the thalamus, hypothalamus, and pineal gland.
  4. The midbrain or mesencephalon contains centers for visual and auditory reflexes and correlating information about muscle tone, posture, and visual reflexes; it also contains cranial nerve nuclei, an important part of the reticular activating system.
  5. The pons (pons varolii), located between the midbrain and the medulla, assists in rhythmic discharge of the respiratory center of the medulla, chewing, facial expressions, and eye movement; it contains cranial nerve nuclei and important centers for rapid eye movement (REM) sleep.
  6. The medulla or medulla oblongata connects the pons with the spinal cord. Functions of the medulla include the following:
     Cardiac center: Regulates heartbeat
     Vasomotor center: Regulates blood pressure
     Respiratory center: Regulates breathing
     Other functions include control of coughing, sneezing, swallowing, and vomiting.
  7. The cerebellum, located in the posterior cranial fossa of the skull, is the second largest segment of the brain; it contains centers for balance, equilibrium, muscular coordination, posture, and balance. The cerebellum controls subconscious movements of skeletal muscle, input from proprioceptors, feedback loops, posture, and future positioning, and it regulates sensations of anger and pleasure.
  8. The reticular formation and the reticular activating system, which form the primitive inner core of the spinal cord and brainstem, are involved in the regulation of respiration, blood pressure, heart rate, endocrine secretions, conditioned reflexes, learning, and consciousness.
  9. The meninges, or membranes, consist of the dura mater, arachnoid mater, and pia mater. The three spaces created by the meninges are as follows:
     Epidural space between cranial bones and dura mater
     Subdural space between dura and arachnoid mater
     Subarachnoid space between arachnoid and pia mater that ends at the vertebral level
  10. Vessels of the brain include the internal carotid system and the vertebrobasilar artery, which connect (anastomose) at the midbrain as the circle of Willis, ensuring blood flow to the brain despite occlusion of the carotid or basilar arteries. Venous drainage from the brain occurs through several veins, as well as through the dural sinuses—spaces in the dura that drain to the internal jugular veins.
- The spinal cord conducts nerve impulses and is a center for spinal reflexes; 31 pairs of peripheral spinal nerves connect the spinal cord and brain with all areas of the body. The white matter on the outside of the spinal cord is made up of myelinated nerve fibers called tracts, which ascend to and descend from the brain. Ascending tracts conduct impulses up the spinal cord to the brain, transmitting pain, temperature, and positional information. Descending tracts conduct impulses from the brain down the cord, sending effector information to muscles and glands. The gray matter on the inside of the spinal cord forms an H pattern.
- Common pathologic conditions of the central nervous system are as follows:
  1. Cerebrovascular accident (CVA), or stroke, is an umbrella term that covers disorders such as aneurysms, blood clots, and hemorrhages. When a stroke occurs, an artery in the brain is occluded or closed off from a blood clot, which is called a thrombus.
  2. An aneurysm is a weakening and bulging of an artery.

3. A blood clot may break away from a particular part of the body and travel to the brain, causing a stroke or cerebrovascular accident.
4. CNS trauma may occur when a concussion causes a brief loss of consciousness or a state of confusion after a head injury. A contusion is a bruise of the brain. Intracranial bleeding is called intracerebral hemorrhage or hematoma.
5. Cerebral palsy is a general term for brain damage before, during, or shortly after birth.
6. Seizure in epilepsy is characterized by an abrupt alteration in brain function, ranging from a mild behavior change to a general convulsion.
7. Primary tumors form from the neuroglia, membrane tissues, and blood vessels associated with the neuron. Most brain tumors do not originate in the brain. They are metastatic from malignant tumors elsewhere in the body.
8. Spinal cord injury can result in a number of neurologic deficits.
9. Central sensitization is known as an increased central neuronal responsiveness and causes hyperalgesia, allodynia, and referred pain and hyperalgesia across multiple spinal segments, leading to chronic widespread pain.

- Drugs influence the central nervous system. Stimulants include caffeine, nicotine, the amphetamines, and cocaine. Depressants are alcohol, narcotics, minor tranquilizers, and barbiturates. Hallucinogens include lysergic acid diethylamide (LSD), phencyclidine (PCP), peyote, and marijuana.
- Many physiologic effects of therapeutic massage are caused by interaction with functions of the central nervous system. Research has shown that applying massage effectively has beneficial effects on the central nervous system and associated neurotransmitters.
- Competence in the interpretation of symptoms and behaviors related to the central nervous system is necessary for determining the factors that are causing the distressing symptoms. Competency also is displayed in the selection of appropriate methods to encourage a return to effective functioning in the system or to create outcomes of relaxation and well-being. Therapeutic benefit from massage is measured by achievable outcomes and is related directly to the ability to use clinical reasoning skills and to solve problems. Massage methods are modified as necessary to meet the goals of the client.
- Knowledge of the central nervous system helps the massage professional to practice safely and to refer clients with conditions contraindicated for massage.

Factual Recall Questions

1. A function of neuroglia is to _____.
   a. Transmit signals to the cell body
   b. Carry signals away from the cell body
   c. Conduct signals from one neuron to another
   d. Support and protect neurons
2. Neurilemma is formed by _____.
   a. Schwann cells
   b. Myelin
   c. Dendrites
   d. Axons
3. Neurons that conduct signals to the central nervous system are called _____.
   a. Sensory
   b. Motor
   c. Associative
4. When a neuron is positively charged on the outside of the cell membrane and negatively charged on the inside, this is called _____.
   a. Saltatory conduction
   b. Membrane potential
   c. Action potential
5. Nerve axon repair in the peripheral nervous system is produced by _____.
   a. Oligodendrocytes
   b. Synaptic vesicles
   c. Neurilemma
   d. Endoplasmic reticulum
6. Action potential between neurons occurs across the synaptic cleft because of _____.
   a. Neurotransmitters
   b. Postsynaptic membrane
   c. Anterograde transport
   d. Nodes of Ranvier
7. The neurotransmitter that primarily excites the skeletal muscles is _____.
   a. Dopamine
   b. Acetylcholine
   c. Cholecystokinin
   d. Somatostatin
8. The portion of the brain that interprets sensory data and compares them against past memories and experiences is the _____.
   a. Ventricles
   b. Pineal body
   c. Cerebrum
9. The structure that connects the right and left hemispheres of the cerebrum is the _____.
   a. Basal ganglia
   b. Sulcus
   c. Corpus callosum
   d. Longitudinal fissure
10. The primary area of the brain that would process the pain/pleasure aspect of massage is the _____.
    a. Frontal lobe
    b. Parietal lobe
    c. Temporal lobe
    d. Occipital lobe
11. Activities that occur in the cerebrum after sensory signals are received and before motor responses are sent are called _____.

a. Integrative functions
b. Convolutions
c. Inhibitory functions

12. Conscious awareness of the environment is related to what structural and functional area of the brain?
    a. Primary motor cortex
    b. Reticular activating system
    c. Sensory-associated cortex

13. The areas of the brain responsible for motor sequencing, posture in relationship to the environment, and processing of spatial relations are the _____.
    a. Limbic lobes
    b. Temporal lobes
    c. Frontal lobes
    d. Parietal lobes

14. Uncontrolled emotional display may indicate problems with what brain area?
    a. Basal ganglia
    b. Left hemisphere of the cerebrum
    c. Limbic system
    d. Primary motor area

15. Which of the following drugs is a central nervous system depressant?
    a. Cocaine
    b. Caffeine
    c. Alcohol
    d. Amphetamines

16. Which brain area regulates vital life functions such as heart rate, blood pressure, and breathing?
    a. Midbrain
    b. Pons
    c. Cerebellum
    d. Medulla oblongata

17. Pleasure states experienced during massage that support mind/body health are processed in what area of the diencephalon?
    a. Thalamus
    b. Pineal body
    c. Meninges
    d. Midbrain

18. A massage session that incorporates rocking affects the vestibular system, including labyrinthine righting reflexes. Which brain area also is stimulated to coordinate appropriate posture?
    a. Cerebellum
    b. Pons
    c. Motor descending tracts
    d. Sensory ascending tracts

19. The protective membrane that adheres to the brain is the _____.
    a. Dura mater
    b. Arachnoid mater
    c. Epidural mater
    d. Pia mater

20. Which of the following is most involved in pain mechanisms?
    a. Histamine

b. Substance P
c. Acetylcholine

Application/Concept Identification and Clinical Reasoning/Synthesis Questions

1. Which of the following best describes the nervous system and the endocrine system?
   a. Predictable physiologic outcomes are constant.
   b. Feedback loops do not affect outcomes.
   c. Linear pathways of effect are constant.
   d. Both are systems of control.

2. Sensory stimulation of massage causes a chemical change in neurons. This change is called _____.
   a. Action potential
   b. Refractory period
   c. Depolarization
   d. Saltatory conduction

3. Which phase of nerve signal conduction is related to muscle energy methods that use some sort of muscle contraction to prepare the muscle to relax and lengthen?
   a. Action potential
   b. Refractory period
   c. Depolarization
   d. Saltatory conduction

4. A person is clumsy and has a dull or foggy mind in terms of understanding information and making decisions. Which of the following neurotransmitters may be involved?
   a. Norepinephrine
   b. Histamine
   c. Glutamate
   d. Dopamine

5. Neurotransmitters work in excitatory and inhibitory pairs. Which of the following would provide a balancing action for enkephalin?
   a. Somatostatin
   b. Substance P
   c. Serotonin

6. A massage client reports that after the massage they had some itchy areas of skin and clothes felt rough against the skin. Which neurotransmitter may be involved?
   a. Histamine
   b. Acetylcholine
   c. Epinephrine

7. A client reports before the massage that their mind is agitated, they feel as though they want to scream, and they are talking loudly and pacing. After the massage, the client feels calmer and wants a nap. Which neurotransmitter is largely responsible for the mood change?
   a. Norepinephrine
   b. Dopamine
   c. Serotonin
   d. Substance P

8. The purpose of therapeutic (feel good) pain during massage to manage undesirable pain is to stimulate which neurotransmitters?

a. Serotonin and endorphin
b. Epinephrine and histamine
c. Acetylcholine and dopamine
d. Histamine and substance P

9. States of higher consciousness are related to _____.
   a. Alertness with relaxation
   b. Decreased health states
   c. Increased sympathetic arousal
   d. Depression with pain

10. Why do the primary motor and the primary somesthetic sensory areas of the brain interfere with the ability to successfully self-massage areas of the back and limbs?
    a. The largest sensory and motor awareness is in these areas.
    b. Distribution of sensory and motor function to the hands is too small to stimulate sensation.
    c. Distribution of sensory and motor function is larger to the hands than to the back and limbs.
    d. The back and limbs have a predominance of sensory distribution over the motor distribution of the hands.

11. Massage sensations travel on which spinal cord tracts?
    a. Sensory ascending
    b. Motor descending
    c. Corticospinal
    d. Lateral reticulospinal

12. Which pathologic process would benefit the most from massage facilitating the movement of body fluids?
    a. Upper motor neuron injury
    b. Lower motor neuron injury
    c. Aneurysm
    d. Chorea

13. Research indicates that massage increases the availability of the following neurotransmitters: norepinephrine, serotonin, and dopamine. Which central nervous system disorder would be most benefited by massage?
    a. Stroke
    b. Cerebral palsy
    c. Depression
    d. Schizophrenia

14. A client has essential tremor. Which of the following is most correct regarding treatment application?
    a. Stress reduction massage will have a significant effect.
    b. Massage will have little effect.
    c. Massage with medication should reverse the condition.
    d. The associated headache is reduced by massage.

15. A client has a spinal cord injury that has resulted in paralysis, but the client can walk with difficulty. Which of the following describes the client's condition?
    a. Monoplegia
    b. Paraplegia
    c. Quadriplegia
    d. Hemiplegia

16. A client fell and sustained a blow to the head. The client was a bit confused at the time and the next day had a headache. Which of the following is the most accurate description of the client's condition?
    a. Aneurysm
    b. Contusion
    c. Transient ischemic attack
    d. Concussion

17. A medication that would stimulate epinephrine also could cause _____.
    a. Enhanced sleep
    b. Weakening of skeletal muscles
    c. An increase in serotonin
    d. An increase in dopamine

Exercise

Using the previous questions as examples, write at least three more questions. Develop plausible wrong answers and be sure that the correct answer is clearly correct. Then write a rationale for each question. The more questions you write, the better you will understand the material.

PERIPHERAL NERVOUS SYSTEM

Review Tips

Massage interacts extensively with the peripheral nervous system by introducing various stimuli that target sensory receptors. How these stimuli are introduced and how the body processes them through feedback mechanisms lead to many of the benefits of massage. For this reason, the content on the peripheral nervous system may appear in questions that are about massage benefits or that describe how massage methods are applied. Questions are often of the concept identification type.

Terminology is important as always. An effective study approach, in addition to reading glossaries and looking up the definitions of terms, is to list each of the massage methods and techniques and then describe how they are used to influence the peripheral nervous system.

Review the content in your textbook and Appendix A that lists pathologic conditions related to the body system and associated indications and contraindications for massage. Massage examinations tend to target safe practice content. As a result, the appropriateness of massage for various pathologic conditions is emphasized.

Quick Content Review

Understanding how the peripheral nervous system works specifically influences the massage practitioner's ability to plan and conduct an effective massage session. The massage applications and outcomes that the client experiences from the massage session depend on the practitioner's knowledge of the physiologic effects of massage methods. Having an understanding of the normal function and pathology of the peripheral nervous system helps the massage professional make appropriate decisions regarding indications and contraindications for massage.

- The peripheral nervous system consists of neurons outside the central nervous system. The afferent (sensory) division consists of nerves that link sensory receptors with the CNS. The efferent, or motor, division consists of nerves that link the CNS to effectors outside the CNS. The somatic nervous system is made up of nerves that keep the body in balance with its external environment by transmitting impulses between the CNS and the skeletal muscles and skin.

- The ANS connects the CNS to the glands, heart, and smooth muscles to maintain the internal body environment. The sympathetic nervous system functions when the body is under stress by producing fight-flight-freeze responses. The parasympathetic nervous system functions under normal body conditions and is the energy conservation and restorative system associated with what commonly is called the relaxation response.

- A nerve is a group of peripheral nerve fibers, or axons, wrapped together. Twelve pairs of cranial nerves originate from the olfactory bulbs, thalamus, visual cortex, and brainstem. Thirty-one pairs of spinal nerves originate in the spinal cord and emerge from the vertebral column. Mixed nerves contain both sensory and motor nerves.

- A plexus is a network of intertwining nerves that innervates a particular region of the body. The four nerve plexuses are the cervical plexus, the brachial plexus, the lumbar plexus, and the sacral plexus.

- A dermatome is a cutaneous (skin) part supplied by a single spinal nerve. A myotome is a skeletal muscle or group of muscles that receives motor axons from a given spinal nerve.

- Mechanical receptors are sensory receptors that detect changes in pressure, movement, or temperature or other mechanical forces. Thermal receptors are sensory receptors that detect changes in temperature. Nociceptors are sensory receptors that detect noxious stimuli. Proprioceptors are sensory receptors that provide the body with information about position, movement, muscle tension, joint activity, and equilibrium.

- A reflex in the physiologic or functional unit of nerve function is an involuntary action. The stretch reflex results when stretching of a muscle elicits a protective contraction of that same muscle. The tendon reflex operates as a feedback mechanism to control muscle tension by causing muscle relaxation. The flexor (withdrawal) and crossed extensor reflexes are polysynaptic reflex arcs. When these reflexes are stimulated, an entire area on one side of the body (withdrawal reflex) or specific areas on both sides of the body (crossed extensor reflex) are affected.

- Cranial nerves and the general function of each are listed here:
    1. Cranial nerve I: The olfactory nerves are sensory and transmit taste and smell information directly to the cerebrum.
    2. Cranial nerve II: The optic nerves are sensory and transmit visual information (e.g., visual acuity, pupillary reaction, visual fields) to the thalamus.
    3. Cranial nerve III: The oculomotor nerves are sensory and motor nerves; they originate in the midbrain and transmit information about eye movement.
    4. Cranial nerve IV: The trochlear nerves arise in the midbrain and are composed primarily of motor nerves that contain few sensory neurons. These nerves innervate the muscles of the eyeball.
    5. Cranial nerve V: The trigeminal nerves arise in the pons and contain sensory neurons for the head, face, skin of the face, and corneas; they also contain motor neurons for mastication (chewing).
    6. Cranial nerve VI: The abducens nerves arise in the pons and contain numerous motor neurons that innervate eye muscles; they also consist of sensory neurons that provide information about eye movement.
    7. Cranial nerve VII: The facial nerves arise in the pons and contain sensory neurons for taste and motor neurons for facial expression, tear production, and salivation.
    8. Cranial nerve VIII: The vestibulocochlear (acoustic or auditory) nerves arise in the pons and are sensory nerves for hearing and equilibrium.
    9. Cranial nerve IX: The glossopharyngeal nerves arise in the medulla; they contain sensory neurons for taste and motor neurons for saliva production, swallowing, and the gag reflex.
    10. Cranial nerve X: The vagus nerves arise in the medulla, with some motor axons originating in the pons. They contain sensory neurons for the pharynx, larynx, trachea, heart, carotid body, lungs, bronchi, esophagus, stomach, small intestine, and gallbladder. Motor neurons carry impulses to the pharyngeal and laryngeal muscles, where they control swallowing and thoracic and abdominal viscera; they also carry impulses to the heart and other body organs, where they control the heart rate and other visceral activities. Most motor fibers of the vagus nerves are autonomic (parasympathetic) fibers.
    11. Cranial nerve XI: The accessory nerves arise in the medulla and contain mainly motor neurons for speaking, turning the head, and moving the shoulders (they supply the larynx, pharynx, trapezius muscles, and sternocleidomastoid muscles).
    12. Cranial nerve XII: The hypoglossal nerves arise in the medulla and contain mostly motor neurons, which innervate the tongue and throat.

- Each spinal nerve attaches to the spinal cord by means of two short roots. The dorsal root is sensory, and the ventral root is motor.

- The four nerve plexuses are the cervical plexus, brachial plexus, lumbar plexus, and sacral plexus; nerves T2 through T12 do not form a plexus.

- The two divisions of the ANS are sympathetic and parasympathetic.

1. Sympathetic stimulation: Neurotransmitter is usually norepinephrine; adrenergic.

2. Parasympathetic stimulation: Neurotransmitter is acetylcholine; cholinergic.

Cardiovascular System

- Cardiac muscle
  1. Sympathetic: Increased rate and strength of contraction (beta-receptors)
  2. Parasympathetic: Decreased rate and strength of contraction
- Smooth muscle of blood vessels
  1. Sympathetic: Skin blood vessels—constriction (alpha-receptors)
  2. Parasympathetic: No effect
- Skeletal muscle of blood vessels
  1. Sympathetic: Dilation (beta-receptors)
  2. Parasympathetic: No effect
- Abdominal blood vessels
  1. Sympathetic: Constriction (alpha-receptors)
  2. Parasympathetic: No effect
- Blood vessels of external genitals
  1. Sympathetic: Constriction (alpha-receptors)
  2. Parasympathetic: Dilation of blood vessels, causing erectile tissues to engorge

Smooth Muscle of Hollow Organs and Sphincters

- Bronchioles
  1. Sympathetic: Dilation (beta-receptors)
  2. Parasympathetic: Constriction
- Digestive tract (except sphincters)
  1. Sympathetic: Decreased peristalsis (beta-receptors)
  2. Parasympathetic: Increased peristalsis
- Sphincters of digestive tract
  1. Sympathetic: Constriction (alpha-receptors)
  2. Parasympathetic: Relaxation
- Urinary bladder
  1. Sympathetic: Relaxation (beta-receptors)
  2. Parasympathetic: Contraction
- Urinary sphincters
  1. Sympathetic: Constriction (alpha-receptors)
  2. Parasympathetic: Relaxation

Eye

- Iris
  1. Sympathetic: Contraction of radial muscle; dilated pupil
  2. Parasympathetic: Contraction of circular muscle; constricted pupil
- Ciliary body
  1. Sympathetic: Relaxation; accommodates for far vision
  2. Parasympathetic: Contraction; accommodates for near vision

Glands

- Sweat glands
  1. Sympathetic: Increased sweat (neurotransmitter: acetylcholine)
  2. Parasympathetic: No effect
- Lacrimal glands
  1. Sympathetic: No effect
  2. Parasympathetic: Increased secretion of tears

- Digestive (e.g., salivary, gastric)
  1. Sympathetic: Decreased secretion of saliva and gastric secretions
  2. Parasympathetic: Increased secretion of saliva
- Pancreas (including islets)
  1. Sympathetic: Decreased secretion
  2. Parasympathetic: Increased secretion of pancreatic juice and insulin
- Liver
  1. Sympathetic: Increased glycogenolysis (conversion of glycogen to glucose) (beta-receptors); increased blood sugar level
  2. Parasympathetic: No effect
- Adrenal medulla
  1. Sympathetic: Increased epinephrine secretion
  2. Parasympathetic: No effect
- Hairs (pilomotor muscles)
  1. Sympathetic: Contraction produces goose pimples, or piloerection (alpha-receptors)
  2. Parasympathetic: No effect
- A third division of the autonomic system is described as the enteric division that controls the visceral functions of the gastrointestinal tract.

The Five Basic Senses

- *Taste:* The four primary taste sensations are sweet, sour, salty, and bitter. Most chemical receptors for the sense of taste are located on the tongue; a few are located in the cheeks and on the floor of the mouth.
- *Smell:* Also called olfaction, this sense relies on chemical receptors located in the roof of the nasal cavity. Smell centers are interconnected with the limbic system and therefore have emotional and behavioral implications.
- *Hearing:* The ear is a complex of three structures, all of which are necessary for the process of hearing.
- *Vision:* The eyes, the organs of vision, are contained within protective bony cavities of the skull called orbits. The eye perceives light in the form of colors ranging from violet to red. Six small muscles attached to each eye affect movement.
- Two other important sense processes are the vestibular sense and the proprioceptive sense.
- The vestibular sense creates awareness of oneself and one's position in the environment. The vestibular sensors are found within the inner ear and continuously monitor head movements. These sensors then report the head's position and direction of movement to the brain where it is processed and the body is told how to react. Another function of these sensors is to control movement of the eyes to compensate for movement of the head, stabilizing vision.
- The proprioceptive sense is the ability to feel, understand, and visualize the body and the ability to plan body movements and positioning without the use of vision or touch. The proprioceptive sensors are located throughout the body within the joints and muscles and monitor and

send information to the brain related to the stretching and compression of the body, which is translated into an overall understanding of the body's location, forces being applied, directional movement, and speed.

Pathologic Conditions

- Pathologic conditions of the peripheral nervous system include nerve root compression, disk herniation, Bell's palsy, Guillain—Barré syndrome (infectious polyneuritis), herpes zoster (shingles), herpes types 1 and 2, multiple sclerosis, depression, anxiety, entrapment and compression, neuropathy, trigeminal neuralgia (tic douloureux), headache from muscle tension, and vertigo.

Factual Recall Questions

1. Peripheral nerves that innervate the muscles and skin are known as _____.
   a. Visceral
   b. Afferent
   c. Somatic
   d. Thermal
2. A bundle of axons and dendrites that carry sensory or motor signals is called a _____.
   a. Neuron
   b. Nerve
   c. Dermatome
   d. Plexus
3. The connective tissue covering that surrounds the fasciculus is called _____.
   a. Endoneurium
   b. Epineurium
   c. Perineurium
   d. Meninges
4. What cranial nerve affects visceral function?
   a. Vagus nerve
   b. Hypoglossal
   c. Trigeminal
   d. Trochlear
5. The dorsal root ganglion contains cell bodies of _____.
   a. Sensory neurons
   b. Motor neurons
   c. Mixed nerves
   d. Cranial nerves
6. The phrenic nerve is part of which plexus?
   a. Cervical
   b. Brachial
   c. Lumbar
   d. Sacral
7. The obturator nerve is found in which plexus?
   a. Cervical
   b. Brachial
   c. Lumbar
   d. Sacral

8. Changes in blood pressure are monitored by _____.
   a. Exteroceptors
   b. Proprioceptors
   c. Visceroreceptors
   d. Nociceptors
9. Reflexes most often are processed in which part of the central nervous system?
   a. Cerebrum
   b. Ventricles
   c. Dura
   d. Spinal cord
10. Mechanical receptors that provide information about position and movement are called _____.
    a. Reciprocal receptors
    b. Thermal receptors
    c. Proprioceptors
    d. Externoreceptors
11. The portion of the ANS that supports energy conservation is the _____.
    a. Parasympathetic
    b. Central
    c. Somatic
    d. Sympathetic
12. The thoracolumbar division of the ANS contains ganglia located _____.
    a. Near the spine
    b. At the effector organs
    c. In the spinal column
    d. In the cranial and sacral areas
13. The release of epinephrine into the body is called _____.
    a. Parasympathetic dominance
    b. Adrenergic stimulation
    c. Sympathetic inhibition
14. The primary neurotransmitter of the parasympathetic system is _____.
    a. Acetylcholine
    b. Epinephrine
    c. Norepinephrine
    d. Adrenaline
15. The bones in the ear that respond to vibration of the tympanic membrane are called _____.
    a. Pinnae
    b. Ossicles
    c. Cochleae
    d. Corti
16. When vision records a change in the environment, a signal is sent to which part of the brain?
    a. Frontal lobe
    b. Cerebellum
    c. Ventricles
    d. Sulcus
17. Righting reflexes combine information from vision and the vestibular mechanisms to maintain _____.
    a. Baroreceptors

b. Equilibrium
c. Sclera
d. Vertigo

18. Which of the following senses exerts the strongest influence on the emotional limbic system?
    a. Smell
    b. Taste
    c. Hearing
    d. Sight

19. Which of the following is a structure of the nose?
    a. Ciliary body
    b. Canthus
    c. Turbinate
    d. Sclera

20. Which of the following best respond to massage methods that move the joints?
    a. Free nerve endings
    b. Dermatomes
    c. Thermal receptors
    d. Proprioceptors

21. Which of the following are viral diseases of the nervous system?
    a. Herpes and vertigo
    b. Polio and neuralgia
    c. Entrapment and herpes
    d. Herpes and polio

Application/Concept Identification and Clinical Reasoning/Synthesis Questions

1. A client is experiencing radiating pain in the abdomen and buttocks. Which of the following statements is most correct?
   a. Client has impingement of the femoral nerve in the sacral plexus.
   b. Client has compression of the thoracodorsal nerve.
   c. Client's symptoms involve the lumbar plexus.
   d. Client's symptoms involve the brachial plexus.

2. During assessment, the massage therapist notices that the client has dilated pupils. The most logical cause of this condition is that the client _____.
   a. Is experiencing sympathetic dominance
   b. Is experiencing parasympathetic dominance
   c. Has a somatic dysfunction

3. A client is sensitive to scents and can get anxious if the smell of something is unpleasant. This reaction is explained by the fact that sense of smell _____.
   a. Is controlled by the vagus nerve
   b. Is an aspect of the limbic system
   c. Affects the vestibular process

4. If a client complains of pain in the skin areas of the buttocks and into the lateral side of the leg, which plexus is a potential site of nerve impingement?
   a. Cervical
   b. Brachial
   c. Lumbar
   d. Sacral

5. Pain, tingling, and numbness in the arm and hand may result from nerve damage in which plexus?
   a. Cervical
   b. Brachial
   c. Lumbar
   d. Sacral

6. During massage, pain that is unrelated to specific symptoms radiates around the ear. This indicates excessive pressure on which nerve?
   a. Great auricular
   b. Thoracodorsal
   c. Medial cutaneous

7. A client complains of discomfort in the region of the low back and buttocks. Which dermatome nerve distribution might indicate where the nerve impingement is located?
   a. C7
   b. T2
   c. C6
   d. L2

8. During the history interview, a client reports that they almost fell down the stairs but was able to regain balance. What type of reflex action was required to accomplish this?
   a. Monosynaptic
   b. Polysynaptic
   c. Patellar
   d. Withdrawal

9. A client is having difficulty being comfortable with the touch of draping material during the massage. The client may be displaying a reduced ability of sensory receptors to _____.
   a. Send impulses
   b. Adapt to sensation
   c. Remain monosynaptic

10. The sensory receptors most affected by deep compression and slow gliding strokes are _____.
    a. Pacinian corpuscles
    b. Root hair plexuses
    c. Merkel disks
    d. Ruffini end organs

11. Which of the following receptors is most likely to adapt and cease responding to sustained compression during massage on one specific area of the body?
    a. Meissner corpuscles
    b. Free nerve endings
    c. Intrafusal fibers
    d. Nociceptors

12. A compressive massage method is applied to the belly of a muscle with the intent of reducing a muscle spasm brought on by a cramp. The receptors most affected are _____.
    a. Joint kinesthetic
    b. Golgi tendon organ
    c. Muscle spindles
    d. Meissner corpuscles

13. As slow, deep gliding is applied to the left upper thigh, the practitioner notices twitching of the muscles in the

back of the opposite leg. What type of reflex has been stimulated?
a. Stretch
b. Tendon
c. Ipsilateral
d. Contralateral

14. A client requests an outcome from the massage session that includes a good night's sleep and less fidgeting. The massage session would need to be designed to accomplish what?
a. Cranial sacral dominance
b. Parasympathetic inhibition
c. Sympathetic inhibition

15. The massage method that most affects the inner ear balance mechanisms is _____.
a. Tapotement
b. Compression
c. Friction
d. Rocking

16. A client indicates in the history interview of being prone to motion sickness. Which massage methods should the therapist avoid?
a. Active joint movement
b. Stretching
c. Rocking

17. A client is complaining of difficulty hitting a golf ball and describes a sense that their timing is off. This could occur as the result of a disruption in what type of reflex?
a. Conditioned reflex
b. Tendon reflex
c. Stretch reflex

18. A client reports that in the past few weeks they have been prone to headaches when in bright light. The client also reports an increase in workload. What function of the ANS might be responsible for the client's sensitivity to light?
a. Parasympathetic dilation of the pupil
b. Sympathetic dilation of the pupil
c. Parasympathetic contraction of the pupil
d. Sympathetic contraction of the pupil

19. A client complains of radiating pain down the arm into the elbow and fingers. The client has not been evaluated by a physician, so a referral is indicated. Which diagnosis by the physician would be most helped by massage?
a. Guillain–Barré syndrome
b. Brachial plexus entrapment
c. Cervical plexus compression
d. Osteoporosis and osteoarthritis

20. A client reports that they have herpes zoster and is experiencing pain. Which of the following would be the best massage approach?
a. A full-body, 1-hour massage with attention to standard precautions that uses tapotement, active joint movement, and frictioning methods
b. A full-body massage lasting 1½ hours that avoids the area of the rash and actively engages the client in muscle energy lengthening and stretching

c. A seated massage that lasts 15 minutes
d. A full-body, 1-hour massage that avoids the area of the rash with attention to universal precautions and a focus on relaxation

21. A client seeks massage after receiving a diagnosis of neuralgia in the left leg. Which of the following would be a realistic therapeutic massage outcome?
a. Reduction of pain and regeneration
b. Long-term symptom decrease
c. Short-term pain management

22. A client is complaining of a recent inability to sleep and a feeling of agitation, and reports concern over a change in management systems at work. The physician's diagnosis was exogenous anxiety. Which of the following treatment plans is most appropriate?
a. Mild exercise program, therapeutic massage, and a medication such as imipramine to control symptoms
b. A hypoventilation syndrome management program, including massage and chiropractic manipulation
c. A mild exercise program, cognitive behavioral therapy, short-term use of diazepam, and relaxation massage
d. Therapeutic massage, meditation, increase in caffeine consumption, and bed rest

Exercise

Using the previous questions as examples, write at least three more questions. Develop plausible wrong answers and be sure that the correct answer is clearly correct. Then write a rationale for each question. The more questions you write, the better you will understand the material.

ENDOCRINE SYSTEM

Review Tips

The content on the endocrine system discusses the control mechanisms of the body. This material lends itself to the case study type of question because hormones influence how people behave. As always, there are terms that you should memorize and be able to use correctly, or you will not be able to interpret the questions or identify the correct answer.

Review the content in your textbook that lists pathologic conditions related to the body system and indications and contraindications for massage. Massage examinations tend to target safe practice content. As a result, the appropriateness of massage for various pathologic conditions is emphasized.

Quick Content Review

- The traditional endocrine glands are the pituitary, thyroid, parathyroid, adrenal, pineal, and thymus; also included are the pancreas, ovaries, testes, and hypothalamus. Many other organs and tissues in the body also have the ability to secrete hormones.

- Hormones mobilize the defenses of the body against stressors; maintain electrolytes, water, and nutrient balance in the blood; and regulate cellular metabolism and energy balance. They direct the creation of the form, especially during reproduction, growth, and development.
- The main difference between hormones and neurotransmitters is location. When they are found in the bloodstream or in a tissue, they are called hormones. When found in the synapses, they are referred to as neurotransmitters.
- The endocrine system may seem removed from the therapeutic application of massage, but massage powerfully interacts with the endocrine system, a major system of control.
- Endocrine functions coordinate most body functions with the nervous system.
- The main differences between endocrine system and nervous system control are speed and duration of effect. The nervous system is fast acting with a short duration of effect, whereas the endocrine system is slow acting with a long duration of effect.
- The concentration of a hormone in the blood is determined by its rate of release and speed of inactivation and removal from the body. The term *half-life* describes the time required for half of the hormone to be eliminated from the bloodstream.
- Hormones are secreted by endocrine glands and other specialized cells into the bloodstream to bind to specific receptors on or in their target cells. In a lock-and-key mechanism, hormones bind only to receptor molecules that fit them exactly.
- The hypothalamus is the link between the body/mind and nerve/endocrine function. During stress, it translates nerve impulses into hormone secretions by endocrine glands. The pituitary, or hypophysis, is located in the head at about eye level. It sits in a recessed area in the sphenoid bone and secretes hormones that regulate growth, fluid balance, lactation, and childbirth.
- The thyroid gland lies on the trachea below the thyroid cartilage. It consists of a right and a left lobe connected by a bridge (isthmus), resulting in a butterfly shape. It regulates metabolism in the body by maintaining an adequate amount of oxygen consumption at the cellular level.
- The parathyroid glands are made up of four round, pea-sized bodies located on the posterior surface of the thyroid lobes. Their hormone, parathormone, when combined with vitamin D, decreases the amount of calcium excreted, causes the release of calcium from bone, and absorbs more calcium from the gastrointestinal tract, resulting in increased blood levels of calcium and phosphorus.
- The pancreas is a long, slender gland located behind the stomach. It is both an exocrine and an endocrine gland.
- The two adrenal glands are located on top of each kidney. Each gland consists of an outer layer called the cortex and an inner portion called the medulla.

- The testes and the ovaries are the male and female gonads. They are located in the pelvic cavity and produce sex hormones identical to those of the adrenal cortex.
- The pineal gland, a tiny gland inside the brain within the diencephalon, is surrounded by pia mater. The complete functions of this gland have not been identified. Serotonin, norepinephrine, dopamine, histamine, and other neurotransmitters and hormones have been identified from this gland, but its major function seems to be to secrete melatonin. The gland is light sensitive and is involved in regulating the rhythmic patterns of the body.
- The thymus gland is located deep to the sternum and mediastinum of the thorax and between the lungs at the level of the fourth and fifth thoracic vertebrae. Often considered part of the lymphatic system and identified as the master gland of the immune system, it does have endocrine secretions.
- Pathology of the endocrine system involves hypersecretion and hyposecretion of hormones. Hypersecretion, the release of too much hormone, often is caused by tumors, immune system dysfunction (autoimmunity), and failure of feedback mechanisms to regulate secretion. Many factors can cause a gland to reduce its hormonal output. Hyposecretion may be caused by tumors, tissue death, or abnormal operation of the regulatory feedback loops. Abnormal immune function also can reduce hormonal output, as well as insensitivity of the target cells to tropic hormones.

Factual Recall Questions

1. Which of the following most accurately describes hormones?
   a. Secreted from exocrine glands
   b. Found in the synapse
   c. Transported in the blood
2. A primary action of hormones is _____.
   a. Increasing or decreasing cellular processes
   b. Supporting positive feedback control of homeostasis
   c. Inhibiting synaptic uptake of neurotransmitters
3. Hypersecretion refers to what effect on endocrine secretion?
   a. Normal decrease
   b. Abnormal decrease
   c. Normal increase
   d. Abnormal increase
4. Which of the following translates nerve impulses into hormone secretions by endocrine glands?
   a. Limbic system
   b. Pituitary gland
   c. Hypothalamus
   d. Adrenal glands
5. The pituitary gland is a primary source of which type of hormone?
   a. Tropic
   b. Melatonin

c. Adrenergic

d. Pitocin

6. Which of the following hormones extends the fight-or-flight response produced by the sympathetic ANS?

a. Epinephrine

b. Amylin

c. Aldosterone

7. What two endocrine glands secrete androgens?

a. Adrenal glands and pituitary

b. Ovaries and thyroid

c. Pineal and adrenal glands

d. Testes and adrenal glands

8. Which of the following endocrine glands is most sensitive to light and dark cycles?

a. Adrenal

b. Parathyroid

c. Pineal

d. Thymus

9. Which of the following is the most common tissue hormone?

a. Prostaglandin

b. Cholecystokinin

c. Atrial natriuretic factor

Application/Concept Identification and Clinical Reasoning/Synthesis Questions

1. Which of the following best explains the massage influence on the endocrine system?

a. Stimulation of mechanoreceptors

b. Decrease in lymphatic stagnation

c. Influence on autonomic nervous system

d. Direct release of hormones

2. An elderly client has been more alert and has gained a bit of weight since receiving massage. Which of the following is the most logical explanation?

a. Massage stimulates the hypothalamus.

b. Excessive pituitary function is inhibited.

c. The pancreas increases insulin output.

d. Thyroid function increases melatonin production.

3. A client complains of dry skin, joint pain, and edema. Which of the following endocrine functions should the client have checked by a physician?

a. Glucagons

b. Androgen

c. Thymosin

d. Thyroid

4. A client has a chronic inflammatory condition that is helped somewhat by aspirin. Why is this the case?

a. Prostaglandins, which are tissue hormones, are involved.

b. Progesterone, which is an androgen, needs to be inhibited.

c. Pituitary hormones are overactive.

5. A client is experiencing lingering anxiety from a minor auto accident 4 hours ago. What difference between the nervous system and the endocrine system would explain this condition?

a. The nervous system is short acting and the endocrine system is long acting.

b. The endocrine system is short acting and the nervous system is long acting.

c. The nervous system transports hormones more consistently through blood and tissues.

d. Endocrine system neurotransmitters have a long duration of effect, and hormones are short acting.

6. Which of the following anterior pituitary hormones can be influenced positively by cold hydrotherapy applications?

a. Melanocyte-stimulating hormone

b. Follicle-stimulating hormone

c. Thyroid-stimulating hormone

7. Which of the following statements is most accurate about type 2 diabetes?

a. A disruption of insulin production occurs in the islet cells of the pituitary gland.

b. Insulin is a powerful diuretic, so increased edema is a warning sign of diabetic coma.

c. Insulin is released when levels of blood sugar, amino acids, and fatty acids rise.

d. Glucagon facilitates the ability of insulin to transport glucose across the cell membrane.

8. Which hormone most supports the resistance phase of Selye's general adaptation response?

a. Progesterone

b. Cortisol

c. Noradrenaline

d. Melatonin

9. Prolonged effects of lingering, unresolved stress can predispose a person to type 2 diabetes because _____.

a. Cortisol supports a rise in blood levels of glucose, fatty acids, and amino acids

b. Glucocorticoids reduce the activity of aldosterone, causing a predisposition to ketoacidosis

c. Catecholamines inhibit the sympathetic dominance pattern, resulting in excessive parasympathetic control over digestive processes

d. Stress shuts down the production of adrenal cortex hormones, putting additional strain on the pancreas for glucose production

10. A female client is experiencing some increase in coarse facial hair and acne. Which of the following hormones may be involved?

a. Androgen

b. Estrogen

c. Progesterone

d. Endorphin

11. An elderly client with a history of slow tissue healing and gradual weight loss begins to stabilize weight and exhibit enhanced healing of skin abrasions after receiving a weekly massage for 3 months. The most likely explanation for this outcome is that massage _____.

a. Influences positive feedback mechanisms to decrease adrenal output
b. Supports hypothalamic release of growth hormone—releasing hormone
c. Changes sleep patterns to increase dopamine influence

12. A 38-year-old client describes symptoms of constipation, increased edema, sensitivity to cold, muscle and joint pain, and hair loss. The client indicates that life stress has increased and is tired and seems unable to cope as effectively as before. On the basis of these symptoms, which condition might suggest the need for referral?
a. Exophthalmos
b. Hypothyroidism
c. Hyperthyroidism
d. Hypocalcemic tetany

13. A client who is a marathon runner developed an inflammatory condition of the knee. As part of the treatment process, the client received an injection of corticosteroid into the area of the knee. The client wishes to have a deep massage in the area to reduce pain. Why is this inappropriate?
a. The massage could decrease the inflammatory response and concentrate medication at the injection site.
b. Deep massage increases the potential for localized inflammation and would disturb the action of the medication.
c. Deep massage would increase the tension of the muscles, causing instability, and inflammation would decrease.
d. Because massage increases the tendency toward tissue repair, excessive scarring could result.

14. A client has just experienced a job shift change from days to nights and is having difficulty adjusting to the sleep pattern. Which endocrine gland initially might be affected, and which treatment approach would be most beneficial?
a. Pineal gland; a massage that focuses on sympathetic stimulation with active participation by the client
b. Adrenal glands; a massage that generates localized inflammatory areas, as is performed with direct pressure and friction on trigger points
c. Thymus gland; a massage that uses sufficient pressure but pain-free compression and rhythmic gliding methods to support parasympathetic dominance
d. Pineal gland; a massage that uses sufficient pressure but pain-free compression and rhythmic gliding methods to support parasympathetic dominance

15. By supporting restorative sleep, on which of the following does massage have the most direct effect?
a. Antidiuretic hormone
b. Cortisol
c. Luteinizing hormone
d. Oxytocin

Exercise

Using the previous questions as examples, write at least three more questions. Develop plausible wrong answers and be sure that the correct answer is clearly correct. Then write a rationale for each question. The more questions you write, the better you will understand the material.

SKELETAL SYSTEM

Review Tips

This content focuses on the general structure of the skeletal system and the specific anatomy of the bones of the body. The information will appear in questions that target joints, muscles, biomechanics, assessment, and various injuries and pathologic conditions. Use the study tools in this text and the flashcards. Questions that specifically target this content include factual recall and the case study type of question about injury or disease.

The various activities review and integrate data, so the names, shapes, and functions of bones are familiar. Information about the skeleton is important for studying the way the body moves. A strong foundation that consists of the names of bones and the locations of bony landmarks will make studying the joints and muscles much easier.

Quick Content Review

- The seven main functions of the skeletal system are as follows:
  1. Supports soft tissues and serves as a framework for the entire body
  2. Provides attachment points for muscles and ligaments
  3. Protects delicate internal organs such as the brain, spinal cord, heart, and lungs
  4. Works as levers to provide movement initiated by the attached muscles
  5. Stores calcium, phosphorus, and other minerals for release to the body as needed
  6. Stores lipids in bone marrow for use as energy
  7. Serves as the production site for blood cells (hematopoiesis) in the red marrow
- Bones are hard, dense, and slightly elastic organs of the skeleton. They have their own system of blood, lymphatic vessels, and nerves. Bones are composed chiefly of bone tissue, called osseous tissue. Two-thirds of bone tissue are composed of inorganic mineral, which gives rigidity, and one-third is composed of organic components, which provide elasticity. Bones have a piezoelectric quality. The structure and function of bones are connected intrinsically. Bones remodel themselves constantly, depending on functional demand.

- The process that creates the skeleton is called ossification. Ossification is a two-part process: chondroblasts, or cartilage-forming cells, create the cartilage model of bones. Bone-building cells, called osteoblasts, develop bone tissue from the cartilage model. Shortly after birth, calcification takes place. This hardening of the bones, called osteogenesis, occurs as calcium salts are deposited in the gel-like matrix of forming bones. Osteocytes are mature bone cells that maintain the bone throughout the lifetime.
- Compact (dense) bone has little space between its tissues. This hard portion of the bone makes up the main shaft of the long bones and the outer layer of other bones. The osteocytes in this type of bone are located in concentric rings around a central haversian canal, through which nerves and blood vessels pass.
- Spongy (cancellous) bone has larger spaces between cells than compact bone, which makes cancellous bones lighter. This type of bone consists of an irregular meshing of small, bony plates, called trabeculae, and is found at the ends of the long bones or at the center of other bones. In some bones, the trabecular spaces are filled with red marrow, which produces blood cells. Bones contain red marrow and yellow marrow.
- Except for the ends that form joints, bones are covered with a thin membrane of connective tissue, called periosteum. A thinner membrane, the endosteum, lines the marrow cavity of a bone; it too contains cells that aid in the growth and repair of bone tissue. Bones of a synovial or movable joint make physical contact at their cartilaginous ends, which is called articular (or hyaline) cartilage.
- The six shapes of bones are as follows:
  1. Flat bones: Generally these bones are more flat than round. Examples are the ribs and skull bones.
  2. Irregular bones: These bones have two or more complex shapes within the same bone structure. Examples are the vertebrae and scapula.
  3. Long bones: Longer in one axis than another, these bones are characterized by a medullary cavity, a hollow diaphysis (shaft) of compact bone, and at least two epiphyses, which are active in the growth of long bones. Most of the bones of the arms and legs are long bones; the hollow structure of the diaphysis offers the advantages of strength and a lightweight. Examples are the femur and ulna.
  4. Short bones: Shaped like long bones but much smaller, these bones make up the structures of the hands and fingers and the feet and toes. This shape of bone also can be classified as a long bone. An example is the metacarpals.
  5. Cube-shaped bones (sometimes classified as short bones): These bones are predominantly cancellous, with a thin cortex of compact bone and no cavity. Examples are the wrist and ankle bones.
  6. Sesamoid bones: Round bones that often are embedded in tendons and joint capsules. An example is the patella.

Bony Landmarks

Depressions and Openings

- Canal: A tunnel or tube in bone. An example is the carotid canal in the temporal bone.
- Fissure: A groove or slit between two bones. An example is the orbital fissure of the sphenoid bone.
- Foramen: An opening in a bone. An example is the vertebral foramen of the spinal column, through which the nerves pass.
- Fossa: A shallow depression in the surface or at the end of a bone. Examples are the infraspinous and supraspinous fossae of the scapula.
- Groove: A depression in the bone that holds blood vessels, nerves, or tendons. Examples are the radial groove of the humerus.
- Meatus: A tunnel or canal found in a bone. An example is the canal in the skull from the external ear to the eardrum.
- Notch: An indentation or large groove. Examples are the greater and lesser sciatic notches of the ilium.
- Sinus: Air cavity within a bone. Examples are the frontal sinuses.

Processes That Form Joints

- Condyle: A rounded projection at the end of a bone that articulates with other bones to form a joint. An example is the medial condyle of the femur.
- Head: A rounded projection found on top of the neck of a bone. An example is the head of the femur.
- Facet: A smooth, flat surface. An example is the facet of a rib or vertebra.
- Process: Any prominent, bony growth that projects. An example is the olecranon process of the ulna.
- Trochlea: A pulley-shaped structure. An example is the trochlea of the humerus.

Processes to Which Tendons and Ligaments Attach

- Crest: A ridge on a bone. An example is the iliac crest.
- Epicondyle: A projection above a condyle. An example is the medial epicondyle of the femur.
- Line: A ridge that is smaller than a crest. An example is the linea aspera of the femur.
- Spinous process, spine, or spina: A sharp, bony, or slender projection. An example is the spinous process of the vertebral column or scapular spine.
- Trochanter: One of two large, bony processes found only on the femur. An example is the greater or lesser trochanter.
- Tubercle: A small, rounded process. An example is the adductor tubercle of the femur.
- Tuberosity: A large, rounded protuberance. An example is tibial tuberosity.
- The two divisions of the skeleton are the axial skeleton and the appendicular skeleton:
  1. The axial skeleton, which forms the axis of the body, consists of the head, vertebral column (spine), and ribs and sternum and provides the body with form and protection. The shoulder and hip girdles, which

have similar structures, are the connectors to the axial skeleton.

2. The appendicular skeleton is composed of the limbs of the body and their attachments. The long bones of the upper and lower limbs, in combination with the muscles, provide fine and gross motor movements. Similar in design, these long bones are the humerus, radius, ulna, and the femur, tibia, fibula. In the same manner, the short carpals of the wrist and the tarsals of the ankle provide the flexibility needed in the hands and feet.

- The endosteum is a thin membrane of connective tissue that lines the marrow cavity of a bone. An endoskeleton is found inside the human body; it accommodates growth.
- The periosteum is a thin membrane of connective tissue that covers bones except at the articulations. The piezoelectric quality of bones allows them to deform slightly and vibrate when electrical currents pass through them.
- Sesamoid bones are round bones that often are embedded in tendons and joint capsules. The largest of these is the patella.
- Spongy bone is also known as cancellous bone.
- Trabeculae represent an irregular meshing of small, bony plates that make up spongy bone. The spaces are filled with red marrow.
- A bone fracture is treated by reduction, which means that the broken ends are pulled into alignment. In general, acute fracture healing has five stages: hematoma formation, cellular proliferation, callous formation, ossification, and remodeling. A hematoma accumulates in the medullary canal and surrounds soft tissue in the first 48—72 hours.

Factual Recall Questions

1. Which of the following is *not* a function of bone?
   a. Storing minerals
   b. Producing blood cells
   c. Generating heat
   d. Storing lipids
2. A type of bone that develops in a tendon or joint capsule is called _____.
   a. Sesamoid
   b. Flat
   c. Irregular
   d. Compact
3. Which aspect of bone structure provides the elastic quality of bone?
   a. Inorganic mineral
   b. Organic material
   c. Trabeculae
   d. Endoskeleton
4. The main component of bone that has the piezoelectric quality is _____.
   a. Compact bone
   b. Cancellous bone
   c. Red marrow
   d. Collagen

5. The external connective tissue covering of bone is called the _____.
   a. Exoskeleton
   b. Endoskeleton
   c. Periosteum
   d. Endosteum
6. The continual changing of bone in response to functional demands is called _____.
   a. Remodeling
   b. Oppositional growth
   c. Haversian
   d. Articulation
7. Which type of bone contains trabeculae?
   a. Compact
   b. Cancellous
   c. Osteon
8. Which of the following bone types contains a diaphysis?
   a. Flat
   b. Irregular
   c. Long
   d. Sesamoid
9. Which of the following is a depression on a bone?
   a. Condyle
   b. Fossa
   c. Line
10. Which of the following bones is located in the appendicular skeleton?
    a. Ethmoid
    b. Clavicle
    c. Sternum
11. Which suture joins the parietal bones and occipital bone?
    a. Squamous
    b. Coronal
    c. Lambdoidal
    d. Sagittal
12. Which of the following bones forms the structure of the nose?
    a. Vomer
    b. Zygomatic
    c. Sphenoid
13. Which bone has a superior articular facet?
    a. Cervical vertebra
    b. Occipital
    c. Thoracic vertebra
    d. Carpal
14. Which of the following landmarks is located on the humerus?
    a. Glenoid fossa
    b. Xiphoid process
    c. Radial styloid
    d. Olecranon fossa
15. The coracoid process is located on which bone?
    a. Scapula
    b. Sternum
    c. Femur
    d. Talus

16. When the posterior cervical area is palpated, the fibrous structure felt is the _____.
    a. Sacrotuberous ligament
    b. Odontoid process
    c. Nuchal ligament
17. The costal angle is located on which bone?
    a. Sternum
    b. Clavicle
    c. Atlas
    d. Rib
18. The foot typically contains how many bones?
    a. 31
    b. 26
    c. 12
19. Which sequence of terms refers to bony landmarks?
    a. Trabeculae, lacunae, crest
    b. Epicondyle, sulcus, fissure
    c. Periosteum, osteon, trochanter
    d. Sesamoid, axial, meatus
20. Which sequence of terms names axial skeleton bones?
    a. Coccyx, occipital, sternum
    b. Rib, sacrum, tibia
    c. Femur, clavicle, ulna
    d. Vertebra, mandible, ilium
21. Which of the following are bony landmarks of the humerus?
    a. Radial tuberosity and styloid process
    b. Iliac fossa and coracoid process
    c. Olecranon fossa and lesser tubercle
    d. Intercondylar fossa and intertrochanteric line
22. Which of the following is located in the vertebral column?
    a. Manubrium
    b. Lamina
    c. Vertebral border
    d. Scaphoid
23. Which of the following is part of the pelvis?
    a. Fovea
    b. Triquetrum
    c. Trochlear notch
    d. Acetabulum
24. When the area over the vertebral column is palpated, the structure most prominently felt is the _____.
    a. Centrum
    b. Spinous process
    c. Annulus fibrosus
    d. Pedicle

Application/Concept Identification and Clinical Reasoning/Synthesis Questions

1. Which spinal deformity exhibits concavity in the lumbar and convexity in the thorax?
    a. Scoliosis
    b. Scurvy

c. Whiplash
d. Hyperlordosis

2. A client experienced an accident in which the trunk was thrust into extension. Which of the following structures might have been injured?
    a. Deltoid ligament
    b. Anterior longitudinal ligament
    c. Anterior superior iliac spine
    d. Linea aspera
3. A young male client is experiencing a growth spurt and complains that the bones in the legs ache. What is responsible for this long bone growth?
    a. Increased testosterone
    b. Increased estrogen
    c. Decreased estrogen
    d. Decreased testosterone
4. If an intervertebral disk rupture occurs, what is the possible outcome?
    a. Narrowed disk space caused by leakage of the nucleus pulposus
    b. Narrowed intervertebral space due to rupture of the fontanel
    c. Impingement of the nerve from pressure exerted by the sella turcica
    d. Increased space in the foramen as it impinges on the spinal cord
5. A client complains of pain in the lower back. Observation indicates an excessive lumbar curve. This is called _____.
    a. Scoliosis
    b. Hypokyphosis
    c. Hyperlordosis
    d. Spondylosis
6. A female client, age 67, has a history of smoking. This could indicate the need for caution with compressive force used during massage for which reason?
    a. Osteonecrosis
    b. Osteomyelitis
    c. Osteoarthritis
    d. Osteoporosis
7. A client complains of pain in the tibia. The client completed a marathon 24 hours before the massage session began. What contraindication to massage may account for the pain?
    a. Stress fracture
    b. Compound fracture
    c. Dislocation
    d. Whiplash

Exercise

Using the previous questions as examples, write at least three more questions. Develop plausible wrong answers and be sure that the correct answer is clearly correct. Then write a rationale for each question. The more questions you write, the better you will understand the material.

JOINTS

Review Tips

The content on joints is more complex than the study of the skeletal system alone because you must be able to identify the parts as well as the function of each joint. The body includes various types of joints. It is necessary to gain an understanding of specific pathologic conditions related to each joint.

Because so many factors are involved in joint structure and function, it is easy to write many different types of questions that cover this content. The data can be represented in all three question types.

Study strategies include flashcards, labeling activities, examples, and metaphors. Building simple models with clay, wood, hinges, and various types of craft materials or even structural toys, such as Tinker toys or Legos, is another excellent study strategy.

Quick Content Review

An articulation, or joint, is the point at which two or more bones meet to connect parts and allow movement within the body. The main parts of a joint are bones, ligaments, cartilage, and, in synovial joints, a joint capsule. Various types of movements occur at joints in response to muscle contraction. A comprehensive understanding of joint structure and function is necessary for the effective practice of therapeutic massage for the joints. One can use massage methods to support joint health and obtain benefits when managing joint dysfunction.

The health and strength of joint structures depend on a certain amount of stress and strain. Cartilage and bone nutrition and growth depend on joint movement and muscle contraction. Cartilage nutrition depends on joint movement through a full range of motion to ensure that all articular cartilage receives the nutrients necessary for health. Ligaments and tendons depend on a normal amount of stress and strain to maintain and increase strength. Bone density and strength increase as a result of the stress and strain created by muscle and joint activity. In contrast, bone density and strength decrease when stress and strain are absent. Without stress and strain, the joints do not function well, but with too much stress and strain, a pathologic condition may develop.

- Elementary principles of joint design are as follows. Some joints provide stability. Some joints provide mobility. The structure of the joint determines the function of the joint. A breakdown or change in any joint structure affects the entire joint function. The design of a joint depends on its function. Each part of the joint has a specific function that is essential to the whole function of the joint. Complex joints are more likely to malfunction than simple joints. Effective functioning of the whole body depends on the integrated action of many joints. Generally, stability must be achieved before mobility is possible. Most joints serve a dual function of mobility and stability. Simple joints provide more stability. Complex joints provide more mobility.
- The two main types of joints are synarthroses and diarthroses.
- Synarthroses are nonsynovial, limited-movement joints consisting of fibrous joints and cartilaginous joints.
- Diarthroses are synovial, freely movable joints, which consist of the following:
  1. A joint capsule formed of fibrous tissue
  2. Hyaline cartilage that covers the joint surfaces
  3. A joint cavity enclosed by the joint capsule
  4. A synovial membrane that lines the inner surface of the capsule and secretes synovial fluid
  5. Synovial fluid that forms a lubricating film over the joint surfaces
- Types of synovial joints include the following:
  1. Hinge joints allow flexion and extension movements in one direction, changing the angle of bones at the joint, similar to a door hinge.
  2. Pivot joints allow rotation around the length of the bone.
  3. Condyloid (condylar) joints allow movement in two directions, but one motion predominates.
  4. A saddle joint is convex in one plane and concave in the other; these surfaces fit together like a rider on a saddle.
  5. A ball-and-socket joint allows movement in many directions around a central point.
  6. Gliding joints, also known as synovial plane joints, allow only a gliding motion in various planes.
- Synarthrosis is a nonsynovial joint with limited movement.
- A suture is a synarthrotic joint in which two bony components are united by a thin layer of dense fibrous tissue.
- A symphysis is a cartilaginous joint in which two bony components are joined directly by fibrocartilage in the form of a disk or plate.
- A synchondrosis is a joint in which the material used to connect the two components is hyaline growth cartilage.
- Syndesmosis is a fibrous joint in which two bony components are joined directly by a ligament, cord, or aponeurotic membrane.
- Bursae are flat sacs of synovial membrane in which the inner sides of the sacs are separated by a fluid film. Bursae are located where moving structures are apt to rub.
- Arthrokinematics refers to movements of joint surfaces. A roll refers to the rolling of one joint surface on another. Gliding refers to the gliding of one component over another. Spin refers to a rotation of the movable component.
- Osteokinematics refers to the movement of bones rather than the movement of articular surfaces.
- Range of motion is a measurement in degrees from the anatomical position and indicates the functional ability of movement for a particular joint. Active and passive joint movement assess for the range of motion of a joint.
- The three categories of range of motion are anatomic, physiologic, and pathologic. Anatomic range of motion refers to

the amount of motion available to a joint within the anatomic limits of the joint structure. Anatomic range of motion may extend the limits of available range of motion to the point where joint injury can occur. Therefore, many joints have established a physiologic range of motion set by the nervous system from information provided by joint sensory receptors. Usually, this physiologic range of motion is somewhat less than the anatomic range of motion, which prevents a joint from being positioned where injury could occur. Pathologic range of motion occurs when motion at a joint fails to reach the normal physiologic range or exceeds normal anatomic limits of motion. Two main pathologic conditions are hypomobility and hypermobility.

- Hypermobility occurs when the range of motion of a joint is greater than normally would be permitted by the structure. It results in instability.
- Hypomobility occurs when the range of motion of a joint is less than normally would be permitted by the structure. It results in restricted range of motion.
- The joint capsule is a connective tissue structure that indirectly connects the bony components of a joint.
- Joint play is the involuntary movement that occurs between articular surfaces (this has nothing to do with the range of motion of a joint produced by muscle contraction). Joint play is an essential component of joint motion and must occur for the joint to function normally. Optimally, a joint has a sufficient amount of play to allow normal motion of the joint. If the supporting joint structures are lax, the joint may have too much play and may become unstable. If the joint structures are tight, too little movement occurs between articular surfaces, and the amount of motion is restricted. Structures that contribute to joint stability include bone shape, ligaments, joint capsule, fibrocartilaginous rings, tendons, fasciae, and muscles.
- A closed kinematic chain occurs when joints of the human body are linked together into a series in such a way that motion at one of the joints is accompanied by motion at an adjacent joint.
- An open kinematic chain occurs when the ends of the limbs or parts of the body are free to move without causing motion at another joint.
- The close-packed position of a synovial joint is the only position in which the surfaces fit together precisely and maximum contact occurs between opposing surfaces. Because joint surfaces are compressed, they permit no movement, and the joint possesses its greatest stability.
- The least-packed position is the position of a synovial joint at which the joint capsule is most lax. Joints tend to assume this position to accommodate the increased volume of synovial fluid which becomes present when inflammation occurs.
- Collagen is a fibrous tissue that provides stability to connective tissue structures.
- Elastin is a fibrous tissue that has elastic properties and allows flexibility in connective tissue structures.
- Fibrocartilage is a connective tissue that permits little motion in joints and structures. It is found in such places as intervertebral disks, and it forms the ears.

- Hyaline cartilage is the thin covering of articular connective tissue that is found on the ends of bones in freely movable joints in the adult skeleton.
- Pathologic conditions of joints and general treatment protocols used for intervention include the following:
  1. Joint disorders fall into the following categories: injury, immobilization, and repetitive overuse.
  2. Joint injuries usually are classified as dislocations and sprains.
  3. A dislocation is a dislodging of the joint parts.
  4. A sprain is the wrenching of a joint with rupture or tearing of the ligaments.
- Immobilization can be caused by a cast or other form of external restraining mechanism; it may occur as a reaction to pain and inflammation or as the result of paralysis. Detrimental effects of immobilization include development of fibrofatty connective tissue within the joint space; adhesions between the folds of the synovial membrane; atrophy of cartilage; regional osteoporosis; weakening of ligaments at insertion sites; and a decrease in water content of articular cartilage, tendons, ligaments, and the joint capsule. Swelling or immobilization of a joint also inhibits and weakens the muscles surrounding the joint, thereby making the joint unable to function normally and placing it at high risk for additional injury.
- Repetitive overuse results from constant static stress on the joints, as occurs with prolonged standing, sitting, or squatting; it can damage joint structures. Ligaments subjected to constant tensile loads creep and can undergo excessive lengthening.
- Cartilage subjected to constant compressive loading also can creep and may undergo excessive deformation. Joints and their supporting structures, when subjected to repetitive loading, can be injured and may fail because they do not have time to recover their original dimensions before they are subjected to another loading cycle.
- Therapeutic massage is helpful in the management of compensatory patterns that may develop as the result of casting and other forms of immobilization. Although direct work over an area involved in an active healing process is contraindicated, massage and other forms of soft tissue work, coupled with movement therapies, can ease the tension and possible pain that may be felt in the rest of the body as the result of changes in movement, sleeping position, and so forth.
- Rest, rehabilitative exercise, ergonomically correct equipment, and education are used to treat and manage overuse syndromes. Therapeutic massage can both restore and manage some types of connective tissue dysfunction. Movement modalities can be used to balance movement function and to reduce tension patterns.

Factual Recall Questions

1. The most complex joint design is likely to function in _____.

a. Stability
b. Viscoelasticity
c. Mobility

2. Principles and characteristics of joint design include all of the following except _____.
   a. The design of a joint depends on its function
   b. The breakdown of any joint structure will affect the entire joint function
   c. Generally, stability must be achieved before mobility
   d. Most joints serve only one function—stability or mobility

3. What type of cartilage is found in joints that function primarily for mobility?
   a. White fibrocartilage
   b. Hyaline cartilage
   c. Yellow fibrocartilage
   d. Elastic cartilage

4. An important component of connective tissue that supports pliability is _____.
   a. Water
   b. Synovial fluid
   c. Colloid
   d. Viscosity

5. The property of connective tissue that causes it to modify in the direction of the force applied and then slowly return to the original state is called _____.
   a. Plastic range
   b. Fibrous
   c. Creep

6. Which of the following joint types has the most limited mobility?
   a. Syndesmosis
   b. Amphiarthrosis
   c. Cartilaginous
   d. Diarthrosis

7. Which of the following is not a characteristic of a synovial joint?
   a. A joint capsule formed of fibrous tissue
   b. Bones separated by fibrocartilage
   c. Hyaline cartilage covering the joint surfaces

8. Which of the following joint structures is highly innervated and serves as a source of sensory data related to the movement and position of a joint?
   a. Stratum synovium
   b. Articular cartilage
   c. Stratum fibrosum

9. The accessory movements at a joint that describe how articulating surfaces move within the joint capsule and contribute to joint play are called _____.
   a. Close-packed position
   b. Arthrokinematics
   c. Osteokinematics

10. The close-packed position of a joint can be described as the _____.
    a. Convex surface fitting minimally into the concave surface

b. Position in which spin, roll, and slide most easily occur
c. Position with the most joint play
d. Convex surface fitting with maximum contact into the concave surface

11. Which of the following describes a neurologic protective mechanism for normal joint function?
    a. Anatomic range of motion
    b. Physiologic range of motion
    c. Joint play
    d. Osteokinematics

12. In which of the following joints does the least amount of bone structure create the anatomic range of motion limits?
    a. Elbow
    b. Hip
    c. Ankle
    d. Knee

13. Active joint movement is used to assess the range of motion of the foot. Which is the most correct term to use when describing a portion of this activity?
    a. Elevation
    b. Retraction
    c. Eversion

14. The term used to describe the movement of the scapula toward the spine is _____.
    a. Rotation
    b. Retraction
    c. Protraction

15. What type of joint is a ball-and-socket joint considered to be?
    a. Pivot
    b. Biaxial
    c. Gliding
    d. Multiaxial

16. The name for the association between joints as they function in relationship to each other is _____.
    a. Joint play
    b. Osteokinematics
    c. Kinematic chains
    d. Diarthrosis

17. The function of joints that often results in a compensation pattern in one joint when a change in function occurs in another joint is called the _____.
    a. Closed kinematic chain
    b. Open kinematic chain
    c. Loose-packed position
    d. Close-packed position

18. The two articulating bones of the temporomandibular joint are the _____.
    a. Temporal and maxilla
    b. Mandible and maxilla
    c. Mandible and temporal
    d. Temporal and zygomatic

19. The glenohumeral joint exhibits extensive mobility because it has _____.

a. Range-of-motion limits provided primarily by soft tissue

b. Physiologic limits to range of motion provided for a loose fit between the humerus and the clavicle

c. A biaxial joint structure, which allows movement in three planes

d. A ball-and-socket joint structure, which allows movement in only two planes

20. Which movement is allowed at the sternoclavicular joint?
a. Flexion
b. Rotation
c. Inversion
d. Extension

21. The coracoclavicular ligament indirectly assists in stabilizing what joint?
a. Glenohumeral
b. Temporomandibular
c. Sternoclavicular
d. Acromioclavicular

22. Which of the following joints allows for pronation and supination?
a. Humeroulnar
b. Radioulnar
c. Humeroradial
d. Radiocarpal

23. Wrist movement is greatest in flexion and extension because the joint_____.
a. Capsule is loose in superior and inferior directions
b. Type is a hinge joint
c. Capsule is loose laterally and medially

24. The joint at which the fingers join the body of the hand is called the _____.
a. Distal interphalangeal
b. Proximal interphalangeal
c. Metacarpophalangeal
d. Intercarpal

25. The articulating bones of the sacroiliac joint are the sacrum and the _____.
a. Ischium
b. Ilium
c. Acetabulum
d. Pubis

26. Which of the following joints is responsible for helping the vertebral column to remain relatively still during walking?
a. Symphysis pubis
b. Sacral lumbar
c. Labrum
d. Sacroiliac

27. Which fibrocartilaginous structure allows greater surface contact of the femur on the tibia?
a. Cruciate
b. Labrum
c. Patella
d. Meniscus

28. The most stable position of the ankle joint is _____.
a. Plantar flexion
b. Plantar rotation

c. Full dorsiflexion
d. Rotated eversion

29. Which of the following joints allows rotation as a motion pattern?
a. Atlantooccipital
b. Atlantoaxial
c. Intervertebral
d. Costovertebral

30. Which two joints are most active during breathing?
a. Intervertebral and costovertebral
b. Vertebral arch and chondrosternal
c. Costochondral and intervertebral
d. Costovertebral and costochondral

31. The action of the ribs during inspiration is that they are _____.
a. Lowered
b. Raised
c. Protracted

32. Which of the following pairs of joint movements are opposites?
a. Retraction, protraction
b. Plantar flexion, pronation
c. Horizontal adduction, diagonal adduction

Application/Concept Identification and Clinical Reasoning/Synthesis Questions

1. Massage methods that move the body most influence which of the following?
a. Synarthrosis joints
b. Interosseous membranes
c. Synovial joints
d. Interosseous ligaments

2. A client reports that they sprained their knee when hit on the lateral side, resulting in a convex position of the medial collateral ligament. Which of the following stains best describes the injury to this ligament?
a. Shear
b. Compression
c. grade 1
d. Tension

3. Which of the following would describe the movement of the ribs during inspiration?
a. Rotated
b. Depressed
c. Fixed
d. Elevated

4. Joint function results from a relationship between _____.
a. Bones and landmarks
b. Stability and mobility
c. Articulations and diarthroses

5. Joints in which stability is reduced because of increased laxity of supportive ligaments also exhibit an increase in _____.
a. Joint play
b. Hypomobility
c. Muscle relaxation

6. A client sprained a joint in one finger. What is going to be the most comfortable position for this joint, and why?
   a. The close-packed position, because this is the most stable position of the joint
   b. The loose-packed position, so that movement can occur most easily
   c. The least-packed position, to accommodate swelling
   d. The close-packed position, to accommodate increased synovial fluid

7. Which of the following best describes the action used during passive joint movement to assess range of motion of the arm during circumduction?
   a. Bending movement that decreases the angle of a joint
   b. Movement of arm medially toward the midline of the body
   c. Twisting and turning of a bone on its own axis
   d. Combined movements of flexion, extension, abduction, and adduction to create a cone shape

8. During assessment, what instructions should be given to the client to provide the most external rotate the hip?
   a. Please move your leg so that you cross it over the other leg at the ankles.
   b. Please straighten your legs and turn the entire leg so that you point your toes toward each other.
   c. Please straighten your legs and turn the entire leg so that you point your toes away from each other.
   d. Please bring your knee toward your chest.

9. Should an injury occur to the sternoclavicular joint that limits its range of motion, what other structure would be affected?
   a. Radius
   b. Olecranon
   c. Scapula
   d. Deltoid ligament

10. A client continues to sprain the ankles. The massage professional notices that the client wears boots with a 2-inch heel. This contributes to potential injury because the _____.
    a. Heel positions the ankle in dorsiflexion, making the ankle joint less stable.
    b. Heel positions the ankle in plantar flexion, making the ankle joint less stable.
    c. Weight is shifted to the ball of the foot, creating an open kinematic chain.
    d. Inferior tibiofibular joint is extended when the heel is raised, creating instability.

11. Which movement of the vertebral joints is best stabilized by the anterior longitudinal ligament?
    a. Extension
    b. Flexion
    c. Rotation

12. The loose-packed position of the hip joint consists of _____.
    a. Flexion, abduction, and lateral rotation
    b. Extension, adduction, and medial rotation
    c. Flexion, adduction, and lateral rotation
    d. Extension, abduction, and lateral rotation

13. If the leg is fixed and the pelvis moves forward into anteversion, what is the result?
    a. Increased kyphosis
    b. Increased lordosis
    c. Decreased lordosis
    d. Decreased scoliosis

14. The most stable position of the knee joint is in _____.
    a. Slight flexion
    b. Full hyperextension
    c. Locked extension
    d. Locked flexion

15. A client was playing football when tackled. Pressure was put on the lateral side of the left knee. Which ligament would have received the most extensive strain?
    a. Lateral collateral
    b. Medial collateral
    c. Posterior cruciate
    d. Posterior meniscofemoral

16. Which of the following pathologic conditions of the joints responds most positively to massage?
    a. Dislocation
    b. Rheumatoid arthritis
    c. Lateral epicondylitis
    d. Kyphosis

17. A client has been participating in a stretching program for longer than a year. Initially, the program was helpful, but during the past 3 months, the program has become more aggressive, and the client is complaining of joint pain. Which alteration in connective tissue may explain what has occurred?
    a. The client has experienced a rupture in connective tissue structures and has developed lax ligaments.
    b. The client has exceeded the limits of the elastic range of the tissue, consistently deformed the tissue in the plastic range, and developed lax ligaments.
    c. An avulsion failure of connective tissue has occurred, resulting in decreased mobility.
    d. Tissue has become dehydrated, increasing creep tendency and contributing to stability provided by muscle contraction.

18. A client is complaining of a feeling of shortening and pulling in the area of the low back and sacroiliac joints. Assessment indicates decreased pliability in the connective tissue structures in this area. Which of the following massage applications is most appropriate to achieve an increase in short-term mobility without compromising stability or creating a remodeling process of the tissue?
    a. Massage methods that slowly introduce creep, increasing pliability at the plastic range of the tissue
    b. Therapeutic inflammation coupled with stretching to exceed the plastic range of the tissue
    c. Elongation stretching to breach the plastic range of the tissue, creating inflammation to restore an appropriate creep pattern

d. Abrupt bending of the connective tissue to support the increase in ligament laxity, thereby increasing mobility

19. A hypermobile knee joint has been diagnosed. Which of the following would be part of an appropriate treatment plan?
    a. Extend the elastic range of connective tissue structures by altering the plastic range.
    b. Elongate the plastic component of connective tissue in the direction of the shortening.
    c. Restore pliability to the connective tissue texture.
    d. Manage muscle contraction around the joint using standard massage methods.

20. A client is experiencing muscle spasms and reduced mobility around a shoulder joint that has a history of dislocation. Which of the following applications of massage would be best to use in assisting this client?
    a. Increase the plastic range of the ligament structures and the stretched tense muscles.
    b. Use friction on tendons and ligaments, and then incorporate a stretching program to increase flexibility.
    c. Reduce muscle spasms to the point that mobility is supported but stability is not compromised.
    d. Use massage methods and stretching to eliminate muscle spasms.

21. A client has a history of a broken wrist. The wrist was in a cast for an extended period because bone repair was slower than normal. The client now is experiencing a decrease in range of motion of the wrist. What might be the cause?
    a. Hypomobility due to contracture
    b. Hypomobility due to reduced muscle tension
    c. Hypermobility due to increased muscle tension
    d. Hypermobility due to increased anatomic range of motion

22. During the history interview, a client reports experiencing a disk herniation posterior in the low back. Which type of injury and what likely location would be indicated?
    a. Extension injury at the sacrolumbar junction
    b. Flexion injury at T12
    c. Flexion injury at the lumbosacral junction
    d. Extension injury at the thoracolumbar junction

23. A client has received a diagnosis of degenerative joint disease. Conservative treatment measures are indicated. Which of the following treatment plans is most appropriate?
    a. Bed rest with over-the-counter antiinflammatory medication
    b. Cortisone injections and moderate exercise
    c. Ice, regular intense exercise, and connective tissue massage
    d. Ice alternated with heat, moderate exercise, general massage, and counterirritation ointments

24. A client has a sore shoulder from a work-related repetitive overuse injury. The client has held the shoulder in the least-packed position with a sling for longer than 3 months. Now the client is experiencing reduced range of motion. Which of the following benefits the most from massage?
    a. Protective muscle splinting
    b. Nerve impingement
    c. Arthritis
    d. Adhesive capsulitis

25. A joint is exhibiting the ability to move normally in the first 90 degrees of flexion, which is determined to be a 10% limitation of the possible expected range of motion (ROM). What should the ROM of the joint be?
    a. 45 degrees of extension
    b. 100 degrees of flexion
    c. 80 degrees of abduction

26. The assessment form indicates that a client has a bilateral anterior tilt of the pelvis. Which of the following would explain best what the massage therapist would see and feel during physical assessment?
    a. One hip is lower than the other.
    b. The client is twisted to the left.
    c. The client is flexed at the hips.
    d. The scapula has retracted.

Exercise

Using the previous questions as examples, write at least three more questions. Develop plausible wrong answers and be sure that the correct answer is clearly correct. Then write a rationale for each question. The more questions you write, the better you will understand the material.

MUSCLES

Review Tips

The content related to muscles is complex. It is important to know muscle structure, location, and function, as well as functional muscle groups (agonist, antagonist, synergist), innervations, and pathologic conditions. Muscle consists largely of connective tissue; therefore, you must grasp the nature of connective tissue types and function. It is more accurate to call what is commonly named *muscle* the *muscle organ* since it is a collection of tissues that work together for a particular function. The function of muscle cells is to actively shorten and pull the connective tissue network to produce movement. Muscle function is not isolated but an integrated system which works together to provide stability and movement.

The following information and suggestions can make this study less confusing. Muscle names can provide clues about location, function, and shape. Nerves often are named to reflect their location. For example, the ulnar nerve is located adjacent to the ulna bone, and the thoracodorsal nerve is located in the posterior thorax.

Function involves joints, so muscle function often is described with the terms *flexion, extension, rotation, adduction,* and *abduction.* Other movement terms used to describe muscle functions are *medial, lateral, depression, elevation,* and *tilt.* Types of muscle function are concentric, which produces (accelerates) movement; eccentric, which controls (decelerates) movement; and isometric, which stabilizes.

Most examinations do not ask specific questions about the exact attachments of muscles because textbooks do not agree. However, some questions of this type may be included, and it is necessary for you to comprehend this information so you can understand muscle function. You must know bony landmarks to learn muscle attachments. Attachment terminology is changing. The shift is being made from origin and insertion to proximal and distal attachment. The proximal attachment (typically the old origin description) is described as "from," and the distal attachment (old insertion terminology) is described as "to."
- From-proximal-origin
- To-distal-insertion

Adding to the confusion is the fact that different textbooks and atlases describe attachments in different ways.

A great way to study muscles—location and function—is to build models. You can obtain skeletal models inexpensively at a store that carries educational supplies, or you can order them online. Then use a modeling compound (e.g., clay, Play-Doh) to build the muscles. Coloring books are helpful. Because muscles and massage so often are connected, it is common to find muscle system terminology in many of the questions on massage examinations. This is especially common in questions of the case study type. This content can appear in all three types of multiple-choice questions.

Quick Content Review

- The functions of muscles include producing movement, generating heat, maintaining posture, and stabilizing joints. All three types of muscle tissue provide the movement necessary for survival. Skeletal muscle moves the limbs. Skeletal, cardiac, and smooth muscle will produce movements such as those involved in breathing, heartbeat, digestion, and elimination. The relative constancy of the internal temperature of the body is maintained in a cool external environment by the "waste" heat generated by muscle tissue during contraction. Maintenance of a stable body posture is the primary function of the musculoskeletal system. The dynamic tension of muscle contraction opposes the forces of gravity. Stability of joint structures is an often overlooked function of muscle. Especially in the more mobile joints, which by nature have a loose structural design, the dynamic and static contraction of muscles surrounding the joint provides external stability, supporting the structures of the joint itself.
- The three types of muscle tissue are skeletal, cardiac, and smooth.

- Skeletal muscle fibers are long cylindrical, tapered cells that have cross-striations caused by the contractile structures inside. Skeletal muscles contain white, red, and intermediate muscle fibers. Each muscle fiber is wrapped by several different layers of connective tissue.
- Cardiac muscle is found in only one organ of the body, the heart. Cardiac muscle fiber does not taper like skeletal muscle fiber but instead forms strong, electrically coupled junctions (intercalated disks) with other fibers. Cardiac muscles form a continuous contractile band around the heart.
- Smooth muscle consists of small, tapered cells with single nuclei. Because the myofilaments are not organized into sarcomeres, they exhibit greater freedom of movement and can contract a smooth muscle fiber to shorter lengths than can be done in skeletal and cardiac muscle.
- Dynamic force produces movement in or of an object.
- Static force applied to an object does not produce movement.
- Elasticity is the ability of a muscle to recoil and resume its original resting length after it is stretched. Applying force is called loading, and releasing force is called unloading.
- Excitability is the ability of a muscle to receive and respond to a stimulus.
- Extensibility is the ability of a muscle to be stretched or extended.
- Contractility is the ability of a muscle to shorten forcibly upon adequate stimulation.
- The all-or-none response occurs when a muscle contraction is initiated and all muscle fibers contract to their full ability, or they do not contract at all.
- The threshold stimulus is the stimulus at which the first observable muscle contraction occurs.
- Maximum stimulus is the point at which all the motor units of a muscle have been recruited and the muscle is unable to increase in strength.
- Tone is the state of slight contraction in all skeletal muscle that enables the muscle to respond to stimulation.
- A motor unit consists of the muscle fibers innervated by a single motor neuron.
- Oxygen debt is the extra amount of oxygen that must be taken in to convert lactic acid to glucose or glycogen.
- The types of skeletal muscle fibers are as follows:
  1. Fast-twitch (white) fibers that contract more rapidly and forcefully are larger than red fibers and belong to larger motor units that activate when the nervous system demands rapid, powerful motion. They do not require much oxygen to contract and are considered anaerobic. White fibers fatigue quickly.
  2. Slow-twitch (red) fibers are smaller, contract more slowly and weakly, and belong to smaller motor units that respond during slower, delicate movements. Red fibers contain much larger quantities of myoglobin, require the presence of oxygen for contraction, and are considered aerobic. They do not fatigue quickly and can hold a contraction for

a long period, making them highly efficient in muscles that maintain posture.

3. Intermediate fibers combine the qualities of red and white fibers, allowing a rapid, moderately forceful contraction and providing moderate fatigue resistance.

- An agonist is a muscle that causes or controls joint motion through a specified plane of motion and is known as a primary or prime mover.
- An antagonist is a muscle that usually is located on the opposite side of the joint from the agonist and that has the opposite action. Agonist and antagonist muscles can contract together at the same time in what is called a co-contraction.
- Synergist muscles aid or assist the action of the agonists but are not primarily responsible for the action; synergists are known as guiding muscles.
- A fixator is a stabilizing muscle that is located at a joint and contracts to fixate, or stabilize, an area, enabling another limb or body segment to exert force and move.
- Deep fascia forms a coarse sheet of fibrous connective tissue that binds muscles into functional groups and forms partitions, called intermuscular septa, between muscle groups.
- A trigger point, as described by Janet Travell, is a hyperirritable locus within a taut band of skeletal muscle, located in the muscular tissue or in its associated fascia, or in both places. The spot is painful on compression and can evoke characteristic referred pain and autonomic phenomena. Lengthening involves neurochemical responses of the muscle fiber. Stretching involves a mechanical force directed toward altering connective tissue structure. The exact physiology of the trigger point concept is unknown.
- According to Myers, tensegrity refers to structures that maintain their integrity primarily through a balance of continuous tensile forces acting on the structure.
- Research has identified that fascia is innervated and contains contractile cells. Muscular system pathology is usually interconnected with nervous system, circulatory system, joint function, and connective tissue function more than pathology of the muscle cell.

Factual Recall Questions

1. Muscle uses which of the following to produce mechanical energy to exert force?
   a. Myoglobin
   b. Adenosine triphosphate
   c. Perimysium
2. Which of the characteristics of muscle tissue is demonstrated by muscles shortening?
   a. Excitability
   b. Contractility
   c. Extensibility
   d. Elasticity
3. The structural units of contraction in skeletal muscle fibers are called _____.
   a. Myoglobins
   b. Myofibrils
   c. Sarcomeres
   d. Fascicles
4. The attachment of myosin to cross-bridges on actin requires which substance?
   a. Calcium
   b. Hemoglobin
   c. Collagen
   d. Potassium
5. Delicate and precise movements such as those seen in the eye muscles are possible because_____.
   a. Multiple sensory neurons innervate the muscles
   b. Large motor units exist in the muscle
   c. The muscle fibers in a motor unit are clustered together
   d. A motor unit consists of a few muscle fibers
6. Anatomically, a strong correlation has been noted between the locations of motor points, acupuncture points, and _____.
   a. Motor end plates
   b. Tendons
   c. Trigger points
   d. Mitotic units
7. The ability of muscles to maintain a certain level of tautness is called _____.
   a. Threshold stimulus
   b. Tone
   c. Treppe
   d. All-or-none response
8. Vascular structures in muscles are characterized as _____.
   a. Limited to the muscular aponeurosis
   b. Abundant and designed to accommodate stretch
   c. Found mainly in the epimysium
   d. Abundant within the ligament structures
9. The connective tissue aspect of muscles is characterized as _____.
   a. The active contractile unit
   b. The main heat-producing structure
   c. Responsive to adenosine triphosphate
   d. Inseparable and continuous with muscle fibers
10. Intermuscular septa are formed primarily from _____.
    a. Deep fascia
    b. Epimysium
    c. Perimysium
11. The long head of biceps brachii attachment at the radial tuberosity is an example of _____.
    a. An origin
    b. An insertion
    c. A direct attachment
    d. A proximal attachment
12. If a strong and sustained contraction without extensive movement is required, which of the following muscle shapes provides the best design?
    a. Parallel
    b. Pennate
    c. Circular

13. Which of the following muscle types has the ability to contract to produce peristalsis?
    a. Cardiac
    b. Circular
    c. Smooth
    d. Pennate
14. A client is complaining of an ache in the eye, ear, and scalp, especially above the ear. Assessment would reveal a trigger point in which of the following muscles?
    a. Orbicularis oculi
    b. Buccinator
    c. Risorius
    d. Occipitofrontalis
15. Which of the following is a muscle of mastication?
    a. Platysma
    b. Lateral pterygoid
    c. Orbicularis oris
16. The muscles of the anterior triangle of the neck as defined by the sternocleidomastoid have a primary function of _____.
    a. Assisting in swallowing
    b. Providing cervical extension
    c. Stabilizing capital rotation
    d. Providing neck flexion
17. Compression by which of the following muscle groups against the brachial nerve plexus often refers pain to the pectoralis, to the rhomboid area, and into the arm and hand?
    a. Splenius capitis and splenius cervicis
    b. Erector spinae
    c. Scalene
18. The abdominal and psoas muscles are the major antagonists for which of the following muscles?
    a. Splenius capitis
    b. Longissimus thoracis
    c. Intertransversarii thoracis
19. A client complains of difficulty achieving a full and deep breath. Assessments indicate exhalation is normal. Lifting of the ribs is restricted during inhalation. Which muscle may be involved?
    a. Diaphragm
    b. Serratus posterior inferior
    c. Internal intercostals
    d. External intercostals
20. A client complains of low back pain that increases with coughing. Assessment indicates tenderness in the deep lumbar area with referred pain to the gluteal area, particularly around the sacroiliac joint. Which muscle is likely to be involved?
    a. Quadratus lumborum
    b. Iliacus
    c. Semispinalis
21. Which of the following muscles has its origin at the crest of the pubis and pubic symphysis and its insertion at the cartilage of the fifth, sixth, and seventh ribs and at the xiphoid process?
    a. Pyramidalis

b. External oblique
    c. Rectus abdominis
    d. Transversus abdominis
22. Which of the following muscles would be innervated by the perineal division of the pudendal nerve?
    a. Levator ani
    b. Cremaster
    c. Longus colli
23. Which of the following muscles of scapular stabilization contains three distinct parts with distinct functions, allowing the muscle to be an antagonist to itself?
    a. Serratus anterior
    b. Trapezius
    c. Pectoralis minor
    d. Rhomboid major
24. Assessment indicates that the left scapular area is rounded forward and protracted. Which of the following muscle pairs is likely to be tense and shortened?
    a. Trapezius and rhomboideus minor
    b. Levator scapulae and supraspinatus
    c. Pectoralis minor and serratus anterior
    d. Teres minor and infraspinatus
25. Assessment indicates that a client has a bilateral medially rotated humerus. The subscapularis muscles are tight and short and contain trigger points. Which of the following muscles is likely to be inhibited?
    a. Anterior deltoid
    b. Pectoralis major
    c. Teres major
    d. Infraspinatus
26. A client is having difficulty raising the arm to comb the hair. Which of the following muscles is likely to be tight and short?
    a. Coracobrachialis
    b. Biceps brachii
    c. Latissimus dorsi
27. Which muscle is attached to the distal half of the anterior surface of the humerus, medial and lateral intermuscular septa, and coronoid process and tuberosity of the ulna?
    a. Brachioradialis
    b. Pronator teres
    c. Supinator
    d. Brachialis
28. Which of the following muscles is synergistic to triceps brachii?
    a. Supinator
    b. Pronator quadratus
    c. Anconeus
29. The ability to execute a coordinated and accurate pattern of movement requires cooperation among various muscle groups called _____.
    a. Myotatic units
    b. Sarcomeres
    c. Reflex arcs
30. The polysynaptic reflex that coordinates muscle action on both sides of the body is the _____ reflex.

a. Stretch
b. Flexor
c. Tendon

31. Which of the following muscles is located in the thenar eminence?
a. Opponens digiti minimi
b. Opponens pollicis
c. Lumbricales

32. Which of the following muscles extends and laterally rotates the hip joint with lower fibers, assists in adduction of the hip with the femur fixed, and assists in extension of the trunk?
a. Gluteus medius
b. Piriformis
c. Gluteus maximus
d. Tensor fasciae latae

33. When the layering of muscles from superficial to deep is considered, which of the following is the deepest layer?
a. Gluteus medius
b. Tensor fasciae latae
c. Gluteus maximus
d. Piriformis

34. Observation and assessment of a client indicate that the left leg is externally (laterally) rotated. Which of the following muscles may be tense and shortened?
a. Gemellus superior
b. Gracilis
c. Pectineus

35. Which of the following pairs consists of muscles that are synergistic with each other?
a. Biceps femoris and gluteus maximus
b. Adductor brevis and gluteus medius
c. Semimembranosus and obturator externus
d. Piriformis and semitendinosus

36. If the legs are fixed, which of the following is a flexor of the hip that assists in flexion of the torso to the thigh?
a. Vastus lateralis
b. Vastus medialis
c. Sartorius
d. Semitendinosus

37. A client complains of difficulty extending the knee. Which muscle group is likely to be tense and short?
a. Adductor
b. Quadriceps femoris
c. Anterior leg
d. Hamstring

38. When beginning flexion, a client feels a "catch" sensation in the back of the knee. The physician says the joint is normal and indicates that this is a muscular problem. Which muscle is likely to be involved?
a. Peroneus brevis
b. Tibialis posterior
c. Popliteus

39. Muscles located in which part of the body are most responsible for dorsiflexion?
a. Anterior leg
b. Posterior leg

c. Lateral arm
d. Medial arm

40. A dancer is finding it difficult to sustain movement that requires them to be on their toes. Which muscle may be inhibited?
a. Plantar interossei
b. Soleus
c. Extensor digitorum

41. Which of the following muscles plantar flexes the ankle and assists with knee flexion?
a. Tibialis posterior
b. Tibialis anterior
c. Peroneus longus
d. Plantaris

42. If the gastrocnemius is tight and short, which of the following muscles is likely to be inhibited?
a. Soleus
b. Tibialis anterior
c. Flexor hallucis longus
d. Flexor digitorum longus

43. Which of the following muscles has its attachment on the great toe?
a. Flexor digitorum brevis
b. Quadratus plantae
c. Flexor hallucis brevis

44. Which of the following medications likely would be prescribed for tendonitis?
a. Antibiotic
b. Muscle relaxant
c. Anticoagulant
d. Antiinflammatory

45. A client is taking an over-the-counter analgesic. What concern would the massage professional have while providing massage?
a. Feedback mechanisms for pain will be altered.
b. Blood pressure may fall dangerously low.
c. The infection may be spread.

46. Which of the following conditions presents regional contraindications for massage?
a. Postpolio syndrome
b. Myositis ossificans
c. Muscular dystrophy
d. Myasthenia gravis

47. If the major function of a muscle is to stabilize, then which of the following muscle functions is involved?
a. Isometric
b. Concentric
c. Eccentric

Application/Concept Identification and Clinical Reasoning/Synthesis Questions

1. If the concentric function of a muscle is extension and lateral flexion, then which of the following is the eccentric function of that same muscle?
a. Stabilizes the adjacent joint

    b. Elevates and rotates the area

    c. Restrains flexion and controls extension

    d. Assists extension and lateral flexion

2. If the concentric function of a muscle is to extend and laterally rotate the thigh at the hip joint, which of the following would be synergist and antagonist muscles?

    a. Hamstrings and iliopsoas

    b. Quadratus femoris and fibularis

    c. Popliteus and plantaris

    d. Quadratus lumborum and transverse abdominis oblique

3. What relationship do the tibialis anterior and extensor digitorum longus have?

    a. They are located in the thigh.

    b. These muscles are synergists to each other.

    c. These muscles are concentric eccentric antagonists.

4. If the attachment of a muscle is located closer to the torso and would be listed as *from* in attachment description, which of the following is being described?

    a. Distal insertion

    b. Distal origin

    c. Proximal origin

5. A client complains of fatigue and muscle soreness after attempting to push a car that was stuck. Which of the following best describes this action?

    a. No movement was produced, so static force was generated.

    b. Dynamic force was used because the car did not move.

    c. Static force produced movement and energy expenditure.

    d. Because the car did not move, little energy was expended.

6. During assessment, the massage professional realizes that a client has extremely mobile joints. Which muscle functions would seem to be impaired?

    a. Production of movement

    b. Generation of heat

    c. Maintenance of posture

    d. Stabilization of joints

7. A client was a sprinter in high school track and was effective during short and quick runs. Now, 10 years later, the client lacks the endurance to run 5 miles as part of a fitness program. The client is in good physical condition with little apparent reason for the difficulties. The most plausible explanation for the client's condition is that the client has _____.

    a. An abundance of slow-twitch fibers in relationship to fast-twitch fibers

    b. An enhanced ability to manage oxygen debt

    c. Legs with a genetic tendency toward a makeup of a greater number of white anaerobic fibers

    d. Increased slow-twitch fibers in the postural muscles

8. A client is complaining of tender areas in the postural muscles along the spine. Assessment indicates a series of trigger points in these muscles. The massage professional must determine how much compressive force should be applied to the trigger points, and how long the contraction should be held. This decision will be affected by the fact that these muscles _____.

    a. Contain a greater number of slow-twitch red fibers that are fatigue resistant

    b. Are prone to oxygen debt

    c. Have an abundance of fast-twitch and intermediate fibers

    d. Require a maximum stimulus to respond to treatment

9. A client complains of a sensation of thickness and stiffness in the myofascial structures of the body. Slow, sustained stretching provides the greatest benefit. The most plausible reason for this effect is the _____.

    a. Neuromuscular unit is deprived of calcium, allowing actin and myosin to disengage

    b. Viscous nature of connective tissue responds to this method by becoming more pliable

    c. Colloid connective tissue ground substance decreases water binding with these methods

    d. Compression against the capillaries promotes blood flow

10. A client is complaining of pain when straightening the elbow. Palpation of triceps brachii at the musculotendinous junction indicates greater tenderness at the insertion when the muscle is activated. The most likely reason for this is the insertion is the _____.

    a. Fixed attachment and tenderness is enhanced during movement

    b. Proximal attachment and is straining at the intermuscular septa

    c. Highly innervated and stimulated belly of the muscle

    d. More movable attachment, so it would produce enhanced tenderness upon motion

11. A client is experiencing a limitation in range of motion of the hip into abduction. Assessment indicates shortening and tension in the adductor group of muscles. Which of the following is the most likely source of the limited range of motion?

    a. Agonists

    b. Synergists

    c. Antagonists

    d. Fixators

12. A client unexpectedly lifted a box that was much too heavy. Now the client is experiencing residual weakness in the biceps and brachialis muscles and tension in the triceps muscle group. Which of the following reflexes best explains this situation?

    a. Stretch

    b. Tendon

    c. Withdrawal

    d. Crossed extensor

13. A client's job requires that they perform the same repetitive lift and hand squeeze task. This person has been doing this job for 8 months. In the beginning, their arms were sore and a bit swollen, but that went away. Over the past 3 months, pain and tension in the arms have returned and have begun to increase. Which of the following best describes the client's current condition?

a. Chain reaction has occurred in myotatic units.

b. Pain has increased tension or spasm, which has increased pain.

c. Joint restriction and fascial shortening have decreased mobility.

14. Which of the following conditions is most likely to benefit directly from a nonspecific general massage session?

a. Contusion

b. Anterior compartment syndrome

c. Muscle tension headache

d. Spasticity

15. Two clients describe accidents in which the muscles of their upper thigh were cut and now have healed. Client A demonstrates a mobile scar with near-normal function. Client B exhibits tissue rigidity and reduced movement. What is the most plausible explanation?

a. Client A limited exercise and kept the area tightly wrapped during the healing process.

b. Client B had increased satellite cell activity during healing, causing increased scar tissue.

c. Client A exercised during healing to stimulate satellite cells.

d. Client B experienced increased circulation and reduced adhesions.

16. A client has been working on a project that required gripping a hammer for an extended period. Now the client is complaining of weakness when attempting to extend the wrist. Which of the following is the most likely explanation?

a. The flexor muscle group of the hand and wrist increased tone levels, resulting in inhibition of the extensor group of muscles in the forearm.

b. The flexor digitorum superficialis and profundus are weak from fatigue, so the wrist extensors have been facilitated.

c. The deep layer of the posterior wrist extensor group is antagonistic to the superficial layer of this same muscle group, resulting in weakness in the wrist extensors.

17. A client with fibromyalgia has been referred from the physician for massage. A treatment plan has been requested for approval before treatment begins. Which of the following would be the most appropriate approach?

a. General massage with active-assisted joint movement and stretching

b. Local massage to the back with friction methods to active tender points

c. Localized massage to the feet and ischemic compression to active trigger points

d. General massage to support restorative sleep and symptomatic pain management

Exercise

Using the previous questions as examples, write at least three more questions. Develop plausible wrong answers and be sure that the correct answer is clearly correct. Then write a rationale for each question. The more questions you write, the better you will understand the material.

BIOMECHANICS

Review Tips

The content on biomechanics combines previous information to promote an understanding of how the body maintains posture and produces movement. This area consists of new terminology that must be understood. The content provides the foundation for assessment procedures. Assessment is necessary to determine indications and contraindications for massage.

This material often is presented in the style of concept identification and clinical reasoning and synthesis questions. The terminology often is tested through factual recall and comprehension questions.

An effective study strategy is to explain a concept in words different from those in the text, or to give an example of what the text is talking about, or to develop a metaphor about the content. As for the previous parts, look up any terminology you do not understand, and make sure you know why the wrong answers are wrong.

Quick Content Review

- Biomechanics is the study of mechanical actions as applied to living bodies. Kinesiology is the study of movement that emerges and blends the knowledge of anatomy, physiology, physics, and geometry and relates them to human movement. Dynamic systems can be divided into kinetics and kinematics. Kinetics involves the forces that cause movement, whereas kinematics refers to the time, space, and mass aspects of a moving system.

- Movement is a fundamental characteristic of human behavior that is accomplished through the contraction of skeletal muscles acting within a system of levers and pulleys.

- In biomechanical terms, the concept of center refers to the center of gravity—that is, the midpoint or center of weight of a body or object. Any loss of biomechanical stability, as occurs with a missing limb or altered posture, alters not only the total body weight distribution but also the center of gravity.

- External forces that act on the body include gravity and those forces generated by the interaction of the body with external forces, such as lifting a box or managing an umbrella in the wind. Therapeutic massage attempts to alter body function by exerting external forces to generate internal forces, which then effect change in the homeostatic mechanisms of the body.

- Inertia is the reluctance of matter to change its state of motion. Any irregularly paced or multidirectional activity is costly in terms of energy reserves.

- Acceleration, which may be defined as the rate of change in velocity, occurs in the same direction as the force that caused it.
- Balance is the ability to control equilibrium. Equilibrium refers to a state of zero acceleration in which no change in the speed or direction of the body occurs.
- Static equilibrium occurs when the body is at rest or is completely motionless.
- Dynamic equilibrium occurs when all of the applied or internal forces that act on the moving body are in balance, resulting in movement with unchanging speed or direction.
- Stability is resistance to change in the acceleration of a body or resistance to the disturbance of the equilibrium of a body.
- The kinetic chain is made up of the myofascial system (muscle, ligament, tendon, and fascia), the articular (joint) system, and the nervous system. If one or more of these systems do not work efficiently, compensations and adaptations occur in the remaining systems, leading to stress in the body and eventually resulting in the development of dysfunctional patterns. All functional movement patterns involve acceleration provided by concentric contractions, stabilization provided by isometric contractions, and deceleration provided by eccentric action. All three actions occur with each movement pattern at every joint in the kinetic chain and in all three planes of motion.
- The basic principles of biomechanics are as follows:
  1. A person has balance when the center of gravity falls within the base of support. Balance is in direct proportion to the size of the base of support. The larger the base of support, the greater is the balance. Balance depends on the weight or mass. The greater the weight, the greater is the balance.
  2. A person has balance depending on the height of the center of gravity. The lower the center of gravity, the greater is the balance. Balance depends on where the center of gravity is in relation to the base of support. The balance is less if the center of gravity is near the edge of the base. However, when anticipating an oncoming force, stability may be improved by placing the center of gravity closer to the side of the base of support expected to receive the force. In anticipation of an oncoming force, stability may also be increased by enlarging the size of the base of support in the direction of the anticipated force. Equilibrium may be enhanced by increasing the friction between the body and the surface it contacts. Rotation about an axis is easier to balance. A bike that is moving is easier to balance than a bike that is stationary.
  3. Human beings move about on two legs composed of three segments each: the thigh, lower leg, and foot. Atop the two legs are the trunk, head, and arm unit. The arm unit is used as a counterbalance and for momentum and moves opposite the leg movement. This pattern is linked in the contralateral reflex arc mechanism.
  4. Flexion and extension of the hip joints cause some rotation in the lumbar spine; to keep the head facing forward and the eyes level, the thorax and cervical spine rotate in the opposite direction. This action is coordinated by reflex patterns that coordinate upright posture in gravity and righting reflexes that keep the eyes on a level plane and the head oriented to the trunk. Reciprocal movements of the upper and lower limbs occur simultaneously with right upper limb flexion at the shoulder joint coordinated with flexion at the left hip joint. Normally, the shoulder joint starts to flex or extend slightly before the same movement occurs in the elbow joint. These movements again serve to keep the head and trunk oriented and to counterbalance the body weight in gravity.
  5. The three main dysfunctional biomechanical patterns are neuromuscular, myofascial, and joint related that can occur as stage 1, 2, or 3 dysfunctional patterns.

Factual Recall Questions

1. What type of action occurs when the muscle lengthens while under tension, changes in tension occur to control the descent of resistance, and joint angle increases?
   a. Isometric eccentric
   b. Isotonic concentric
   c. Isometric concentric
   d. Isotonic eccentric
2. The amount of force on a specific area is called _____.
   a. Pressure
   b. Inertia
   c. Acceleration
   d. Center of gravity
3. A person who is maintaining an upright posture while reaching for an object is displaying _____.
   a. Static balance
   b. Dynamic balance
   c. Static equilibrium
4. Which of the following statements would describe the least amount of balance?
   a. Greater weight centered over a large base of support
   b. The center of gravity outside the base of support
   c. A low center of gravity with rotation around the axis
5. Because the body movements of the limb most often require rapid movement and attachments of the muscles are close to the joint, which lever type is found most often?
   a. First-class
   b. Second-class
   c. Third-class
6. During normal gait, when one foot is in contact with the floor, this is called the _____.
   a. Stance phase
   b. Double stance
   c. Swing phase
   d. Double swing

7. Which of the following aspects of the gait cycle would result in the most concentric contraction of the plantar flexors?
   a. Heel strike
   b. Midstance
   c. Toe-off preswing
   d. Midswing

8. A reversible limitation of range of movement that occurs as a result of change in connective tissue following long-term muscle spasms is called _____.
   a. Nonoptimal motor function
   b. Capsular pattern
   c. Regional postural muscular imbalance
   d. Functional block

9. During joint movement and muscle strength assessment, it is important to isolate the movement to the jointed area that is being assessed. This is called _____.
   a. Force
   b. Resistance
   c. Balance
   d. Stabilization

10. Wrist flexion has a normal range of 0 to 80 degrees. A client is assessed with a range of motion of 100 degrees. This jointed area would be considered _____.
    a. Balanced
    b. Hypermobile
    c. Hypomobile

11. The typical range of motion in extension for the lumbar spine is _____.
    a. 25 degrees
    b. 5 degrees
    c. 40 degrees

12. A client is having difficulty moving the head into cervical extension beyond 10 degrees. Which of the following cervical flexor muscles may be restricting mobility?
    a. Longissimus capitis
    b. Sternocleidomastoid
    c. Splenius capitis

13. A client is unable to rotate the cervical area to turn the head past 20 degrees to the left. Muscle testing should indicate what?
    a. Even strength on both sides
    b. Increased tension in the right cervical rotators
    c. Weakness in the right cervical rotators
    d. Increased strength in the cervical flexors

14. Which of the following muscles is able to affect the sternoclavicular joint indirectly?
    a. Anterior deltoid
    b. Triceps brachii
    c. Pectoralis minor
    d. Pectoralis major

15. The primary function of the shoulder girdle muscles that have attachments at the axial skeleton, the scapula, and the clavicle is _____.
    a. Extension of the shoulder joint

b. Stability of the scapula
c. Mobility of the humerus

16. A client has elbow flexion of 90 degrees. This is considered _____.
    a. Normal
    b. Hypermobility
    c. Hypomobility

17. How is the area positioned and where is resistance applied when a muscle test for normal function of the wrist flexors is performed?
    a. Elbow is flexed, and resistance is applied against the forearm.
    b. Wrist is flexed, and resistance is applied against the palm of the hand.
    c. Elbow is extended, and resistance is applied against the palm of the hand.
    d. Wrist is flexed, and resistance is applied against the dorsal side of the hand.

18. Concentric contraction occurs in which muscles when the thigh is flexed toward the trunk?
    a. Hamstrings
    b. Gluteus maximus
    c. Iliopsoas
    d. Vastus lateralis

19. A client lying prone is unable to lift the thigh off the table when attempting hip extension. Which muscle is unable to contract effectively?
    a. Sartorius
    b. Adductor magnus
    c. Rectus femoris
    d. Semimembranosus

20. A massage practitioner wishes to assess the ability of the knee to move into slight internal and external rotation. How should the knee be positioned?
    a. Full extension
    b. 5 degrees of hyperextension
    c. 30 degrees of flexion
    d. 10 degrees of flexion

21. The sequence of muscle contraction determined by the nervous system to produce optimal movement is called a _____.
    a. Stabilization action
    b. Gait action
    c. Firing pattern
    d. Lower crossed syndrome

22. If during assessment, the rhomboid muscles, posterior deltoid, and infraspinatus muscle test as inhibited, which of the following most logically is indicated?
    a. Lower crossed syndrome
    b. Myofascially related dysfunction
    c. Gait assessment
    d. Upper crossed syndrome

23. Which of the following muscle joint complexes would have 80 degrees of internal rotation?
    a. Knee

b. Shoulder

c. Cervical area

d. Trunk

24. When a joint is moved so that the joint angle is decreased, what is occurring?

a. Prime movers and the synergist concentrically contract. The antagonist eccentrically functions while lengthening to allow movement.

b. Prime movers concentrically contract with the antagonist so that synergists lengthen to allow movement.

c. Movement occurs as the antagonist contracts and prime movers eccentrically control the movement.

Application/Concept Identification and Clinical Reasoning/Synthesis Questions

1. Which of the following is likely to result in joint-related dysfunction?

a. Constant loading of a joint

b. Generalized edema

c. Closed kinematic chain

2. An example of a core stabilizing inner unit muscle would be?

a. Latissimus dorsi

b. Adductor longus

c. Quadriceps

d. Transversus abdominis

3. Which of the following would be considered a fulcrum?

a. Quadriceps muscles

b. Radius

c. Deltoid ligament

d. Glenohumeral joint

4. When carrying a massage table from the car to the office, what is the responsibility of the muscles?

a. Create a lever to distribute the load

b. Exert effort to move the load

c. Provide a fulcrum for the lever

d. Maintain static balance

5. During normal gait in the adult, lumbar rotation is countered by cervical spine rotation in the opposite direction to _____.

a. Keep the eyes on a level plane and the head oriented forward with the trunk

b. Maintain same-side counterbalance action of the arms and legs

c. Coordinate the lever action of the elbows with that of the knees

6. After tripping down a staircase, but not falling, a client describes a sudden onset of pain during twisting and reaching movements. Which type of biomechanical dysfunction is most likely to be occurring?

a. Neuromuscular

b. Myofascial

c. Joint related

7. A massage professional positions the client's body to assess the strength of the hip flexors. Which is the correct position for the hand that is applying resistance?

a. Near the hip

b. At the ankle

c. At the distal end of the femur

d. On the tibia

8. A client is experiencing an upper chest breathing pattern. Which of the following may test as short and too strong from this type of breathing?

a. Diaphragm

b. Suprahyoid group

c. Scalene group

d. Infraspinatus

9. A client complains of pain and tension in the lower back more to the left side. Physical assessment indicates that the pelvis is elevated on the left compared with the right. The client also indicates difficulty raising the left arm over the head. Which of the following muscles may be involved?

a. Psoas major

b. Rectus abdominis

c. Latissimus dorsi

d. Semispinalis

10. If the scapula remains fixed and immobile, what would result at the glenohumeral joint?

a. Range of motion would be limited.

b. Internal and external rotation would be enhanced.

c. Flexion would be unaffected.

11. The glenohumeral joint is a good example to describe which of the following correct biomechanical principles?

a. When mobility increases, stability also increases.

b. When stability is less, mobility decreases.

c. As mobility increases, stability decreases.

12. A client is unable to turn the palm up past 45 degrees. Which of the following movements is hypomobile?

a. Supination

b. Pronation

c. Flexion

d. Extension

13. A client is lying supine, and observation indicates that the left leg is rotated internally. What should muscle testing reveal?

a. Muscles that externally rotate the hip are short, and muscles that internally rotate the hip are inhibited.

b. Muscles that externally rotate the hip are inhibited, and muscles that internally rotate the hip are overly strong.

c. Gluteus medius should test weak.

d. Adductor longus should test weak.

14. The knee is placed in extension, and the client is asked to hold this position. Resistance is applied to the concentrically contracting muscles. Pain and weakness are felt. What is a logical explanation for this?

a. Hamstring muscle group is weak.

b. Q angle is being altered in a lateral direction by contraction of the vastus medialis.

c. Popliteus muscle has been unable to unlock the screw-home mechanism.

d. Quadriceps muscle group is unable to hold a contraction effectively against resistance.

15. A client experienced a second-degree ankle sprain when the foot was forced into inversion. Which of the following muscles would have experienced an extension injury?

a. Fibularis longus

b. Soleus

c. Flexor digitorum longus

d. Interossei

16. An individual was running up the stairs carrying a heavy briefcase in the left hand. Later that day, the person felt increased tension in the left biceps brachii. Two days later, during a regular massage session, the client describes weakness and heaviness in one leg when walking up stairs or a hill. If normal gait reflexes are functioning, where would assessment likely find an inhibited muscle pattern?

a. Right arm extensors

b. Left hip flexors

c. Right hip flexors

d. Left hip extensors

17. A client experienced an auto accident 4 years ago that resulted in a bulging disk at L4. The injury has since healed with minimum difficulty. During assessment, palpation indicates a moderate decrease in pliability of the lumbar dorsal fascia and mild shortening in the lumbar muscles. Forward flexion and rotation of the lumbar area are impaired mildly. Massage was focused to reduce muscle shortening in the lumbar area and increase connective tissue pliability. Immediately after the massage, the client reported increased mobility, but within 15 minutes began to complain of lower back pain. What is the most likely explanation for this occurrence?

a. A shift of the condition from second-degree functional stress to first-degree functional tension

b. Increase in stability around the past injury

c. Stabilization in the area around the past injury

d. Destabilization of resourceful compensation in the lumbar area around the past injury

18. A client complains of joint pain in the knee, and assessment indicates hypermobility with pain on passive movement. Which of the following would be the most appropriate treatment plan?

a. Local muscle energy work and lengthening of the extensors and flexors of the knee

b. General massage with regional contraindications to the knee area and referral for more appropriate diagnosis of possible capsular dysfunction

c. Referral for diagnosis before any massage

d. General massage with attention to friction methods at the joint capsule

19. A client is experiencing pain with any activity involving external or lateral rotation of the right shoulder. Range of motion is limited to 40 degrees. This condition has been coming on gradually. Muscle testing indicates weakness when resistance is applied to move the shoulder from external rotation to internal rotation. Shortening in the muscles of internal rotation is evident. Which of the following would be the most logical treatment plan?

a. Muscle energy methods to support lengthening of the infraspinatus and methods to increase tone in the subscapularis

b. Deep massage to the rhomboid muscles and stretching of the lumbar fascia

c. Traction of the scapulothoracic junction

d. Massage to reduce tension in the pectoralis major and latissimus dorsi, with percussion to increase tone in the infraspinatus and teres major

Exercise

Using the previous questions as examples, write at least three more questions. Develop plausible wrong answers and be sure that the correct answer is clearly correct. Then write a rationale for each question. The more questions you write, the better you will understand the material.

INTEGUMENTARY, CARDIOVASCULAR, LYMPHATIC, AND IMMUNE SYSTEMS

Review Tips

Knowledge of the integumentary, cardiovascular, lymphatic, and immune systems usually is tested with factual recall and comprehension questions. Also, pathologic conditions for each of these systems are targeted in examination questions. A common focus of question development is to connect the anatomy and physiology of each body system to a specific application of massage. The classic example of this is massage targeted to influence cardiovascular and lymphatic function.

As explained previously, you must know the definition of each term and must be able to use each term correctly. More complex questions use the terminology in the question and possible answers, and unless you can decipher the language, you will not know what the question or the provided answers mean. There is no easy way to study terminology. Using flashcards, reading glossaries, and doing labeling exercises reinforce the definitions of various terms. Use the study tools in this guide, and make sure that when you read your textbooks, you know what the words mean. Also make sure that you understand the meaning of general language used to write the questions. If you are not sure of the meaning of a word, look it up in the dictionary.

Quick Content Review

- The integument is made up of the skin and its appendages: hair, sebaceous glands, sweat glands, nails, and breasts.
- The epidermis is the outer layer of skin; it consists of sub-layers called strata. Four or five layers of strata make up the outer layer of skin, depending on location on the body.
- The dermis, the inner layer of skin, is much thicker than the epidermis and is composed of dense connective tissue that contains collagen and elastin fibers. The various appendages of the skin originate in the dermis and push upward through the epidermis. Blood vessels and nerves are present in the dermis but not in the epidermis. Subcutaneous tissue, which is located below the dermis, is also called superficial fascia. It consists of loose connective tissue and contains fat (adipose) tissue as well.
- The cardiovascular system is a transport system composed of the heart, blood vessels, and blood. It functions to bring nutrients to the tissues and to remove waste products from them.
- One part of the cardiovascular system, the heart, is a hollow, muscular pump about the size of a closed fist. It is located in the mediastinum, which is the space between the lungs. The pericardium is a sac that surrounds the heart. It secretes a lubricating fluid that prevents friction caused by movement of the heart.
- The two small, thin-walled upper chambers of the heart are the right and left atria. They are separated by the thin interatrial septum. The two large lower chambers are the left and right ventricles. Their thick walls are separated by the interventricular septum.
- The cardiac cycle is the sequence of events in one heartbeat. It consists of diastole and systole. The average person has 60–70 cardiac cycles per minute. The number of cardiac cycles in 1 minute is known as the heart rate.
- The vascular system, which is the other part of the cardiovascular system, consists of blood vessels that carry blood from the heart to the lungs and body tissues and back to the heart in a continuous cycle.
- Arteries are blood vessels that transport blood from the heart; these branch off into smaller and smaller arteries. The smallest of the arteries are called the arterioles.
- Capillaries are the tiny blood vessels located between the arterioles and the veins.
- Veins function to collect blood from the capillaries and transport the blood back to the heart. The smallest of the veins are the venules. The veins get larger as they get closer to the heart. The largest veins return blood to the right atrium of the heart.
- Blood pressure is the amount of pressure exerted by the blood on the walls of the blood vessels. The maximum pressure is called systolic pressure; this occurs when the ventricles contract. Diastolic pressure occurs when the ventricles relax. Blood pressure is measured with a sphygmomanometer, a cloth-covered rubber bag that is wrapped around the arm over the brachial artery. Blood pressure is highest during contraction of the heart (systole), which produces systolic blood pressure. Blood pressure is lowest when the heart is relaxing (diastole), which produces diastolic pressure.
- The hepatic portal system begins in the capillaries of the digestive organs and ends in the portal vein. Portal blood, which contains substances absorbed by the stomach and intestines, is passed through the liver, which absorbs, excretes, or converts nutrients and toxins. Restriction of outflow through the hepatic portal system can lead to portal hypertension.
- Blood is a form of connective tissue. It transports nutrients to the individual cells and removes waste products. The cellular components of blood are red blood cells, white blood cells, and platelets. Blood cells float in a thick, straw-colored fluid called plasma. All blood cells are formed in the red bone marrow. Red blood cells, or erythrocytes or red blood corpuscles, constitute more than 90% of the formed elements in blood. Their function is to transport oxygen to the cells and carbon dioxide away from the cells. White blood cells are also known as leukocytes, or white blood corpuscles. Their white color is due to a lack of hemoglobin. Thrombocytes, or platelets, are the smallest cellular elements of the blood. They are important in the blood-clotting process. A special protein, called fibrin, is formed to seal damaged blood vessels by trapping red blood cells, platelets, and fluid to form a clot. This protein also anchors the clot in place.
- The term *arteriosclerosis* means hardening of the arteries and refers to arteries that have become brittle and have lost their elasticity. Although the condition has several causes, the most common and important cause is atherosclerosis, the deposit of fatty plaques in medium-sized and large arteries.
- The lymphatic system collects accumulated tissue fluids from the entire body and returns them to the blood circulation. The system goes one way, beginning in the tissues and ending in the blood vessels. The lymphatics work as an active part of immunity by filtering and destroying foreign substances and microorganisms. Foreign particles and pathogenic bacteria are screened out by lymph nodes that are spaced along the course of the vessels. The lymph nodes also play an active role in digestion by absorbing fats from the small intestine.
- The tiny lymph capillaries are open-ended channels found in the tissue spaces of the entire body except for the brain, spinal cord, and cornea.
- Interstitial fluid surrounds and bathes every cell. It helps transport nutrients and oxygen and remove waste. Lymph capillaries collect the interstitial fluid. Once in the capillaries, the fluid is called lymph. They join to form larger lymph vessels that look like veins but have thinner, more

transparent walls. Like veins, they have valves to prevent backflow.

- Immunity is a complex response which networks all body systems to eliminate any pathogen, foreign substance, or toxic material that may cause damage to the body. The immune system is not a specific structural organ system but rather a functional system. The immune system protects the body directly by cell attack and indirectly by release of mobilizing chemicals and protective antibody molecules. Lymphocytes are the cells of specific immunity because they recognize and destroy specific molecules and have the ability to remember a particular pathogen.

Factual Recall Questions

1. The outer layer of the skin is called the_____.
   a. Epidermis
   b. Dermis
   c. Superficial fascia

2. Which of the following produces dark pigment in the skin?
   a. Dermis
   b. Stratum corneum
   c. Adipose
   d. Melanocytes

3. Erector pili muscles are attached to_____.
   a. Nails
   b. Hair
   c. Fat cells
   d. Lunula

4. Sebum is produced by _____.
   a. Sweat glands
   b. Mammary glands
   c. Sebaceous glands

5. Sweat produced by which of the following glands has the strongest odor?
   a. Eccrine
   b. Apocrine
   c. Ceruminous
   d. Sebaceous

6. What is the first heart chamber to receive blood from the superior and inferior venae cavae?
   a. Right ventricle
   b. Right atrium
   c. Left ventricle
   d. Left atrium

7. Which portion of the cardiac cycle involves relaxation of the ventricles during filling?
   a. Sinoatrial node
   b. Systole
   c. Atrioventricular bundle
   d. Diastole

8. Which of the following is a contagious skin disease?
   a. Impetigo
   b. Alopecia

c. Scleroderma
   d. Vitiligo

9. Which of the following benign skin growths has the greatest potential for becoming malignant?
   a. Angioma
   b. Mole
   c. Lipoma
   d. Freckle

10. A massage professional identifies a few small lumps in the axillary area of a female client. What might be a pathologic concern?
    a. Basal cell carcinoma
    b. Candidiasis
    c. Psoriasis
    d. Fibrocystic disease

11. The heart muscle is called _____.
    a. Pericardium
    b. Myocardium
    c. Epicardium
    d. Endocardium

12. Which of the following heart valves controls the flow of blood from the left ventricle into the aorta?
    a. Atrioventricular
    b. Mitral
    c. Tricuspid
    d. Semilunar

13. Which of the following vessels carries blood to the lungs?
    a. Aorta
    b. Superior vena cava
    c. Pulmonary trunk
    d. Inferior vena cava

14. During a general massage, the massage practitioner notices that the dorsalis pedis pulse is weaker on the left. Where is the practitioner palpating?
    a. Upper arm
    b. Wrist
    c. Knee
    d. Ankle

15. A client reports that they commonly have a blood pressure of 90/50 mm Hg. What would this condition be called?
    a. Tachycardia
    b. Hypertension
    c. Hypotension
    d. Bradycardia

16. Applying deep pressure during massage to the neck near sternocleidomastoid could compress which artery?
    a. Basilar
    b. Carotid
    c. Axillary

17. Deep extended pressure behind the knee is contraindicated by potential damage to which artery?
    a. Celiac
    b. Femoral
    c. Popliteal
    d. Tibial

18. Which of the following veins is located in the arm?
    a. Basilic
    b. Jugular
    c. Renal
    d. Iliac
19. A client has undergone surgery for varicose veins in the legs. Which vein was removed?
    a. Azygos
    b. Brachiocephalic
    c. Hepatic
    d. Saphenous
20. Which of the following contributes to hematopoiesis?
    a. Erythrocyte
    b. Monocyte
    c. Stem cell
    d. Thrombocyte
21. Which of the following results from a temporary deficiency or diminished supply of blood to a tissue?
    a. Aneurysm
    b. Embolus
    c. Thrombus
    d. Ischemia
22. A pulmonary embolism may begin as _____.
    a. Deep vein thrombosis
    b. Hemophilia
    c. Angina pectoris
    d. Arrhythmia
23. Interstitial tissue fluid that has moved into open-ended capillaries is called _____.
    a. Lymphocytes
    b. Lymph
    c. Plasma
    d. Fibrin
24. Both lymphatic ducts empty lymph into the _____.
    a. Mediastinal nodes
    b. Subclavian veins
    c. Mesenteric artery
    d. Cisterna chyli
25. Which of the following stores lymphocytes and blood?
    a. Thymus
    b. Peyer's patches
    c. Bone marrow
    d. Spleen
26. Which of the following is considered contagious?
    a. Hodgkin disease
    b. Mononucleosis
    c. Leukemia
    d. Lymphoma
27. Which results from having had the measles as a child?
    a. Nonspecific immunity
    b. Immune deficiency
    c. Specific immunity
    d. Phagocytosis
28. Antigens are destroyed or suppressed by _____.
    a. The thymus
    b. Antibodies

c. Nonspecific immunity
d. Lymph nodes
29. The immune function of mucus occurs because it _____.
    a. Is sticky
    b. Creates inflammation
    c. Performs phagocytosis
    d. Washes pathogens from the body
30. Allergy is a condition of _____.
    a. Immune system suppression
    b. Lack of T-cell activity
    c. Overactive immune response
    d. Immune deficiency
31. What is the contribution of the urinary system to immune function?
    a. Protective acid balance
    b. Mechanical barrier
    c. Development of lymphocytes
32. Which of the following is considered sterilization for aseptic pathogen control?
    a. Iodine application
    b. Chlorine solution
    c. Alcohol wipes
    d. Extreme heat
33. The most likely transmission route for human immunodeficiency virus (HIV) and hepatitis is _____.
    a. Handshaking
    b. Body fluids
    c. Environmental contact
    d. Droplets in the air
34. Which of the following is a result of congestive heart failure?
    a. Edema
    b. Cerebral atherosclerosis
    c. Aortic aneurysm
35. A ventricular thrombus is located where?
    a. Leg
    b. Brain
    c. Heart
    d. Kidney
36. Which of the following is an autoimmune disorder?
    a. Callus
    b. Stress fracture
    c. Ganglion
    d. Rheumatoid arthritis

Application/Concept Identification and Clinical Reasoning/Synthesis Questions

1. Which of the following are aspects of the venous pump?
    a. Capillaries and arteries
    b. Breathing and muscle contraction
    c. Bradycardia and arrhythmia
2. Which aspect of lymphatic circulation is affected most by skin stretching?
    a. Lymphatic plexuses

b. Superficial lymphatic circulation

c. Deep lymphatic circulation

d. Movement of lymph through nodes

3. Which of the following functions of the integumentary system is supported by maintenance of sanitary procedures?

a. Protecting against water loss

b. Detecting sensory stimuli

c. Preventing entry of bacteria and viruses

4. A massage practitioner notices that a client's skin has a yellowish gold color. This is an indication of _____.

a. Cyanosis

b. Anemia

c. Fever

d. Jaundice

5. A client has a history of heart attack and has reduced blood flow to the heart. Which of the following vessels is most involved?

a. Coronary

b. Left external carotid

c. Celiac

d. Renal

6. A client complains of pooling of blood in the lower extremities. Which of the following circumstances would be a likely cause?

a. Increased walking

b. Lying with the feet above the heart

c. Standing still for extended periods

7. Which of the following would be an indication for referral?

a. A radial pulse of 85 beats per minute

b. A femoral pulse of 55 beats per minute

c. A carotid pulse of 70 beats per minute

d. A dorsalis pedis pulse of 52 beats per minute

8. After a 1-hour massage focused on relaxation, a client becomes dizzy when sitting up. What is the likely cause?

a. Stimulation of baroreceptors

b. Increase in sympathetic stimulation

c. Pulse rate of 65 beats per minute

d. Decrease in parasympathetic tone

9. Massage that provides a pumping compression to the foot encourages lymphatic flow because the _____.

a. Palmar plexus is stimulated

b. Parotid nodes are drained

c. Plantar plexus is stimulated

d. Axillary nodes are drained

10. A client has been experiencing ongoing work and family stress and cannot seem to recover from an upper respiratory infection. The most logical cause is that ongoing stress _____.

a. Increases natural killer cells

b. Supports the development of autoimmune disease

c. Suppresses T-cell activity

d. Decreases cortisol secretion

11. A client is immune suppressed. The physician has approved massage therapy. The most appropriate approach is general massage with _____.

a. Specific use of stimulation techniques to encourage sympathetic dominance

b. Focus on aggressive lymphatic drainage

c. Active stretching to encourage parasympathetic dominance

d. Support for nonspecific homeostatic regulation and restorative sleep

Exercise

Using the previous questions as examples, write at least three more questions. Develop plausible wrong answers and be sure that the correct answer is clearly correct. Then write a rationale for each question. The more questions you write, the better you will understand the material.

RESPIRATORY, DIGESTIVE, URINARY, AND REPRODUCTIVE SYSTEMS

Review Tips

Knowledge of the respiratory, digestive, urinary, and reproductive systems usually is tested through factual recall and comprehension questions. Pathologic conditions for each of these systems are targeted in examination questions. Another focus of question development is to connect the anatomy and physiology of each body system to specific applications of massage. The classic example is massage targeted to influence the respiratory and digestive systems. Massage during pregnancy requires an understanding of the gestation and birthing processes, so this content does appear in examination questions.

As explained previously, you must know the definition of each term and must be able to use each term correctly. More complex questions use the terminology in the question and possible answers, and unless you can decipher the language, you will not know what the question or the provided answers mean. Use the study tools in this guide, and make sure that when you read your textbooks, you know what the words mean. Also make sure that you understand the meaning of general language used in the questions. If you are not sure of the meaning of a word, look it up in the dictionary.

Quick Content Review

- Respiration is the movement of air into and out of the lungs, the exchange of oxygen and carbon dioxide between the lungs and the blood, and the exchange of oxygen and carbon dioxide between blood and body tissues.

- The lower two-thirds of the external nose is composed mostly of cartilage. The upper third, or bridge of the nose, is formed from two small hard nasal bones. The tip of the nose is the apex, and the nostrils are the nares. The nasal cavity is the actual space inside the external and internal nose structures. It is separated into left and right sides by the septum, a partition composed of cartilage and bone. At the upper portion of the nasal cavity, three thin curled bones—the turbinates, or conchae—project inward from the two outer walls. Venous areas called swell bodies are located on the turbinates.

- The sinuses are four groups of air-filled spaces that open into the frontal, ethmoid, sphenoid, and maxillary bones of the skull. The nasopharynx is the continuation of the nasal cavity into the throat, or pharynx. The larynx, or voice box, connects the pharynx to the trachea. Its structure consists of cartilage, ligaments, connective tissue, muscles, and vocal cords. The vocal cords and the spaces between the cords are located inside the glottis.

- The trachea, or windpipe, is the main airway to the lungs. It is a 4- to 5-inch tube that begins at the glottis and ends at the junction of the two main bronchi near the level of the sternal angle.

- The two lungs are the primary organs of respiration. These soft, spongy, highly vascular structures are separated into left and right lungs by the mediastinum. The diaphragm is a dome-shaped sheet of muscle attached to the thoracic wall that separates the lungs and the thoracic cavity from the abdominal cavity.

- During the seconds before a breath is taken, the pressure inside the lungs and that outside the body are equal, whereas the pressure inside the pleural space is slightly lower. When inhalation begins, the external intercostal muscles between the ribs contract, lifting the lower ribs up and out. This creates a vacuum that expands the lungs, causing the pressure inside the lungs to decrease. The diaphragm moves down, increasing the volume of the pleural cavities and decreasing the pressure even further. Elastic fibers in the alveolar walls stretch, permitting expansion of the air sacs. The lungs draw in air until the pressure is equal again.

- During exhalation, pressure inside the pleural cavity increases; the external intercostals, diaphragm, and alveolar walls relax; the volume inside the lungs decreases; and the pressure in the lungs increases until it again equals the air pressure. The respiratory rate in adults is about 12–16 breaths per minute. In the newborn, the respiratory rate is about 35 and gradually decreases to adult values at about age 20. Emotions are a powerful stimulus for respiratory change. Fear, grief, and shock slow the respiratory rate; anger and sexual arousal increase the respiratory rate.

- The digestive tract consists of the mouth, pharynx, esophagus, stomach, small intestine, large intestine, rectum, and anus. Accessory structures include the salivary glands, pancreas, liver, and gallbladder. Digestion begins in the mouth and ends in the small intestine and is accompanied by digestive enzymes (protein catalysts) that split large substances into small ones. The gastrointestinal tract contains glands that secrete mucus and digestive enzymes.

- The abdomen, or abdominal cavity, contains the major organs of digestion. The cavity is lined with a mucous membrane, the peritoneum, the function of which is to prevent friction.

- Products of digestion are propelled along the tract from the esophagus to the anus by the rhythmic contraction of smooth muscle called peristalsis. Digestive secretion generally refers to the release of various substances from the exocrine glands that serve the digestive system. Digestive secretion includes the release of saliva, gastric juice, pancreatic juice, bile, and intestinal juice.

- The citric acid cycle is the main pathway by which energy in food is released by cells to manufacture their own energy-rich ATP.

- The four essential steps in the process of digestion are as follows:
  1. Ingestion: Food entering the mouth.
  2. Digestion: The mechanical and chemical breakdown of food from its complex form into simple molecules.
  3. Absorption: These simple molecules are moved from the digestive tract to the circulatory or lymphatic system; vitamins and minerals are absorbed in the small intestine; amino acids, simple sugars, and small fatty acids pass through the intestinal villi into the bloodstream; the larger fatty acids are reconstituted to fats in the intestinal wall and pass into the lymphatic system; capillaries of the intestinal villi become venules and then veins; and finally, the large portal vein carries absorbed nutrient molecules to the liver. The liver converts these substances into compounds required for bodily functions.
  4. Elimination (egestion): Removal and release of solid waste products from food that cannot be digested or absorbed.

- The main food groups are proteins, carbohydrates, and fats.
  1. Proteins are large, high-molecular-weight substances that contain carbon, hydrogen, oxygen, nitrogen, and smaller amounts of other elements. Proteins break down into amino acids. The body uses 24 amino acids for its metabolic requirements. Dietary proteins include animal products and bean and grain combinations. Proteins are the chief structural components of the body.
  2. Carbohydrates: Complex carbohydrates are long chains of glucose molecules found in rice and vegetables. Glucose is the main fuel for the manufacture of ATP in the cell. Sugars are converted to glucose in the liver.
  3. Fats: In addition to serving as a reservoir of stored energy, fats are essential components of the cell membrane and myelin sheath of the nerve fiber. Dietary fats are found in nuts, seeds, oils, and animal products.

- The urinary system includes the kidneys, ureters, and bladder.

1. Kidneys: The kidneys are reddish brown, bean-shaped organs located on the posterior wall of the abdomen against the back body wall musculature, just above the waist. The kidneys are embedded in fat and are located about the spinal level of T11 to L3 on each side of the vertebral column. The right kidney is lower than the left because of its displacement by the liver. An adrenal gland sits on top of each kidney.

2. Ureters: Ureters are two narrow tubes that extend from the kidney and connect to the bladder. The two ureters lie anterior to the psoas muscles.

3. Bladder (urinary bladder): The urinary bladder, a reservoir for urine, is a muscular, baglike organ that lies in the pelvis.

4. Urethra: The urethra is the tube that carries urine from the bladder. The opening at the end of the urethra is called the meatus.

- In the average person, the kidneys filter about 100 L of blood per day, reabsorbing 99 L of filtrate and leaving about 1 L of urine.

- Water is a constituent of all living things. The water content of the tissues of the body varies. Adipose tissue (fat) has the lowest percent of water; the skeleton has the second lowest water content.

- The male and female reproductive systems are as follows:

1. The male reproductive system consists of the testicles, epididymis, vas deferens, ejaculatory duct, urethra, penis, and scrotum. The testicles contain tiny seminiferous tubules that produce sperm. The prostate gland surrounds the urethra and produces a milky alkaline fluid.

2. The female reproductive system is designed for childbearing. The system consists of two ovaries, two fallopian tubes, a uterus, and a vagina. Also included in the system are the external genitalia and mammary glands. The ovaries are solid glands that produce the hormones estrogen and progesterone. The external female genitalia are known collectively as the vulva.

- Pregnancy

1. Gestation takes approximately 38–40 weeks and is divided into trimesters. At the beginning of the second trimester, the baby weighs almost 2 ounces. The bones are growing and the muscle movement is increasing. The last trimester is mostly a weight-gaining and maturing process that prepares the baby for life outside the womb. Various physiologic changes occur for the pregnant individual during these periods as well. The first trimester is a time of radical hormonal changes. Changes may consist of moodiness, fatigue, possible back pain, constipation, and energy-level changes. In the second trimester, appetite increases, blood volume increases, and the body places additional workload on all physiologic functions. The last trimester finds the person heavy with the baby, and posture changes are evident. Internal organs are crowded. Physiologic systems are strained by sustaining the pregnant individual and baby. The connective tissue structure of the body is altered by softening, to allow for the expansion needed for the birth. This is a time of rest and waiting.

2. The hormone oxytocin stimulates contraction of the uterus. Prelabor can begin at any point in the last few weeks or last days of pregnancy. The cervix at this stage softens and may start to thin out a little, which allows it to dilate (open up) slightly. As the baby's head presses down against the amniotic membranes that contain fluid, the membranes may break, producing what is known as "breaking the water." This is the classic prelabor symptom.

Factual Recall Questions

1. Which of the following is a mechanical action of inhalation and exhalation that draws oxygen into the lungs and releases carbon dioxide into the atmosphere?
   a. Breathing
   b. External respiration
   c. Internal respiration

2. The nasal cavity is separated into right and left portions by the _____.
   a. Nares
   b. Sinuses
   c. Ethmoid
   d. Septum

3. The air sacs in the lungs are called _____.
   a. Epiglottis
   b. Bronchioles
   c. Lobes
   d. Alveoli

4. A client is displaying behavior consistent with sympathetic nervous system dominance. What would be the state of the bronchioles?
   a. Bronchodilation
   b. Bronchoconstriction
   c. Pneumothorax
   d. Hyperventilation

5. Why would a person with a spinal cord injury at C6 be able to breathe without a ventilator?
   a. The intercostal nerves exit at C5.
   b. The phrenic nerve originates at C3.
   c. The mediastinum is intact.
   d. The pleural cavity is innervated at C1.

6. The external intercostal muscles create a vacuum in the thorax because the _____.
   a. Upper ribs expand
   b. Ribs are pulled together
   c. Lower ribs are lifted up and out
   d. Diaphragm muscle arches upward

7. Which of the following is contagious?
   a. Tuberculosis
   b. Hay fever
   c. Emphysema
   d. Cystic fibrosis

8. What supports addictive behavior related to food consumption?
   a. Need for nutrients
   b. Pleasure sensations
   c. Energy requirement
9. The abdominal cavity is lined by a mucous membrane called the _____.
   a. Peritoneum
   b. Synovium
   c. Omentum
   d. Mesentery
10. The enzyme amylase found in saliva is part of the digestive process for _____.
    a. Proteins
    b. Fats
    c. Lipids
    d. Carbohydrates
11. The folds in the stomach that expand when food is ingested are called _____.
    a. Bolus
    b. Rugae
    c. Chyme
    d. Pylorus
12. Which portion of the small intestine contains ducts from the liver, gallbladder, and pancreas?
    a. Ileum
    b. Jejunum
    c. Duodenum
    d. Mesentery
13. Which of the following acts as a digestive organ and also detoxifies the blood?
    a. Pancreas
    b. Stomach
    c. Liver
    d. Gallbladder
14. A major function of the large intestine is to _____.
    a. Absorb water
    b. Concentrate bile
    c. Remove and store glycogen
    d. Convert amino acids
15. Which of the following structures of the colon also contains lymphatic tissue?
    a. Cecum
    b. Appendix
    c. Ascending colon
    d. Sigmoid colon
16. The food source that breaks down into amino acids is _____.
    a. Protein
    b. Carbohydrate
    c. Fat
17. Which of the following pathologic conditions of the digestive system affects the liver?
    a. Cystic fibrosis
    b. Diverticular disease
    c. Cirrhosis
    d. Gastritis
18. Which of the following conditions is contagious?
    a. Appendicitis
    b. Hepatitis
    c. Reflux esophagitis
    d. Irritable bowel syndrome
19. Which of the following conditions is considered a medical emergency and requires immediate referral?
    a. Gastroenteritis
    b. Peptic ulcer disease
    c. Inflammatory bowel disease
    d. Strangulated hernia
20. Micturition is _____.
    a. Parasympathetic action to void urine
    b. Sympathetic action to increase the retention of feces
    c. Movement of blood through the nephrons
21. When stretch receptors signal that the bladder needs to empty, what muscle contracts?
    a. Pectineus
    b. Coccygeus
    c. Pyramidalis
    d. Detrusor
22. Cystitis is _____.
    a. Inflammation of the medulla of the kidney
    b. Infection of the glomerulus
    c. Bladder infection
    d. Obstruction of the urethra
23. Erectile tissue is able to become firmer because _____.
    a. This tissue becomes engorged with blood
    b. Muscles contract, stiffening the tissue
    c. The tissue absorbs water from the lymph
    d. Smooth muscles encircle the tissue, acting as a sphincter
24. Which of the following secretes a lubricating fluid in the female external genitalia?
    a. Fundus
    b. Bartholin gland
    c. Clitoris
    d. Symphysis pubis
25. During sexual development in the female, which occurs last?
    a. Hypothalamus matures.
    b. Estradiol is produced.
    c. Adrenal cortex hormone signals pubic hair growth.
    d. Ovulation
26. The alkaline role of semen is to _____.
    a. Stimulate orgasm
    b. Counteract the acidic nature of vaginal fluid
    c. Thin the protective coating of the ovum
    d. Lubricate the ejaculatory duct
27. Which of the following sexually transmitted diseases has a bacterial origin?
    a. Genital warts
    b. Herpes genitalis

   c. Gonorrhea

   d. Hepatitis B

28. A 56-year-old male client complains of difficulty voiding urine. What would be the most likely diagnosis from his physician?

   a. Endometriosis

   b. *Trichomoniasis* vaginitis

   c. Bartholin cyst

   d. Benign prostatic hyperplasia

29. The amount of energy expended by the body at any given time is called _____.

   a. Citric acid cycle

   b. Total metabolic rate

   c. Basal metabolic rate

   d. Digestion

30. Most body water is located in _____.

   a. Interstitial fluid

   b. Lymph

   c. Intracellular fluid

   d. Plasma

31. Force exerted by water is called _____.

   a. Hydrostatic pressure

   b. Dehydration

   c. Osmosis

   d. Electrolyte balance

32. Which of the following is a medical emergency?

   a. Lactation

   b. Vaginitis

   c. Ectopic pregnancy

   d. Prelabor

Application/Concept Identification and Clinical Reasoning/Synthesis Questions

1. During the first trimester, progesterone increases. Which of the following results can therapeutic massage directly and mechanically influence?

   a. Increased urination

   b. Constipation

   c. Nausea

   d. Lymphatic stagnation

2. A client complains of a congested nose and low back stiffness. What is the logical connection between the two?

   a. Respiratory mucus is too thin and allows bacteria to enter the body, causing a kidney infection.

   b. Swell bodies in the nose are unable to function properly, so normal movement during sleep is disrupted.

   c. Olfactory nerves are increasing parasympathetic arousal, causing an increase in muscle tension.

   d. Nasal congestion is blocking the sinus cavities and the inner ear, changing muscle tone in the lower extremities.

3. During assessment, a client is observed with mild tachypnea, tension in the muscles of the neck and shoulder, and nervousness. Which of the following is the most likely reason?

   a. Nitrogen levels have risen and oxygen levels have decreased, creating a decrease in tidal volume.

   b. Oxyhemoglobin is saturated with carbon dioxide, and the muscles display tetany.

   c. An increase in carbon dioxide in the blood is triggering sympathetic activation.

   d. Oxygen levels have increased and carbon dioxide levels have dropped, predisposing to a breathing pattern disorder.

4. Massage methods that modulate the breathing rhythm also _____.

   a. Predispose a person to pulmonary embolism

   b. Suppress treatment for sleep apnea

   c. Interact with the autonomic nervous system

   d. Interfere with most meditation methods

5. A client has severely limited all dietary fat. Which of the following might occur?

   a. Inability to digest protein

   b. Difficulty with hormone production

   c. Interference with the absorption of water-soluble vitamins

6. Appropriate massage for the colon begins at the _____.

   a. Ascending colon, ends at the rectum, and moves toward the cecum

   b. Sigmoid colon and ends at the cecum, with directional flow toward the rectum

   c. Rectum and ends at the cecum, with directional flow toward the cecum

   d. Splenic flexure and ends at the hepatic flexure, with directional flow toward the sigmoid colon

7. Massage may be contraindicated for those with renal insufficiency because massage _____.

   a. Causes an increase in blood pressure

   b. Increases blood volume through the kidneys

   c. Spreads bacteria through the urinary system

   d. Increases the difficulty with incontinence

8. Thirty minutes into a relaxation massage, a male client has an erection. What is the most logical reason for this response?

   a. The client has been "sexualizing" the massage.

   b. Erection is a parasympathetic response.

   c. Stimulation of the skin shifts blood flow.

   d. Activation of sympathetic reflexes triggers the response.

9. If a client is in the second trimester of a pregnancy, the application of massage _____.

   a. Will be most comfortable if it is given with the client prone

   b. Will be most comfortable if the client is positioned on their side

   c. Of the feet is contraindicated

   d. Should focus most on lymphatic drainage

10. During massage, a lactating client experiences the let-down response. The most likely cause is that massage _____.

a. Stimulates the release of oxytocin
b. Stimulates the production of testosterone
c. Decreases colostrum
11. A client with a diagnosis of asthma is referred for massage. What would be the most likely benefits of massage?
 a. Activation of the sympathetic nervous system that would support bronchoconstriction
 b. Reduction in anxiety and increased mobility of the ribs
 c. Stimulation of the client's ability to inhale but inhibition of excessive exhalation
 d. Increase in the tone of respiratory muscles, supporting effective exhalation
12. A regular client reports various digestive upsets, including dry mouth and constipation. The physician who wants a treatment plan and justification has cleared the client for massage. Which of the following would be the best plan to submit to the physician?
 a. Stimulating massage coupled with instruction on self-help breathing, producing an increase in oxygen and a decrease in carbon dioxide to support ongoing ANS sympathetic dominance
 b. General massage combined with deep massage to the colon to suppress peristalsis and break down concentrated fecal matter
 c. General massage focused to generate relaxation with diaphragmatic breathing and rhythmic stroking to the colon to stimulate peristalsis
 d. General massage to create parasympathetic dominance and lymphatic drainage, with visceral massage to the liver to increase detoxification and support upper chest breathing
13. A client is experiencing weakness and exhaustion; impaired concentration, memory, and performance; disturbed sleep; and emotional sweating. A complete physical has ruled out any existing pathologic condition. Stress is indicated as a probable cause. The treatment plan that would most likely reverse the stress response is massage to_____.
 a. Promote lymphatic drainage and stimulate arterial circulation
 b. Support proper breathing function and reverse breathing pattern disorder

c. Reduce scar tissue and prevent adhesions
d. Stimulate an increase in heart rate and blood pressure
14. A couple has experienced difficulties conceiving a third child. The doctors can find no reason for the difficulties. The couple asks whether massage could be of help. The answer is yes. The most logical justification is that massage can _____.
 a. Assist in the success of sexual intercourse by encouraging adrenaline secretion
 b. Increase the rate of ovulation by stimulating the hypothalamus to secrete follicle-stimulating hormone
 c. Encourage more efficient homeostatic mechanisms in the body, thereby promoting general health, including fertility
 d. Increase the levels of testosterone, prolactin, and progesterone, thus promoting ovulation
15. A massage therapist feels restless on days off and finds it difficult to sleep. The most logical reason for this phenomenon is that providing massage _____.
 a. Usually promotes a parasympathetic response in the client and the practitioner; on days without performing massage, the practitioner fails to stimulate relaxation responses as effectively.
 b. Is fatiguing; on days off, the massage practitioner has more energy.
 c. Interferes with natural entrainment responses, and on days off, the practitioner is more in tune with biorhythms.
 d. Increases adrenaline and other stimulating hormones and neurotransmitters; when this occurs, hyperventilation syndrome is common, resulting in restlessness and sleep disturbance.

Exercise

Using the previous questions as examples, write at least three more questions, one of each type: factual recall and comprehension, application and concept identification, and clinical reasoning and synthesis. Develop plausible wrong answers and be sure that the correct answer is clearly correct. Then write a rationale for each question. The more questions you write, the better you will understand the material.

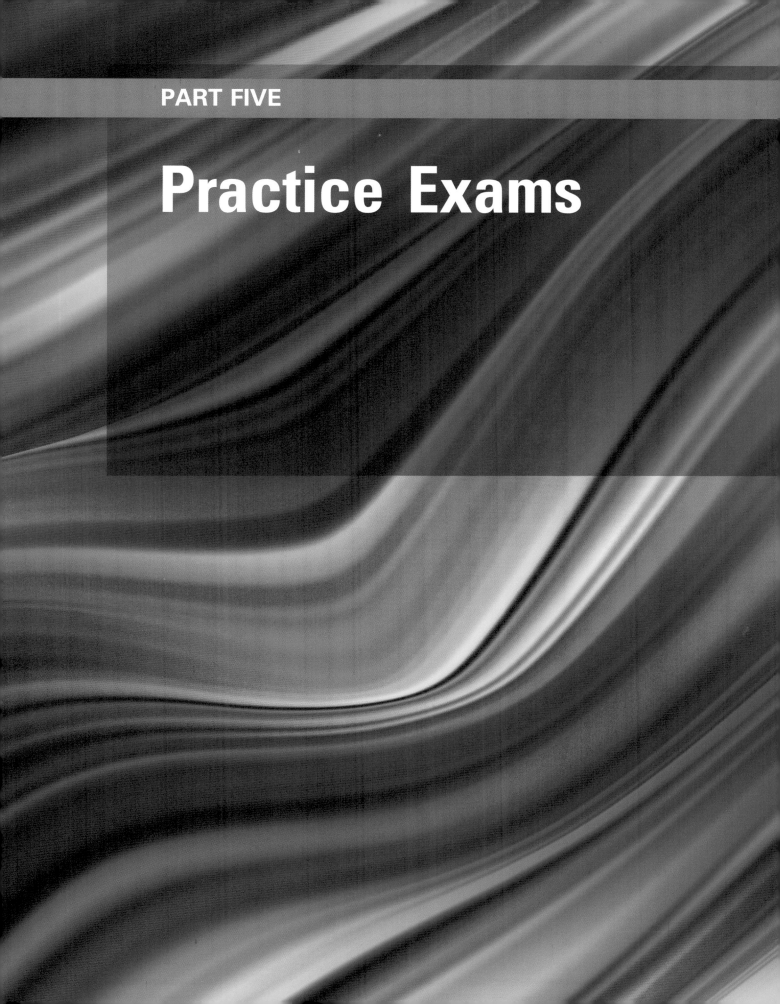

PART FIVE

Practice Exams

CHAPTER 9

Practice Exams

This portion of the review process targets actual exam-taking skills. The questions reflect the writing style and content found on the MBLEx. You will notice that the questions are more concisely written than in previous chapters. Also, the multiple-choice questions are based on three instead of four possible answers. There are five exams with a total of 700 questions. The mock exam is formulated to reflect the actual MBLEX exam with questions in all categories at the proper ratio with a total of 100 questions. The other four practice exams target content areas: anatomy and physiology 150 questions, kinesiology 100, pathology 175, and massage theory and practice 175.

In the answer key is found in Appendix C. Each question has a rationale for why the correct answer is the best answer and why the wrong answers are incorrect. Attempt to understand all aspects of each rationale.

Remember, these specific questions will not be on any licensing exam. No review guide or website presents the actual questions that appear on the exams. Just because you know the answers to all the questions on practice exams does not mean you will pass the licensing exam, or any other certification exam. When practicing, focus less on getting the answers right. Focus more on language and critical thinking.

What the practice exams help you do is develop test-taking skills. Try to complete one question every minute—that is, 60 questions in an hour. It is easy to get stuck on a question and waste time. If you are not able to confidently identify the answer to a particular question in 1 minute, skip it and move on.

Use the Evolve website provided with this review guide to take several additional practice exams. Again, the practice exam study strategy is to develop the ability to complete one question each minute, and to be confident when the question content and type are randomized.

Be smart while you study. Review content multiple times in multiple ways. Practice problem solving. Work on timing.

PRACTICE TEST 1

Mock Exam Modeling the MBLEx—100 Questions

The questions are randomized. The distribution of topics tested will be as follows:

Anatomy and Physiology 11% 11 questions.

Kinesiology 12% 12 questions.

Pathology, Contraindications, Areas of Caution, Special Population 14% 14 questions.

Benefits and Physiological Effects of Techniques that Manipulate Soft Tissue 15% 15 questions.

Client Assessment Reassessment and Treatment Planning 17% 17 questions.

Ethics, Boundaries, Laws, and Regulations 16% 16 questions.

Guidelines for Professional Practice 15% 15 questions.

1. When a massage/bodywork session reduces the client's stress response, what is an effect on arteries?
   a. Vasoconstriction
   b. Increased blood pressure
   c. Decreased arterial pressure

2. A common term used to describe energetic anatomy is
   a. nerve.
   b. meridian.
   c. self-care.

3. The area of the brain involved with control of balance, posture, eye movement, and coordination of movement is the
   a. cerebellum.
   b. medulla.
   c. thalamus.

4. Targeting massage/bodywork application to the shoulder would involve understanding
   a. regional anatomy.
   b. developmental anatomy.
   c. gross anatomy.

5. In what location would pressure applied during massage need to be adapted during the menstrual cycle?
   a. Anterior thorax
   b. Hypogastric
   c. Upper left quadrant

6. What structure allows some materials to enter the cell and keeps others out?
   a. Cytoplasm
   b. Cell membrane
   c. Lysosome

7. How does the stomach support immunity?
   a. Secretion of hydrochloric acid
   b. Suppression of mucus production
   c. Production of antibodies

8. What structure is referred to as the pacemaker of the heart?
   a. Left ventricle
   b. Atrioventricular node
   c. Sinoatrial node

9. What structure lines the abdominopelvic cavity and enfolds the internal organs?
   a. Peritoneum
   b. Pericardium
   c. Visceral

10. A structure that secretes androgens is located in the
    a. cranium.
    b. trunk.
    c. pleura.

11. Muscle spindles are most sensitive to what type of stimulus?
    a. Slow lengthening
    b. Rapid lengthening
    c. Sudden shortening

12. During massage an uptake of interstitial fluid occurs at the
    a. lymph nodes.
    b. ventricles.
    c. lymph capillaries.

13. A massage practitioner is assessing a knee sprain in the subacute healing phase by asking the client to move the knee while the practitioner applies a counter force. The type of joint movement is
    a. passive.
    b. assisted.
    c. resistive.

14. Active movement during a massage session would be used to assess which joint type?
    a. Diarthrosis
    b. Cartilaginous
    c. Syndesmoses

15. When standing still in front of a closed door and pushing on it without it moving, the muscle action is
    a. eccentric.
    b. isotonic.
    c. isometric.

16. What is similar to the social security and Medicare taxes withheld from the pay of most employees?
    a. Income tax
    b. Self-employment tax
    c. Worker's compensation

17. The hip joint is abducted. The massage practitioner asks the client to move the hip toward the midline. How would the muscle group that returns the hip to the anatomical position be functioning?
    a. Shortening
    b. Lengthening
    c. Stabilizing

18. A massage client points to the ischial tuberosity as a location of discomfort. What muscle(s) would the massage practitioner assess in the indicated area?
    a. Sartorius
    b. Quadriceps
    c. Hamstrings

19. The healthcare provider system adopted by the U.S. Department of Health and Human Services as part of the implementation of the Health Insurance Portability and Accountability Act (HIPAA) uses a/n
    a. Employer Identification Number (EIN).
    b. National Provider Identification number (NPI).
    c. Taxpayer Identification Number (TIN).

20. A massage practitioner functioning as sole proprietor is organizing a list of business expenses to inform decisions on fee structure for services. There needs to be sufficient profit from the business to cover personal expenses of $40,000 per year. If the business expenses are $25,000 per year and the person estimates 20 hours of income-producing sessions per week based on 50 working weeks per year, what is the minimum fee for service for each hour?
    a. $90
    b. $50
    c. $65

21. A massage client is asked to abduct the arms. The observed action would be
    a. arms move over abdomen.
    b. arms move toward trunk.
    c. arms move away from trunk.

22. What is an accurate description of flexion at the lumbar spine?
    a. Decreasing lordosis
    b. Increasing lordosis
    c. Decreasing kyphosis

23. What ingredient in a massage lubricant product could produce anaphylaxis?
    a. Alcohol
    b. Water
    c. Nuts

24. An active ingredient in antiseptics is
    a. isopropyl alcohol.
    b. sodium hypochlorite.
    c. quaternary ammonium.

25. A massage practitioner is palpating muscles that are synergists. Where is the assessment occurring?
    a. Latissimus dorsi and teres major
    b. Gluteus medius and adductor magnus
    c. Supraspinatus and pectoralis minor

26. Two regular clients are longtime friends. During the session it is common for the clients to talk to the practitioner about each other. Occasionally they will ask a question about their friend. What is the best response of the massage practitioner?
    a. It makes me nervous when you talk about your friend during the session.
    b. Confidentiality requirements do not allow me to share information about other clients.
    c. I can only answer your question because both of you are friends and clients.

27. Which of the following would be considered sexual harassment?
    a. A coworker gossiping about pay scales
    b. A practitioner explaining sexual boundaries
    c. A client telling inappropriate jokes

28. Contraction of which muscle produces extension of the head?
    a. Longus capitis
    b. Spinalis cervicis
    c. Longus colli

29. The manifestation of disease is best described as
    a. acute episode of a chronic illness.
    b. subjective feelings of discomfort.
    c. signs and symptoms.

30. What is it called when there is a localized abnormal dilation of a blood vessel, usually an artery, which creates a weakness in the wall of the vessel?
    a. Aneurysm
    b. Cerebrovascular accident (CVA)
    c. Edema

31. A joint classified based on function would be
    a. symphyses.
    b. synarthrosis.
    c. synovial joint.

32. While performing a postural analysis with a massage client, the practitioner identifies that the palms of client's hands are facing the greater trochanter. What muscle is short?
    a. Triceps
    b. Latissimus dorsi
    c. Anterior serratus

33. A massage practitioner talks about personal issues during the massage session, and the client has complained to the desk staff. This is an example of
    a. breach in confidentiality.
    b. fostering dual relationships.
    c. breach of professional boundaries.

34. The treatment room has a mirror on the wall that can reflect the client's body during the session. The massage practitioner looks into the mirror as the client moves the drapes to change position and will occasionally see portions of the body undraped. This is
    a. sexual misconduct.
    b. therapeutic alliance.
    c. values conflict.

35. Lack of exercise during an illness may cause skeletal muscle to undergo
    a. hypertrophy.
    b. atrophy.
    c. regeneration.

36. What condition is caused by a virus?
    a. Hepatitis
    b. MRSA
    c. Thrush

37. A massage client indicates on the intake that they have a hernia just below the rib cage and above the abdomen. What type of hernia would this be?
    a. Umbilical
    b. Hiatal
    c. Inguinal

38. If a massage client has autonomy in a healthcare relationship, it means
    a. ability to pay for services.
    b. self-determination.
    c. right to medical insurance.

39. A high school football player was diagnosed with an anterior shoulder dislocation following a tackle. Which of the following nerves is most likely damaged in this scenario?
    a. Radial
    b. Median
    c. Axillary

40. When a massage practitioner refuses to perform a method that is contraindicated, which ethical principle is upheld?
    a. Proportionality
    b. Nonmaleficence
    c. Justice

41. A transient decrease in blood pressure that occurs when a massage client sits up after the session is known as
    a. orthostatic hypotension.
    b. myocardial ischemia.
    c. vasodilation.

42. When developing a massage care plan for a client with an injury to the medial collateral ligament of the knee, when does the inflammatory phase of healing begin?
    a. 2—3 weeks after injury
    b. First days after injury
    c. 4—6 weeks after injury

43. A massage method that presses, twists, and rolls soft tissue is
    a. kneading.
    b. vibration.
    c. gliding.

44. Which of the following diseases has as primary symptoms tremor and rigidity?
    a. Multiple sclerosis
    b. Alzheimer's disease
    c. Parkinson's disease

45. An area where applied pressure during the massage is adapted to target skin and superficial facia to protect deeper structures from compression is the
    a. anterior triangle of the neck.
    b. plantar aspect of the foot.
    c. anterior thigh.

46. A massage practitioner prefers to work with clients who are experiencing limited ability to perform activities of daily living. How would the practitioner market to this client population?
    a. Describe how massage therapy supports a meditation practice for stress management
    b. Focus on outcome goals related to improved mobility
    c. Promote a facility that offers amenities and ambiance for a soothing experience

47. The massage practitioner performs postassessment to
    a. determine scope of practice.
    b. identify contraindications.
    c. evaluate response to previous treatment.

48. A bodywork approach that targets connective tissue by modifying application to glide superficial tissue is
    a. lymphatic drainage.
    b. polarity therapy.
    c. myofascial release.

49. The approach to care that acknowledges the whole person is
    a. biopsychosocial.
    b. based on fixed outcomes.
    c. population specialization.

50. What massage method is applied with the lightest pressure range?
    a. Kneading
    b. Holding
    c. Shaking

51. Beneficial results experienced by clients related to soft-tissue methods applied during massage are primarily from
    a. fluid exchange in the blood and lymph systems.
    b. biomechanical changes in posture.
    c. regulatory mechanisms of the nervous system.

52. What condition could a client experience with the most potential for massage/bodywork benefit and the fewest cautions?
    a. Pancreatitis
    b. Tension headache
    c. Pulmonary edema

53. What is an evidence-informed benefit of massage therapy for a client diagnosed with cancer?
    a. Detoxing the body of cancer cells
    b. Increasing the action of chemotherapy
    c. Reducing pain and anxiety

54. How does the outcome for the session influence the sequence of the massage session?
    a. A session based on improved mobility is interspersed with assessment and interventions.
    b. An outcome based on stress management will require a longer session and participation by the client.
    c. An outcome targeting systemic pain management will result in shorter, more frequent sessions.

55. What condition requires the massage practitioner be most cautious with pressure intensity during method application?
    a. Plantar fasciitis
    b. Diverticulosis
    c. Rheumatoid arthritis

56. Selective serotonin reuptake inhibitors (SSRIs) are generally prescribed for which condition?
    a. Depression
    b. Hypertension
    c. Diabetes

57. What massage method is indicated as an intervention when a small local area is targeted?
    a. Joint movement
    b. Friction
    c. Gliding

58. The most consistent research finding related to massage therapy benefits is
    a. decreased response of somatic reflex regulation.
    b. changes in systemic blood flow.
    c. modulation in the autonomic nervous system.

59. An example of a bodywork method that combines hydrotherapy and thermotherapy is
    a. hot stones.
    b. warm foot soak.
    c. counterirritant ointment.

60. A client indicates on the health history form that they have diabetes. What would be the next best action the massage practitioner takes?
    a. Ask clarifying questions about medication
    b. Refer client to a practitioner who works in a medical setting
    c. Proceed with posture and gait assessment

61. A massage client requests moderate pressure and tissue elongation. What combination of methods will best accomplish this result?
    a. Friction combined with vibration
    b. Compression combined with gliding
    c. Kneading combined with shaking

62. What is the most biologically plausible effect of soft-tissue manipulation on fascia?
    a. Releases fascial adhesions
    b. Changes the length of collagen fibers
    c. May promote sliding in the fascial layers

63. Methods applied during massage that twist tissue specifically create what type of soft-tissue deformation?
    a. Shear
    b. Torsion
    c. Compression

64. An immediate effect of a cold pack is
    a. histamine response.
    b. vasodilatation.
    c. vasoconstriction.

65. A massage practitioner notices a client has an altered gait and walks with a limp. What assessment type is providing this information?
    a. Orthopedic tests
    b. Visual
    c. Muscle strength

66. A client demonstrates a movement that is difficult for them to perform. What form of assessment is the massage practitioner performing?
    a. History
    b. Postural
    c. Visual

67. A bodywork form using compression over loose clothing is
    a. shiatsu.
    b. Swedish.
    c. manual lymph drain.

68. What is the massage practitioner performing when applying pressure in an area without movement?
    a. Compression
    b. Drag
    c. Friction

69. When a massage practitioner uses palpation to assess the client, they are
    a. touching the client.
    b. assessing activities of daily living.
    c. taking an accurate history.

70. Observation of a client's symmetry in the sagittal plane would be a form of
    a. treatment planning.
    b. postural assessment.
    c. documentation.

71. Discussion of the health history with the massage client is necessary to
    a. refer to other health professionals.
    b. determine session time.
    c. identify contraindications.

72. A client asks why a health history is taken prior to the session. What is the best response by the massage practitioner?
    a. State legislation mandates that all clients complete a form with contact information
    b. Decisions based on the information provided help determine contraindications and adaptations to care
    c. Client files include a health history form, informed consent form, and SOAP notes

73. During the session, the massage practitioner identifies a rash on the back of the client's legs. This was not disclosed prior to the session. The practitioner discusses the finding with the client. The client indicates that this occurs when they shave their legs. The client is a long-distance bicyclist and wants the hamstring area addressed. What is the initial dilemma faced by the practitioner?
    a. Explaining to the client the area needs to be avoided
    b. How to adapt to work on the area
    c. Evaluating if the rash is a local contraindication

74. A client has been diagnosed with an inflamed gallbladder diagnosed as chronic cholecystitis and will be undergoing surgery in a week. They would like a massage therapy session for stress. What is the most logical approach?
    a. The client could receive a modified session with appropriate adaption
    b. The practitioner would need to postpone the session
    c. The client's doctor would need to provide specific treatment directions

75. A client fell and hit their head when leaving home to receive their the bodywork session. There is a noticeable bump on the head and the client indicates they experienced visual disturbances right after the fall that cleared within minutes. They drove alone to the facility. They indicate they feel fine except for a dull headache and are ready for the session. What is the next action for the massage practitioner to take?
    a. Provide the session and call emergency contact on file so they can take them home
    b. Explain that head injury is serious and that they should immediately seek medical assessment
    c. Perform a balance assessment and assess to make sure eye pupils are equal. Then address headache

76. A massage practitioner is communicating with a client about evidence-informed practice related to client requested outcomes. This is considered an aspect of
    a. professional boundaries.
    b. dealing with conflict.
    c. realistic session goals.

77. A client with a gift card for a massage therapy session is unsure what to expect during and after the session. The client has not had a massage previously. Which outcome would be best for the practitioner to suggest for this client for the first session?
    a. Well-being
    b. Pain relief
    c. Increased mobility

78. What position of the massage client supports reduction of simple edema in the foot?
    a. Supine with lower legs elevated
    b. Supine with knees bent and heels on the table
    c. Prone with lower legs flat on the table

79. A client is seeking massage therapy for stress management and neck stiffness. The client is uncomfortable prone. The thought process of the practitioner is to use the side-lying position to best access the thorax and cervical area. What is the practitioner doing?
    a. Performing an intake assessment
    b. Developing a treatment strategy
    c. Determining outcome goals

80. A client prefers to remain clothed during the session. The massage practitioner informs the client that this is possible and requests the client to wear loose clothing to the session. How has the practitioner adapted for this client?
    a. Focusing on head, hands, and feet which clothing does not cover
    b. Using primarily compression methods
    c. Formulated a treatment strategy over clothing

81. A client's demeanor reminds a massage practitioner of a difficult coworker evoking an emotional response. This is an example of
    a. countertransference.
    b. transference.
    c. dual relationship.

82. A massage practitioner has a friend who is also a client and hesitates raising the fee rate for them. This is an example of
    a. power differential.
    b. transference.
    c. dual relationship.

83. A massage practitioner advises a client to take a certain medication. This is a violation of
    a. scope of practice.
    b. dual relationship.
    c. emotional boundaries.

84. Two self-employed massage practitioners are each renting a room in a larger wellness center. One practitioner wants to charge $75 per session and the other $95 per session. What best describes the ethical dilemma?
    a. Confidentiality
    b. Differing credentials
    c. Interest conflict

85. A massage practitioner is employed by a chiropractic office along with four other individuals performing a variety of bodywork services. One practitioner has a personality conflict with a coworker and tends to talk about this in the break room. What ethical principle is violated?
    a. Respect for others
    b. Beneficence
    c. Justice

86. What is the best action if a massage client asks for their spine to be adjusted?
    a. Include methods with spinal adjustment potential
    b. Explain limits of scope of practice
    c. Indicate that spinal adjustment naturally occurs

87. A practitioner has just graduated from their massage training program. The next step required for professional practice is
    a. investigating forms of business structures.
    b. meeting all jurisdictional requirements for legal practice.
    c. developing marketing for the target market.

88. A massage practitioner is employed by a physical therapist. The patient requests specific stretching for a shoulder issue. What is the most appropriate action for the practitioner?
   a. Include stretching as requested
   b. Perform more specific assessment
   c. Refer to the physical therapist

89. A massage practitioner wants to practice in a home office. What is required?
   a. Compliance with local zoning and business licensing
   b. Limited liability corporation business structure
   c. Health department inspection

90. What is an ethical issue related to legislated draping regulations in massage practice?
   a. Respect
   b. Autonomy
   c. Veracity

91. What has the most potential for harm if used incorrectly?
   a. Air purifiers
   b. Disinfectants
   c. Antiseptic

92. The massage facility parking area should
   a. be adjacent to a designated smoking area.
   b. have adequate lighting.
   c. have multiple trash receptacles.

93. What is the best explanation for concern when using the hands to apply massage methods?
   a. The intrinsic muscles in the hands attach at the elbow joint leading to repetitive strain
   b. The structure of the joints in the fingers cannot be stabilized
   c. Repetitive pushing and pulling actions increase injury potential in the small structures

94. A biomechanical issue that occurs when the massage practitioner applies long gliding methods using the hand or forearm is
   a. movement of the glenohumeral joint beyond 45% of flexion.
   b. inability to lock knee joints during trunk flexion.
   c. repetitive strain injury from movement of the forearm in supination/pronation.

95. An indication that the massage table height is too low is
   a. feet positioned shoulder width apart.
   b. trunk flexion beyond 30 degrees.
   c. standing on balls of the feet.

96. A massage client is immunocompromised due to a medication used to control an autoimmune condition. What should be used to protect the client during the session?
   a. Smock
   b. Face shield
   c. Mask

97. Which business structure uses the social security number for federal tax purposes?
   a. Sole proprietor
   b. Corporation
   c. Partnership

98. An advantage of employment at a franchise-based massage business is
   a. brand recognition.
   b. adaptable service fees.
   c. lead therapist on staff.

99. Which tax form would an employee of a wellness center receive at the end of the calendar year?
   a. 1099-NEC
   b. W-4
   c. W-2

100. What client record is completed for each client visit?
   a. Session documentation
   b. Treatment plan
   c. Informed consent

PRACTICE TEST 2

Just Anatomy and Physiology—150 Questions

This practice exam targets ANATOMY and PHYSIOLOGY. The questions are written in the MBLEx style. There are 150 questions. Effective study involves understanding all the terminology and how the concepts relate. Understand why the incorrect answers are not the best response to the question. The questions are clustered by content area to help identify topics that need additional study.

System Structure
1. What plane divides the body into front and back regions?
   a. Transverse (horizontal)
   b. Frontal (coronal)
   c. Midsagittal (median)

2. Which of the following terms refers to the foot?
   a. Pedal
   b. Cervical
   c. Femoral

3. When a part of the body is on the side away from the midline, it is referred to as
   a. lateral.
   b. caudal.
   c. dorsal.

4. Targeting massage/bodywork application to the knee would involve understanding
   a. developmental anatomy.
   b. regional anatomy.
   c. gross anatomy.

5. A massage client indicates on the health history form they have been diagnosed with coronary artery disease and have had stents placed. Knowledge in what area is needed to determine contraindications?
   a. Pathophysiology
   b. Systemic physiology
   c. Metabolism

6. Very light pressure (level 1) applied during the massage session would directly contact which tissue type?
   a. Connective
   b. Epithelial
   c. Muscle

7. Fascia is what type of tissue?
   a. Connective
   b. Epithelial
   c. Muscle

8. When the massage/bodywork application targets fluid movement, which body systems are targeted?
   a. Renal and digestive
   b. Integumentary and exocrine
   c. Cardiovascular and lymphatic

9. Which of the following is a type of cartilage?
   a. Collagen
   b. Adipose
   c. Hyaline

10. Of the various types of muscle tissue, which type is the main focus of massage/bodywork?
    a. Smooth
    b. Cardiac
    c. Skeletal

11. Massage/bodywork designed to generally influence the whole person would target which level of body organization?
    a. System level
    b. Organism level
    c. Organ level

12. The chemical processes in the body that release energy as complex compounds are broken down into simpler ones are called
    a. catabolism.
    b. causation.
    c. anabolism.

13. Homeostasis is an example of
    a. correlation.
    b. physiology.
    c. collagen.

14. What structure allows some materials to enter the cell and keeps others out?
    a. Cell membrane
    b. Cytoplasm
    c. Lysosome

15. The jelly-like substance that carries particles around the cell is
    a. cell membrane.
    b. endoplasmic reticulum.
    c. cytoplasm.

Circulation

16. What structure is a key part of the heart's electrical system?
    a. Atrioventricular node
    b. Sinoatrial node
    c. Atria

17. The blood vessels that deliver oxygen and nutrients to the heart muscle are the
    a. carotid.
    b. coronary.
    c. vena cava.

18. What chamber of the heart pumps blood to the lungs?
    a. Right ventricle
    b. Left atrium
    c. Left ventricle

19. What blood vessel brings oxygen-rich blood from the lungs to the heart?
    a. Vena cava
    b. Aorta
    c. Pulmonary vein

20. What chamber of the heart receives all the blood from the body that is oxygen depleted?
    a. Left ventricle
    b. Left atrium
    c. Right atrium

21. Where is the heart located?
    a. Myocardium
    b. Mediastinum
    c. Pericardium

22. What is the relationship of the heart to the diaphragm?
    a. The heart position stabilizes the diaphragm
    b. Diaphragmic movement aids mitral valve function
    c. The heart lies on top of the diaphragm

23. If the intent of the massage method application is to target intermittent compression over a major artery, where would be the location of practitioner's hands?
    a. Anterior medial thigh distal to the groin
    b. Plantar aspect of the foot
    c. Between the scapula from C7 to T5

24. What enters the superior and inferior venae cavae?
    a. Brachiocephalic fluid
    b. Arterial blood
    c. Deoxygenated blood

25. Blood cell development in red marrow is called
    a. hematopoiesis.
    b. phagocytosis.
    c. thrombophlebitis.

26. When a massage/bodywork session reduces the client's stress response, what is an effect on arteries?
    a. Decreased arterial pressure
    b. Increased blood pressure
    c. Vasoconstriction

Digestive

27. The hormones ghrelin and leptin affect
    a. menstruation.
    b. hunger sensations.
    c. bone healing.

28. The liver belongs to which system?
    a. Digestive
    b. Lymphatic
    c. Respiratory

29. The gastrointestinal tract is also called the
    a. omentum.
    b. alimentary canal.
    c. mesentery.

30. What structure lines the abdominal cavity and enfolds the internal organs?
    a. Viscera
    b. Pericardium
    c. Peritoneum

31. The segment of the small intestine which receives partially digested food from the stomach is the
    a. duodenum.
    b. jejunum.
    c. ileum.

32. What digestive organ could be injured by excessive pressure during a massage method application on the abdomen?
    a. Cecum
    b. Liver
    c. Pylorus

33. What type of acid is found in the stomach?
    a. Nitric acid
    b. Sulfuric acid
    c. Hydrochloric acid

34. Where is bile made?
    a. Liver
    b. Gallbladder
    c. Pancreas

35. How does the stomach support immunity?
    a. Secretion of hydrochloric acid
    b. Suppression of mucus production
    c. Production of antibodies

36. Numerous microorganisms colonizing the human gastrointestinal tract are called
    a. mucus.
    b. gastric juices.
    c. microbiota.

Endocrine

37. Which hormone would be most affected when sympathetic autonomic nervous system activation is reduced as the client relaxes during a massage/bodywork session?
    a. GABA
    b. Oxytocin
    c. Adrenaline

38. The endocrine gland located in the cervical area is the
    a. thyroid.
    b. pancreas.
    c. pineal.

39. A structure that secretes androgens is located in the
    a. cranium.
    b. trunk.
    c. pleura.

40. The use of percussion over the sternum of an adolescent client could affect the
    a. hypothalamus.
    b. pituitary.
    c. thymus.

41. What endocrine function is the central stress response system?
    a. Hypothalamic—pituitary—gonadal axis
    b. Hypothalamic—pituitary—adrenal axis
    c. Hypothalamic—pituitary—thyroid axis

42. The presence or absence of what structure classifies a gland as endocrine or exocrine?
    a. Ducts
    b. Blood vessels
    c. Islets

43. Which of the following hormones is regulated directly by the hypothalamus?
    a. Thyroxin
    b. Cortisol
    c. Prolactin

44. The difference between endocrine glands and exocrine glands is
    a. endocrine glands secrete hormones.
    b. endocrine glands secrete saliva.
    c. endocrine glands secrete mucus.

45. Cross communication networks among the endocrine system and nervous system involve the
    a. circadian rhythms.
    b. hypothalamus.
    c. pineal gland.

Integumentary

46. The hypodermis is directly below what layer of skin?
    a. Dermis
    b. Epidermis
    c. Stratum germinativum

47. What structure does the massage practitioner directly contact?
    a. Dermis
    b. Stratum corneum
    c. Interstitium

48. Where on the body are sebaceous glands located?
    a. Soles of the feet
    b. Shoulders
    c. Palms of the hands

49. Located in hairy areas of the body are
    a. proprioceptors.
    b. endocrine organs.
    c. apocrine glands.

50. A massage method using contact on the skin surface to produce a sliding of superficial tissue on deeper structures targets the
    a. interstitium.
    b. chyme.
    c. alveoli.

51. Pressure applied specifically to affect the skin during massage is the primary stimulus for
    a. visceral pain.
    b. muscle tone.
    c. touch sensation.

52. How does the integumentary system directly function as part of the immune system?
    a. Absorbs sunlight and synthesizes vitamin D
    b. Functions as a physical barrier to pathogens
    c. Excretes waste products into the sweat

53. The large onion-shaped receptors that are found deep in the dermis and in subcutaneous tissue which respond to deep pressure during massage application are
    a. Pacinian corpuscles.
    b. Merkel discs.
    c. Ruffini's corpuscle.

54. Massage application to what area stimulates the most sensory receptors of the skin?
    a. Abdomen
    b. Back
    c. Hands

Lymphatic

55. The tonsils belong to which system?
    a. Lymphatic
    b. Integumentary
    c. Digestive

56. Which of the following is the lymphoid organ that is a reservoir for red blood cells and filters organisms from the blood?
    a. Appendix
    b. Spleen
    c. Pancreas

57. Uptake of interstitial fluid occurs at the
    a. lymph nodes.
    b. ventricles.
    c. lymph capillaries.

58. The relationship of interstitial fluid and lymph is
    a. interstitial fluid becomes lymph when collected by lymphatic vessels.
    b. lymph is the fluid that fills the interstitial spaces.
    c. lacteals filter interstitial fluid which then becomes lymph.

59. Lymphatic fluid begins as interstitial fluid and is reintroduced into the blood as
    a. enzymes.
    b. lymphocytes.
    c. plasma.

60. Manual rhythmic pumping massage methods used on the thorax are similar to
    a. smooth muscle peristalsis.
    b. breathing to support lymphatic flow.
    c. neuroregulation of the cardiac cycle.

61. Lymph moving from the calf toward the abdomen would first pass through what group of lymph nodes?
    a. Popliteal
    b. Superficial cubital
    c. Inguinal

62. Lymph is initially formed from
    a. urine.
    b. interstitial fluid.
    c. cytoplasm.

63. What is within lymphatic vessels and organs that acts to defend the body against disease?
    a. Erythrocytes
    b. Lymphocytes
    c. Platelets

64. The lymph within lymphatic vessels is eventually emptied into the blood stream via the
    a. hepatic veins.
    b. subclavian arteries.
    c. subclavian veins.

65. The special lymphatic capillaries responsible for the absorption of fats, known as lacteals, can be found in the
    a. intestinal villi.
    b. esophagus.
    c. stomach.

66. Which of following massage methods would most support uptake of interstitial fluid into the lymph capillaries located in the superficial tissues?
    a. Friction
    b. Percussion
    c. Gliding

Muscular

67. What muscle shape produces a strong contraction over a short range of motion?
    a. Convergent pennate
    b. Pennate
    c. Parallel

68. An efferent neuron and the grouping of muscle fibers innervated by the neuron is a
    a. motor unit.
    b. plexus.
    c. sarcomere.

69. Muscle groups interconnected neurologically so movement occurs in a coordinated manner are
    a. threshold stimulus.
    b. crossed extensor reflexes.
    c. myotatic units.

70. Peristalsis is the main function of
    a. skeletal muscle.
    b. smooth muscle.
    c. cardiac muscle.

71. Skeletal muscle contraction begins at the
    a. actin filaments.
    b. cross-bridges.
    c. neuromuscular junction.

72. When muscle tissue shortens but no movement occurs, the action is called
    a. isometric.
    b. concentric.
    c. eccentric.

Nervous

73. What system detects sensations and controls most functions?
    a. Nervous
    b. Cardiovascular
    c. Immune

74. The sternocleidomastoid muscle is innervated by the
    a. subcostal nerve.
    b. suprascapular nerve.
    c. accessory nerve.

75. What is the basic functional unit of the nervous system?
    a. Neuroglia
    b. Neuron
    c. Nerve

76. A bundle of sensory and motor axons wrapped in fibrous connective tissue is called a
    a. neuron.
    b. ganglion.
    c. mixed nerve.

77. Which part of the brain ensures that the heart continues to beat and maintains breathing?
    a. Medulla
    b. Cerebrum
    c. Cerebellum

78. What is the thalamus's primary function?
    a. Involved in emotional reactions with motivated behavior
    b. Contributes to sense of balance and coordination
    c. Relays sensory messages to the cerebral cortex

79. What is the pituitary gland's primary function?
    a. Releases hormones and regulates endocrine glands
    b. Contributes to sense of balance and coordination
    c. Relays sensory messages to the cerebral cortex

80. Which part of the brain maintains postural balance?
    a. Medulla
    b. Cerebellum
    c. Limbic

81. The primary function of the limbic system is
    a. releasing hormones and regulating endocrine glands.
    b. emotional reactions with motivated behavior.
    c. storage of new information in memory.

82. Injury to the Broca's area in the left frontal lobe would
    a. interfere with the ability to talk.
    b. prevent storage of new information in memory.
    c. prevent comprehension of speech.

83. The primary function of the hippocampus is
    a. speech comprehension.
    b. the ability to talk.
    c. storage of new information in memory.

84. The, axillary, radial, median, and ulnar nerves are
    a. located in the leg.
    b. branches of the brachial plexus.
    c. impinged in cervicogenic headaches.

85. How many pairs of spinal nerves emerge from the spinal cord?
    a. 18
    b. 12
    c. 31

86. What nerve innervates the deltoid muscles?
    a. Axillary
    b. Musculocutaneous
    c. Ulnar

87. Which bony structure protects the spinal cord from damage?
    a. Vertebral column
    b. Skull
    c. Ribcage

88. A massage client indicates "pins and needles" sensation on the side of their foot. What nerve may be involved?
    a. Radial
    b. Tibial
    c. Thoracodorsal

89. Knee pain would most often be related to the
    a. fibular (peroneal) nerve.
    b. median nerve.
    c. pudendal nerve.

90. What nerve lies adjacent to the femoral artery?
    a. Obturator
    b. Saphenous
    c. Accessory

91. Afferent neuron impulses move into the central nervous system along
    a. descending tracts.
    b. neurolemma.
    c. ascending tracts.

92. Which of the following is the point at which an impulse is transmitted from one neuron to another neuron?
    a. Synapse
    b. Dendrite
    c. Glial cell

93. Nerve impulse conduction occurs fastest in
    a. unmyelinated nerve fibers.
    b. myelinated nerve fibers.
    c. neuroglia.

94. What is the correct sequence of events in a reflex?
    a. Stimulus—sensory neuron—motor neuron—action
    b. Stimulus—motor neuron—sensory neuron—action
    c. Action—sensory neuron—motor neuron—stimulus

95. A massage client would first respond to the application of moderate pressure during a session as a
    a. reticular activation.
    b. motor response.
    c. sensory stimulus.

96. The medulla oblongata is continuous with which structure?
    a. Frontal cortex
    b. Spinal cord
    c. Corpus callosum

97. Which part of a neuron does the myelin sheath cover?
    a. Synapse
    b. Dendrites
    c. Axon

Reproduction

98. The prostate is part of the
    a. male reproductive system.
    b. female reproductive system.
    c. digestive system.

99. Which hormone has the primary responsibility of developing and maintaining female sexual characteristics?
    a. Testosterone
    b. Estrogen
    c. Thyroxine

100. In what location would pressure applied during massage need to be adapted during the menstrual cycle?
    a. Hypogastric
    b. Anterior thorax
    c. Upper left quadrant

101. A major difference in reproductive system anatomy is
    a. only males make testosterone.
    b. only males have gonads.
    c. female organs are primarily located inside the body.

102. The relationship between the endocrine system and reproductive system is
    a. neurotransmitters.
    b. hormones.
    c. corpus callosum.

103. When during the menstrual cycle is the egg released?
    a. Ovulation
    b. Menopause
    c. Menstruation

104. The contraction rate during labor and delivery of a baby are a/n
    a. negative feedback loop.
    b. action potential.
    c. positive feedback loop.

Respiratory

105. What is located lateral to the mediastinum?
    a. Kidneys
    b. Heart
    c. Lungs

106. Which term means between the ribs?
    a. Intercostal
    b. Costovertebral
    c. Metacarpal

107. What is the name of the membrane that surrounds each lung?
    a. Mucus
    b. Pleura
    c. Serous

108. Where does the trachea branch into the bronchi?
    a. Distal end
    b. Proximal end
    c. Larynx

109. When percussion methods are used to target lung function, the massage application is focused at which location?
    a. Dorsal cavity
    b. Rib cage
    c. Right lower quadrant

110. What is the correct branching order into the lungs?
    a. Bronchioles, trachea, bronchi
    b. Trachea, bronchi, bronchioles
    c. Trachea, bronchioles, bronchi

111. What gas is a waste product of respiration?
    a. Hydrogen
    b. Methane
    c. Carbon dioxide

112. How is waste carbon dioxide expelled from the body?
    a. Through expiration
    b. Through inspiration
    c. By peristalsis

113. What is anaerobic respiration?
    a. Respiration with oxygen
    b. Respiration without carbon dioxide
    c. Respiration without oxygen

114. What are alveoli?
    a. Air sacs in the lungs
    b. Coverings of the lungs
    c. Hollow tubes leading to the lungs

115. What substance builds up in muscle during anaerobic exercise?
    a. Nitric oxide
    b. Lactic acid
    c. Glucose

116. Contraction of the diaphragm causes which action to take place?
    a. Micturition
    b. Inspiration
    c. Peristalsis

117. Why is the alveolar surface moist?
    a. To aid blood flow in the intestines
    b. To support the ability to swallow
    c. To aid the diffusion of gases in the alveoli

118. Which of these are accessory respiratory muscles?
    a. Serratus anterior
    b. Obturator internus
    c. Diaphragm

119. Which compound in the blood carries oxygen?
    a. Platelets
    b. Fibrin
    c. Hemoglobin

120. What function does the mucus in the trachea serve?
    a. Aid diffusion of gases in the lung
    b. Trap foreign particles
    c. Increase blood flow to the alveoli

121. The scalene muscles are accessory muscles to which action?
    a. Inspiration
    b. Expiration
    c. Vomiting

122. Increasing blood concentration of carbon dioxide causes
    a. carbon monoxide poisoning.
    b. stimulation of cough reflex.
    c. increase in respiratory rate.

123. What does the pressure in the lungs do during expiration?
    a. Increases
    b. Expands the ribs
    c. Decreases

124. What causes an oxygen debt in the body?
    a. Anaerobic exercise
    b. Aerobic exercise
    c. Endurance exercise

125. What involves both somatic and autonomic regulation?
    a. Chewing
    b. Breathing
    c. Jumping

126. Assessment of a massage client's breathing rate indicates breathing that is deeper and more rapid than normal. This would be considered
    a. hyperventilation.
    b. tachycardia.
    c. bradypnea.

Skeletal

127. The tibia is part of the
    a. axial skeleton.
    b. pelvic girdle.
    c. appendicular skeleton.

128. What is the common name of the sternum?
    a. Breastbone
    b. Collarbone
    c. Shoulder blade

129. What is the sheath of connective tissue enveloping the bone except at articulation?
    a. Diaphysis
    b. Endosteum
    c. Periosteum

130. What is part of a vertebra?
    a. Epicondyle
    b. Pedicle
    c. Malleolus

131. The term used to describe where bones meet to form a joint is
    a. articulation.
    b. ligament.
    c. bursa.

132. When palpating the anterior aspect of the leg, just inferior to the joint line, the massage practitioner should be able to locate the
    a. fibular shaft.
    b. medial malleolus.
    c. tibial tuberosity.

133. What bone type is found within a tendon?
    a. Sesamoid
    b. Flat
    c. Irregular

134. A massage client recently donated bone marrow. What area would be considered an area of caution?
    a. Ilium
    b. Calcaneus
    c. Clavicle

135. A function of bone marrow is
    a. tendon attachment.
    b. hematopoiesis.
    c. protection of brain.

136. The boney structure that protects the lungs is the
    a. xiphoid process.
    b. shoulder girdle.
    c. thoracic cage.

Special Senses

137. Vestibulo-ocular reflex involves
    a. mitral valve and nose.
    b. eyes and ears.
    c. ear drum and nares.

138. The semicircular canals are found
    a. in the ear.
    b. in the eye.
    c. in the nose.

139. Moving the head during the massage session influences
    a. nociceptors.
    b. swallowing.
    c. vestibular function.

140. Odors are detected by
    a. proprioceptors.
    b. chemical receptors.
    c. mechanoreceptors.

141. A massage client has issues with depth perception which involves the
    a. eyes.
    b. ears.
    c. nose.

142. A client informs the massage practitioner that they are often dizzy. What is this sensation related to?
    a. Olfactory nerves
    b. The back of the tongue
    c. The inner ear

Urinary

143. A primary function of the kidney is
    a. elimination of solid waste.
    b. removal of dead blood cells.
    c. blood pressure regulation.

144. What is the structure that collects urine in the body?
    a. Bladder
    b. Ureter
    c. Urethra

145. Which body system filters the blood and eliminates wastes in liquid form?
    a. Lymphatic system
    b. Urinary system
    c. Endocrine system

146. Where are the kidneys located?
    a. The back wall of the abdominal cavity
    b. Above and behind the pubic bone
    c. Anterior to the ilium

147. An organ of the urinary system is the
    a. spleen.
    b. adrenal.
    c. kidney.

148. Applying pressure during the massage session distal to the umbilicus and proximal to the pubic bone may cause discomfort related to the
    a. stomach.
    b. bladder.
    c. gallbladder.

149. The detrusor muscle is found in the
    a. bladder.
    b. uterus.
    c. prostrate.

150. The potential need of a client to urinate during the massage session related to the autonomic nervous system is
    a. an enteric response.
    b. a parasympathetic response.
    c. a sympathetic response.

PRACTICE TEST 3

Just Kinesiology—100 Questions

1. The observable actions in the transverse plane when the massage practitioner performs joint movement assessment are
   a. flexion or extension.
   b. adduction or abduction.
   c. medial or lateral rotation.

2. Muscles that are shaped like tubes, located on the anterior and posterior aspects of the body and can flex and extend a joint, function primarily in the
   a. frontal plane.
   b. transverse plane.
   c. sagittal plane.

3. When standing still in front of a closed door and pushing on it without it moving, what muscle action is occurring?
   a. Isometric
   b. Isotonic
   c. Eccentric

4. Muscles working together concentrically to produce a movement would be the prime mover and
   a. antagonist.
   b. synergist.
   c. fixator.

5. A massage client is having difficulty bending forward and then standing. Dysfunction is occurring in the
   a. sagittal plane.
   b. transverse plane.
   c. frontal plane.

6. A muscle that is shaped like a triangle with fiber oriented diagonally and functioning in the frontal plane would be best designed to
   a. function as a sphincter.
   b. adduct or abduct.
   c. flex or extend.

7. The hip joint is flexed. How would the muscle group that returns the hip to the anatomical position be functioning as the hip returns to the anatomical position?
   a. Shortening
   b. Lengthening
   c. Stabilizing

8. What muscle assists the prime mover and functions to stabilize the moving joint?
   a. Fixator
   b. Antagonist
   c. Synergist

9. When a hinge joint is flexed, the action of the muscles controlling the motion is
   a. pennate.
   b. eccentric.
   c. isometric.

10. A muscle functioning as an agonist would be acting
    a. antagonistically.
    b. eccentrically.
    c. concentrically.

11. Strain applied to a ligament is monitored by
    a. neuromuscular spindles.
    b. joint kinesthetic receptors.
    c. lamellar corpuscles.

12. Mechanical receptors that provide information about body position and movement are
    a. proprioceptors.
    b. nociceptors.
    c. tactile receptor.

13. Elongation of a muscle combined with moderate pressure in the belly of the muscle would primarily stimulate
    a. free nerve endings.
    b. Golgi tendon receptors.
    c. spindle cells.

14. Muscle spindles are most sensitive to what type of stimulus?
    a. Rapid lengthening
    b. Slow lengthening
    c. Sudden shortening

15. A massage client indicates stiffness with pain especially when sitting on a hard chair. What muscles are being compressed?
    a. Hamstrings
    b. Quadriceps
    c. Sartorius

16. A massage client is having difficulty moving their little toe. What muscle is directly involved?
    a. Flexor hallucis brevis
    b. Flexor digiti minimi brevis
    c. Extensor hallucis brevis

17. What two muscles are synergists?
    a. Supraspinatus and pectoralis minor
    b. Gluteus medius and adductor magnus
    c. Latissimus dorsi and teres major

18. What muscle functions as an antagonist to vastus lateralis?
    a. Biceps femoris short head
    b. Gracilis
    c. Rectus femoris

19. A client complains of discomfort at the lateral aspect of the scapula, inferior to the glenoid cavity when they extend their elbow. What is the most logical reason for this symptom?
    a. The triceps brachii proximal attachment is at the infraglenoid tubercle of the scapula
    b. The lateral supracondylar ridge is the proximal attachment site of the brachioradialis
    c. The trapezius muscles elevate the shoulder girdle, adduct, depress, and rotate the scapula

20. What is the distal attachment of the brachioradialis?
    a. Lateral supracondylar ridge of the humerus
    b. Distal styloid process of the radius
    c. Base of the fifth metacarpal

21. What is the distal attachment of the triceps brachii?
    a. Infraglenoid tubercle of the scapula
    b. Radial tuberosity and bicipital aponeurosis of the forearm
    c. Olecranon process of ulna

22. A massage client indicates tenderness when the temporalis muscle is massaged. Additional assessment involves the massage practitioner asking the client to activate the muscle by
    a. protruding the lower lip.
    b. elevating and retracting the mandible.
    c. medially rotating the eyes.

23. An action of the levator scapulae is to
    a. laterally rotate and flex the head.
    b. pull the scalp backward.
    c. elevate the scapula and help retract it.

24. During postural assessment, the massage practitioner notices the client has an elevated left shoulder. In addition to a short levator scapula what other synergist should be assessed?
    a. Lower trapezius
    b. Middle trapezius
    c. Upper trapezius

25. What is the deepest muscle that acts on the atlanto-occipital joint?
    a. Rectus capitis lateralis
    b. Splenius capitis
    c. Sternocleidomastoid

26. Which muscle group would be the most difficult to massage?
    a. Plantar muscles
    b. Muscles of mastication
    c. Suboccipital muscles

27. Actions of the splenius capitus include the ability to
    a. elevate and draw the angle of the mouth laterally.
    b. extend and laterally flex the neck.
    c. rotate the head to the opposite side and flex the neck.

28. How does the action of the scalenus posterior relate to inspiration?
    a. Elevates the second rib
    b. Stabilizes xiphoid
    c. Antagonist to external intercostals

29. An abductor is a skeletal muscle that
    a. moves a limb in the median plane.
    b. moves a limb away from the midline.
    c. moves a limb toward the midsagittal plane.

30. Where would massage be applied to address the muscles that work together to extend the head?
    a. Occipital bone
    b. Sternum
    c. Mandible

31. Muscles that attach to the ribs and pubis with parallel fibers would produce what action when acting concentrically?
    a. Rotation of hip
    b. Extension of lumbar spine
    c. Flexion of the trunk

32. A muscle with a diagonal fiber direction with attachments at the pubis and the linea aspera of the femur would primarily be considered a/n
    a. abductor.
    b. adductor.
    c. flexor.

33. A muscle shaped like a rectangle with horizontal fiber direction that functions in the transverse plane is
    a. quadratus plantae.
    b. quadratus lumborum.
    c. quadratus femoris.

34. A pennate muscle that functions at the elbow is
    a. interossei.
    b. brachialis.
    c. triceps.

35. Active movement to palpate the muscle which proximally attaches on the distal posterior femur would be
    a. knee flexion.
    b. hip extension.
    c. shoulder adduction.

36. A massage client indicates limitation of movement during internal rotation of the glenohumeral joint. Palpation identifies tenderness at the lesser tubercle. What structure is involved?
    a. Ligamentum nuchae
    b. Subscapularis muscle
    c. Shaft of the clavicle

37. While performing a postural analysis, the massage practitioner observes that the palms of client's hands are facing the greater trochanter. What muscle is short?
    a. Latissimus dorsi
    b. Triceps
    c. Anterior serratus.

38. What muscles are involved in forced expiration and defecating?
    a. Superior and inferior gemelli
    b. Gluteus maximus and medius
    c. Levator ani and coccygeus muscles

39. Contraction of which muscle produces extension of the neck?
    a. Longus capitis
    b. Spinalis cervicis
    c. Longus colli

40. The movement of the sole of the foot toward the median plane is
    a. inversion.
    b. rotation.
    c. abduction

41. What type of cartilage is normally found on joint surfaces?
    a. Fibrocartilage
    b. Hyaline cartilage
    c. Elastic cartilage

42. A massage practitioner is performing active joint movement assessment of shoulder abduction. The observed action would be
    a. arms move over abdomen.
    b. arms move toward trunk.
    c. arms move away from trunk.

43. What is an accurate description of flexion at the lumbar spine?
    a. Decreasing kyphosis
    b. Increasing lordosis
    c. Decreasing lordosis

44. Lifting the shoulders toward the ears is an example of
    a. elevation.
    b. extension.
    c. eversion.

45. The zero position for measuring joint range of motion for most joints is based on which of the following?
    a. Ideal alignment
    b. Anatomic position
    c. Sagittal plane

46. What is the name for moving the shoulders caudally?
    a. Depression
    b. Contraction
    c. Abduction

47. Movement produced voluntarily at a joint would be considered
    a. arthrokinematics.
    b. osteokinematic.
    c. equilibrium.

48. Which of the following is the ability of the massage client to voluntarily move a limb through an arc of movement?
    a. Passive range of motion
    b. Manual muscle testing
    c. Active range of motion

49. What is the term for the property of joints that allows the joint surfaces to glide, roll, and spin on each other allowing functional range of motion?
    a. Accessory motion
    b. Oscillatory motion
    c. Linear motion

50. Synovial joint movement is
    a. controlled by the vagus nerve.
    b. under somatic nervous system control.
    c. considered primarily involuntary.

51. In addition to flexion and extension, what other joint movement occurs at the knee?
    a. Adduction
    b. Rotation
    c. Nutation

52. What joint occurs between the axial and appendicular skeleton?
    a. Glenohumeral
    b. Atlantoaxial joint
    c. Sacroiliac

53. The massage practitioner would palpate the deltoid ligament at the
    a. hip.
    b. elbow.
    c. ankle.

54. A massage client is asked to perform circumduction. What joint type is being assessed?
    a. Ball and socket
    b. Hinge
    c. Gliding

55. A massage client informs the practitioner that they have been doing exercises focusing on frontal plane movement. What movements would the massage practitioner include in assessment?
    a. Adduction/abduction
    b. Flexion/extension
    c. Medial/lateral rotation

56. A massage practitioner is reviewing charts prior to a session and notices the abbreviation ROM? What would be the most common interpretation?
    a. Range of motion
    b. Repair of muscles
    c. Restriction of movement

57. The massage practitioner is assessing the ulnar collateral ligament. Where would palpation be located?
    a. Lower limb
    b. Upper limb
    c. Thorax

58. A massage client is experiencing knee joint issues involving the articular cartilage. What fluid would be affected?
    a. Plasma fluid
    b. Lymph fluid
    c. Synovial fluid

59. The multifidus muscle provides stabilization to which joints?
    a. Carpal joints
    b. Spinal joints
    c. Acromioclavicular joints

60. An example of a uniaxial joint is the
    a. hip.
    b. jaw.
    c. elbow.

61. The sutures of the skull are considered
    a. diarthrosis joints.
    b. fibrous joints.
    c. ellipsoid joints.

62. A massage practitioner is performing passive joint movement during the session to assess range of motion. A movement that combines flexion, extension, adduction, and abduction would be used to assess which joint?
    a. Acetabulofemoral joint
    b. Tibiofibular joint
    c. Tibiofemoral joint

63. The massage practitioner would use active movement to assess which joint type?
    a. Syndesmoses
    b. Cartilaginous
    c. Diarthrosis

64. A joint classified based on function would be
    a. synovial.
    b. symphyses.
    c. synarthrosis.

65. Which joint allows protraction and retraction?
    a. Sternoclavicular
    b. Sternochondral
    c. Tibiofibular

66. Zygapophyseal joints are considered
    a. saddle joints.
    b. gliding joints.
    c. pivot joints.

67. The joints of the fingers and toes are classified as
    a. synovial.
    b. syndesmosis.
    c. synarthrosis.

68. How is range of motion assessed?
    a. Movement
    b. Palpation
    c. Pain scale

69. Joint range of motion is described as
    a. a method used to stretch muscles.
    b. the amount of motion available at a specific joint.
    c. the degree of flexibility in soft tissue.

70. A joint's range of motion is measured in
    a. pounds.
    b. weight.
    c. degrees.

71. Typical range of motion of the elbow out of the anatomical position is
    a. 0 to 150 degrees.
    b. 0 to 45 degrees.
    c. 80 to 0 degrees.

72. Typical range of motion of the hip joint into hyperextension is
    a. 0 to 30 degrees.
    b. 0 to 5 degrees.
    c. 0 to 110 degrees.

73. When a client lifts their chin up away from their chest, as if beginning to nod "yes," and the cervical spine is not extended, what is the typical range of motion?
    a. 45 to 0 degrees
    b. 0 to 15 degrees
    c. 0 to 5 degrees

74. The typical range of motion of the shoulder from anatomical position into abduction without movement of the scapula is
    a. 90 to 5 degrees.
    b. 180 to 0 degrees.
    c. 0 to 30 degrees.

75. What joint would have a range of motion of adduction 45 to 0 degrees?
    a. Wrist
    b. Hip
    c. Knee

76. A massage practitioner is assessing an ankle sprain in the subacute healing phase by asking the client to move the ankle while the practitioner applies a counter force. The type of joint movement is
    a. assisted.
    b. resistive.
    c. passive.

77. A massage client demonstrates to the practitioner the available range of motion of the wrist without discomfort. This is what type of assessment?
    a. Assisted joint movement
    b. Passive joint movement
    c. Active joint movement

78. A client is resting comfortably during the session and the practitioner moves the ankle through the available range of motion. This is considered
    a. passive.
    b. resistant.
    c. assisted.

79. The massage practitioner moves the elbow joint along with a client actively moving the same joint. This is considered
    a. isometric joint movement.
    b. resistive joint movement.
    c. assisted joint movement.

80. When a person is in a relaxed standing posture, supporting the gravitational line with the normal knee-locked position, which muscle is used for balance?
    a. Pectoralis major
    b. Gastrocnemius
    c. Middle trapezius

81. Three main types of proprioceptors are muscle spindles, tendon organs, and _____.
    a. cervical/lumbar plexuses
    b. spinal nerves
    c. joint kinesthetic receptors

82. A massage client has been working on a project that required gripping a hammer for an extended period. Now the client is complaining of weakness when attempting to extend the wrist. Which of the following is the most likely explanation?
    a. The flexor muscle group of the hand and wrist increased tone levels, resulting in inhibition of the extensor group of muscles in the forearm
    b. The flexor digitorum superficialis and profundus are weak from fatigue, so the wrist extensors have been facilitated
    c. The deep layer of the posterior wrist extensor group is antagonistic to the superficial layer of this same muscle group, resulting in weakness in the wrist extensors

83. A compressive massage method is applied to the belly of a muscle with the intent of reducing a muscle spasm brought on by a cramp. The receptors most affected are
    a. joint kinesthetic.
    b. Golgi tendon organ.
    c. muscle spindles.

84. A massage client complains of pain and tension in the lower back, more to the left side. Physical assessment indicates that the pelvis is elevated on the left compared to the right. The client also reports difficulty raising the left arm over the head. Which of the following muscles may be involved?
    a. Psoas major
    b. Rectus abdominis
    c. Latissimus dorsi

85. If the scapula remains fixed and immobile, what would be the result at the glenohumeral joint?
    a. Range of motion would be limited
    b. Internal and external rotation would be enhanced
    c. Flexion would be unaffected

86. During muscle strength testing, the flexors and extensors of the elbow seem equally strong. Why is this a dysfunctional pattern?
    a. Gait patterns should inhibit flexors
    b. Flexors should be about 25% stronger than extensors
    c. Extensors should be 30% stronger than adductors

87. Which of the following is produced voluntarily?
    a. Joint play
    b. Arthrokinematic movement
    c. Osteokinematic movement

88. A client exhibits increased internal rotation of the right shoulder. Which of the following is the most appropriate massage approach for reversing this condition?
    a. Friction and traction to the external rotators
    b. Muscle energy methods and elongation of the internal rotators
    c. Compression and tapotement to the internal rotators

89. A massage client is experiencing a limitation in range of motion of the hip into abduction. Assessment indicates shortening and tension in the adductor group of muscles. Gluteus medius muscle tests as weak. Which of the following are most likely the source of the weakness and limited range of motion?
    a. Agonists
    b. Synergists
    c. Antagonists

90. Contraction of the external intercostal muscles creates a vacuum in the thorax because the
    a. upper ribs expand.
    b. ribs are pulled together.
    c. diaphragm muscle arches upward.

91. Joints in which stability is reduced because of increased laxity of supportive ligaments will exhibit an increase in
    a. joint play.
    b. hypomobility.
    c. muscle relaxation.

92. Should an injury to the sternoclavicular joint limit its range of motion, what other structure will be affected?
    a. Radius
    b. Olecranon
    c. Scapula

93. A massage client sprained the joint in one of the fingers. What is going to be the most comfortable position for the joint, and why?
    a. Close-packed position, because this is the most stable position of the joint
    b. Loose-packed position, so that movement can occur most easily
    c. Least-packed position, to accommodate swelling

94. During assessment, what instructions should be given to the massage client to rotate the hip externally?
    a. Please move your leg so that you cross it over the other leg at the ankles
    b. Please straighten your legs and turn the entire leg so that you point your toes toward each other
    c. Please straighten your legs and turn the entire leg so that you point your toes away from each other.

95. When a muscle group is located on the anterior aspect of the torso and functions in the sagittal plane, where would the antagonist group be located?
    a. Posterior torso
    b. Lateral thigh
    c. Upper limb.

96. The opponens pollicis is in a functional muscle group with what other muscle?
    a. Flexor pollicis brevis
    b. Opponens digiti minimi
    c. Flexor digitorum profundus

97. Which of the following muscles crosses two joints and functions as both a flexor and extensor?
    a. Vastus lateralis
    b. Rectus femoris
    c. Soleus

98. A massage client complains of a stiff IT band since beginning a new exercise program. What concentric movement would be involved?
    a. Trunk flexion
    b. Plantar flexion
    c. Hip extension

99. A client complains of restricted breathing and a catch in their side after pushing a car that was stuck in a ditch. Which muscle should be evaluated?
    a. Adductor magnus
    b. Anterior serratus
    c. Psoas

100. A massage client complains of a headache on the lateral sides of the skull. They recently purchased new glasses which feel somewhat tight. What muscles would be involved?
    a. Temporalis
    b. Masseter
    c. Pterygoid

PRACTICE TEST 4

Pathology, Contraindications, Areas of Caution, Special Populations—175 Questions

1. Which is the single most effective deterrent to the spread of disease?
   a. Proper hand washing
   b. Linen sterilization
   c. Sanitizing equipment

2. The manifestation of disease is best described as
   a. feelings of discomfort.
   b. signs and symptoms.
   c. acute episode of a chronic illness.

3. Which of the following is a systemic sign of a disease?
   a. Fever
   b. Swelling of the knee
   c. Rash on face

4. What is it called when there is a localized abnormal dilation of a blood vessel, usually an artery, which creates a weakness in the wall of the vessel?
   a. Edema
   b. CVA
   c. Aneurysm

5. Which describes a chronic condition?
   a. Temporary
   b. Continuous
   c. Acute

6. Lack of exercise during an illness may cause skeletal muscle to undergo
   a. regeneration.
   b. hypertrophy.
   c. atrophy.

7. Thoracic outlet syndrome is a compression of a nerve or blood vessel in what area?
   a. Neck and shoulder
   b. Lumbar spine
   c. Posterior knee

8. Pathology can be described as
   a. stages in tissue healing.
   b. disruption in homeostasis.
   c. acquired immune response.

9. Abnormal cellular change that can become cancerous is
   a. hyperplasia.
   b. paresthesia.
   c. hyperalgesia.

10. A massage client describing fatigue related to recovery from injuries received in a car accident is indicating reduced
    a. allodynia.
    b. resilience.
    c. stress.

11. A condition caused by bacteria is a/n
    a. contusion.
    b. allergy.
    c. infection.

12. The experience of increased sensation sensitivity experienced as pain is
    a. ultradian rhythm.
    b. salutogenesis.
    c. hyperalgesia.

13. Pain that is not originating from the somatic structures but may refer to the surface of the body in typical patterns is
    a. visceral pain.
    b. joint pain.
    c. connective tissue pain.

14. A massage client that heals quickly from an injury and recovers quickly from an illness has
    a. decreased immune response.
    b. robust adaptive capacity.
    c. resilience decline.

15. A restorative care approach for a long-term care plan would indicate the massage client is
    a. prone to infection.
    b. exhibiting stress symptoms.
    c. generally healthy.

16. A condition commonly encountered by a massage practitioner is
    a. phantom pain.
    b. bone cancer.
    c. upper respiratory infection.

17. A client with a progressive autoimmune condition often experiences
    a. reduced adaptive capacity.
    b. resilient homeostasis.
    c. normal biological rhythms.

18. Increasing levels of adaptive demand predispose an individual to
    a. health.
    b. stress.
    c. congenital disease.

19. What is a common underlying cause of chronic disease?
    a. Inflammation
    b. Resilience
    c. Restorative sleep

20. Where do insulin-dependent massage clients have a local contraindication?
    a. Medical port
    b. Cervical spine
    c. Injection site

21. In what situation is inflammation most productive?
    a. Diabetes
    b. Injury healing
    c. Multiple sclerosis

22. What condition requires the massage practitioner be most cautious with pressure intensity in the limbs during method application?
    a. Rheumatoid arthritis
    b. Diverticulosis
    c. Plantar fasciopathy

23. What is a noncontagious skin condition?
    a. Herpes simplex
    b. Psoriasis
    c. Hepatitis

24. What degenerative condition is common in clients 65—80 years old?
    a. Pancreatitis
    b. Osteoarthrosis
    c. Meningitis

25. During the massage session, a client experiences shortness of breath and altered mental status. This is a/n
    a. negative feedback loop.
    b. emotional response.
    c. medical emergency.

26. The most common condition encountered by the massage practitioner related to diabetes is
    a. obesity.
    b. depression.
    c. cancer.

27. What sign would indicate the massage practitioner should refer to the client's physician?
    a. Anxiety
    b. Nausea
    c. Rash

28. What condition involves occlusion in an artery?
    a. Myocardial infarction
    b. Peripheral neuropathy
    c. Parkinson's disease

29. A massage client indicates they have a condition related to their spine. What might this be called?
    a. Preeclampsia
    b. Spondylolisthesis
    c. Cystic fibrosis

30. What condition is caused by bacteria?
    a. Scabies
    b. Tuberculosis
    c. Infectious mononucleosis

31. The massage practitioner notices that a client's skin color and whites of the eyes look yellow. This is a common sign of
    a. vitiligo.
    b. cyanosis.
    c. liver disease.

32. On the history form a massage client indication they have condition is caused by a virus. What condition would they be experiencing?
    a. Hepatitis
    b. MRSA
    c. Thrush

33. The spread of pathogens by coughing or sneezing is considered
    a. direct contact transmission.
    b. vector transmission.
    c. droplet transmission.

34. Which of the following suffixes indicate a sensitivity to pain?
    a. -algesia
    b. -itis
    c. -asthenia

35. The client informs the massage practitioner that they have a hernia just below the rib cage and above the abdomen. What type of hernia would this be?
    a. Inguinal
    b. Umbilical
    c. Hiatal

36. A massage client diagnosed with olecranon bursitis might experience discomfort at which joint in the body?
    a. Ankle
    b. Elbow
    c. Hip

37. A client indicates the outcome of the massage session is stress management. What is a common stress symptom to be addressed during the session?
    a. Disturbed sleep
    b. Lumbar pain
    c. Joint stiffness

38. Pediculosis is a condition related to
    a. bad breath.
    b. lice.
    c. athletes' foot.

39. Which of the following is a grade II muscle strain?
    a. Complete tearing of the muscle with complete strength loss
    b. Tearing of a few muscle fibers without strength loss
    c. Moderate and incomplete tearing of muscle fibers with some strength loss

40. Where is a muscle strain on the biceps brachii most likely to occur?
    a. Midpoint of the muscle belly
    b. Musculotendinous junction
    c. Spine of the scapula

41. During an intake interview, the client informs the massage practitioner they have a torticollis affecting their right side. The massage therapist should notice what postural change in the region?
    a. Right side bending of the head and left rotation of the chin
    b. Right side bending of the torso and right rotation of the pelvis
    c. Left side bending head and right rotation of the shoulder

42. Which of the following defines an avulsion fracture?
    a. A fracture caused by repeated low-force trauma
    b. One fragment of the bone is driven into another
    c. A sudden muscular contraction with the ligament pulling away from the bone

43. A massage client describes an anterior shoulder disloca-
    tion related to a fall. Which of the following nerves is
    most likely damaged in this scenario?
    a. Radial
    b. Median
    c. Axillary

44. An irritation of the fluid-filled sacs that decrease fric-
    tion between structures in the body is
    a. bursitis.
    b. nerve entrapment.
    c. tendinopathy.

45. A massage client had a laceration anterior to the medial
    malleolus, which required stitches and now is com-
    plaining of pain along the medial border of the foot.
    Which nerve is most likely involved?
    a. Saphenous nerve
    b. Axillary nerve
    c. Intermediate dorsal cutaneous nerve

46. Respirations less than 10 breaths/minute in a resting
    adult are considered which of the following?
    a. Hypoventilation
    b. Tachypnea
    c. Bradypnea

47. A sprain occurs when what structure is injured?
    a. Tendon
    b. Ligaments
    c. Muscle

48. A resting pulse of more than 100 beats/minute is
    considered
    a. bradycardia.
    b. tachycardia.
    c. tachypnea.

49. A concern a massage practitioner may have when a
    client sits up after laying on the massage table for an
    hour is called
    a. orthostatic hypotension.
    b. myocardial ischemia.
    c. vasodilation.

50. Which of the following is most likely to be increased
    with infection?
    a. Red blood cells
    b. White blood cells
    c. Platelets

51. A myocardial infarction is the result of damage to the
    a. Purkinje fibers.
    b. pulmonary veins.
    c. coronary arteries.

52. Which of the following describes lymphedema?
    a. Pathologic accumulation of protein-rich fluid in the
       tissue
    b. Accumulation of lymphocytes in the blood and
       tissues
    c. Leakage of red blood cells into the surrounding
       tissue

53. What type of hernia occurs when a sac formed from the
    peritoneum and intestines pushes outward through the
    abdominal wall?
    a. Femoral
    b. Inguinal
    c. Umbilical

54. What is the most common osteoporosis-related
    fracture?
    a. Rib fracture
    b. Vertebral compression fracture
    c. Metacarpal fracture

55. Where would a massage practitioner observe for an
    outbreak of herpes simplex virus type 1 skin lesions?
    a. Genitals
    b. Foot
    c. Mouth

56. What type of benign soft-tissue tumor is usually seen in
    the popliteal area?
    a. Baker's cyst
    b. Lipoma
    c. Nevus

57. A massage practitioner works with distance runners. What
    type of fracture most commonly occurs in this
    population?
    a. Greenstick fracture
    b. Compound fracture
    c. Stress fracture

58. A massage client has injured the medial collateral liga-
    ment of the knee. When does the inflammatory phase
    of healing begin?
    a. 2—3 weeks after injury
    b. First days after injury
    c. 4—6 weeks after injury

59. What age group is most likely to suffer from Osgood–Schlatter syndrome?
    a. Adolescents
    b. Toddlers
    c. Infants

60. What is the major sign or symptom of meningitis?
    a. Confusion
    b. Tinnitus
    c. Headache

61. What is the most common type of dementia?
    a. Alzheimer's disease
    b. Frontotemporal dementia
    c. Lewy body dementia

62. A massage practitioner is concerned about a client that is showing signs of Parkinson's disease. What sign did the practitioner notice?
    a. Neuropathy
    b. Tremor
    c. Edema

63. A client complains of dizziness when getting off the treatment table. The massage practitioner notices nystagmus. What should the massage practitioner do?
    a. Return client to the supine position
    b. Walk slowly with the client
    c. Help the client sit down

64. A massage client indicates they have a condition classified as a primary headache. What diagnosis do they have?
    a. Headache associated with increased blood pressure
    b. Migraine headaches
    c. Headache associated with fever

65. Which of the following diseases has as primary symptoms of tremor and rigidity?
    a. Parkinson's disease
    b. Alzheimer's disease
    c. Multiple sclerosis

66. A client has a Morton's neuroma. Where is caution for massage application indicated?
    a. Fourth and fifth metatarsal heads
    b. Second and third metatarsal heads
    c. Third and fourth metatarsal heads

67. During both observation and palpation assessment, the massage practitioner identifies abnormal accumulation of tissue fluid in the lower legs. This condition is called
    a. edema.
    b. dilatation.
    c. emesis.

68. Which of the following terms means pain along the course of a nerve?
    a. Neuroplasticity
    b. Neuralgia
    c. Neuroglia

69. A massage practitioner is volunteering at a marathon. The weather is hot and humid. What medical emergency might occur?
    a. Orthopnea
    b. Hyperthermia
    c. Hypothermia

70. Which term means a sticking together of two structures that are normally separated?
    a. Diaphoresis
    b. Anaphylaxis
    c. Adhesion

71. A massage practitioner notices a client's skin color is slightly bluish. This condition is
    a. xanthosis.
    b. erythrocytosis.
    c. cyanosis.

72. Which of the following is a lesion of the mucous membrane of the stomach?
    a. Gastric ulcer
    b. Hiatal hernia
    c. Gastroesophageal reflux

73. Recurrent attacks of drowsiness and sleep is
    a. narcolepsy.
    b. epilepsy.
    c. polydipsia.

74. A client asks if massage can help recovery from a stroke. To find more information, the massage practitioner might use what term?
    a. Myocardial infarction
    b. CVA
    c. Angina pectoris

75. Which term indicates severe chest pain caused by insufficient blood supply?
    a. Mitral valve prolapse
    b. Aortic stenosis
    c. Angina pectoris

76. A massage client indicates on the health history they have cirrhosis. This is a disease of which organ?
    a. Gallbladder
    b. Liver
    c. Colon

77. A massage practitioner observes a wound as a result of skin being scraped or rubbed away by friction. The term used to chart this finding is
    a. incision.
    b. contusion.
    c. abrasion.

78. Which of the following is an infectious condition that usually occurs on the trunk of the body?
    a. Shingles
    b. Diuresis
    c. Myelitis

79. Which term means a cavity that contains pus?
    a. Abscess
    b. Cellulitis
    c. Acne

80. When is inflammation most productive for tissue healing?
    a. 1—7 days postinjury
    b. 21—36 days postinjury
    c. 14—21 days postinjury

81. In which stage of healing does the body produce new capillaries?
    a. Inflammation
    b. Proliferation
    c. Remodeling

82. What is the immediate response of the blood vessels to injury?
    a. Capillary density
    b. Vasodilation
    c. Vasoconstriction

83. Aggressive contraction of a wound occurs during what phase of wound healing?
    a. Proliferative phase
    b. Inflammatory phase
    c. Maturation phase

84. At what stage of tissue healing should pain be minimal?
    a. Subacute
    b. Remodeling
    c. Acute

85. A massage client sprained their ankle 6 weeks ago. What would indicate a normal healing process?
    a. Localized aching and edema postactivity
    b. Ability to fully resume preinjury activity levels
    c. Reduced pain and more confident movement

86. Areas on the body that are vulnerable to injury related to pressure applied during the bodywork method application are
    a. endangerment sites.
    b. visceral referred pain locations.
    c. enamel and dentin.

87. Which condition might a neurologist refer for massage?
    a. Primary hyperaldosteronism
    b. Epilepsy
    c. Emphysema

88. With what condition could a client experience the most potential for massage/bodywork benefit and the fewest cautions?
    a. Pulmonary edema
    b. Pancreatitis
    c. Tension headache

89. An area where pressure applied during massage is adapted to target skin and superficial facial to protect deeper structures from compression is the
    a. plantar aspect of the foot.
    b. anterior triangle of the neck.
    c. anterior thigh.

90. The inguinal triangle is considered an endangerment site because of what structures?
    a. Carotid artery, jugular vein, and vagus nerve
    b. Popliteal artery and vein, and tibial nerve
    c. External iliac artery, femoral artery, and femoral nerve

91. The ulnar nerve, and radial and ulnar arteries could be injured when aggressive bodywork methods are applied at the
    a. medial epicondyle of the humerus.
    b. posterior triangle of the neck.
    c. inguinal triangle.

92. During massage application, caution is required in the area of the 12th rib because of the
    a. saphenous vein.
    b. brachial plexus.
    c. kidneys.

93. What structures are located in the cervical, axilla, and inguinal areas that are considered cautionary related to pressure application?
    a. Lymph nodes
    b. Carotid arteries
    c. Styloid processes

94. A client asks the massage practitioner to use deep friction between the biceps and triceps muscles. The practitioner states this is contraindicated because
    a. this is the popliteal fossa.
    b. the area is the location of the median nerve.
    c. the femoral artery is located in the area.

95. During massage application, the location of the descending aorta requires caution when applying pressure on the
    a. axilla area.
    b. umbilicus area.
    c. lateral epicondyle.

96. The massage practitioner suspects a client may be experiencing venous thromboembolism. What action should the practitioner take?
    a. Stop the session, talk with client about the advisability of continuing the session
    b. Stop the session, call emergency services and wait with client until ambulance arrives
    c. Stop the session, explain why, and refer the client to their physician or emergency room

97. What situation requires immediate calling of emergency services and waiting with the client until first responders arrive?
    a. Signs of a stroke
    b. Potential concussion
    c. Symptoms of rhabdomyolysis

98. Symptoms of reexperiencing events, avoidance, numbing, and hyperarousal indicate potential
    a. biological rhythms feedback.
    b. posttraumatic stress disorder.
    c. stress coping adaptability.

99. A biologically plausible massage-related outcome goal indicated for anxiety and sleep disorders is
    a. stress management.
    b. inflammation reduction.
    c. functional mobility.

100. What illness can be caused by bacteria, virus, or fungus?
    a. Pneumonia
    b. Raynaud disease
    c. Sickle cell disease

101. Massage practitioners often work with clients diagnosed with multicausal and often chronic nonproductive patterns that interfere with well-being, activities of daily living, and productivity. These conditions can be classified as
    a. peripheral and central sensitization.
    b. neuromatrix theory of pain.
    c. pain and fatigue syndromes.

102. A contagious condition is
    a. tinea corporis.
    b. angioma.
    c. seborrheic keratosis.

103. A common musculoskeletal injury is a
    a. spina bifida.
    b. cellulitis.
    c. contusion.

104. A client indicates they have an injury. What condition might the massage client be experiencing?
    a. Atherosclerosis
    b. Concussion
    c. Prostatitis

105. Where would a gastric ulcer be found?
    a. Cecum
    b. Duodenum
    c. Stomach

106. What is the name of a digestive disease in which pouches within the large bowel wall become inflamed?
    a. Diverticulitis
    b. Pancreatitis
    c. Appendicitis

107. The most difficult bone injury to diagnosis is a
    a. stress fracture.
    b. compound fracture.
    c. spiral fracture.

108. A hiatal hernia is the protrusion of which of the following into the thorax?
    a. The duodenum
    b. The upper part of the stomach
    c. The transverse colon

109. Blackheads can result from a blockage of which of the following glands?
    a. Sudoriferous
    b. Sebaceous
    c. Ceruminous

110. A client has muscle atrophy of the entire arm. The massage practitioner asks if the client had an injury in what area?
    a. Sacral plexus
    b. Pharyngeal plexus
    c. Brachial plexus

111. Which pathological condition often progresses for decades and is a caution for massage?
    a. Osteoporosis
    b. Osteomyelitis
    c. Osteogenesis imperfecta

112. A massage client has an exaggerated lateral curve of the spine? This condition is
    a. lordosis.
    b. scoliosis.
    c. kyphosis.

113. A massage client asks the massage practitioner to avoid an area on their arm with a first-degree burn. What sign would the practitioner notice during observation assessment?
    a. Reddening of skin
    b. Blisters on skin
    c. Skin is charred

114. During palpation assessment, a massage practitioner identifies an excessive accumulation of fluid in tissues of the client's ankles and would chart the condition as possible
    a. infarction.
    b. aneurysm.
    c. edema.

115. A massage practitioner is explaining to the client findings from joint movement assessment and potential for a referral. What condition would indicate need for referral?
    a. Anatomical barrier
    b. Bone to bone end feel
    c. Soft-tissue approximation

116. How is an ulcer defined?
    a. An area of destroyed mucous membrane and an open sore or lesion
    b. A wound that occurs when skin, tissue, and/or muscle is torn or cut open
    c. A protrusion of the stomach into the diaphragm

117. What type of joint would be affected by rotator cuff tendinitis?
    a. Fibrous joint
    b. Synovial joint
    c. Cartilaginous joint

118. Inflammation of a vein is called
    a. vasodilatation.
    b. varicose veins.
    c. phlebitis.

119. What cranial nerve is involved with tic douloureux?
    a. Olfactory
    b. Optic
    c. Trigeminal

120. What is an evidence-informed benefit of massage therapy for a client receiving oncology care?
    a. Reducing pain and anxiety
    b. Increasing the action of chemotherapy
    c. Detoxing the body of cancer cells

121. What is a common concern for the massage practitioner when working with athletes?
    a. Endocrine disorders
    b. Joint injury
    c. Autoimmune conditions

122. When evaluating joint movement in an athlete for areas of hyper- or hypomobility, what needs to be considered before determining appropriateness of intervention?
    a. Type of counterirritant ointment used
    b. Travel schedule of the athlete
    c. Effects of sport specific training

123. Skin injury related to sliding on a surface is a/an
    a. contusion.
    b. puncture.
    c. abrasion.

124. An over-the-counter medication often used by sport and tactical athletes is
    a. NSAIDs.
    b. muscle relaxers.
    c. diuretics.

125. Common in individuals that participate in physically demanding sports or work activities is
    a. illness.
    b. trauma.
    c. depression.

126. A client participates in a contact sport such as American football. What is the most common sport injury this client may have which will require adaptation during the massage session?
    a. Contusion
    b. Puncture
    c. Blister

127. When adapting massage application for those who participate in physically demanding work or sports, most injures are considered
    a. indications for direct work.
    b. regional contraindications.
    c. general contraindications.

128. A client who is a distance runner describes muscle soreness, decreased joint flexibility, and general fatigue 24 hours after activity. What is the most likely cause?
    a. Ankle sprain
    b. New equipment
    c. Over exertion

129. A massage client tripped on an extension cord in their hallway and hurt their ankle. What is the most likely injury?
    a. Sprain
    b. Fracture
    c. Dislocation

130. A stretch, tear, or rip in the muscle or adjacent tissue, such as fascia or tendons, is called a/n
    a. sprain.
    b. avulsion.
    c. strain.

131. A client who is a firefighter has a muscle strain in their forearm diagnosed as grade 2. What would the massage practitioner expect to identify in the soft-tissue structures surrounding the area?
    a. Observable defect in the area
    b. Cocontraction muscle guarding
    c. Loss of muscle function

132. A client has been diagnosed with inflammation of the synovial sheath surrounding a tendon and reports that the physician indicates the massage practitioner should avoid massage in the area for the next few days. What is the most likely diagnosis?
    a. Tenosynovitis
    b. Tendinitis
    c. Tendinosis

133. The most serious heat-related condition is
    a. heat exhaustion.
    b. heatstroke.
    c. heat cramps.

134. Pregnancy is generally considered a hypercoagulable state, which means
    a. increased fatigue.
    b. development of gestational diabetes.
    c. blood clots more readily than normal.

135. A client in the postpartum period shows the massage practitioner a bulge in their abdomen along the line of the linea alba. The practitioner would refer for what condition?
    a. Inguinal hernia
    b. Diastasis recti
    c. Prolapsed uterus

136. Why is pregnancy a risk factor for deep-vein thrombosis?
    a. Hypercoagulability
    b. Gestational diabetes
    c. Preeclampsia

137. The most common adaptation during the second half of a normal pregnancy is
    a. avoiding work on the legs.
    b. positioning and bolstering.
    c. increasing the duration of the session.

138. What is it called when the body returns to a nonpregnant state?
    a. Transition
    b. Trimester
    c. Postpartum

139. Hormone fluctuation in the postpartum period can cause
    a. depression.
    b. preeclampsia.
    c. menopause.

140. The permission of a parent or guardian is required to work with
a. disabilities.
b. cancer patients.
c. minors.

141. A client who is 84 years old would require the massage practitioner to
a. research about physical effects of aging.
b. learn specific methods for this population.
c. gain a specific certificate for practice.

142. A client had a minor surgical procedure performed 2 days ago. A major concern for the massage practitioner is
a. pain management.
b. scar tissue.
c. infection potential.

143. In what situation would general contraindications for massage treatment exist?
a. Chronic illness
b. Acute illness
c. Acute injury

144. A primary outcome of massage for those experiencing an acute condition is
a. pain management.
b. improved mobility.
c. faster wound healing.

145. Acute care assumes that the person has a
a. physician.
b. current injury or illness.
c. diagnosis.

146. At which stage of the recovery process of a soft tissue injury is massage locally contraindicated?
a. Remodeling stage
b. Proliferation stage
c. Acute inflammatory stage

147. When a part of the body is avoided during a massage session what exists?
a. Absolute contraindication
b. Regional contraindication
c. Systemic contraindication

148. An absolute contraindication means
a. no bodywork is performed.
b. localized areas are avoided.
c. methods are adapted.

149. Massage application needs to be adapted in the advanced stages of osteoporosis because
a. the joint surface is necrotic.
b. tendons become fibrotic.
c. bones are brittle.

150. A caution for massage application that can become a contraindication due to inflammation of a vein causing pain and swelling is called
a. phlebitis.
b. embolus.
c. hematoma.

151. A massage practitioner might refer for diagnosis if they observe excessive accumulation of fluid in tissue spaces, mostly common in the extremities. This condition is likely
a. hematoma.
b. edema.
c. aneurysm.

152. Which of the following is an endangerment site requiring cautions and adaptation during massage application?
a. Plantar surface of foot
b. Axilla
c. Forearm

153. A massage client has dermatitis which is inflammation of the
a. joints.
b. nerves.
c. skin.

154. Edema is indicated by pressing an area, removing the finger, and observing if the
a. indentation remains.
b. skin springs back.
c. area flushes red.

155. What structure under the upper right part of the abdomen may be at risk from excessive pressure applied in the area?
a. Aorta
b. Ulnar nerve
c. Liver

156. Botulinum toxin injections are used in children with cerebral palsy for which of the following?
a. To reduce fibrosis
b. To reduce spasticity
c. To increase circulation

157. A massage client informs the massage practitioner that they may need to use the restroom because they take a medication that increases urination called a
    a. diuretic.
    b. diuresis.
    c. glomerulus.

158. A client has a condition called atrial fibrillation. What medication might they be taking that could require the massage therapist to adapt the session?
    a. Atorvastatin
    b. Aspirin
    c. Warfarin sodium

159. SSRIs are generally prescribed for which condition?
    a. Depression
    b. Hypertension
    c. Diabetes

160. Which drug class is used to reduce or prevent clotting in the blood?
    a. Antihistamines
    b. Anticoagulants
    c. Diuretics

161. A client inhales a beta agonist to relieve asthma symptoms which may result in a/n
    a. increase in heart rate.
    b. few moments of incoordination.
    c. decrease in blood pressure.

162. A class of medications used to treat angina are
    a. proton pump inhibitors.
    b. nitrates.
    c. bronchodilators.

163. If a massage client is taking a narcotic pain medication (codeine, Vicodin, or Darvocet), which type of approach should be used with caution?
    a. Reflexology
    b. Relaxation massage
    c. Deep-tissue massage

164. Which of the following medications is an opioid?
    a. Ibuprofen
    b. Acetaminophen
    c. Codeine

165. Which drug class is used to reduce hypertension by decreasing water and electrolytes in the kidneys?
    a. Diuretics
    b. Beta-blockers
    c. Antiarrhythmics

166. What is the most common drug administration route?
    a. Topical
    b. Oral
    c. Injection

167. Which would be considered the trade name of the drug?
    a. Tylenol
    b. Acetaminophen
    c. Metformin

168. Which of the following would be classified as a cardiovascular medication?
    a. Antihypertensive
    b. Steroids
    c. Antibiotics

169. The medication classification used in pain management is
    a. antiparkinsonism.
    b. analgesics.
    c. antitussives.

170. A type of medication that is used for respiratory conditions is
    a. bronchodilators.
    b. anticonvulsants.
    c. antidepressants.

171. A client indicates on the massage therapy intake form that they are prescribed steroids. Which type of condition would the client most likely be experiencing?
    a. Hormonal
    b. Cardiovascular
    c. Autoimmune

172. A client takes an antidepressant medication. What would be a common side effect?
    a. Dry mouth
    b. Muscle weakness
    c. Joint pain

173. A client has been diagnosed with epilepsy since childhood. The condition would be controlled with what medication classification?
    a. Antihistamine
    b. Anticonvulsant
    c. Antineoplastic

174. What adaptation would be most indicated for a massage client diagnosed with gastroesophageal reflux disease?
    a. Client positioning
    b. Massage duration
    c. Pressure depth

175. A client has been taking antiviral medications for several years. What is the most like condition being treated?
    a. MRSA
    b. HIV
    c. PTSD

PRACTICE TEST 5

Theory and Practice of Massage and Bodywork—175 Questions

1. Perceived reduction in pain related to soft-tissue manipulation is most likely related to
   a. increase sympathetic arousal.
   b. the relaxation response.
   c. localized circulatory changes.

2. The most consistent research finding related to massage therapy benefits is
   a. modulation in the autonomic nervous system.
   b. changes in systemic blood flow.
   c. decreased response of somatic reflex regulation.

3. What is the most logical reason for potential changes in local blood flow related to soft-tissue manipulation?
   a. Interstitial fluid movement from compression
   b. Fibroblast proliferation due to inflammation
   c. Vasodilation related to nitric oxide and histamine

4. What is the most biologically plausible effect of soft-tissue manipulation on fascia?
   a. Releases fascial adhesions
   b. Changes the length of collagen fibers
   c. May promote sliding in the fascial layers

5. Soft tissue manipulation may alter short-term pain perception through
   a. hyperstimulation analgesia.
   b. fascial reorganization.
   c. increased systemic circulation.

6. Beneficial results of soft tissue methods experienced by massage clients appear to be primarily through
   a. biomechanical changes in posture.
   b. regulatory mechanisms of the nervous system.
   c. fluid exchange in the blood and lymph systems.

7. Mechanical forces introduced into soft tissue may influence body-wide movement capacity by
   a. changing the pull muscles place on fascia.
   b. creating inflammation.
   c. creating fibrotic changes in the joint capsule.

8. A hormone related to safe touch is
   a. leptin.
   b. melatonin.
   c. oxytocin.

9. The approach to massage/bodywork care that acknowledges the whole person is
   a. biopsychosocial.
   b. based on fixed outcomes.
   c. population specialization.

10. What is as important as methods used in achieving a massage client's outcomes?
    a. Education qualification
    b. Therapeutic alliance
    c. Practice setting

11. A massage method that presses, twists, and rolls soft tissue is
    a. kneading.
    b. vibration.
    c. gliding.

12. A massage client asks if any methods can have a pulling sensation during the session. What method can create this effect?
    a. Oscillation
    b. Kneading
    c. Hacking

13. A massage client requests a calming outcome from the session and wishes to remain clothed. What method best meets these criteria?
    a. Gliding
    b. Rocking
    c. Tapotement

14. What is the massage practitioner performing when applying pressure in an area without movement?
    a. Friction
    b. Drag
    c. Compression

15. A massage client requests moderate pressure and tissue elongation in the posterior thigh area. What combination of methods will best accomplish this result?
    a. Compression combined with gliding
    b. Friction combined with vibration
    c. Kneading combined with shaking

16. What method typically is applied with a lubricant?
    a. Holding
    b. Compression
    c. Gliding

17. What method is indicated as an intervention when a small local area is targeted?
    a. Gliding
    b. Joint movement
    c. Friction

18. Methods that twist tissue specifically create what type of soft tissue deformation?
    a. Torsion
    b. Shear
    c. Compression

19. A practitioner applies pressure perpendicular to and in the middle of soft-tissue attachments. The result is the area experiences combined loading becoming compressed on one side and elongated on the other. The resulting tissue deformation is best described as
    a. torsion stress.
    b. bending stress.
    c. tensile stress.

20. What method can be used to assess range of motion?
    a. Joint movement
    b. Traction
    c. Vibration

21. What method is applied with the lightest pressure range?
    a. Kneading
    b. Holding
    c. Shaking

22. When providing a general massage therapy session with a relaxation outcome,
    a. the protocol is rhythmic and smoothly applied.
    b. frequent pre- and postassessments are performed.
    c. the client is initially positioned prone.

23. General sequence of massage method application is
    a. anterior-lateral-ventral.
    b. supine-prone-seated.
    c. superficial-deeper-superficial.

24. How does the outcome for the session influence the sequence of the session?
    a. An outcome based on stress management will require a longer session and participation by the client
    b. A session based on improved mobility is interspersed with assessment and interventions
    c. An outcome targeting systemic pain management will result in shorter more frequent sessions

25. Thermotherapy provides benefit because of the
    a. mechanical response of force application.
    b. physiological response to temperature changes.
    c. psychological response to compassionate communication.

26. A complementary approach based on water is
    a. hydrotherapy.
    b. cupping.
    c. percussion tools.

27. Cryotherapy benefit is related to
    a. sauna.
    b. water.
    c. cold temperature.

28. An example of a method that combines hydrotherapy and thermotherapy is
    a. warm foot soak.
    b. hot stones.
    c. counterirritant ointment.

29. What is the reason hydrotherapy and thermotherapy are applied together?
    a. Water is a solvent
    b. Water can be many temperatures
    c. Water is the easiest application

30. When applying an ice pack,
    a. wrap the ice pack in a cloth to protect the skin.
    b. cover the ice pack with a warm towel.
    c. leave in place for 30 minutes.

31. Contrast thermotherapy is
    a. using hot water immersion.
    b. alternating hot and cold applications.
    c. alternating between a wet and dry sauna.

32. Cold applications in a targeted area can
    a. penetrate into deep muscle layers.
    b. lead to shock.
    c. shift pain perception.

33. If a cold application is left on the skin for an extended time, what could occur?
    a. Frostbite
    b. Ulcer
    c. Anaphylaxis

34. A safety concern related to thermotherapy is
    a. bruising.
    b. burns.
    c. vasodilation.

35. An immediate effect of a cold pack is
    a. histamine response.
    b. vasodilatation.
    c. vasoconstriction.

36. A bodywork form using compression over loose clothing is
    a. manual lymph drain.
    b. Swedish.
    c. Shiatsu.

37. A manual therapy approached used by massage practitioners that targets connective tissue is
    a. myofascial release.
    b. polarity therapy.
    c. lymphatic drainage.

38. Passive treatment in this system includes terms like effleurage, pétrissage, and tapotement:
    a. neuromuscular therapy.
    b. Swedish massage.
    c. myofascial release.

39. A bodywork form considered modern and western is
    a. neuromuscular therapy.
    b. classical massage.
    c. Thai massage.

40. A study that performs a systematic review using defined statistical methods to combine the findings of several primary studies is called a
    a. clinical trial.
    b. case report.
    c. meta-analysis.

41. Which touch modality is based on the premise that change can be affected in different parts of the body by working the corresponding reflex areas in the feet, hands, or ears?
    a. Polarity therapy
    b. Reflexology
    c. Shiatsu

42. A client asks why a health history is taken prior to the session. The best response is
    a. state legislation mandates that all clients complete a form with contact information.
    b. decisions based on the information provided help determine contraindications and adaptations.
    c. client files include a health history form, informed consent form, and SOAP notes.

43. Discussion of the health history with the client is necessary to
    a. refer to other health professionals.
    b. determine session time.
    c. identify contraindications.

44. When a massage practitioner uses palpation to assess the client, they are
    a. touching the client.
    b. assessing activities of daily living.
    c. taking an accurate history.

45. When the bodywork session outcome targets improved movement, what will be included in the session?
    a. Hot packs
    b. Range of motion assessment
    c. Side-lying positioning

46. During the session, the massage practitioner identifies a rash that was not disclosed by the client prior to the session. What is the initial dilemma faced by the practitioner?
    a. How to adapt to work on the area
    b. Determining if the rash is a local contraindication
    c. Explaining to the client the area needs to be avoided

47. The method used to assess for range of motion is
    a. percussion.
    b. kneading.
    c. joint movement.

48. During the massage session intake interview, the client informs the massage practitioner they are experiencing lower back discomfort. In what section of the SOAP notes would this go?
    a. S
    b. O
    c. P

49. A client indicates on the health history form that they have diabetes. What would be the next action the massage practitioner takes?
    a. Ask clarifying questions about medication
    b. Refer client to a practitioner who works in a medical setting
    c. Proceed with posture and gait assessment

50. A client has been diagnosed with an inflamed gallbladder diagnosed as chronic cholecystitis and will be undergoing surgery in a week. They would like a massage therapy session for stress. What is the most logical approach?
    a. The client's doctor would need to provide specific treatment directions
    b. The practitioner would need to postpone the session
    c. The client could receive a modified session with appropriate adaption

51. A massage practitioner notices that a regular client, age 82, has increased edema in their legs. How would this situation affect the session?
    a. Additional communication is needed to determine if the session can occur or if referral is indicated
    b. The session cannot be performed and emergency services should be contacted
    c. The legs can be bolstered to promote fluid movement with lymphatic drain methods used

52. A client fell and hit their head when leaving for the bodywork session. There is a noticeable bump on the head and the client indicates they experienced visual disturbances that cleared within minutes. They drove alone to the facility. They indicate they feel fine except for a dull headache and are looking forward to the session. What is the next action to take?
    a. Provide the session and call emergency contact on file so they can take them home
    b. Explain that head injury is serious and that they should immediately seek medical assessment
    c. Perform a balance assessment and observe if eye pupils are equal

53. A client's demeanor reminds a massage practitioner of a sibling evoking an emotional response. This is an example of
    a. dual relationship.
    b. transference.
    c. countertransference.

54. A massage practitioner has been working with a family member providing therapeutic massage. When adjusting fees schedules, the massage practitioner hesitates raising the fee rate for them. This is an example of
    a. transference.
    b. dual relationship.
    c. power differential.

55. If a massage practitioner refuses to perform a method that is contraindicated for a client's condition and recommends referral to the person's medical team for recommendations, which ethical principle is upheld?
    a. Nonmaleficence
    b. Proportionality
    c. Justice

56. A massage practitioner advises a client to take an over-the-counter medication for allergies. This is a violation of
    a. emotional boundaries.
    b. dual relationship.
    c. scope of practice.

57. A massage practitioner has been asked to speak with the business owner concerning a client complaint. The concern is of an ethical nature. Which of the issues would be most likely?
    a. The client indicated that the massage practitioner had an unpleasant body odor
    b. The client felt that the massage practitioner was soliciting them for a cash tip in exchange for sexual acts
    c. The client indicated that the massage practitioner was complaining during the session about how they were paid

58. If a massage client has autonomy in a healthcare relationship, this means
    a. self-determination.
    b. ability to pay for services.
    c. right to medical insurance.

59. What is the best action if a massage client asks for their neck to be cracked during the session?
    a. Include methods with spinal adjustment potential
    b. Explain limits of scope of practice
    c. Indicate that spinal adjustment naturally occurs

60. A massage practitioner is an employee of a chiropractor. The practitioner finds out that a newly hired massage practitioner is receiving a higher per client fee than they are. What is the most professional action for the massage practitioner to take?
    a. Schedule a meeting with the chiropractor to discuss the situation
    b. Ignore the situation and look for a different position
    c. Discuss the situation with the newly hired practitioner

61. What situation would involve a "zero tolerance policy" with the massage session terminated and the client dismissed?
    a. Client consistently arriving late for appointments
    b. Client being frustrated by the cancellation policy
    c. Client removing draping material exposing their body

62. When does a massage practitioner explain all policies to the client so the client can make an informed decision about receiving massage therapy services?
    a. When a policy violation occurs
    b. Initial intake interview
    c. Included on professional website

63. A client feels as if the massage practitioner was sexually inappropriate during the session and reports the situation to the business manager. What event would justify the client's feelings and action?
    a. The massage practitioner's groin area repeatedly makes contact with the client's body during the session
    b. The massage practitioner failed to explain that the business policy is for clients to wear undergarments covering the gluteal and pelvic area during the session
    c. The massage practitioner talked about non–massage-related topics throughout the session

64. A massage studio focusing on wellness has a zero tolerance policy. Which of the following would be considered sexual harassment?
    a. A practitioner explaining sexual boundaries
    b. A client repeatedly telling inappropriate jokes
    c. A coworker gossiping about pay scales

65. A self-employed massage practitioner has had a new massage franchise open near their practice and is experiencing conflicting feelings. Some of their clients have gotten massage sessions at the franchise when unable to book with them. The feedback to the massage practitioner from these clients is that the facility is professionally run and massage therapists competent. What conflict type best describes what the massage practitioner is experiencing?
    a. Data conflict
    b. Interest conflict
    c. Relationship conflict

66. What is an ethical issue related to legislated draping regulations?
    a. Veracity
    b. Autonomy
    c. Respect

67. The receptionist in a large massage practice has a personality conflict with one of the massage staff. The business owner is generally happy with the performance of the receptionist but recently has been reviewing the schedule to make sure all massage staff are being booked for sessions according to policy. What is the ethical concern of the business owner?
    a. Justice
    b. Beneficence
    c. Fidelity

68. When using a plug-in table warmer, what causes the most concern related to safety of the practitioner?
    a. Air quality
    b. Potential burns
    c. Tripping hazard

69. Air quality in a treatment room would be most affected by
    a. essential oils.
    b. hypoallergenic lotion.
    c. location in facility.

70. The purpose of lubricant use during the massage session is to reduce
    a. inflammation.
    b. drag on the skin.
    c. skin flaking.

71. What treatment table type requires safety inspection of hinges and cables?
    a. Portable
    b. Hydraulic
    c. Stationary

72. What has the most potential for harm if used incorrectly?
    a. Antiseptic
    b. Air purifiers
    c. Disinfectants

73. What is a safety concern when choosing lubricants used during the massage session?
    a. Cost
    b. Allergens
    c. Manufacturer

74. What ingredient in a product used during the bodywork session could produce anaphylaxis?
    a. Alcohol
    b. Water
    c. Nuts

75. When ordering supplies for use during the massage session, be aware of
    a. volume cost discounts.
    b. product reviews.
    c. expiration date.

76. A primary concern when purchasing equipment to use during the massage session is
    a. ability to disinfect as needed.
    b. storage convenience.
    c. manufactures warranty.

77. What is an additional use of pillowcases when preparing for the session?
    a. Cleaning the table and counters
    b. Covering bolsters and supports
    c. Replacing trash receptacle

78. If the massage practitioner has a contagious illness spread by respiratory droplets, they
    a. work if face mask and gloves are used.
    b. do not work until the illness is resolved.
    c. avoid working with anyone immune compromised.

79. What is safe to apply to the skin?
    a. Sterilant
    b. Disinfectant
    c. Antiseptic

80. The material used for draping supplies
    a. needs to be able to withstand disinfecting when laundered.
    b. would be able to be efficiently folded and stored.
    c. should have an antimicrobial coating.

81. An active ingredient in antiseptics is
    a. isopropyl alcohol.
    b. sodium hypochlorite.
    c. quaternary ammonium.

82. Which method destroys all organisms using heat?
    a. Sanitization
    b. Disinfection
    c. Sterilization

83. Disinfectants applied to surfaces have a required
    a. dilution ratio.
    b. contact time.
    c. ingredient list.

84. Disinfecting tools used during a session is intended to
    a. kill germs on surfaces or objects.
    b. remove dirt and impurities from surfaces or objects.
    c. lower the number of germs on surfaces or objects to a safe level.

85. What is used when cleaning?
    a. Bleach
    b. Soap and water
    c. Hydrogen peroxide

86. A facility risk assessment is
    a. an inspection by Occupational Safety and Health Administration (OSHA).
    b. a process when potential safety concerns are identified.
    c. when control measures to reduce risks are implemented.

87. What is a strategy to avoid contamination of products used during the massage session?
    a. Limit type of product used
    b. Adding disinfectant to product
    c. Single-use containers

88. What item is a safety risk in the professional facility?
    a. Extension cords
    b. Ventilation fan
    c. Air filter

89. What hazardous chemicals are most likely encountered by a massage practitioner?
    a. Fire extinguishers
    b. Oil-based lubricants
    c. Cleaning products

90. The facility parking area should
    a. be adjacent to a designated smoking area.
    b. have adequate lighting.
    c. have multiple trash receptacles.

91. A tiled entry way in the facility can become a safety hazard when
    a. wet.
    b. small.
    c. near carpet.

92. A coworker has been frustrated and angry over events at work and in their personal life. Should this situation escalate there is a potential for
    a. workplace hazard.
    b. sexual harassment.
    c. workplace violence.

93. A massage practitioner suspects a client is under the influence of alcohol. The best action to take is
    a. communicating with the client.
    b. continue with the session.
    c. refuse to provide the session.

94. What is the field of study that focuses on the adaptation of equipment for safety of the practitioner?
    a. Kinesiology
    b. Biomechanics
    c. Ergonomics

95. If a client threatens to harm themselves or others, the massage practitioner has an ethical and legal duty to
    a. discuss this information with the client's family.
    b. report this information to the authorities.
    c. discuss this information with a mentor or supervisor.

96. A biomechanical concern related to use of the thumb to apply soft-tissue methods is
    a. sustaining a stable position.
    b. instability of the hinge joint.
    c. compression of the carpal joints.

97. What is the best explanation for concern when using the hands to apply massage methods?
    a. The structure of the joints in the fingers cannot be stabilized.
    b. Repetitive pushing and pulling actions increase injury potential in the small structures.
    c. The intrinsic muscles in the hands attached at the elbow joint leading to repetitive strain.

98. A biomechanical issue that occurs when the practitioner applies long gliding methods using the hand or forearm is
    a. repetitive strain injury from movement of the forearm in supination/pronation.
    b. inability to lock knee joints during trunk flexion.
    c. movement of the glenohumeral joint beyond 45% of flexion.

99. Which of the following actions has the greatest potential for injury when providing bodywork sessions?
    a. Long stroke length with feet in a symmetrical stance
    b. Compression using the palm with 15 degrees of trunk flexion at the hip
    c. Feet positioned in asymmetrical stance while providing short excursion gliding

100. Applying what method has the greatest potential for repetitive strain injury in the forearm near the elbow?
    a. Gliding
    b. Kneading
    c. Compression

101. An indication that the table height is too low is
    a. trunk flexion beyond 30 degrees.
    b. feet positioned shoulder width apart.
    c. standing on balls of the feet.

102. When considering the workspace what is an ergonomic factor?
    a. Number of rooms available
    b. Availability of reception staff
    c. Sufficient space to move around the treatment table

103. An indication that the table height is too high is
    a. flexed knees.
    b. elevated shoulders.
    c. feet flat on floor.

104. Safe adaptation to allow more pressure delivery during the massage session is to
    a. change to symmetrical stance.
    b. use increased upper body strength.
    c. shift center of gravity forward from the feet.

105. A client has a noncontagious skin condition, but there are areas of broken skin. The massage practitioner would use
    a. face shield.
    b. protective gloves.
    c. gown.

106. What type of personal protective equipment protects against spread of airborne pathogens?
    a. Mask
    b. Gown
    c. Gloves

107. Which condition requires using gown, gloves, and mask?
    a. Hyperlipidemia
    b. Chronic obstructive pulmonary disease (COPD)
    c. Methicillin-resistant *Staphylococcus aureus* (MRSA)

108. When the schedule for the day has multiple massage clients, what form of protective equipment prevents contamination of clothing?
    a. Gowns and smocks
    b. Safety boots and coverings
    c. Masks and gloves

109. Being attentive to personal and professional boundaries is a type of
    a. self-care.
    b. palliative approach.
    c. client intervention.

110. A massage practitioner evaluates increasing the number of clients they schedule each week versus having more recreational time. This is an example of
    a. maximizing income potential.
    b. work/life balance.
    c. professional disclosure.

111. A massage client is immunocompromised due to a medication used to control an autoimmune condition. What should be used to protect the client from airborne pathogens during the session?
    a. Face shield
    b. Mask
    c. Smock

112. What situation would indicate use of a face shield?
    a. The practitioner has allergies
    b. A client has an upper respiratory infection
    c. Using disinfecting chemicals

113. A practitioner is feeling fatigued and anxious even through their client schedule is full with a waiting list. The practitioner may be experiencing
    a. motivation.
    b. illness.
    c. burnout.

114. A client requests the practitioner use deep pressure with the thumbs. The massage practitioner explains that this type of application puts them at risk and does not perform the methods as requested. The practitioner demonstrated
    a. limits of scope of practice.
    b. attention to injury prevention.
    c. application of ergonomics.

115. A massage practitioner is applying for a position that allows scheduling flexibility even though they declined a job that paid more but required working evenings. The practitioner is demonstrating
    a. self-care.
    b. target marketing.
    c. fiscal responsibility.

116. A massage practitioner has converted a mobile practice to a solo office practice. What piece of equipment can now be used to prevent injury?
    a. Air filter
    b. Hot towel cabbie
    c. Electric lift table

117. A principle of draping is
    a. the body is covered except areas being worked on.
    b. a blanket is needed during the session.
    c. sheets are the preferred material.

118. An alternative to draping during the massage session is
    a. using disposable materials.
    b. working over clothing.
    c. working on a mat.

119. A massage client has sensitive skin and experiences contact dermatitis from many laundry detergents. How would the practitioner approach this situation?
    a. Purchase the linens and detergent used by the client
    b. Work with minimal draping
    c. Discuss alternatives with the client

120. A client indicates they are hot and want less draping during the session. An appropriate reply is
    a. draping can be removed if underwear remains on.
    b. draping is required.
    c. draping is required but can be modified.

121. A client is concerned about feeling exposed during the session since this has occurred once before. How would the massage practitioner respond?
    a. What would make you most comfortable?
    b. The drape is always secure
    c. A blanket can be added for additional coverage

122. A business that is owned and operated by one person only is a
     a. sole proprietorship.
     b. partnership.
     c. corporation.

123. The draping method at an employee's work setting is different than how the massage practitioner was trained. What is the practitioner's appropriate response?
     a. I prefer to use my own draping approach
     b. I will need to be trained in the draping method
     c. The client guides my draping methods

124. Choosing a specific group of people or demographics to build a client base is a/n
     a. income projection.
     b. target market.
     c. business plan.

125. A massage business determines a fee for services by investigating
     a. income tax rate.
     b. business loans.
     c. demographics.

126. To be reimbursed by a health insurance company requires a/n
     a. National Provider Identification Number.
     b. Employer Identification Number.
     c. Taxpayer Identification Number.

127. A plan for using income is a/n
     a. budget.
     b. expense report.
     c. income statement.

128. Which business structure is able to file federal tax using an individual's social security number?
     a. Corporation
     b. Sole proprietor
     c. Partnership

129. What identifier allows the IRS to track wages and other payments from the business to the business's employees and owners?
     a. Social Security Number
     b. Doing Business As Registration
     c. Employer Identification Number

130. The healthcare provider identification system adopted by the U.S. Department of Health and Human Services as part of the implementation of the Health Insurance Portability and Accountability Act (HIPAA) uses a/n
     a. Employer Identification Number.
     b. National Provider Identification (NPI) Number.
     c. Taxpayer Identification Number.

131. What federal tax identification number is used for businesses?
     a. National Provider Identification Number
     b. Sales Tax Number
     c. Employer Identification Number

132. When investigating use of social media for business, what element is needed?
     a. Software
     b. Blog
     c. Website

133. Business risk analysis is a
     a. process that identifies issues that could cause problems.
     b. tax audit for payroll taxes.
     c. plan for reducing improper client behavior.

134. Using social media as a business platform needs to
     a. be provided by a company specializing in development.
     b. reflect the professional nature of the business.
     c. contain access to multiple advertising outlets.

135. A massage practitioner is determining their fee structure for services. Personal expenses are $40,000 per year. If the business overhead expenses are $25,000 per year and the person estimates 20 hours of income-producing sessions per week based on 50 working weeks per year, what is the minimum fee for service for each hour?
     a. $65
     b. $50
     c. $90

136. Determining the demographics of the target market for a wellness-based business related to setting fees would require identifying
     a. number of single-family households.
     b. distance from location.
     c. average yearly income.

137. An employer is estimating the total cost of paying all the employees. This is called the
    a. tax burden.
    b. wage/labor burden.
    c. cost benefit ratio.

138. A business plan that pairs the objectives of a business with the needs of the customer is the
    a. facility plan.
    b. exit plan.
    c. strategic plan.

139. Attending to business operations that are not specifically related to the massage therapy practice is
    a. office management.
    b. client records completion.
    c. ergonomics and biomechanics.

140. Maintaining the safety of the practice facility is an example of
    a. fiscal responsibility.
    b. office management activities.
    c. activities of daily living.

141. A client posts a social medial review mentioning how friendly and helpful the front desk staff was during their visit to the business. This individual was complimenting the
    a. the massage therapist.
    b. spa attendant.
    c. receptionist.

142. A marketing advantage a franchise-based massage business has that a self-employed massage therapist may not initially have when opening a new massage office is
    a. brand recognition.
    b. adaptable service fees.
    c. lead therapist on staff.

143. Participating in local professional groups is a form of
    a. risk management.
    b. social media.
    c. networking.

144. Advertising for a sole practitioner working part time from their home office can be effectively provided by
    a. radio advertisements.
    b. word of mouth.
    c. social media advertisements.

145. The marketing function of a website is
    a. to convince website visitors to become customers.
    b. provides an online scheduler.
    c. dispenses health-related information.

146. A strategy for preparing for an interview is
    a. preparing a market evaluation.
    b. learning about the business.
    c. organizing accounting records.

147. A massage practitioner is preparing for a career change from sole practice to employee at a chiropractic center. Discussion with the office manager about the potential for being hired is the
    a. application.
    b. interview.
    c. job search.

148. What document is used to provide information related to work experience?
    a. W-4
    b. Cover letter
    c. Resume

149. During an interview for a position at a wellness center, the massage practitioner provides an alternative work schedule. After discussion, an agreement on a different work schedule was reached. What occurred?
    a. Negotiation
    b. Marketing
    c. Budgeting

150. Once the decision to hire a massage practitioner is made, the next step is
    a. organizing the treatment room.
    b. developing promotional material to fill the schedule.
    c. completing employment forms for payroll taxes.

151. Which tax form would a massage practitioner working for a chiropractor receive at the end of the calendar year?
    a. 1099-NEC
    b. W-4
    c. W-2

152. What client record is completed for each massage client visit?
    a. Session documentation
    b. Treatment plan
    c. Informed consent

153. A client reports they have moved to a different location. What form is updated?
    a. Assessment
    b. Intake
    c. Treatment plan

154. What business records are the responsibility of an employee?
    a. Hours worked
    b. Supply expenses
    c. Rental expenses

155. The form W-4 informs the employer about
    a. eligibility for workplace benefits.
    b. income tax to withhold from employees' wages.
    c. access to unemployment insurance.

156. A massage practitioner is leaving an employment situation at a resort spa and is opening a mobile-based massage business. What taxes will they need to pay that cover social security and Medicare?
    a. Income tax
    b. Self-employment tax
    c. Worker's compensation

157. Who is eligible for unemployment compensation?
    a. Employees
    b. Self-employed
    c. Independent contractors

158. Who is responsible for paying federal and state unemployment tax?
    a. Independent contractor
    b. Self-employed
    c. Employer

159. What covers employees if injured on the job?
    a. Social security
    b. Medicare
    c. Workers' compensation

160. A business conducted from a residence may be eligible for some tax deductions if
    a. it is regularly and exclusively used as principal place of business.
    b. it has barrier-free access and adjacent restrooms.
    c. it meets zoning requirements.

161. An energetic-based system that might be incorporated into a client session is
    a. lymphatic drainage.
    b. muscle energy technique.
    c. therapeutic touch.

162. What area is most difficult to support with research?
    a. Biofields
    b. Pain
    c. Endocrine response

163. A common term used for energetic anatomy is
    a. nerve.
    b. meridian.
    c. self-care.

164. A quantified outcome goal is that the massage client will
    a. increase range of motion 15 degrees.
    b. be able to resume normal work activities.
    c. need to be reassessed in 12 sessions.

165. Which of the following is an example of condition management?
    a. Restoring a client's range of motion to its preinjury state
    b. Assisting the client in learning to walk again
    c. Maintaining the existing physical compensation patterns

166. A person who is experiencing an impingement in the cervical plexus would have which symptoms?
    a. Shoulder pain, chest pain, arm pain, wrist pain, and hand pain
    b. Headaches, neck pain, and breathing difficulties
    c. Gluteal pain, leg pain, genital pain, and foot pain

167. The most effective massage methods used to work on nerve impingement syndromes are
    a. percussion and shaking.
    b. muscle energy techniques and lengthening.
    c. rapid deep compression.

168. The massage therapist has been running behind and the next client has been waiting for 15 minutes. It is most important that the massage therapist
    a. maintain scheduled appointments on time.
    b. have materials and activities available for clients to entertain themselves.
    c. make sure sheets and linens are changed and equipment is disinfected between massages.

169. A massage professional wants to know whether an office that is being considered for rental is located in an appropriate business district. Where would this information be found?
    a. Facility rental agreement
    b. Local zoning office
    c. State licensing bureau

170. A massage practitioner has been experiencing increasingly severe low back pain and works in a full-time practice that cares for 20 clients per week. What could the massage practitioner do to reduce back strain?
    a. Bend the knees past 25 degrees while performing massage
    b. Raise the table height to prevent torso bending
    c. Keep the head forward and down to change the center of gravity

171. A massage professional is feeling strain in the knees. Which of the following is the most logical cause?
    a. Performing massage on hard floors
    b. Working with clients in the side-lying position
    c. Keeping the knees flexed and static

172. A massage practitioner has been seeing the same client weekly for 3 months. This client often discusses personal issues with the massage practitioner. During the previous session, the massage professional provided some reading information to help the client and talked with the client about how the practitioner had dealt with a similar issue. The client has canceled the following two appointments. What is the most logical cause?
    a. Feedback about the massage broke down

    b. Conversation with the client overshadowed the massage session
    c. Gender issues are influencing the session

173. The massage therapist should stay in the massage room and assist which of the following clients onto and off of the massage table?
    a. A client in the first trimester of pregnancy
    b. A 65-year-old man with diabetes
    c. An elderly woman with high blood pressure

174. Which of the following methods is most beneficial for abdominal massage performed to encourage fecal movement within the large intestine?
    a. Gliding
    b. Holding position
    c. Percussion

175. If using foot reflexology theory, where would the massage practitioner focus massage on the foot to affect the neck?
    a. Heel
    b. Tips of the toes
    c. Base of the large toe

Indications and Contraindications to Massage

Because each situation is different, it is difficult to make recommendations regarding when to give a massage and when not to give one. Each situation should be evaluated so it can be determined whether massage is indicated or contraindicated. Since this review system targets entry-level licensure, the recommendations provided are conservative. The existence of contraindications does not always mean that therapeutic massage is inappropriate. What most contraindications require is caution, which may call for modification of the massage treatment and, in some cases, supervision by and cooperation with the client's healthcare team. The clinical reasoning model is a valuable tool for making decisions about contraindications. This appendix presents two models of a guideline system that can be used for determining the indications and contraindications for massage. Specific conditions, symptoms, indications, and contraindications for massage follow. Use a medical dictionary to look up unfamiliar terms.

THE ONTARIO MODEL

The following are absolute contraindications (CIs) to massage (meaning massage treatment should not be given).

General Contraindications

1. Acute-stage pneumonia
2. Advanced kidney failure (modified treatment may be possible with medical consent)
3. Advanced respiratory failure (modified treatment may be possible with medical consent)
4. Diabetes with complications (e.g., gangrene, advanced heart or kidney disease, very high or unstable blood pressure)
5. Eclampsia-toxemia in pregnancy
6. Hemophilia

7. Hemorrhage
8. Liver failure (modified treatment may be possible with medical consent)
9. Post cerebrovascular accident (cerebrovascular accident [CVA], stroke), condition not yet stabilized
10. Post myocardial infarction (myocardial infarction [MI], heart attack), condition not yet stabilized
11. Severe atherosclerosis
12. Severe hypertension (if unstable)
13. Shock (all types)
14. Significant fever (higher than 101°F [38.3°C])
15. Some acute conditions that require first aid or medical attention:
    - Anaphylaxis
    - Appendicitis
    - CVA
    - Diabetic coma, insulin shock
    - Epileptic seizure
    - MI
    - Pneumothorax, atelectasis
    - Severe asthma attack, status asthmaticus
    - Syncope (fainting)
16. Some highly metastatic cancers not judged to be terminal
17. Systemic contagious/infectious conditions

Local (Regional) Contraindications

1. Acute flare-up of inflammatory arthritis (e.g., rheumatoid arthritis, systemic lupus erythematosus, ankylosing spondylitis, Reiter syndrome); may be general CI, depending on case
2. Acute neuritis
3. Aneurysms deemed life-threatening (e.g., of the abdominal aorta); may be general CI, depending on location
4. Ectopic pregnancy
5. Esophageal varicosities (varices)
6. Frostbite

7. Local contagious condition
8. Local irritable skin condition
9. Malignancy (especially if judged unstable)
10. Open wound or sore
11. Phlebitis, phlebothrombosis, arteritis; may be general CI if located in a major circulatory channel
12. Recent burn
13. Sepsis
14. Temporal arteritis
15. 24–48 hours after antiinflammatory treatment (target tissue and immediate vicinity)
16. Undiagnosed lump

General Conditions

The following conditions require an awareness of the possibility of adverse effects from massage therapy. Substantial treatment adaptation may be appropriate. Medical consultation often is needed.

1. Any condition of spasticity or rigidity
2. Asthma
3. Cancer (including finding appropriate relationships to other current treatments)
4. Chronic congestive heart failure
5. Chronic kidney disease
6. Client taking antiinflammatory drugs, muscle relaxants, anticoagulants, analgesics, or any other medications that alter sensation, muscle tone, standard reflex reactions, cardiovascular function, kidney or liver function, or personality, behavior, or reasoning ability
7. Coma (may be absolute CI, depending on cause)
8. Diagnosed atherosclerosis
9. Drug withdrawal
10. Emphysema
11. Epilepsy
12. Hypertension
13. Immunosuppressed client
14. Inflammatory arthritis
15. Major or abdominal surgery
16. Moderately severe or juvenile-onset diabetes
17. Multiple sclerosis
18. Osteoporosis, osteomalacia
19. Pregnancy and labor
20. Post MI
21. Post CVA
22. Recent head injury

Local (Regional) Conditions

1. Acute disk herniation
2. Aneurysm (may be general CI, depending on location)
3. Any acute inflammatory condition
4. Any antiinflammatory treatment site
5. Any chronic or long-standing superficial thrombosis
6. Buerger disease (may be general CI if unstable)

7. Chronic arthritic conditions
8. Chronic abdominal or digestive disease
9. Chronic diarrhea
10. Contusion
11. Endometriosis
12. Flaccid paralysis or paresis
13. Fracture (while casted and immediately after cast removal)
14. Hernia
15. Joint instability or hypermobility
16. Kidney infection, stones
17. Mastitis
18. Minor surgery
19. Pelvic inflammatory disease
20. Pitting edema
21. Portal hypertension
22. Prolonged constipation
23. Recent abortion/vaginal birth
24. Trigeminal neuralgia

Other Important Considerations

1. Massage therapists are expected to know how and when to consult with physicians and other health professionals.
2. Most emotional or psychiatric conditions affect massage treatment. Individual decisions must be made according to case circumstances and, in many instances, medical advice. Medications may be a factor.
3. The client may be allergic to certain massage oils and creams or to cleansers or disinfectants used on sheets and tables. Therefore, it is crucial to ask clients about any allergies before the treatment is performed.
4. The presence of pins, staples, or artificial joints may alter treatment indications.
5. The massage therapist should be aware of the role of common chronic conditions that affect public health (e.g., cardiovascular disease, cancer, substance abuse, chronic mental diseases).

The local health department can provide additional information on public mental health services, environmental hazards, occupational health, and various healthcare organizations available in the community.

THE OREGON MODEL: INDICATIONS AND CONTRAINDICATIONS BY BODY SYSTEM

The Oregon Board of Massage developed this extensive list. However, the board made no specific recommendations regarding indications or contraindications for massage. The descriptions of disease processes and the massage recommendations were added by this author, using a very conservative approach. If an indication for massage is not listed for a disease process, massage has no direct benefit; such cases are designated *N/A*. This textbook reviews basic massage procedures. Advanced training in the medical application of massage, as well as direct supervision by a physician, chiropractor, physical therapist, psychologist, dentist, podiatrist, or other healthcare professional, will greatly expand the application of massage in rehabilitative situations.

The Integumentary System

Assessment parameters include color (e.g., pallor, jaundice, cyanosis, erythema, mottling), texture (e.g., dry, moist, scaly), scars (normal and keloid), vascularity (e.g., dilated veins, angiomas, varicosities, ecchymoses, petechiae, purpura), temperature, rashes, lesions, nail condition, hair condition, contour, hydration, and edema.

Deviations that suggest the need for evaluation and referral include lumps or masses, rashes of unknown origin, lesions, burns, urticaria, itching of unknown origin, cyanosis, jaundice, ulcerations, multiple bruises, and petechiae.

Specific Disease Processes and Bacterial Conditions
- Carbuncle
  - *Definition/symptoms:* Mass of connected boils
  - *Indications:* Massage may increase systemic circulation and may assist healing
  - *Contraindications:* Refer client to physician; regional; avoid affected area
- Cellulitis
  - *Definition/symptoms:* Inflammation of subcutaneous tissue with redness and swelling
  - *Indications:* Avoid
  - *Contraindications:* Regional; may be associated with erysipelas, a contagious condition; refer client to physician
- Folliculitis
  - *Definition/symptoms:* Inflammation of hair follicle
  - *Indications:* Massage may enhance systemic circulation and assist healing
  - *Contraindications:* Regional; refer client to physician; avoid affected area
- Furuncle (boil)
  - *Definition/symptoms:* Pus-filled cavity formed by infection of hair follicle
  - *Indications:* Massage may enhance systemic circulation and assist healing
  - *Contraindications:* Regional; refer client to physician; avoid affected area
- Impetigo
  - *Definition/symptoms:* Highly contagious bacterial skin infection that occurs most often in children; begins as a reddish discoloration and develops into vesicles with a yellow crust
  - *Indications:* Massage may enhance systemic circulation and assist healing
  - *Contraindications:* Regional; refer client to physician; avoid affected area

- Syphilis
  - *Definition/symptoms:* Primary stage: a usually painless lesion (chancre) present on exposed skin; secondary stage: begins about 2 months after chancre disappears and produces a variety of symptoms, including skin rash
  - *Indications:* N/A
  - *Contraindications:* General; rash is contagious; refer client to physician .

Viral Conditions
- Bell palsy
  - *Definition/symptoms:* Infection of seventh cranial nerve; primary symptom is paralysis of facial features, including the eyelids and mouth
  - *Indications:* Relaxation massage may facilitate healing
  - *Contraindications:* Regional; refer client to physician for diagnosis
- Herpes simplex
  - *Definition/symptoms:* Acute viral disease marked by groups of watery blisters on or near mucous membranes
  - *Indications:* Recurrence is stress induced; massage may reduce stress levels
  - *Contraindications:* Regional; contagious; avoid affected area
- Herpes zoster (shingles)
  - *Definition/symptoms:* Viral infection that usually affects the skin of a single dermatome; produces a red, swollen plaque that ruptures and crusts
  - *Indications:* Condition is painful; general massage may ease pain
  - *Contraindications:* Regional; avoid affected area; may need to refer client to physician
- Warts
  - *Definition/symptoms:* Usually benign, excess cell growth of the skin
  - *Indications:* N/A
  - *Contraindications:* Regional; avoid affected area; contagious; may become malignant; if any changes in wart occur, refer client to physician

Fungal Conditions
- Ringworm, athlete's foot, fungal infection of the nails
  - *Definition/symptoms:* Scaly and crusty cracking of the skin
  - *Indications:* Keep area dry; do not use lubricants
  - *Contraindications:* Regional; do not use lubricants near the area because fungi thrive in a moist environment

Allergic Reactions
- Atopic dermatitis (eczema)
  - *Definition/symptoms:* Common inflammation of the skin marked by papules, vesicles, and crusts
  - *Indications:* Symptom of an underlying condition; refer client to physician for diagnosis

- *Contraindications:* Regional; avoid affected area
- Contact dermatitis
  - *Definition/symptoms:* Inflammation that occurs in response to contact with an external agent
  - *Indications:* Use unscented lubricants (scents often cause allergic reactions)
  - *Contraindications:* Regional; avoid affected area
- Urticaria (hives)
  - *Definition/symptoms:* Red, raised lesions caused by leakage of fluid from skin and blood vessels; primary symptom is severe itching
  - *Indications:* Do not use scented products; hives may have an emotional component
  - *Contraindications:* Regional; avoid affected area

Benign Conditions

- Mole
  - *Definition/symptoms:* Pigmented, fleshy growth of skin
  - *Indications:* Watch for any change in a mole; refer client to physician if a change is noted
  - *Contraindications:* Regional; avoid mole
- Psoriasis
  - *Definition/symptoms:* Chronic inflammation of the skin; probably genetic; symptoms include scaly plaque and excessive growth rate of epithelial cells
  - *Indications:* May be stress induced; massage reduces stress
  - *Contraindications:* Regional; avoid affected area
- Scleroderma
  - *Definition/symptoms:* Autoimmune disease that affects blood vessels and connective tissue of the skin; primary symptom is hard, yellowish skin
  - *Indications:* N/A
  - *Contraindications:* Regional (except in systemic cases); refer client to physician

Malignant Conditions

- Skin cancer
  - *Definition/symptoms:* Squamous cell carcinoma, basal cell carcinoma, melanoma, Kaposi's sarcoma
  - *Indications:* N/A
  - *Contraindications:* Watch for any change in a mole or existing skin condition; if this occurs, refer client to physician immediately

The Skeletal System, Muscular System, and Articulations

Assessment parameters include range of motion, swelling, masses, deformity, pain or tenderness, temperature, crepitus, spasm, paresthesia, pulses, skin color, paralysis, atrophy, and contracture.

Deviations that suggest the need for evaluation and referral include malalignment of an extremity, asymmetry of musculoskeletal contour, progressive or persistent pain, masses or progressive swelling, numbness or tingling with loss of function, diminished or absent peripheral pulses, pallor or coolness of one extremity, redness or increased temperature of one extremity, and differences in size of extremities.

Specific Disease Processes

- Atonicity (flaccidity)
  - *Definition/symptoms:* Reduced ability or inability of the muscle to contract (hypotonicity)
  - *Indications:* Massage to tone; relaxation of opposing muscle groups
  - *Contraindications:* Regional; refer client to physician for diagnosis before proceeding
- Contracture
  - *Definition/symptoms:* Fixed resistance to passive stretching of muscles; usually the result of fibrosis or tissue ischemia
  - *Indications:* Massage and stretch
  - *Contraindications:* Do not stretch past fixed barrier
- Convulsion
  - *Definition/symptoms:* Sudden, involuntary series of muscle contractions, sometimes called a seizure
  - *Indications:* N/A
  - *Contraindications:* Refer client to physician immediately
- Fibrillation
  - *Definition/symptoms:* A small, local contraction of muscle that is invisible under the skin; results from spontaneous, synchronous activation of single muscle cells
  - *Indications:* Massage, direct pressure
  - *Contraindications:* If continuous, refer client to physician for diagnosis
- Hypertonicity
  - *Definition/symptoms:* Increased muscle tone
  - *Indications:* Massage and stretch
  - *Contraindications:* Recurrence without explanation; refer client to physician for diagnosis
- Spasms (cramp)
  - *Definition/symptoms:* Sudden, painful onset of muscle contraction
  - *Indications:* Use reciprocal inhibition; push muscle belly together and slowly stretch
  - *Contraindications:* If recurring and transient, refer client to physician
- Tic
  - *Definition/symptoms:* Spasmodic twitching; often occurs in the face
  - *Indications:* May be stress induced; massage is beneficial in reducing stress
  - *Contraindications:* Refer client to physician for diagnosis to rule out underlying pathologic condition

Soft Tissue Injuries

- Dislocation
  - *Definition/symptoms:* Displacement of a bone within a joint
  - *Indications:* N/A
  - *Contraindications:* Immediately refer client to physician

- Sprain
  - *Definition/symptoms:* Traumatic injury of ligaments that form a skeletal joint; may involve injury (strain) of muscles or tendons
  - *Indications:* RICE (rest, ice, compression, elevation), first aid, gentle massage, and range of motion facilitate healing
  - *Contraindications:* Regional; all traumatic injuries should be evaluated by a physician
- Strain
  - *Definition/symptoms:* Traumatic injury caused by overstretching or overexertion of muscle or tendon tissue
  - *Indications:* RICE, first aid, gentle massage, and range of motion may facilitate healing
  - *Contraindications:* Regional; all traumatic injuries should be evaluated by a physician
- Subluxation
  - *Definition/symptoms:* Any deviation from the normal relationship in which the articular cartilage is touching any portion of its mating cartilage
  - *Indications:* Massage may help relieve muscle spasm
  - *Contraindications:* Refer client to physician

Infectious Processes

- Osteomyelitis
  - *Definition/symptoms:* Bacterial infection of the bone; symptoms include deep pain and fever
  - *Indications:* N/A
  - *Contraindications:* General; immediately refer client to physician; difficult to diagnose and treat

Inflammatory Processes

- Ankylosing spondylitis
  - *Definition/symptoms:* Chronic inflammatory disease; can be progressive; usually involves the sacroiliac joint and spinal articulations; cause is unknown and appears to be genetic; if progressive, calcification of the joints and articular surfaces occurs; begins with feelings of fatigue and intermittent low back pain; synovial tissue around the involved joints becomes inflamed; heart disease also may occur
  - *Indications:* Massage may be helpful under direct supervision of a physician
  - *Contraindications:* General; refer client to physician; avoid any area of inflammation
- Bursitis
  - *Definition/symptoms:* Inflammation of bursa
  - *Indications:* Massage may take pressure off joint by relaxing and normalizing surrounding musculature; ice
  - *Contraindications:* Regional; avoid affected area; work above and below jointed area
- Fibromyalgia
  - *Definition/symptoms:* General disruption in connective tissue muscle component; symptoms include tender point activity; vague symptoms of pain and fatigue

- *Indications:* Massage may be beneficial; work with client's physician if clearance for massage has been given
- *Contraindications:* General; refer client to physician for diagnosis before performing massage; do not use therapeutic inflammation methods
- Gouty arthritis
  - *Definition/symptoms:* Metabolic condition in which sodium urate crystals trigger a chronic inflammatory process, often in joints of the great toe
  - *Indications:* Dietary adjustment necessary
  - *Contraindications:* Regional; avoid area of inflammation
- Lupus erythematosus
  - *Definition/symptoms:* Chronic inflammatory disease that affects many body tissues; common symptom is a red rash on the face
  - *Indications:* Massage may be beneficial under physician's close supervision
  - *Contraindications:* General; systemic disease
- Osgood-Schlatter disease
  - *Definition/symptoms:* Osteochondrosis (inflammation of bone and cartilage) of the tibial tuberosity
  - *Indications:* N/A
  - *Contraindications:* Regional; avoid affected area
- Rheumatoid arthritis
  - *Definition/symptoms:* Autoimmune inflammatory joint disease characterized by synovial inflammation that spreads to other tissues
  - *Indications:* Stress responsive; massage can be helpful under medical supervision if clearance for massage has been given
  - *Contraindications:* General; refer client to physician for diagnosis before performing massage; do not use therapeutic inflammation methods
- Tendonitis
  - *Definition/symptoms:* Inflammation of tendon and tendon-muscle junction
  - *Indications:* Massage may assist healing; ice
  - *Contraindications:* Regional; avoid affected area; work above and below the area
- Tenosynovitis
  - *Definition/symptoms:* Inflammation of tendon sheath, usually from repetitive movement
  - *Indications:* Massage may relieve muscle hypertension and may assist healing of area; ice
  - *Contraindications:* Regional; avoid affected area; work above and below the area

Compression Processes

- Carpal tunnel syndrome
  - *Definition/symptoms:* Inflammation in tendon sheaths in the carpal tunnel that creates pressure on the median nerve; symptoms include weakness and tingling in the hand
  - *Indications:* Symptoms often are confused with thoracic outlet syndrome; massage is proving to be beneficial

- *Contraindications:* Regional; refer client to physician for diagnosis

Degenerative Processes

- Muscular dystrophy
  - *Definition/symptoms:* A group of muscle disorders characterized by atrophy of skeletal muscle without nerve involvement
  - *Indications:* Massage is beneficial; work closely with client's physician if clearance for massage has been given
  - *Contraindications:* General
- Osteoarthritis
  - *Definition/symptoms:* Degenerative joint disease of the articular cartilage; age and joint damage are risk factors
  - *Indications:* Massage is beneficial
  - *Contraindications:* Regional; avoid area of inflammation
- Osteoporosis
  - *Definition/symptoms:* Loss of minerals and collagen from bone matrix, resulting in reduced volume and strength of skeletal bone
  - *Indications:* Gentle massage is beneficial; use care and caution
  - *Contraindications:* General

Abnormal Spinal Curve

- Kyphosis
  - *Definition/symptoms:* Abnormal increased convexity of the thoracic spine
  - *Indications:* Massage is beneficial as part of the treatment plan
  - *Contraindications:* Regional; in severe cases, proceed after obtaining physician's recommendation
- Lordosis
  - *Definition/symptoms:* Abnormal increased concavity in the curvature of the lumbar spine
  - *Indications:* Massage is beneficial as part of the treatment plan
  - *Contraindications:* Regional; in severe cases, proceed after obtaining physician's recommendation
- Scoliosis
  - *Definition/symptoms:* Lateral curve of vertebral column
  - *Indications:* Massage is beneficial as part of the treatment plan
  - *Contraindications:* Regional; in severe cases, proceed after obtaining physician's recommendation

Disordered Muscular Processes

- Low back pain
  - *Definition/symptoms:* May be of many varieties: muscular, nerve entrapment, or disk problem
  - *Indications:* Massage can be beneficial as part of the treatment plan
  - *Contraindications:* Regional; important to refer client to physician to rule out serious condition of the spine or viscera

- Spasmodic torticollis
  - *Definition/symptoms:* A contracted state of the cervical muscles that causes pain and rotation of the head
  - *Indications:* Massage is beneficial
  - *Contraindications:* Regional; refer client to physician for diagnosis to rule out serious disease
- Temporomandibular joint (TMJ) dysfunction
  - *Definition/symptoms:* Dysfunction in the TMJ; pain and muscle contraction
  - *Indications:* Massage is beneficial; work closely with dentist and physician
  - *Contraindications:* Regional if painful

Neurologic Conditions

Assessment parameters include mental status, the presence of involuntary movements, coordination and balance, muscle tone and strength, and changes in sensory perception (i.e., touch, pain, temperature, vibration, position sense, hearing, and vision).

Deviations that suggest the need for evaluation and referral include inequality of pupil size; diplopia; abnormal Babinski's sign (extensor plantar response); seizures (partial or generalized); significant personality changes; changes in sensorium; progressively worsening or persistent headache; temporary loss of speech, vision, or motion; triad of fever, headache, and nuchal rigidity; vomiting; and change in pupil size with head injury.

Specific Disease Processes

- Dyskinesia
  - *Definition/symptoms:* Impairment of the power of voluntary movement, resulting in fragmentary or incomplete movement and possibly pain
  - *Indications:* Massage is beneficial as part of a physician-directed treatment plan
  - *Contraindications:* General; refer client to physician for diagnosis and treatment plan
- Dystonia
  - *Definition/symptoms:* Disordered, random tonicity of muscles
  - *Indications:* Massage is beneficial as part of a physician-directed treatment plan
  - *Contraindications:* General; refer client to physician for diagnosis and treatment plan
- Insomnia
  - *Definition/symptoms:* Inability to sleep or interrupted sleep
  - *Indications:* Massage is beneficial
  - *Contraindications:* Regional; refer client to physician for specific diagnosis to rule out serious underlying condition
- Peripheral neuropathy
  - *Definition/symptoms:* General functional disturbances or pathologic changes in the peripheral nervous system caused by diabetic neuropathy, ischemic neuropathy, or

traumatic neuropathy; symptoms include numbness, burning, and pain

- *Indications:* Massage is beneficial as part of the treatment plan
- *Contraindications:* General; refer client to physician for diagnosis to determine underlying condition

- Tinnitus
  - *Definition/symptoms:* Noise in the ear; symptoms include ringing, buzzing, roaring, and clicking
  - *Indications:* N/A
  - *Contraindications:* Regional; refer client to physician for specific diagnosis
- Vertigo
  - *Definition/symptoms:* Sensation of movement, not to be confused with dizziness
  - *Indications:* N/A
  - *Contraindications:* General; usually symptomatic of underlying condition; physician's diagnosis required

Vascular Processes

- Cerebrovascular accident (CVA)
  - *Definition/symptoms:* Stroke; a disturbance in cerebral circulation; major causes include atherosclerosis (thrombosis), embolism, hypertensive intracerebral hemorrhage, or ruptured saccular aneurysm; symptoms differ depending on where the disturbance in circulation occurs; general symptoms include weakness or paralysis of the arm or leg, headache, numbness, blurred or double vision, and confusion or dizziness; often only one side is affected; symptoms persist for at least 24 hours, usually much longer
  - *Indications:* Massage may be beneficial during recovery under physician's supervision and during long-term care for continued support
  - *Contraindications:* Refer client to physician for diagnosis
- Headache
  - *Definition/symptoms:* Pain or dull ache in the head and upper neck; can have a variety of causes such as muscle tension, sinus pressure, pinched nerve, vascular disruption (e.g., migraine headache, cluster headaches), and toxins
  - *Indications:* Massage may be beneficial
  - *Contraindications:* Refer all clients with a persistent, severe headache to physician for specific diagnosis
- Head injury
  - *Definition/symptoms:* Contusion (bump on the head); laceration (cut or break in the skin); subdural and epidural injury may produce disorientation, nausea, and uneven pupil dilation
  - *Indications:* Immediately refer client to physician if any of the signs listed previously are noted
  - *Contraindications:* General; all traumatic injuries must be evaluated by a physician
- Transient ischemic attack (TIA)
  - *Definition/symptoms:* Episodes of neurologic dysfunction that usually are of short duration (a few minutes) but may persist for 24 hours; reversible; symptom

pattern is the same with each attack because the same vessel is involved; small strokes, seizures, migraine symptoms, postural hypotension, and Stokes-Allen syndrome may be misdiagnosed as TIAs
  - *Indications:* Massage may be beneficial under physician's supervision
  - *Contraindications:* Refer client to physician for diagnosis

Infectious Processes

- Conjunctivitis
  - *Definition/symptoms:* Inflammation or infection of mucous membranes of the eye
  - *Indications:* N/A
  - *Contraindications:* Regional; refer client to physician; may be contagious; avoid affected area
- Parkinson disease
  - *Definition/symptoms:* Nervous disorder characterized by abnormally low levels of the neurotransmitter dopamine, resulting in involuntary trembling and muscle rigidity
  - *Indications:* Massage is beneficial as part of a physician-directed treatment plan
  - *Contraindications:* General
- Poliomyelitis
  - *Definition/symptoms:* Viral infection of nerves that control skeletal muscles
  - *Indications:* Massage is beneficial as part of a physician-directed treatment plan
  - *Contraindications:* General
- Postpolio syndrome
  - *Definition/symptoms:* Symptoms of fatigue and general muscle weakness appear years after poliomyelitis has been resolved
  - *Indications:* Massage is beneficial as part of a physician-directed treatment plan
  - *Contraindications:* Regional; refer client to physician for specific diagnosis

Neuromuscular Processes

- Multiple sclerosis
  - *Definition/symptoms:* Primary disease of the central nervous system marked by degeneration of myelin
  - *Indications:* Massage is beneficial as part of a physician-directed treatment plan
  - *Contraindications:* General
- Spinal cord injury
  - *Definition/symptoms:* Traumatic injury or degenerative process of the spinal cord; may result from compression, cut, or tissue replacement in scarring
  - *Indications:* Massage is beneficial as part of a physician-directed treatment plan
  - *Contraindications:* Regional
- Trigeminal neuralgia (tic douloureux)
  - *Definition/symptoms:* Compression or degeneration of fifth cranial nerve; primary symptom is recurring episodes of stabbing pain in the face

- *Indications:* Avoid entire area of trigeminal nerve innervation; massage may trigger pain response
- *Contraindications:* Regional

Miscellaneous Disorders

- Seizure disorders
  - *Definition/symptoms:* Sudden bursts of abnormal neuronal activity that cause temporary changes in brain activity; may vary from mild, affecting conscious motor control or sensory perception, to severe, resulting in convulsion
  - *Indications:* Massage may be beneficial
  - *Contraindications:* General; follow physician's recommendations for massage
- Sleep apnea
  - *Definition/symptoms:* Cessation of breathing during sleep
  - *Indications:* Stress may be a factor; massage is beneficial in reducing stress
  - *Contraindications:* Regional
- Thoracic outlet syndrome
  - *Definition/symptoms:* Compression of brachial nerve plexus; primary symptom is pain that radiates to the shoulder and arm
  - *Indications:* Massage is beneficial as part of the treatment plan
  - *Contraindications:* Regional; refer client to physician for specific diagnosis

Endocrine System

Assessment parameters include fatigue, depression, and changes in energy level, as well as hyperalertness, sleep patterns, and mood. These can affect the skin, hair, and personal appearance.

Deviations that suggest the need for evaluation and referral include cold, clammy skin; numbness of fingers, toes, or mouth; rapid heartbeat; a feeling of faintness; vertigo; tremors and dyspnea (difficulty breathing); thyroid nodule; unusually warm hands and feet; and lethargy.

Specific Disease Processes

- Diabetes mellitus
  - *Definition/symptoms:* Metabolic disorder; body loses the ability to oxidize carbohydrates because of faulty pancreatic activity, especially at the islets of Langerhans, which affects insulin production; symptoms include thirst, hunger, and acidosis; severe symptoms include difficulty breathing and changes in blood chemistry that lead to coma
  - *Indications:* Massage is given under supervision of the primary care physician; it is beneficial for enhancing circulation and reducing stress; exercise also is beneficial
  - *Contraindications:* General; work only under physician's supervision

- Hyperglycemia
  - *Definition/symptoms:* High blood sugar, resulting from inadequate insulin in the blood; symptoms are the same as those for diabetes mellitus
  - *Indications:* See *Diabetes mellitus*
  - *Contraindications:* See *Diabetes mellitus*
- Hypoglycemia
  - *Definition/symptoms:* Low blood glucose, resulting from an excess of insulin in the blood; symptoms include light-headedness, anxiety, and forgetfulness
  - *Indications:* Dietary changes; massage is helpful and may relieve stress
  - *Contraindications:* Refer client to physician to determine the cause of low blood sugar
- Hyperthyroidism
  - *Definition/symptoms:* Overproduction of thyroid hormone; can be caused by a tumor or by problems with the self-regulatory mechanism in the pituitary gland; symptoms include anxiety, bulging eyes, high metabolic rate, and nervousness
  - *Indications:* Massage is beneficial for relaxing the client
  - *Contraindications:* General; work within physician's recommendations
- Hypothyroidism
  - *Definition/symptoms:* Underproduction of thyroid hormone; symptoms include sensitivity to cold, weight gain, fatigue, and dullness
  - *Indications:* Massage is beneficial for stimulating metabolic function
  - *Contraindications:* General; work within physician's recommendations
- Neuropathy
  - *Definition/symptoms:* Functional disturbance or pathologic change in peripheral nervous system; symptoms include numbness, burning, and tingling pain
  - *Indications:* Massage is beneficial under medical supervision; may calm hypersensitive nerves
  - *Contraindications:* General; work under physician's direction

Cardiovascular System

Assessment parameters include skin color and appearance, respiratory rate and effort, condition of nails and nail beds (e.g., clubbing, cyanosis), pain or tenderness, and points of radiation, swelling, and symmetry of chest cavity.

Deviations that suggest the need for evaluation and referral include pulse over 90 or under 60 beats per minute; dyspnea; pitting edema; distended neck veins; glossy appearance of the skin; positive Homans' sign (calf tenderness with dorsiflexion of the foot); asymmetry of limb circumference; red, warm, tender, and hard veins; edema; pain and tenderness of extremity; clubbing of nail beds; chest pain (especially if radiating to left arm); central or peripheral cyanosis; pallor; mottling or cyanosis of a limb; stasis ulcers; and splinter hemorrhages (small red to black streaks under fingernails).

Physiologic Processes

- Anemia
  - *Definition/symptoms:* Reduced red blood cell count or hemoglobin; symptoms include fatigue and pallor
  - *Indications:* Massage can be beneficial as part of the treatment plan
  - *Contraindications:* General; refer client to physician for diagnosis, and proceed under physician's direction
- Aneurysm
  - *Definition/symptoms:* Abnormal widening of the arterial wall; tends to form thrombi and also to burst; a pulsating bulge and pressure are felt with accompanying symptoms of pain
  - *Indications:* N/A
  - *Contraindications:* Regional; immediately refer client to physician; avoid direct heavy pressure into arterial vessels
- Angina pectoris
  - *Definition/symptoms:* Chest pain caused by inadequate oxygen to heart (usually from blocked coronary arteries)
  - *Indications:* Massage is beneficial as part of a lifestyle change
  - *Contraindications:* General; massage is performed under physician's supervision
- Arteriosclerosis and atherosclerosis
  - *Definition/symptoms:* Hardening of the arteries; a type of coronary heart disease; symptoms may be mild to severe; may be mistaken for other problems
  - *Indications:* Massage is beneficial as part of a lifestyle change
  - *Contraindications:* General; perform massage under physician's supervision
- Congestive heart failure
  - *Definition/symptoms:* Left heart failure; inability of the left ventricle to pump effectively; one symptom is increased fluid retention
  - *Indications:* Massage is beneficial in helping diuretics remove excess fluid
  - *Contraindications:* General; must work under physician's supervision; client may have difficulty breathing in a supine position
- Deep vein thrombosis
  - *Definition/symptoms:* Blood clot in deep veins; risk factor for pulmonary embolism (blood clot in the lungs); often asymptomatic; symptoms may include swelling, edema, and pain described as aching and throbbing
  - *Indications:* N/A
  - *Contraindications:* Regional to general, depending on the severity of symptoms; always refer client to physician for unexplained pain; never massage over such areas
- Hemophilia
  - *Definition/symptoms:* Blood clotting disorder; primary symptom is spontaneous bleeding due to an inability to form clots
  - *Indications:* Extremely light energy type of massage given only under physician's direction
  - *Contraindications:* General; work only under physician's supervision

- Myocardial infarction (MI)
  - *Definition/symptoms:* Death of cardiac muscle cells, usually from inadequate blood supply, often from coronary thrombosis or coronary artery disease; symptoms include severe pain in the chest or left arm, difficulty breathing, and weakness
  - *Indications:* During rehabilitation, massage can be beneficial when supervised by a physician
  - *Contraindications:* General; refer client to physician immediately
- Mononucleosis
  - *Definition/symptoms:* Induced by Epstein–Barr virus; symptoms include fever, fatigue, and swollen glands
  - *Indications:* Massage is beneficial as part of the treatment plan; care must be taken with contagious conditions
  - *Contraindications:* General; refer client to physician for specific diagnosis
- Phlebitis
  - *Definition/symptoms:* Inflammation of a vein; may be caused by a blood clot; symptoms include edema, stiffness, and pain; veins may streak red
  - *Indications:* N/A
  - *Contraindications:* Regional to general; see *Deep vein thrombosis*
- Raynaud syndrome
  - *Definition/symptoms:* Arteriospastic condition caused by vasospasms of the small cutaneous and subcutaneous arteries and arterioles; usually activated by cold but can be emotionally triggered; symptoms include skin pallor and pain
  - *Indications:* Care must be taken to avoid triggering the symptoms; interview client carefully; massage may be beneficial for reducing stress
  - *Contraindications:* Refer client to physician for specific underlying diagnosis; condition may be symptomatic of serious disorder
- Syncope
  - *Definition/symptoms:* Sudden loss of strength; fainting; may be caused by a cardiac spasm resulting from closure of coronary arteries
  - *Indications:* N/A
  - *Contraindications:* General; immediately refer client to physician
- Varicose veins
  - *Definition/symptoms:* Enlarged veins in which blood pools; caused by collapse of valve system; tend to form thrombi
  - *Indications:* N/A
  - *Contraindications:* Regional; avoid affected area

Lymphatic and Immune Systems

Assessment parameters include skin color and condition, evidence of eye irritation, lymph nodes, and nasal discharge/irritation.

Deviations that suggest the need for evaluation and referral include a client history of chronic fatigue or recurrent physical ailments (e.g., skin, respiratory, gastrointestinal) in the absence of general illness; history of food intolerance; failure to gain weight; unexplained weight loss; rashes of unknown origin; urticaria; enlarged, tender nodes; and excessive or persistent dryness and scaliness of skin.

Specific Disease Processes

- Allergy
  - *Definition/symptoms:* Hypersensitivity of immune system to relatively harmless environmental antigens; symptoms include increased mucous membrane inflammation, occasionally spastic bladder
  - *Indications:* Massage is beneficial
  - *Contraindications:* Refer client to physician for specific diagnosis
- Autoimmune disease
  - *Definition/symptoms:* Disease in which the immune system attacks the body's own tissues; symptoms include inflammation, fatigue, and allergy
  - *Indications:* Massage is beneficial with physician's recommendation
  - *Contraindications:* General; refer client to physician for specific diagnosis
- Chronic fatigue syndrome
  - *Definition/symptoms:* May be induced by a virus; symptoms include swollen glands, low-grade fever, muscle and joint aches, headache, and fatigue
  - *Indications:* Massage is beneficial
  - *Contraindications:* General; refer client to physician for specific diagnosis
- Human immunodeficiency virus (HIV) infection
  - *Definition/symptoms:* Viral infection transmitted by means of body fluids; causes immunosuppression
  - *Indications:* Massage is beneficial with physician's recommendation; follow antiviral precautions for control of virus; 10% bleach solution; avoid body fluid contact
  - *Contraindications:* General; work with client's physician
- Lymphedema
  - *Definition/symptoms:* Swelling of tissue caused by partial or complete blockage of lymph vessels
  - *Indications:* Massage is beneficial as part of the treatment plan and is given under the supervision of the primary care physician
  - *Contraindications:* Refer client to physician for diagnosis

The Respiratory System

Assessment parameters include the rate and pattern of respiration, chest movement, color, nodes, chest configuration, ease of chest excursions, fremitus, and pain.

Deviations that suggest the need for evaluation and referral include inspiratory flaring of the nostrils; use of accessory muscles; intercostal retractions or bulging; pursed lips on exhalation; splinting; uneven chest movement; altered tactile fremitus/crepitus (increased or decreased); cyanosis or pallor; enlarged, tender nodes; pain with breathing; and a respiratory rate over 20 respirations per minute in the absence of exertion or strong emotion.

Specific Disease Processes

- Asthma
  - *Definition/symptoms:* Recurring muscle spasms in the bronchial wall accompanied by fluid retention and production of mucus; stress-specific condition
  - *Indications:* Massage is beneficial; monitor breathing closely
  - *Contraindications:* Work under direction of client's physician
- Tuberculosis
  - *Definition/symptoms:* Infectious disease caused by *Mycobacterium tuberculosis*; early stage requires testing to reveal infection; advanced cases are marked by lung destruction, coughing, fatigue, weakness, and weight loss; may be confused with bronchitis and pneumonia
  - *Indications:* Droplet transmission; contagious; be aware of sanitation
  - *Contraindications:* General; work only if physician recommends and clears for contagious condition
- Upper respiratory infection (bronchitis, common cold, sinusitis, pneumonia)
  - *Definition/symptoms:* Viral or bacterial in origin; symptoms include increased production of mucus, fever, body aches, and headaches
  - *Indications:* Light massage may be beneficial to ease body ache; avoid heavy pressure; watch for contamination
  - *Contraindications:* Refer client to physician if symptoms are severe or persist longer than 2 weeks

The Digestive System

Assessment parameters include skin; contour of abdomen (flat, rounded, concave, protuberant, distended); symmetry; observable masses; palpable masses; movement; tenderness or pain; and location and contour of umbilicus.

Deviations that suggest the need for evaluation and referral include a history of persistent or recurring nausea or vomiting; abdominal pain of unknown origin; rebound tenderness; epigastric pain that occurs 1–3 hours after meals; rigid or boardlike abdomen (unrelated to callisthenic exercise); persistent or increasing abdominal or epigastric pain; history of blood in stools or vomitus; difficulty swallowing; masses or nodules; enlarged, tender nodes; bulge or swelling in abdomen; change in location or inversion/eversion of umbilicus; and lesions in oral cavity or on lips or tongue.

Specific Disease Processes

- Constipation
  - *Definition/symptoms:* Slow movement of bowels; hard, compacted, dry stool
  - *Indications:* Massage is beneficial; increase fiber and water consumption and moderate exercise; may be drug related

- *Contraindications:* Refer client to physician if severe or persistent or if a mass is felt in the large intestine
- Diarrhea
  - *Definition/symptoms:* Loose bowels; excessive loss of water in stool; can be caused by a virus or bacterium or can be a symptom of other disease processes
  - *Indications:* Loose stool may occur 24 hours after vigorous massage
  - *Contraindications:* Refer client to physician if symptoms persist or dehydration is present
- Flatulence
  - *Definition/symptoms:* Intestinal gas
  - *Indications:* May be diet or stress related; massage may reduce stress
  - *Contraindications:* Refer client to physician if intestinal tract is distended painfully or to rule out severe underlying condition
- Halitosis
  - *Definition/symptoms:* Bad breath; may indicate digestive problems or sinus infection
  - *Indications:* N/A
  - *Contraindications:* Refer client to physician for specific diagnosis

Inflammatory Processes

- Appendicitis
  - *Definition/symptoms:* Inflammation of the mucosal lining of the appendix, caused by trapped food or fecal matter; more common in individuals younger than age 25; symptoms include mild periumbilical pain, nausea, vomiting, increasing pain in the lower right quadrant, muscle spasm, and rebound tenderness
  - *Indications:* N/A
  - *Contraindications:* Immediately refer client to physician
- Cholelithiasis and cholecystitis
  - *Definition/symptoms:* Gallstones formed as a result of inflammation; primary symptom is severe pain in upper abdomen radiating to back and right shoulder
  - *Indications:* N/A
  - *Contraindications:* Immediately refer client to physician
- Cirrhosis of the liver
  - *Definition/symptoms:* Chronic disease that replaces liver tissue with connective tissue; major cause is alcohol consumption; early symptoms include gas, change in bowel habits, slight weight loss, nausea in the morning, and a dull, heavy ache in the right upper quadrant of the abdomen; advanced symptoms include jaundice, peripheral edema, bleeding, and red palms
  - *Indications:* Massage is beneficial in stress reduction and drug withdrawal
  - *Contraindications:* Refer client to physician for diagnosis; work under direction of client's physician
- Colitis
  - *Definition/symptoms:* Inflammatory condition of the large intestine; one type (irritable bowel syndrome) is brought on by stress
  - *Indications:* Painful condition; massage may be helpful in general stress and pain reduction

- *Contraindications:* Immediately refer client to physician; work with chronic conditions under direct supervision of client's physician
- Crohn disease (regional enteritis)
  - *Definition/symptoms:* Chronic relapsing inflammatory disease of the intestinal tract; symptoms include intermittent diarrhea, colicky pain in lower abdomen, fatigue, and low-grade fever
  - *Indications:* Painful condition; massage may be helpful in general stress and pain reduction
  - *Contraindications:* Refer client to physician immediately; with chronic conditions, work under physician's direct supervision
- Diverticulosis
  - *Definition/symptoms:* Formation of small pockets in the large intestine, caused by herniation of the mucosa; if pockets become inflamed, condition is called *diverticulitis*; symptoms include gas, diarrhea, and pain
  - *Indications:* Diet may need adjustment to include more fiber
  - *Contraindications:* Refer client to physician if pain or symptoms persist
- Duodenal ulcer
  - *Definition/symptoms:* Ulcer caused by hyperacidity in duodenal bulb; stress related; symptoms include burning pain that feels better after eating
  - *Indications:* Massage is beneficial for reducing stress; lifestyle and diet changes may be necessary
  - *Contraindications:* Refer client to physician for specific diagnosis; support physician's treatment plan
- Hepatitis
  - *Definition/symptoms:* Infectious disease that has generalized effects on the body but that predominantly affects the liver; type A is common in children and in people living in institutions; it is transmitted by fecal matter, orally through contaminated food and water; usual symptoms are mild and flulike; types B and C affect all age groups and are transmitted through blood, needles, the fecal-oral route, and sexual contact
  - *Indications:* Careful use of aseptic procedures
  - *Contraindications:* General; refer client to physician and work only with physician's recommendation and guidelines concerning contagious condition
- Gastritis
  - *Definition/symptoms:* Acute inflammation of the stomach; a common condition usually caused by irritants such as alcohol or aspirin; symptoms include pain, nausea, and belching
  - *Indications:* Massage is beneficial because gastritis sometimes is stress related, and massage may reduce stress
  - *Contraindications:* Refer client to physician for specific diagnosis
- Hernia
  - *Definition/symptoms:* Protrusion of a loop or piece of an organ or tissue through an abnormal opening; hiatal—protrusion of any structure (usually the esophagus or the end of the stomach) through the hiatus of the diaphragm; inguinal—protrusion through the inguinal

ring, causing swelling of the scrotum and possibly a medical emergency; umbilical—protrusion at the umbilicus; in inguinal and umbilical hernias, weakness in the abdominal wall may be noted
- *Indications:* N/A
- *Contraindications:* Refer client to physician; avoid area
- Pancreatitis
  - *Definition/symptoms:* Inflammation of the pancreas; may be present with diabetes and is aggravated by consumption of alcohol; one symptom is severe abdominal pain
  - *Indications:* Painful condition; massage help to reduce general stress and pain
  - *Contraindications:* Refer client to physician immediately; with chronic conditions, work under client's physician's direct supervision
- Stress ulcer
  - *Definition/symptoms:* Ulcer related to severe stress (e.g., trauma, burns, long-term illness); symptoms similar to those seen in gastritis
  - *Indications:* Massage is beneficial for reducing stress; lifestyle and dietary changes may be necessary
  - *Contraindications:* Refer client to physician for specific diagnosis; support physician's treatment plan
- Ulcer
  - *Definition/symptoms:* Peptic ulcer—break or open sore not covered by protective mucus in the gastrointestinal wall that is exposed to pepsin and gastric juice; often caused by alcohol, pepsin, bile salts, and stress
  - *Indications:* Massage is beneficial for reducing stress levels; lifestyle and dietary changes may be necessary
  - *Contraindications:* Refer client to physician for specific diagnosis; support physician's treatment plan

Metabolism

Assessment parameters include eating patterns, skin, hair, nails, weight and height data, and general health status.

Deviations that suggest the need for evaluation and referral include significant underweight or overweight, evidence of nutritional deficiencies (e.g., dry hair or skin, fatigue), and respiratory problems.

Specific Disease Processes
- Cystic fibrosis
  - *Definition/symptoms:* Inherited disorder that disrupts cell transport and causes exocrine glands to produce thick secretions; thick pancreatic secretions may block the pancreatic duct
  - *Indications:* Massage is beneficial with specific training to loosen mucus with percussive techniques
  - *Contraindications:* General; work under direct supervision of client's physician
- Malnutrition
  - *Definition/symptoms:* Deficiency of calories in general and often in protein; malnutrition may be caused by increased nutrient demand on the body without sufficient food intake (e.g., severe burns, illness, lack of

food, especially protein); symptoms include flaking skin, brittle hair, hair loss, slow-healing sores, bruising, susceptibility to infection, and fatigue; more common in children and the elderly and with drug and alcohol abuse; be aware of eating disorders (*Note:* Malnutrition also can be caused by insufficient or improper digestion and absorption of food)
  - *Indications:* With anorexia or bulimia, massage may be beneficial for reducing stress
  - *Contraindications:* Refer client to physician for diagnosis and treatment plan
- Obesity
  - *Definition/symptoms:* Excess body fat (over 30% of normal body weight); risks of obesity include diabetes, stroke, heart attack, gallstones, and high blood pressure
  - *Indications:* Morbid obesity (over 60% of normal body fat) may cause difficulty in positioning client; fluid retention, risk of blood pressure fluctuation, and interference with breathing are other possible problems; massage position may have to be altered
  - *Contraindications:* Refer client for nutritional and dietary consultation

The Reproductive and Urinary Systems

Assessment parameters include pain (groin, periumbilical, flank, abdominal, dysuria), patterns of urination and output, urine consistency (color, concentration, or hematuria), edema (facial, ankle), weight changes, skin changes, discharge, and masses.

Deviations that suggest the need for evaluation and referral include a history of unusual vaginal, urethral, or nipple discharge; breast, penile, scrotal, or inguinal masses or lumps; genital blisters, lesions, or growths; changes in urinary frequency, output, or control or in urine characteristics; sudden weight gain, abnormal menstrual periods, edema, skin abnormalities, pain or tenderness (costovertebral angle, abdominal area, or low back), masses or lumps, and tender or enlarged nodes.

Specific Disease Processes
- Breast cancer
  - *Definition/symptoms:* Abnormal, malignant tissue growth on or in the breast; most common cause of cancer in women; encourage monthly breast self-examination and regular checkups
  - *Indications:* Be aware of changes in tissue around axillary region
  - *Contraindications:* If changes are noted, refer client to physician; early diagnosis is important
- Dysmenorrhea
  - *Definition/symptoms:* Painful menstruation; may be caused by endometriosis (abnormal growth and distribution of uterine lining); symptoms include heavy periods and clotting
  - *Indications:* Massage is beneficial for reducing stress and pain
  - *Contraindications:* Refer client to physician for diagnosis

- Pelvic inflammatory disease
  - *Definition/symptoms:* Inflammation of the uterus, fallopian tubes, ovaries, and surrounding tissue; infection often is introduced by intercourse; symptoms include pain and tenderness in the lower abdomen, backache, pain during intercourse, heavy periods, and vaginal discharge
  - *Indications:* N/A
  - *Contraindications:* Refer client to physician for diagnosis
- Premenstrual syndrome (PMS)
  - *Definition/symptoms:* Occurs approximately 1 week before onset of period; symptoms include breast tenderness and swelling, fluid retention, headache, irritability, anxiety, depression, and poor concentration
  - *Indications:* Massage is beneficial
  - *Contraindications:* Refer client to physician if symptoms are severe
- Testicular cancer
  - *Definition/symptoms:* Malignant growth in testicle; usually a slow-growing lump
  - *Indications:* N/A
  - *Contraindications:* Refer client to physician immediately if the client mentions such a symptom
- Toxic shock syndrome
  - *Definition/symptoms:* Staphylococcal bacterial infection that can arise from the use of tampons; can be life-threatening; initial flulike symptoms with red rash; can be prevented by changing tampons several times a day (*Note:* This condition has also occurred in women who do not use tampons)
  - *Indications:* N/A
  - *Contraindications:* Immediately refer client to physician
- Urinary tract infection
  - *Definition/symptoms:* Acute pyelonephritis—inflammation of kidney and pelvis; usually occurs in women with abrupt onset of fever, chills, malaise, and back pain, also tenderness on palpation over the costovertebral region; cystitis—affects men and women, usually caused by transmission of bacteria through the urethra following improper cleansing after bowel movement; may cause pain in lower abdomen above pubic bone and low backache
  - *Indications:* N/A
  - *Contraindications:* Refer client to physician for diagnosis and treatment

Sexually Transmitted Diseases

- Genital herpes
  - *Definition/symptoms:* Viral infection; primary symptom is blister-like lesions
  - *Indications:* N/A
  - *Contraindications:* Refer client to physician; follow sanitation requirements
- Gonorrhea
  - *Definition/symptoms:* Bacterial infection; may be asymptomatic, or symptoms may include painful urination and pus or cloudy discharge
  - *Indications:* N/A

- *Contraindications:* Refer client to physician; contagious; follow sanitation requirements
- Human immunodeficiency virus (HIV) infection
  - *Definition/symptoms:* Viral infection transmitted by blood and body fluids
  - *Indications:* Massage is beneficial with physician's recommendation; follow antiviral precautions for control of virus with 10% bleach solution; avoid body fluid contact; immediately wash area thoroughly with antiviral agent should body fluid contact occur
  - *Contraindications:* Refer client to physician for treatment; follow sanitation requirements
- Syphilis
  - *Definition/symptoms:* Bacterial infection; in stage 1, red sore (chancre) appears; in stage 2, flulike symptoms develop; in stage 3, the disease attacks the brain and nervous tissue
  - *Indications:* N/A
  - *Contraindications:* Refer client to physician; contagious; follow sanitation requirements

Psychiatric Disorders

Assessment parameters include general appearance and behavior, perceptions of sensations, mood and affect, thought content, and intellectual capacity.

Deviations that suggest the need for evaluation and referral include marked changes in posture, dress and hygiene, motor activity, and speech and facial expression; lack of orientation to time, place, or person; inappropriate manifestation of anxiety, agitation, anger, euphoria, or depression; presence of hallucinations, delusions, paranoia, and illusions; changes in usual intellectual capacity; or suicidal or homicidal ideation.

Specific Disease Processes

- Anxiety, depression (bipolar or manic/depressive disorders)
  - *Definition/symptoms:* All types of emotionally erratic or unusual behavior may be symptomatic; listen to conversation carefully; often symptoms are subtle and client may try to hide discomfort; symptoms may include anorexia (self-starvation); bulimia (eating and vomiting or laxative abuse); addictive disorders; chemical and compulsive behavior; somatization disorder; manifestation of physical pain or symptoms from emotional causes; and posttraumatic stress disorders, often associated with sexual and physical childhood abuse
  - *Indications:* Massage provided under the direction of a psychiatrist or psychologist is beneficial; always work within the client's, physician's, or counselor's treatment parameters
  - *Contraindications:* Refer client to physician for counseling care; client often will dissociate from the body or will be hypersensitive to stimulation; the therapist must be sensitive to psychiatric issues because often the massage therapist is the first person with whom the client shares these issues; it is important to refer the client for competent counseling and psychiatric care (Table A.1)

| TABLE A.1 | Diseases and Indications and Contraindications for Massage Therapy |

Disease	Indications and Contraindications for Massage Therapy
Alzheimer Disease Progressive mental deterioration with confusion, memory failure, disorientation, restlessness, agnosia, speech, and movement.	• The degeneration of Alzheimer disease may be slowed with therapeutic intervention and medication. • Studies indicate that sensory stimulation modalities such as rhythmic massage and movement may provide calming and orienting influences.
Amyotrophic Lateral Sclerosis (ALS) Also known as Lou Gehrig disease; progressive disease that begins in the central nervous system, involves the degeneration of motor neurons, and eventually results in the atrophy of voluntary muscle.	• Massage is indicated for ALS with caution and under a physician's supervision. • Degrees of pressure and intensity should be adjusted as the disease progresses. • General constitutional methods are indicated.
Aneurysm Weakening and bulging of any artery, including those in the brain.	• Contraindicated; immediately refer client to a physician.
Ankylosing Spondylitis Also called rheumatoid inflammatory disorder; destroys the articular hyaline cartilage, causing the bones to fuse and spinal ligaments to ossify.	• Complex backache involving the joint structures. • Requires the practitioner to incorporate therapeutic massage into a total treatment program supervised by the appropriate healthcare professional.
Anterior Compartment Syndrome Covers the anterior compartment of the leg, interfering with blood flow and compressing the nerves.	• Treatment is contraindicated regionally unless supervised by the diagnosing or treating healthcare provider. • Massage methods may soften the connective tissue sheath, relieving some of the pressure, but could aggravate flow to the area, thus increasing the pressure. • Elevation and ice may help.
Anxiety Endogenous anxiety is a biochemical phenomenon that usually is unrelated to environmental stimuli. Reactive, or exogenous, anxiety is prompted by an anxiety-provoking stimulus such as specific events, situations, relationships, or conflicts.	• Massage and exercise often are effective as part of a comprehensive management strategy for anxiety symptoms.
Bell Palsy Causes partial or total paralysis of the facial muscles on one side as the result of inflammation or injury to the seventh cranial nerve.	• Massage approaches for infectious disease can be supportive and may reduce stress. • The practitioner must gauge the intensity and duration of any therapeutic intervention so that the demand to adapt does not overtax an already stressed system, aggravating the condition. • The "less-is-more" philosophy of intervention, which calls for shorter, more frequent interventions, is often indicated.
Bladder Infection (Cystitis) Bacteria in the bladder spread from the perineal region.	• Therapeutic massage modalities may be useful for pain and stress management but only with the careful supervision of the treating physician. • Acute infectious processes contraindicate massage until the infection has run its course.

Breathing Pattern Disorder
Complex disorder that causes altered breathing function.

- Therapeutic massage approaches and moderate application of movement therapies such as Tai chi, yoga, or aerobic exercise assist with breathing.

Bursitis
Inflammation of the bursae, especially those located between the bony prominences and a muscle or tendon such as in the shoulder, elbow, hip, or knee; usually results from trauma and repetitive use.

- Therapeutic massage can be a beneficial adjunct treatment, especially with symptomatic management of pain in supporting increased range of motion.
- Massage directly over the bursae is contraindicated.

Carpal Tunnel Syndrome
Results from irritation of the meridian nerve as it passes under the transverse carpal ligament into the wrist.

- Various forms of massage application reduce muscle spasm, lengthen shortened muscles, and soften and stretch connective tissue, restoring a more normal space around the nerve and alleviating impingement.

Cervical Cancer
Cervical dysplasia is a change in the cells of the cervix. Some of these abnormal cells can develop into cancerous cells.

- Massage for clients with malignancy is contraindicated unless the appropriate healthcare professional gives approval and supervision.
- As with most chronic illness and pain, therapeutic massage offers generalized support for homeostasis and can offer palliative or comfort care for the maintenance of these conditions.

Chorea
Results from the degeneration of neurons in the basal ganglia.

- Therapeutic massage supports a multidisciplinary treatment.
- The practitioner can manage secondary muscle tension effectively with massage therapy and other forms of soft tissue manipulation.

Cirrhosis
Infiltration of connective tissue into the functioning cells of the liver, causing slow deterioration of the liver.

- Caution is indicated, depending on the degree of liver dysfunction.
- Nonstressful general massage may be beneficial in stress management.

Colon Cancer
Usually affects the lowest part of the rectum.

- Comprehensive stress management programs with medical supervision, including therapeutic massage methods, are often effective in managing these conditions.

Concussion
Brain trauma that may be mild, moderate, or severe.

- Massage and bodywork is an effective part of a supervised comprehensive care program.
- Massage and other forms of bodywork can help manage secondary muscle tension.

Constipation
Difficulty in passing stools or an incomplete or infrequent passage of hard stools.

- After these conditions are diagnosed, stress management can be an important part of ongoing therapeutic management.
- A specific type of massage to the large intestine can assist in managing constipation.
- The method is contraindicated in inflammatory bowel disease, and permission from the client's physician should be obtained for any other conditions.

Contracture
Chronic shortening of a muscle, especially the connective tissue component.

- Gentle, slow intervention using connective tissue methods and stretching may improve contractures.
- Applying massage may prevent or slow the development of a contracture.
- The practitioner must consider the reason for the contracture when developing a treatment plan.

Continued

TABLE A.1	Diseases and Indications and Contraindications for Massage Therapy—cont'd
Disease	**Indications and Contraindications for Massage Therapy**
Contusion Muscle bruise from trauma to the muscles involving local internal bleeding and inflammation.	• Direct work over the area of injury is contraindicated regionally until all signs of inflammation have dissipated.
Cramps Painful muscle contractions; may result from mild myositis or fibromyositis, and can be a symptom of any irritation or of an electrolyte imbalance.	• The practitioner can manage simple cramps or spasms by firmly pushing the belly of the muscle together or by initiating reciprocal inhibition, which involves placing the attachment and insertion of the cramping muscle close together and then contracting the antagonist. • The muscle lengthens gently after the cramp or spasm subsides.
Cystic Fibrosis Genetic disease that involves exocrine gland dysfunction.	• Percussion helps loosen the phlegm but should not be attempted without medical supervision and training.
Depression Associated with a decrease in the neurotransmitters norepinephrine, serotonin, and dopamine.	• Therapeutic massage supports a multidisciplinary treatment of depression because such methods influence serotonin, among other neurotransmitters. • In addition, the practitioner can manage secondary muscle tension effectively with massage therapy and other forms of soft tissue manipulation.
Diabetes Mellitus Results when the pancreas does not produce enough insulin or does not produce any insulin at all.	• A general stress management program supports the management of diabetes. • The practitioner should refer the client for immediate medical care for any noted tissue changes. • In pain management of diabetic neuropathy, massage approaches used as part of a supervised program can prove beneficial for short-term reduction of pain symptoms.
Disk Degeneration Occurs when the fibrocartilage surrounding the intervertebral disk ruptures, releasing the nucleus pulposus, which cushions the vertebrae above and below.	• Various forms of massage are important in managing the muscle spasm and pain; muscle spasms serve a stabilizing and protective function called *guarding*. • Therapeutic intervention seeks to reduce pain and excessive tension and to restore moderate mobility while allowing for the resourceful compensation produced by the muscle tension pattern.
Dislocation Displacement of the bones of a joint; a *subluxation* is a partial dislocation.	• Massage and bodywork are contraindicated locally over a trauma area until healing is complete.
Edema Condition in which excess fluid accumulates within the interstitial spaces.	• General contraindications exist for anyone with kidney disease. • Therapeutic massage tends to increase blood volume through the kidneys via mechanical and reflexive processes. • In the healthy individual, therapy supports the filtration process. • For those with kidney disease, the increased volume can strain kidney function.

Emphysema
Chronic pulmonary disease that is marked by an abnormal increase in the size of air spaces distal to the terminal bronchiole with destruction of the alveolar walls.

- Simple palliative measures to provide comfort and encourage sleep are appropriate.
- In chronic conditions such as emphysema, general stress management and maintenance of normal function of the muscles of respiration are beneficial, again after the appropriate added stress levels caused by massage stimulation are gauged.

Epicondylitis
Inflammation of the epicondyle of the humerus and surrounding tissues.

- Therapeutic massage can be a beneficial adjunct treatment, especially when the symptomatic management of pain supports increased range of motion.

Fibromyalgia
Condition with symptoms of widespread pain or aching, persistent fatigue, generalized morning stiffness, nonrestorative sleep, and multiple tender points.

- General constitutional approaches seem to work best to reduce symptomatic pain reduction and restore the sleep pattern.
- The client should avoid any form of therapy that causes therapeutic inflammation, including intense exercise and stretching programs, until healing mechanisms in the body are functioning.
- If tender points have been injected with antiinflammatory medications, anesthetics, or other substances, the practitioner should not massage over these areas.

Flaccid Muscles
Decreased muscular tone.

- Flaccid or spastic muscles often are associated with motor neuron disorders.
- The reason for the change in tone determines the appropriateness of therapeutic massage.
- These conditions differ from general muscle tension or weakness in that the dysfunction has a physical cause rather than a functional one.

Fracture
Break or rupture in a bone.

- Massage and bodywork are contraindicated locally over a trauma area until healing is complete.
- Light, subtle methods of touch therapy (e.g., gentle laying on of hands) may be beneficial in diminishing pain.
- Stress fractures may not be readily detectable. Referral is indicated if the history points toward a mechanical stress condition such as participation in a recent athletic event.

Gout
Form of arthritis caused by a disturbance in metabolism.

- Massage therapy is contraindicated regionally.

Growing Pains
Occur during growth spurts in children and adolescents, when the bone grows faster than the attached muscles.

- Treatment of local areas may be contraindicated if inflammation is present.
- Methods that do not introduce any sort of therapeutic inflammation often soothe general growing pains.
- The practitioner should avoid intense stretching and frictioning methods.
- Methods that relax and lengthen the muscle and soften the connective tissue are appropriate.

Headache
Pain that occurs in the forehead, eyes, jaw, temples, scalp, skull, occiput, or neck.

- Massage therapy is effective in treating muscle tension headache but much less so with migraine or cluster headaches; it can relieve secondary muscle tension headache caused by the pain of the primary headache.
- Headache often is stress induced; stress management in all forms usually is indicated for chronic headache conditions.

Continued

TABLE A.1	Diseases and Indications and Contraindications for Massage Therapy—cont'd
Disease	**Indications and Contraindications for Massage Therapy**
Hepatitis Infection of the liver.	• Abdominal pain or referred back pain may indicate one of several gastrointestinal disorders; in such cases, referral is necessary for proper diagnosis. • Many gastrointestinal diseases are bacterial or viral and are contagious. • The practitioner should take appropriate precautions to maintain sanitary practice.
Hernia Caused by the weakness of abdominal muscles or protrusion of an abdominal organ (commonly the small intestine) through an opening in the abdominal wall.	• Treatment of a client with a hernia is contraindicated regionally, and referral is indicated for initial diagnosis or for any change in a hernia.
Infectious Arthritis Caused by infections such as rheumatic fever, gonorrhea, and tuberculosis.	• Infectious disease is a contraindication of massage unless the appropriate healthcare professionals directly supervise the massage therapy.
Irritable Bowel Syndrome Also called spastic or irritable colon.	• Most chronic gastrointestinal diseases have a strong correlation to stress. • Comprehensive stress management programs, including therapeutic massage methods, are often effective in managing these conditions.
Joint Injuries Include sprains, fractures, associated strains, and impact trauma.	• Pain and swelling of joint injury can be overcome with judicious and short-term use of pain medication, antiinflammatory medications, and appropriate rehabilitation exercise. • Massage, myofascial release, and trigger point work are often effective after the acute phase (2–3 days). • Although direct work over an area that is actively healing is contraindicated unless supervised, massage and other forms of soft tissue work, coupled with movement therapies, can manage compensatory patterns that develop because of casting and other forms of immobilization.
Kidney Failure Inability of the kidneys to excrete waste products and retain electrolytes. Also known as renal failure.	• General contraindications exist for anyone with kidney disease. • Therapeutic massage tends to increase blood volume through the kidneys via mechanical and reflexive processes. • In the healthy individual, therapy supports the filtration process. • For those with kidney disease, the increased volume can strain kidney function.
Legg–Calvé–Perthes Disease Degeneration and necrosis of the head of the femur, followed by recalcification.	• Necrosis is usually a localized condition that requires regional avoidance of the involved bone area. • Because massage provides the generalized effect of enhanced circulation, indirect benefits might be realized with careful use of these methods; however, because these disorders are pathologic conditions, the primary healthcare provider must give permission for and must supervise any massage.

Lordosis
Accentuation of the normal lumbar curve that develops to compensate for the protuberant abdomen of pregnancy or great obesity.

- Massage therapy modalities are effective in managing backache.
- Benefits are derived from reduction in protective muscle spasm compensation (guarding) and generalized pain-modulating effects.
- Be aware that protective spasm provides stabilization.
- Complex backache involving the joint structures requires that therapeutic massage be incorporated into a total treatment program with supervision provided by the appropriate healthcare professional.

Lymphatic System Disorders
Include edema, cancer, and autoimmune conditions.

- Massage is contraindicated for malignant and infectious conditions until the client's healthcare professional gives approval.
- Modification of massage application is necessary, depending on the type of treatment the client is receiving and the stress and fatigue levels.
- Massage that relaxes the client supports well-being and is helpful.
- The practitioner can manage simple edema with massage application focused to support the lymphatic system; more complicated lymphedema requires support of the appropriate healthcare professional concerning massage application.

Multiple Sclerosis
Disease of autoimmune or viral cause (or both) in which myelin degenerates in random areas of the central nervous system.

- Massage can be an effective part of a comprehensive, long-term care program.
- Stress management is also an important component of an overall care program for any chronic disease.
- Massage and other forms of bodywork can help manage secondary muscle tension caused by alteration of posture and the use of equipment such as wheelchairs, braces, and crutches.
- Because therapeutic massage produces some stress, the practitioner must gauge the intensity and duration of any therapeutic intervention to avoid aggravating the condition.

Muscle Infection
Caused by several bacteria, viruses, and parasites, often producing local or widespread myositis (muscle inflammation).

- Massage therapy is contraindicated until infection is no longer present.

Muscle Strain
Injury to skeletal muscles resulting from overexertion or trauma; can range from mild to moderate to severe.

- Direct work over the area of injury is contraindicated regionally until all signs of inflammation have dissipated.
- The use of ice and gentle range of motion can support healing.
- Methods used to manage distortion in posture resulting from compensation in the rest of the body are helpful.

Muscle Tension Headache
Contracted muscles exert pressure on the nerves and blood vessels in the area, causing pain, which is a dull, persistent ache with feelings of tightness around the head, temples, forehead, and occipital areas.

- Various strategies are available to treat stress-induced muscle tension headaches, including massage.
- Chronic patterns often indicate connective tissue shortening.
- Headaches respond best to whole-body therapy, which not only addresses immediate areas but also relaxes the entire body.

Muscular Dystrophy
Characterized by atrophy of skeletal muscles with no malfunction of the nervous system.

- Careful intervention may slow the atrophy process.
- Passive and active range-of-motion methods directly affect the muscles and joints and aid in the circulation and elimination processes.
- Abdominal massage may help with constipation.
- The practitioner should avoid methods that cause any inflammation.

Continued

TABLE A.1	Diseases and Indications and Contraindications for Massage Therapy—cont'd
Disease	**Indications and Contraindications for Massage Therapy**
Myasthenia Gravis In this autoimmune disease, the immune system attacks muscle cells at the neuromuscular junction and interferes with the action of acetylcholine.	• General constitutional massage methods are indicated. • The practitioner should avoid stressing the system and should work toward general restorative processes that reduce pain, support sleep, and create an overall sense of well-being.
Myelitis Infection of the spinal cord or brainstem (or both).	• Infectious processes are contraindicated for massage intervention unless closely supervised by appropriate medical personnel. • Immediately refer clients with unusual or unexplained stiff neck for diagnosis.
Myofascial System Disorder Pertains to a muscle and its sheath of connective tissue or fascia.	• Intervention focuses on reversing nonproductive processes and supporting resourceful compensation patterns that develop in response to chronic problems. • The goal is to support circulation, connective tissue strength and pliability, and nervous system interaction. • The compression and stroking of massage support circulation. • Connective tissue responds to methods that affect the viscoelastic, plastic, and colloid properties. • Muscle tension patterns respond to compression and drag that stimulate proprioceptors. • Muscle energy methods systematically use contraction and relaxing of muscles combined with lengthening to restore the normal length of muscles. • Trigger points respond to methods that reduce hyperactivity, such as muscle energy methods and compression. • Calming the sympathetic arousal is also necessary.
Myopathy: Metabolic and Toxic Abnormal condition of skeletal muscle characterized by muscle weakness, wasting, and histologic changes within muscle tissue, as seen in any of the muscular dystrophies.	• Treatment for these types of myopathy usually is not contraindicated, as long as the therapeutic approaches are general and focus on supporting body restoration and healing processes. • Massage can support detoxification efforts because these methods enhance circulation. • The practitioner must take care in toxic conditions not to tax an already overloaded system.
Myositis Ossificans Involves an inflammatory process that stimulates the formation of osseous tissue in the fascial components of muscles.	• Treatment is contraindicated regionally.
Neuropathy Inflammation or degeneration of the peripheral nerves.	• Nerve pain is difficult to manage, does not respond well to analgesics, and often is intractable. • Massage, because of the interface with the nervous system, may provide short-term, symptomatic pain relief through shifts in neurotransmitters and stimulation of alternate nerve pathways, resulting in hyperstimulation analgesia and counterirritation. • Any therapy that increases mood-elevating and pain-modulating mechanisms makes coping with nerve pain somewhat easier for short periods.

Osteitis Fibrosa Cystica
Disease in which fibrous tissue and cysts replace bone tissue, making the bones weak and prone to fracture.

- The practitioner must exercise caution before using any massage and bodywork requiring any amount of compressive force on a client with a condition that causes demineralization of bone or that results in brittle, fragile bones.

Osteoarthritis
Degenerative joint disease, osteoarthritis is the breakdown of joints caused by normal wear and tear.

- Because progression and flare-ups of the disease often are stress related, the generalized gentle stress reduction methods provided by massage therapy may be beneficial in long-term management of the condition, if supervised as part of a total care program.
- The practitioner should avoid frictioning techniques and any other forms of bodywork that cause inflammation.
- General systemic changes in the neurotransmitters and hormones that accompany exercise and many forms of bodywork can elevate mood and thus reduce pain perception.

Osteochondritis Dissecans
Condition that affects a joint in which a fragment of cartilage and its underlying bone become detached from the articular surface.

- Massage therapy is contraindicated regionally.

Osteogenesis Imperfecta
Group of hereditary disorders that appear in newborns or young children. The bones are deformed and fragile as a result of demineralization and defective formation of connective tissue.

- The practitioner must exercise caution before using any massage and bodywork requiring any amount of compressive force on a client with a condition that causes demineralization of bone or that results in brittle, fragile bones.

Osteomyelitis
Inflammation in the bone, bone marrow, or periosteum, usually caused by pyogenic (pus-producing) bacteria.

- Massage is contraindicated in infectious disease unless carefully supervised by medical personnel.
- The therapist always must refer clients with vague pain symptoms for proper diagnosis.

Osteonecrosis (Ischemic Necrosis)
Death of a segment of bone, usually caused by insufficient blood flow to a region of the skeleton.

- Necrosis is usually a localized condition that requires regional avoidance of the involved bone area.
- Because massage provides the generalized effect of enhanced circulation, the practitioner might realize indirect benefits with careful use of these methods; however, because these disorders are pathologic conditions, massage must be given only with the permission and supervision of the primary healthcare provider.

Osteoporosis
Bone lacks calcium and other minerals and bone protein.

- The practitioner must exercise caution before using any massage and bodywork requiring any amount of compressive force on a client with a condition that causes demineralization of bone or that results in brittle, fragile bones.

Paget Disease (Osteitis Deformans)
Occurs when the bones undergo normal periods of calcium loss followed by periods of excessive new cell growth.

- The practitioner must exercise caution before using any massage and bodywork requiring any amount of compressive force on a client with a condition that causes demineralization of bone or that results in brittle, fragile bones.

Pancreatitis
Inflammation of the pancreas.

- Abdominal pain or referred back pain may indicate one of several gastrointestinal disorders.
- In such cases, referral is necessary for proper diagnosis.

Continued

TABLE A.1	Diseases and Indications and Contraindications for Massage Therapy—cont'd
Disease	**Indications and Contraindications for Massage Therapy**
Parkinson Disease Disease in which neurons that release the neurotransmitter dopamine in the brain degenerate, thus slowing or stopping its release.	• Because massage has been shown to increase dopamine activity, its use is indicated for managing Parkinson disease and tremor. • In addition, the practitioner can effectively manage secondary muscle tension with massage therapy and other forms of soft tissue manipulation.
Peptic Ulcer Gastric or duodenal ulcer that affects the lining of the esophagus, stomach, or duodenum.	• Abdominal pain or referred back pain may indicate one of several gastrointestinal disorders; in such cases, referral is necessary for proper diagnosis. • Most chronic gastrointestinal diseases have a strong correlation to stress. • Comprehensive stress management programs, including therapeutic massage methods, often are effective in managing these conditions.
Plantar Fasciitis Inflammation of the plantar fascia and surrounding myofascial structures.	• Acute-phase plantar fasciitis responds to rest and ice. • After the inflammation has diminished, soft tissue methods that address the connective tissue and the judicious use of stretching are beneficial.
Poliomyelitis—Postpolio Syndrome Viral infection of the nerves that control skeletal muscle movement. Years later, postpolio syndrome can cause fatigue, muscle aching, and weakness.	• For postpolio syndrome, general constitutional approaches seem to work best to aid in overall pain reduction and restoration of the sleep pattern. • The practitioner should avoid any form of therapy that causes therapeutic inflammation, including intense exercise and stretching programs.
Pregnancy Abnormality and Bleeding During Pregnancy	• Refer the client immediately to the appropriate physician or emergency department.
Regional Enteritis Chronic inflammation of the intestine, most commonly the ileum; also called Crohn disease.	• The intestinal tract is highly responsive to changes in autonomic function and endocrine patterns. • Comprehensive stress management programs, including therapeutic massage methods, often are effective in managing these conditions.
Rheumatoid Arthritis Crippling condition characterized by swelling of the joints in the hands, feet, and other parts of the body as a result of inflammation and overgrowth of the synovial membranes and other joint tissues.	• Because the progression and flare-ups of the disease are often stress related, the generalized gentle stress reduction methods provided by massage therapy may be beneficial in long-term management of the condition, if supervised as part of a total care program. • The practitioner should avoid frictioning techniques and any other forms of bodywork that cause inflammation.
Rotator Cuff Tear Often caused by repeated impingement, overuse, or other conditions that weaken the rotator cuff and eventually cause partial or complete tears.	• Work on acute myofascial tears is contraindicated; however, massage therapy may be indicated in the rehabilitative process and as part of a supervised treatment protocol. • The practitioner can manage and improve compensatory patterns with massage.

Schizophrenia

Most common mental disorder; includes a large group of psychotic disorders characterized by gross distortion of reality.

- Therapeutic massage supports a multidisciplinary treatment approach, for such methods influence neurotransmitters; supervision is necessary.

Sciatica

Inflammation of the sciatic nerve.

- Various forms of massage application reduce muscle spasm, lengthen shortened muscles, and soften and stretch connective tissue, restoring a more normal space around the nerve and alleviating impingement.

Scoliosis

Lateral curvature of the spine, a common abnormality of childhood, especially in females.

- Massage methods help to manage compensatory muscle spasms and connective tissue changes.
- Compressions or joint movements are contraindicated, unless supervised by medical professionals; light, superficial methods may be indicated with supervision.

Shin Splints

Inflammation of the proximal portion of any of the musculotendinous structures originating from the lower part of the tibia.

- Massage approaches may be beneficial as long as they do not increase inflammation and a stress fracture has been ruled out.

Skin Conditions

Contagious: contagious fungi, viral, bacterial, and parasites.
Noncontagious: dermatitis, psoriasis.

- Therapeutic massage usually is not contraindicated in localized skin conditions, but local (regional) avoidance of the affected area is necessary.
- Localized touch can irritate most skin disorders.
- Massage is contraindicated if the skin is inflamed or if the condition is contagious or is transmissible through touch.
- Malignancy is a contraindication unless the appropriate medical personnel supervise the therapy.

Spinal Abnormalities: Scoliosis, Kyphosis, and Lordosis

Abnormal curvatures of the spine may be congenital, may result from paralysis or weakness or tension in spinal muscles, or may result from rapid growth of the body, especially after puberty.

- If skeletal problems create or are part of a permanent condition, supportive care is required.
- Massage methods help to manage compensatory muscle spasms and connective tissue changes.
- Any type of compressive force or joint movement method is contraindicated for fragile skeletal structure, regardless of the cause, unless carefully supervised by appropriate medical professionals.
- Light, superficial methods, such as the gentle laying on of hands used in some forms of touch systems, might be indicated, again with supervision.

Spinal Cord Injury

Any of the traumatic disruptions of the spinal cord that often are associated with extensive musculoskeletal involvement.

- Massage is an effective part of a comprehensive, supervised rehabilitation and long-term care program.
- Massage and other forms of bodywork can help manage secondary muscle tension resulting from alteration of posture and the use of equipment such as wheelchairs, braces, and crutches.
- Specifically focused massage can help in the management of difficulties with bowel paralysis.
- The circulation enhancement of massage can assist in the management of a decubitus ulcer.

Spondylitis

Inflammation of more than one vertebra.

- Massage therapy modalities are effective in managing backache.
- Benefits are derived from reduction in protective muscle spasm compensation (guarding) and generalized pain-modulating effects.
- Be aware that protective spasm provides stabilization.

Continued

TABLE A.1   Diseases and Indications and Contraindications for Massage Therapy—cont'd

Disease	Indications and Contraindications for Massage Therapy
Spondylolisthesis Part of one vertebra moves forward on another.	• Complex backache involving the joint structures requires the practitioner to incorporate therapeutic massage into a total treatment program supervised by the appropriate healthcare professional.
Spondylosis Formation of bony spurs at the disk margin of the vertebral bodies that causes degenerative changes in the intervertebral disks.	• Complex backache involving the joint structures requires the practitioner to incorporate therapeutic massage into a total treatment program supervised by the appropriate healthcare professional.
Stomach Cancer (or Gastric Cancer) Disease in which stomach cells become malignant (cancerous) and grow out of control, forming a tumor.	• Abdominal pain or referred back pain may indicate one of several gastrointestinal disorders; in such cases, referral is necessary for proper diagnosis.
Stroke Sudden loss of neurologic function caused by vascular injury to the brain.	• Stroke is a medical emergency that requires immediate referral. • Massage and bodywork is an effective part of a supervised comprehensive care program. • Massage and other forms of bodywork can help in the management of secondary muscle tension resulting from alterations in posture and the use of equipment such as wheelchairs, braces, and crutches.
Tendonitis or Tenosynovitis Inflammation of a tendon or a tendon sheath.	• Any methods that could increase the inflammatory response are contraindicated for areas of inflammation. • In the acute phase, the use of ice and gentle movement is indicated; chronic conditions may benefit from methods that elongate connective tissue structures, thus relieving friction in the area.
Thoracic Outlet Syndrome Occurs because the brachial plexus and the blood supply of the arm become impinged, resulting in shooting pains, weakness, and numbness.	• Massage methods help relieve muscle impingement of nerves by relaxing and lengthening the muscles.
Thrombosis Formation of a thrombus (blood clot) within the lumen (open cavity) of the blood vessels or heart.	• Thrombosis contraindicates massage; because obstruction could be a medical emergency, immediate referral is indicated.
Thrombus Clot that forms inside a blood vessel.	• Massage therapy is contraindicated regionally and generally because of the potential for moving the clot or for increased bruising from the medication. • Thrombosis can be a medical emergency, and immediate referral is indicated; treatment may include elevation, application of heat packs to the affected area, and use of blood-thinning medications (such as heparin or warfarin).
Torticollis Involves spasm or shortening of one of the sternocleidomastoid muscles; also called wry neck.	• Management of torticollis with massage therapy involves relaxing the neck, releasing trigger points, stretching contracted muscles, and improving range of motion. • Avoidance of pressure on the vessels under the sternocleidomastoid muscle is important.

Tremors
Involuntary muscle twitches.

- Because massage has been shown to increase dopamine activity, it is indicated in the management of tremor.
- The practitioner can manage secondary muscle tension effectively with massage therapy and other forms of soft tissue manipulation.

Tuberculosis
Systemic disease caused by tubercular bacillus.

- Massage is contraindicated in infectious disease unless carefully supervised by medical personnel.
- The therapist always must refer clients with vague pain symptoms for proper diagnosis.

Ulcerative Colitis
Primarily affects the sigmoid colon, with symptoms of lower abdominal pain and bloody diarrhea.

- Abdominal pain or referred back pain may indicate one of several gastrointestinal disorders; in such cases, referral is necessary for proper diagnosis.
- The intestinal tract is highly responsive to changes in autonomic function and endocrine patterns.
- Sympathetic arousal changes peristaltic action and can send the intestinal tract into all kinds of dysfunction.
- Comprehensive stress management programs, including therapeutic massage methods, often are effective in managing these conditions.

Urinary Incontinence
Inability to control urination, most often caused by weak pelvic floor muscles or nerve damage.

- Stress is a contributing factor to incontinence; any form of stress management helps somewhat with stress and urge incontinence.
- The practitioner must consider that incontinent clients require frequent and easy access to the restroom.

Vertebral Subluxation
Muscle spasms (entrapment) and shortening; disk degeneration; disk herniation.

- Various forms of massage are important for managing muscle spasm and pain associated with the aforementioned conditions.
- The student must remember that muscle spasms serve a stabilizing and protective function called *guarding*.
- Without some protective spasm, the nerve could be damaged further, but too much muscle spasm increases the discomfort.
- Therapeutic intervention seeks to reduce pain and excessive tension and to restore moderate mobility while allowing for the resourceful compensation produced by the muscle tension pattern.
- Because low back pain is a common disorder, the massage practitioner must be familiar with its causes and treatment protocols.

Vertigo
Sensation that the body or the environment is spinning or swaying.

- Movement therapies can help or aggravate vertigo; therefore, the practitioner must take care to design an individual therapeutic program that is based on the client's history.
- Massage methods can deal effectively with muscle tension and can diminish anxiety and nausea, but the benefit is temporary because symptoms return with recurrence of vertigo.

Whiplash
Injury to the soft tissues of the neck caused by sudden hyperextension or flexion (or both) of the neck.

- Direct intervention during the acute phase is contraindicated unless closely supervised by a physician or other qualified healthcare professional.
- Massage methods are valuable as part of rehabilitation efforts in the subacute phase and can help restore function if the condition is chronic.
- Extension injury is more severe and requires careful intervention.

Glossary

HOW TO USE THE GLOSSARY TO STUDY

Repetition improves retention. Understanding the language used in test questions is necessary to identify the meaning and then the best answer to a question. Reviewing the glossary helps reinforce the language encountered on exams. Review in chunks of 7—10 terms at a time. Read the term and definition silently and then out loud. Avoid attempts to memorize. Concentrate on recognition and comprehension.

Progress through the glossary over a period of days and weeks. Then repeat.

Abbreviation   Shortened forms of words or phrases.

Abduction   Lateral movement away from the midline of the trunk.

Absorption   Movement of food molecules from the digestive tract to the circulatory or lymphatic system.

Abuse   Exploitation, misuse, mistreatment, molestation, or neglect.

Acetylcholine   Neurotransmitter that stimulates the parasympathetic nervous system and the skeletal muscles and is involved in memory.

Acne   Chronic inflammation of the sebaceous glands and hair follicles caused by interactions between bacteria, sebum, and sex hormones.

Acquired immunodeficiency syndrome   Dysfunction in the immune system, which defends the body against disease. Abbreviated AIDS.

Active joint movement   Movement of a joint through its range of motion by the client.

Active range of motion   Movement of a joint by the client without any type of assistance from the massage practitioner.

Active transport   Transport of substances into or out of a cell with the use of energy.

Active-assisted movement   Movement of a joint in which the client and the therapist produce the motion.

Active-resistive movement   Movement of a joint by the client against resistance provided by the therapist.

Acupressure   Methods used to tone or sedate acupuncture points without the use of needles.

Acupuncture   The practice of inserting needles at specific points on meridians, or channels, to stimulate or sedate energy flow or to regulate or alter body function. A branch of Chinese medicine, acupuncture is the art and science of manipulating the flow of Qi, the basic life force, and Xue, the blood, body fluids, and nourishing essences. Western medicine uses acupuncture primarily to reduce pain. Acupressure, which uses digital pressure, follows the same Asian principles.

Acupuncture point   Asian term for a specific point that correlates with a neurologic motor point.

Acute   Term that describes a condition in which the signs and symptoms develop quickly, last a short time, and then disappear.

Acute disease   Disease that has a specific beginning, as well as signs and symptoms that develop quickly, last a short time, and then disappear.

Acute illness   Short-term illness that resolves by means of the normal healing process and, if necessary, supportive medical care.

Acute pain   Symptom of a disease condition or temporary aspect of medical treatment. Acute pain acts as a warning signal because it can activate the sympathetic nervous system. It usually is temporary and of sudden onset and is easily localized. The client frequently can describe the pain, which often subsides without treatment.

Adaptation   Response to sensory stimulation in which nerve signaling is reduced or ceases.

Adduction   Medial movement toward the midline of the body.

Adenosine triphosphate   Compound that stores energy in the muscles. When adenosine triphosphate is broken down during catabolic reactions, it releases energy. Abbreviated ATP.

Adrenergic   Stimulation of the sympathetic nervous system that causes the release of epinephrine and similar neurotransmitters and hormones.

Aerobic exercise training   Exercise program focused on enhancing fitness and endurance.

Afferent   Toward a center or point of reference.

Afferent nerves   Sensory nerves that link sensory receptors with the central nervous system and transmit sensory information.

Agonist   Muscle that causes or controls joint motion through a specified plane of motion; also known as the primary or prime mover.

Alimentary canal   Tube-shaped portion of the digestive system known as the gastrointestinal tract; the alimentary canal is about 30 feet long and contains several special structures throughout its length.

All-or-none response   Property of a muscle fiber (cell) contraction by which, when contraction is initiated, the fiber contracts to its full ability or does not contract at all.

Allied health   Division of medicine in which the professional receives training in a specific area of medicine to provide support for the physician.

Alopecia   Hair loss or baldness on part or all of the body.

Amphiarthrosis   Slightly movable joint that connects bone to bone with fibrocartilage or hyaline growth cartilage. The two types in the human body are symphyses and synchondroses.

Amyotrophic lateral sclerosis   Progressive disease that begins in the central nervous system and involves the degeneration of motor neurons and the subsequent atrophy of voluntary muscle. Also called Lou Gehrig disease.

Anabolism   Chemical processes in the body that join simple compounds to form more complex compounds of carbohydrates, lipids, proteins, and nucleic acids. These processes require energy supplied by adenosine triphosphate.

Anaplasia   Meaning "without shape," the term describes abnormal or undifferentiated cells that fail to mature into specialized cell types. Anaplasia is a characteristic of malignant cells.

Anatomic barriers   Anatomic structures determined by the shape and fit of bones at the joint.

Anatomic position   Standard position in which the person stands upright with the feet slightly apart, arms hanging at the sides, and palms facing forward with thumbs outward.

Anatomic range of motion   Amount of motion available to a joint based on its structure and determined by the shapes of the joint surfaces, joint capsule, and ligaments, as well as muscle bulk and surrounding musculotendinous and bony structures.

Anatomy   The study of the structures of the body and the relationships of its parts.

Androgens   Male sex hormones.

Anemia   A decrease in the normal number of red blood cells or in the amount of hemoglobin or iron present in the blood.

Aneurysm   A permanent dilation of part of a blood vessel caused by weakness or damage to its structure. The most common sites of aneurysms are the aorta and the arteries of the brain.

Antagonism   Opposition, as when massage produces the opposite effect, such as with medications.

Antagonist   A muscle that usually is located on the opposite side of a joint from the agonist and that has the opposite action. The muscle that opposes movement of the prime movers.

Anterior pelvic rotation   Anterior movement of the upper pelvis; the iliac crest tilts forward in a sagittal plane.

Antibody   A specific protein that is produced to destroy or suppress antigens.

Antigen   Any substance that causes the body to produce antibodies.

Anxiety   A feeling of uneasiness that usually is connected with an increase in sympathetic arousal responses.

Aorta   Large artery that carries oxygen- and nutrient-enriched blood out of the heart.

Apical surface   The surface of epithelial cells that is exposed to the external surface, such as the atmosphere or a passage in the body.

Apocrine   Type of sweat gland that discharges a thicker and more odoriferous form of sweat.

Aponeurosis   Broad, flat sheet of fibrous connective tissue.

Appendicular skeleton   Part of the skeleton that is composed of the limbs and their attachments.

Applied kinesiology   Methods of evaluation and bodywork that use a specialized type of muscle testing and various forms of massage and bodywork for corrective procedures.

Approximation   Technique of pushing muscle fibers together in the belly of the muscle.

Art   Craft, skill, technique, and talent.

Arterial circulation   Movement of oxygenated blood under pressure from the heart to the body through the arteries.

Arterioles   The smallest arteries.

Arteriosclerosis   Term that means "hardening of the arteries"; it is used to refer to arteries that have become brittle and have lost their elasticity.

Artery   Blood vessel that transports oxygenated blood from the heart to the body or deoxygenated blood from the heart to the lungs.

Arthritis   The most common type of joint disorder, *arthritis* literally means "inflammation of the joint."

Arthrokinematic movement   Accessory movement that occurs as the result of inherent laxity or joint play that is present in each joint. Joint play allows the ends of the bones to slide, roll, or spin smoothly onto one another. These essential movements occur passively with movement of the joint and are not under voluntary control.

Articulation   Another word for a joint, the structure created when bones connect to each other.

Ascending tracts   Tracts that carry sensory information to the brain.

Aseptic technique   Procedures that kill or disable pathogens on surfaces to prevent transmission.

Asian approaches   Methods of bodywork that have developed from ancient Chinese methods.

Assessment   The collection and interpretation of information provided by the client, the client's family and friends, the massage practitioner, and referring medical professionals.

Asymmetrical stance   Position in which the body weight is shifted from one foot to the other while standing.

Atherosclerosis Condition in which fatty plaque is deposited in medium-sized and large arteries.

Athlete Person who participates in sports as an amateur or a professional. Athletes require precise use of their bodies.

Atom The smallest particle of an element that retains and exhibits the properties of that element. Atoms are made up of protons, neutrons, and electrons.

Atrium One of two small, thin-walled upper chambers of the heart; the right and left atria are separated by a thin interatrial septum.

Atrophy A decrease in the size of a body part or organ that is caused by a decrease in the size of the cells.

Attachments Connections of skeletal muscles to bones; often referred to as the origin and the insertion.

Autonomic nervous system Division of the peripheral nervous system that is composed of nerves that connect the central nervous system to the glands, heart, and smooth muscles to maintain the internal body environment. The body system that regulates involuntary body functions through the sympathetic "fight-flight-fear response" and the restorative parasympathetic "relaxation response." The sympathetic and parasympathetic systems work together to maintain homeostasis through a feedback loop system.

Autoregulation Control of homeostasis through alteration of tissue or function.

Avulsion Injury to a ligament or tendon that involves tearing off of its attachment.

Axial skeleton The axis of the body; the axial skeleton consists of the head, the vertebral column (the spine), and the ribs and sternum and provides the body with form and protection.

Axon A single elongated projection from the nerve cell body that transmits impulses away from the cell body.

Ayurveda System of health and medicine that grew from East Indian roots.

Bacteria Primitive cells that have no nuclei. Bacteria cause disease by secreting toxic substances that damage human tissues, by becoming parasites inside human cells, or by forming colonies in the body that disrupt normal function.

Balance The ability to control equilibrium. Two types of balance are static or still balance and dynamic or moving balance.

Ball-and-socket joint Joint that allows movement in many directions around a central point. Ball-and-socket joints are ball-shaped convex surfaces that are fitted into concave sockets. This type of joint allows the greatest freedom of movement but is the most easily dislocated.

Basal metabolic rate Rate of energy expenditure of the body under normal, relaxed activities.

Basal surface Tissue surface that faces the inside of the body.

Basement membrane Permeable membrane that attaches epithelial tissues to underlying connective tissues.

Beating Form of heavy tapotement that involves use of the fist.

Benign Term that describes the type of tumor that remains localized within the tissue from which it arose and does not undergo malignant changes. Benign tumors usually grow slowly.

Bias Tendency to favor or be prejudice toward or against something or someone.

Biologic rhythms The internal, periodic timing component of an organism, also known as a biorhythm. Circadian rhythms work on a 24-hour cycle to coordinate internal functions such as sleep. Ultradian rhythms repeat themselves from every 90 minutes to a few hours, whereas seasonal rhythms are annual functions.

Biomechanics The study of mechanical principles, movements, and actions as applied to living bodies.

Biopsychosocial model An interdisciplinary model used in healthcare that looks at the interconnection between biology, psychology, and socio-environmental factors.

Blood pressure Measurement of pressure exerted by the heart on the walls of blood vessels. The highest pressure exerted, which is called systolic pressure, results when the ventricles are contracted. Diastolic pressure, the lowest pressure, occurs when the ventricles are at rest. Blood that is forced into the aorta during systole sets up a pressure wave that travels down the arteries. This wave expands the arterial wall, and expansion can be palpated by pressing the artery against tissue; the waves constitute the pulse rate.

Blood Thick, red fluid that provides oxygen, nourishment, and protection to the cells and carries away waste products. Whole blood consists of two components: formed cellular elements and liquid plasma. Blood is a form of connective tissue.

Body mechanics Use of the body in an efficient and biomechanically correct way.

Body segment Area of the body between joints that provides movement during walking and balance.

Body supports Pillows, folded blankets, foam forms, or commercial products that help contour the flat surface of a massage table or mat.

Body/mind Interaction between thought and physiology that is connected to the limbic system, to the hypothalamic influence on the autonomic nervous system, and to the endocrine system.

Bodywork Term that encompasses all the various forms of massage, movement, and other touch therapies.

Boundary Personal space that exists within an arm's length perimeter. Personal emotional space is designated by morals, values, and experience.

Brain The largest and most complex unit of the nervous system, the brain is responsible for perception, sensation, emotion, intellect, and action.

Brainstem Primitive portion of the brain that contains centers for vital functions and reflex actions, such as vomiting, coughing, sneezing, posture, and basic movement patterns.

Breathing pattern disorders Complex set of behaviors that lead to overbreathing in the absence of a pathologic condition. These disorders are considered a functional syndrome because all body parts are working effectively; therefore, a specific pathologic condition does not exist.

Burnout   Condition that occurs when a person uses up energy more quickly than it can be restored.

Bursa   Flat sac of synovial membrane in which the inner sides of the sac are separated by fluid film. Bursae are located where moving structures are apt to rub.

Bursitis   Inflammation of a bursa.

Callus   Area of thickened, hardened skin that develops in an area of friction or a region of recurrent pressure.

Cancer   Malignant, nonencapsulated cells that invade the surrounding tissue. They often break away, or metastasize, from the primary tumor and form secondary cancer masses.

Capillary   One of the small blood vessels found between arteries and veins that allows the exchange of gases, nutrients, and waste products. The walls of the capillaries are thin, allowing molecules to diffuse easily.

Carbohydrates   Sugars, starches, and cellulose composed of carbon, hydrogen, and oxygen.

Cardiac cycle   Synchronized sequence of events that takes place during one full heartbeat.

Cardiac muscle fibers   Smaller, striated, involuntary muscle fibers (cells) in the heart that contract to pump blood.

Cardiac output   Amount of blood pumped by the left ventricle in 1 minute.

Care or treatment plan   Plan created to achieve therapeutic goals. It outlines agreed-upon objectives; the frequency, duration, and number of visits required; progress measurements; the date of reassessment; and massage methods to be used.

Career   A chosen pursuit; a life's work.

Carotene   Yellow pigment found in the dermis that provides a natural yellow tint to the skin of some individuals.

Cartilage   A form of flexible connective tissue. Types of cartilage include hyaline, fibrocartilage, and elastic cartilage.

Catabolism   Chemical processes in the body that release energy as complex compounds are broken down into simpler ones.

Catecholamines   A group of neurotransmitters that are involved in sleep, mood, pleasure, and motor function.

Cell   Basic structural unit of a living organism. A cell contains a nucleus and cytoplasm and is surrounded by a membrane.

Center of gravity   Imaginary midpoint or center of weight of a body or object, at which the body or the object could balance on a point.

Centering   The ability to focus the mind by screening out sensation.

Central nervous system   The brain and the spinal cord and their coverings.

Cerebellum   The second-largest part of the brain, the cerebellum is involved in balance, posture, coordination, and movement.

Cerebrospinal fluid   Clear, colorless fluid that flows throughout the brain and around the spinal cord, cushioning and protecting these structures and maintaining proper pH balance.

Cerebrum   The largest of the brain divisions, the cerebrum consists of two hemispheres that occupy the uppermost region of the cranium. The cerebrum receives, interprets, and associates incoming information with past memories and then transmits the appropriate motor response.

Certification   Voluntary credentialing process that usually requires education and testing; tests are administered privately or by government regulatory bodies.

Cerumen   Sticky substance released by glands in the ear. Also known as earwax, cerumen protects the ear from the entry of foreign material and repels insects.

Ceruminous glands   Modified apocrine glands found in the external ear canal that secrete cerumen.

Chakra   Energy fields or centers of consciousness within the body.

Challenge   Living each day knowing that it is filled with things to learn, skills to practice, tasks to accomplish, and obstacles to overcome.

Charting   Process of keeping a written record on a client or patient. The most effective charting methods follow clinical reasoning, which emphasizes a problem-solving approach. Many systems of charting are used, but all these models have similar components: POMR (problem-oriented medical record) and SOAP (subjective, objective, analysis, and plan—the four parts of the written record).

Chemical effects   Effects of massage produced by the release of chemical substances in the body. These substances may be released locally from massaged tissue, or they may be released into the general circulation.

Chemical properties   Properties that demonstrate how a substance reacts with other substances or responds to a change in the environment.

Chronic   Term that describes the type of disease that develops slowly and lasts for a long time, sometimes for life.

Chronic disease   Disease with a vague onset that develops slowly and lasts for a long time, sometimes for life.

Chronic illness   Disease, injury, or syndrome that shows little change or slow progression.

Chronic pain   Pain that continues or recurs over a prolonged time, usually for longer than 6 months. Onset may be obscure, and the character and quality of the pain may change over time. Chronic pain usually is poorly localized and is not as intense as acute pain, although for some, the pain is exhausting and depressing. Chronic pain usually does not activate the sympathetic nervous system.

Circulatory   Systems that depend on the pumping action of skeletal muscle (i.e., arterial, venous, lymphatic, respiratory, and cerebrospinal fluid circulatory systems).

Circumduction   Circular movement of a limb, in which the movements of flexion, extension, abduction, and adduction are combined to create a cone shape.

Client information form   Document used to obtain information from the client about health, preexisting conditions, and expectations for the massage.

Client outcome   Results desired from the massage and from the massage therapist.

Client/practitioner agreement and policy statement   A detailed written explanation of all rules, expectations, and procedures for the massage.

Close-packed position   Position of a synovial joint in which the surfaces fit together precisely and maximum contact occurs between opposing surfaces. Compression of joint surfaces permits no movement, and the joint possesses its greatest stability.

Closed kinematic chain   Positioning of joints in such a way that motion at one of the joints is accompanied by motion at an adjacent joint. Also called closed kinetic chain.

Coalition   A group formed for a particular purpose.

Cognition   Conscious awareness and perception, reasoning, judgment, intuition, and memory.

Collagen   Protein substance composed of small fibrils that combine to create the connective tissue of fasciae, tendons, and ligaments. When combined with water, collagen forms gelatin. Collagen accounts for approximately one fourth of the protein in the body.

Collagenous fibers   Strong fibers with little capacity for stretch. They have a high degree of tensile strength, which allows them to withstand longitudinal stress.

Collaterals   Branches from an axon that allow communication among neurons.

Combining vowel   A vowel added between two roots or a root and a suffix to make pronunciation of the word easier.

Comfort barrier   The first point of resistance short of the client's perception of any discomfort at the physiologic or pathologic barrier.

Commitment   Ability and willingness to be involved in what is happening around us so as to have a purpose for being.

Communicable disease   Disease caused by pathogens that are spread easily; a contagious disease.

Compact (dense) bone   The hard portion of bone that protects spongy bone and provides the firm framework of the bone and the body. Osteocytes in this type of bone are located in concentric rings around a central haversian canal, through which nerves and blood vessels pass.

Compensation   Process of counterbalancing a defect in body structure or function.

Compression   Pressure into the body to spread tissue against underlying structures. (This massage manipulation sometimes is classified with pétrissage.) Also, the exertion of inappropriate pressure on nerves by hard tissue (e.g., bone).

Compressive force   Amount of pressure exerted against the surface of the body for the purpose of applying pressure to the deeper body structures; pressure aimed in a particular direction.

Concentric contraction   Action of a prime mover or agonist by which a muscle develops tension as it shortens to provide enough force to overcome resistance, described as positive contraction.

Concentric isotonic contraction   Application of a counterforce by the massage therapist while allowing the client to move, which brings the origin and the insertion of the target muscle together against the pressure.

Condition management   Use of massage methods to support clients who are unable to undergo a therapeutic change but who wish to function as effectively as possible under a set of circumstances.

Condyle   Rounded projection at the end of a bone.

Condyloid (condylar) joint   Joint that allows movement in two directions, with one motion predominating. The joint resembles a condyle, which is a rounded protuberance at the end of a bone that forms an articulation.

Confidentiality   Respect for the privacy of information.

Conflict   An expressed struggle between at least two interdependent parties who perceive incompatible goals, scarce resources, or interference from the other party in achieving their goals.

Connective tissue   The most abundant type of tissue in the body, connective tissue supports and holds together the body and its parts, protects the body from foreign matter, and is organized to transport substances throughout the body.

Contamination   Process by which an object or an area becomes unclean.

Contractility   The ability of a muscle to shorten forcibly upon adequate stimulation. This property sets muscle apart from all other types of tissue.

Contracture   Chronic shortening of a muscle, especially the connective tissue component.

Contraindication   Any condition that renders a particular treatment improper or undesirable.

Control   The belief that we can influence events by the way we feel, think, and act.

Contusion   A bruise.

Corn   A painful, conical thickening of skin over bony prominences of the feet caused by continued pressure and friction on normally thin skin. Soft corns are those located in moist areas, such as between the toes.

Coronary arteries   Arteries that supply oxygenated blood to the heart muscle itself; they are located in grooves between the atria and ventricles and between the two ventricles.

Coronary veins   Veins that return deoxygenated blood from the heart to the right atrium.

Cortisol   A glucocorticoid, also known as hydrocortisone. Levels of stress often are measured by an assessment of cortisol levels. A stress hormone produced by the adrenal glands that is released during long-term stress; an elevated level indicates increased sympathetic arousal.

Counterirritation   Superficial stimulation that relieves a deeper sensation by stimulating different sensory signals.

Counterpressure   Force applied to an area that is designed to match exactly (isometric contraction) or in part (isotonic contraction) the effort or force produced by the muscles in that area.

Countertransference   Personalization of the professional relationship by the therapist, in which the practitioner is unable to separate the therapeutic relationship from personal feelings and expectations for the client.

Cramps   Painful muscle spasms or involuntary twitches that involve the whole muscle.

Cranial nerves Twelve pairs of nerves that originate from the olfactory bulbs, thalamus, visual cortex, and brainstem. They transmit information to and from the sensory organs of the face and the muscles of the face, neck, and upper shoulders.

Craniosacral and myofascial approaches Methods of bodywork that work reflexively and mechanically with the fascial network of the body.

Cream Type of lubricant that is in a semisolid or solid state.

Credential Designation earned by completing a process that verifies a certain level of expertise in a given skill.

Creep The slow movement of viscoelastic materials back to their original state and tissue structure after the release of a deforming force.

Cross-directional stretching Tissue stretching that pulls and twists connective tissue against its fiber direction.

Cryotherapy Therapeutic use of ice.

Cultural appropriation The practice of using or taking something from another culture without giving proper recognition or respect to that culture often found in massage and bodywork modalities.

Cultural competency A set of principles, beliefs, and attitudes about cultural differences and experiences including the willingness to learn about multiple cultures with the intension of respect.

Cultural diversity The existence of a variety of cultural or ethnic groups in an organization.

Culture The arts, beliefs, customs, institutions, and all other products of human work and thought created by a specific group of people at a particular time.

Cupping Type of tapotement/percussion that involves the use of a cupped hand; it often is used over the thorax.

Cutaneous sensory receptors Sensory nerves in the skin.

Cytoplasm Material enclosed by the cell membrane.

Cytoskeleton Framework of proteins inside the cell that provides flexibility and strength.

Cytosol Fluid that surrounds the nucleus or organelles inside the cell membrane.

Database All available information that contributes to therapeutic interaction.

Deep fascia A coarse sheet of fibrous connective tissue that binds muscles into functional groups and forms partitions, called intermuscular septa, between muscle groups.

Deep inspiration Movement of air into the body by hard breathing to meet an increased demand for oxygen. Any muscles that can pull the ribs up are called into action.

Deep transverse friction Specific rehabilitation technique that creates therapeutic inflammation by causing a specific, controlled reinjury of tissues through the application of concentrated therapeutic movement that moves the tissue against its grain over only a small area.

Defensive measures The means by which our bodies defend against stressors (e.g., production of antibodies and white blood cells, behavioral or emotional means).

Degenerative joint disease Progressive change in joint surfaces, commonly called osteoarthritis.

Dendrites Branching projections from the nerve cell body that carry signals to the cell body.

Denial The ability to retreat and to ignore stressors.

Deoxyribonucleic acid Genetic material of the cell that carries the chemical "blueprint" of the body. Abbreviated DNA.

Depression 1. Condition characterized by a decrease in vital functional activity and by mood disturbances of exaggerated emptiness, hopelessness, and melancholy or of unbridled high energy with no purpose or outcome. 2. Downward or inferior movement.

Depth of pressure Compressive stress that can be light, moderate, deep, or varied.

Dermatitis General term for acute or chronic skin inflammation characterized by redness, eruptions, edema, scaling, and itching. The three main types are atopic dermatitis, seborrheic dermatitis, and contact dermatitis. Eczema is a form of dermatitis.

Dermatome Cutaneous (skin) distribution of spinal nerve sensation.

Dermis Inner layer of skin that contains collagen and elastin fibers, which provide much of the structure and strength of the skin; it is much thicker than the epidermis.

Descending tracts Tracts that carry sensory information from the brain to the spinal cord.

Diagnosis Labeling of signs and symptoms by a licensed medical professional.

Diagonal abduction Movement of a limb through a diagonal plane directly across and away from the midline of the body.

Diagonal adduction Movement of a limb through a diagonal plane toward and across the midline of the body.

Diaphragm Dome-shaped sheet of muscle attached to the thoracic wall that separates the lungs and the thoracic cavity from the abdominal cavity. As the chest cavity enlarges, the diaphragm moves downward and flattens to create a vacuum that allows air to flow into the lungs. As the chest contracts and the diaphragm relaxes, the diaphragm arches upward, helping air to flow out of the lungs.

Diarthrosis A freely movable synovial joint.

Diffusion Movement of ions and molecules from an area of higher concentration to one of a lower concentration.

Digestion The mechanical and chemical breakdown of food from its complex form into simple molecules.

Direction The flow of massage strokes from the center of the body outward (centrifugal) or from the extremities inward toward the center of the body (centripetal). Direction can involve circular motions; it can flow from origin to insertion of the muscle, can follow the muscle fibers, or can flow transverse to the tissue fibers.

Direction of ease Position the body assumes with postural changes and muscle shortening or weakening, depending on how it has balanced against gravity.

Disclosure Acknowledging and informing the client of any situation that interferes with or affects the professional relationship.

Disease Abnormality in functions of the body, especially when the abnormality threatens well-being.

Disinfection Process by which pathogens are destroyed.

Disk herniation Pathologic condition that occurs when the fibrocartilage that surrounds the intervertebral disk ruptures, releasing the nucleus pulposus that cushions the vertebrae above and below. Resultant pressure on spinal nerve roots may cause pain and may damage the surrounding nerves.

Dissociation Detachment, discontentedness, separation, isolation.

Dopamine Neurochemical that influences motor activity involving movement (especially learned fine movement, such as handwriting), conscious selectivity (what to pay attention to), mood (in terms of inspiration), and potentially intuition, joy, and enthusiasm. If the dopamine level is low, the opposite effects are seen, such as lack of motor control, clumsiness, inability to decide what to attend to, and boredom.

Dorsal root One of two roots that attach a spinal nerve to the spinal cord.

Dorsiflexion (dorsal flexion) Movement of the ankle that results in movement of the top of the foot toward the anterior tibia.

Dosha Ayurvedic concept that describes chemical processes in the body. The three types are Vata, Pitta, and Kappa.

Drag The amount of pull (stretch) on the tissue (tensile stress).

Drape Fabric used to cover the client and keep the individual warm while the massage is given.

Draping Procedures of covering and uncovering areas of the body and turning the client during the massage.

Draping material Coverings that provide the client with privacy and warmth. The most commonly used coverings are standard bed linens, because they are large enough to cover the entire body and are easy to use for most draping procedures.

Dual role Overlap in the scope of practice, with one professional providing support in more than one area of expertise.

Duration Length of time a method lasts or stays in the same location.

Dynamic force Force applied to an object that produces movement.

Dysfunction In-between state in which one is "not healthy" but also is "not sick" (i.e., experiencing disease).

Eccentric Action of an antagonist by which a muscle lengthens while under tension and changes in tension to control the descent of resistance. Eccentric movements, which may be thought of as controlling movement against gravity or resistance, are described as negative contractions.

Eccentric isotonic contraction Application of a counterforce while the client moves the jointed area, which allows the origin and the insertion to separate. The muscle lengthens against the pressure.

Eccrine Type of sweat gland that releases a watery fluid known as sweat, which cools the body and provides minor elimination of metabolic waste.

Edema Accumulation of abnormal amounts of fluid in tissue spaces.

Efferent Away from a center or point of reference.

Efferent nerves Motor nerves that link the central nervous system to the effectors outside it and transmit motor impulses.

Effleurage Gliding strokes; horizontal strokes applied with the fingers, hand, or forearm that usually follow the fiber direction of the underlying muscle, fascial planes, or dermatome pattern.

Effort Force applied to overcome resistance.

Elastic fibers Connective tissue fibers that are extensible and elastic. They are made of a protein called elastin, which returns to its original length after it is stretched.

Elasticity The ability of a muscle to recoil and resume its original resting length after it is stretched.

Elastin Connective tissue type of fiber that has elastic properties and allows flexibility of connective tissue structures.

Electrical–chemical functions Physiologic functions of the body that rely on or produce body energy; often called *chi*, prana, and meridian energy.

Element Substance that contains only a single type of atom.

Elevation Upward or superior movement.

Elimination (egestion) Removal and release of solid waste products from food that cannot be digested or absorbed.

Employee A person who works for another for a wage.

End feel The perception of the joint at the limit of its range of motion. The end feel is soft or hard. (*See* Joint end feel.)

Endangerment site Any area of the body where nerves and blood vessels surface close to the skin and are not well protected by muscle or connective tissue; therefore, deep, sustained pressure into these areas may damage the vessels and nerves. The kidney area is included because the kidneys are loosely suspended in fat and connective tissue, and heavy pounding is contraindicated in this area.

Endocannabinoid system A biochemical communication system in the human body, which plays an important role in regulating physiology, mood, and everyday experience. CBD, short for cannabidiol, is a chemical compound from the *Cannabis sativa* plant that has become popular as a topical used during massage.

Endocrine gland Ductless gland that secretes hormones directly into the bloodstream.

Endocytosis Cellular process of engulfing particles located outside the cell membrane into a cell through formation of vesicles.

Endogenous Made in the body.

Endoplasmic reticulum Network of intracellular membranes in the form of tubes that is connected to the nuclear membrane.

Endorphins Peptide hormones that mainly work in the way that morphine does to suppress pain. They influence mood, producing a mild euphoric feeling such as that seen in runner's high.

Endoskeleton   The bony support structure found inside the human body that accommodates growth.

Endosteum   Thin membrane of connective tissue that lines the marrow cavity of a bone.

Endurance   A measure of fitness. The ability to work for prolonged periods and the ability to resist fatigue.

Energetic approaches   Methods of bodywork that involve subtle body responses.

Energy   The capacity to work; work is movement of or change in the physical structure of matter.

Enkephalins and endorphins   Neurochemicals that elevate mood, support satiety (reduce hunger and cravings), and modulate pain.

Entrainment   Coordination or synchronization to an internal or external rhythm, especially when a person responds to certain patterns by moving in a manner that is coordinated with those patterns.

Entrapment   Pathologic pressure placed on a nerve or vessel by soft tissue.

Environmental contact   Contact with pathogens found in the environment in food, water, and soil and on various surfaces.

Epicondyle   A bony projection above a condyle.

Epidermis   The outer or top layer of skin composed of sublayers called strata. The epidermis contains no nerves or blood vessels.

Epilepticus   A continuous seizure.

Epinephrine   Catecholamine released by the nervous system and involved in fight-or-flight responses such as dilation of blood vessels to the skeletal muscles. Epinephrine is classified as a hormone when secreted by the adrenal gland.

Epinephrine/adrenaline   Neurochemical that activates arousal mechanisms in the body; the activation, arousal, alertness, and alarm chemical of the fight-or-flight response and of all sympathetic arousal functions and behaviors.

Epithelial tissues   A specialized group of tissues that cover and protect the surface of the body and its parts, line body cavities, and form glands. Epithelial tissue usually is found in areas in which substances move into and out of the body during secretion, absorption, and excretion.

Erythrocytes   Red blood cells that contain hemoglobin and that transport oxygen to the cells and carbon dioxide away from the cells.

Essential touch   Vital, fundamental, and primary touch that is crucial to well-being.

Essential tremor   A chronic tremor that does not proceed from any other pathologic condition.

Ethical behavior   Right and good conduct that is based on moral and cultural standards as defined by the society in which we live.

Ethical decision-making   The application of ethical principles and professional skills to determine appropriate behavior and to resolve ethical dilemmas.

Ethics   The science or study of morals, values, or principles, including ideals of autonomy, beneficence, and justice; principles of right and good conduct.

Etiology   The study of factors involved in the development of disease, including the nature of the disease and the susceptibility of the person.

Eversion   Movement of the sole of the foot outward away from the midline.

Excitability   The ability of a muscle to receive and respond to a stimulus.

Exemption   A situation in which a professional is not required to comply with an existing law because of educational or professional standing.

Exocrine gland   Gland that secretes hormones through ducts directly into specific areas. Exocrine glands constitute part of the endocrine system.

Exocytosis   Movement of substances out of a cell.

Experiment   Method of testing a hypothesis.

Expressive touch   Touch applied to support and convey awareness and empathy for the client as a whole.

Extensibility   The ability of a muscle to be stretched or extended.

Extension   Movement that increases the angle between two bones, usually by movement of the body part back toward the anatomic position.

External respiration   The exchange of oxygen and carbon dioxide between the lungs and the bloodstream.

External rotation   Rotary movement around the longitudinal axis of a bone away from the midline of the body. Also known as rotation laterally, outward rotation, and lateral rotation.

External sensory information   Stimulation from an origin exterior to the surface of the skin that is detected by the body.

Facet   A smooth, flat surface on a bone.

Facilitated diffusion   The transport of substances by carriers to which the substance binds for movement of the substance into a cell along the concentration gradient without energy.

Facilitation   The state of a nerve in which it is stimulated but not to the point of threshold—the point at which it transmits a nerve signal.

Fascia   Fibrous membrane that covers, supports, and separates muscles; subcutaneous tissue that connects the skin to the muscles.

Fascial sheath   Flat sheet of connective tissue that is used for separation, stability, and muscular attachment points.

Feedback   Method of autoregulation that is used to maintain internal homeostasis that links body functions; the noninvasive, continual exchange of information between the client and the professional.

Feedback loop   Self-regulating control system in the body that receives information, integrates that information, and provides a response to maintain homeostasis. Negative feedback reverses the original stimulus, whereas positive feedback enhances and maintains the stimulus.

Fibrocartilage   Connective tissue that permits little motion in joints and structures, is found in places such as the intervertebral disk, and forms our ears.

Fibromyalgia   A syndrome with symptoms of widespread pain or aching, persistent fatigue, generalized morning stiffness, nonrestorative sleep, and multiple tender points.

A disrupted sleep pattern, coupled with the dysfunction of myofascial repair mechanisms, seems to be a factor.

Fibrous joint   Articulation in which fibrous tissue connects bone directly to bone.

Fistula   Tract that is open at both ends through which abnormal connection occurs between two surfaces.

Fitness   General term that is used to describe the ability to perform physical work.

Fixator   One of the stabilizing muscles surrounding a joint or body part that contracts to fixate, or stabilize, the area, enabling another limb or body segment to exert force and move.

Flaccid   Term used to describe a muscle with decreased or absent tone.

Flexion   Movement that decreases the angle between two bones as the body part moves out of the anatomic position.

Fontanels   Areas of the skull of an infant in which bone formation is incomplete. The fontanels allow for compression of the skull as the infant travels through the birth canal and expansion as the brain grows.

Foramen   An opening in a bone, such as the foramen magnum of the skull.

Force   Any push or pull placed on an object in an attempt to affect motion or shape.

Forced expiration   Movement of air out of the body; it is produced by activating muscles that can pull down the ribs and muscles that can compress the abdomen, forcing the diaphragm upward.

Forced inspiration   Movement of air into the body; this occurs when an individual is working hard and needs a great deal of oxygen. It involves not only muscles of quiet and deep inspiration but also muscles that stabilize or elevate the shoulder girdle in an effort to elevate the ribs directly or indirectly.

Fossa   A depression in the surface or at the end of a bone.

Free nerve endings   Sensory receptors that detect itch and tickle sensations.

Frequency   The number of times a method repeats itself within a specified time period.

Friction   Specific circular or transverse movements that do not glide on the skin and that are focused on the underlying tissue.

Frontal (coronal) plane   Vertical plane that divides the body into anterior and posterior (front and back) parts.

Fungi   A group of simple parasitic organisms that are similar to plants but that have no chlorophyll (green pigment). Most pathogenic fungi live on tissues on or near the skin or mucous membranes.

Gait   Rhythmic and alternating motions of the legs, trunk, and arms, resulting in propulsion of the body; the walking pattern.

Gait cycle   Subdivided into the stance phase and the swing phase, this cycle begins when the heel of one foot strikes the floor and continues until the same heel strikes the floor again.

Gallbladder   A small, 3- to 4-inch sac that stores and concentrates bile.

Ganglion   Cystic, round, usually nontender swelling located along a tendon sheath or a joint capsule.

Gate control theory   Hypothetical gating mechanism that functions at the level of the spinal cord; a "gate" through which pain impulses reach the lateral spinothalamic system. Painful impulses are transmitted by large-diameter and small-diameter nerve fibers. Stimulation of large-diameter fibers prevents the small-diameter fibers from transmitting signals. Stimulation (rubbing, massaging) of large-diameter fibers helps to suppress the sensation of pain, especially sharp pain.

General adaptation syndrome   Method the body uses to mobilize different defense mechanisms when threatened by actual or perceived harmful stimuli. Process that calls into play the three stages of response to stress (i.e., the alarm reaction, the resistance reaction, and the exhaustion reaction).

General contraindications   Factors that require a physician's evaluation to rule out serious underlying conditions before any massage is indicated. If the physician recommends massage, the physician must help to develop a comprehensive treatment plan.

Gestation   Period of fetal growth from conception until birth.

Gestures   The way a client touches the body while explaining a problem. These movements may indicate whether the condition is a muscle problem, a joint problem, or a visceral problem.

Gibbus   Angular deformity of a collapsed vertebra, the causes of which include metastatic cancer and tuberculosis of the spine.

Gliding joints   Known also as synovial planes, gliding joints allow only a gliding motion in various planes.

Goals   Desired outcomes.

Golgi tendon receptors   Receptors in the tendons that sense tension.

Gray matter   Unmyelinated nervous tissue, particularly that found in the central nervous system.

Gross anatomy   The study of body structures visible to the naked eye.

Ground substance   Medium in which cells and protein fibers are suspended. Ground substance is usually clear and colorless and has the consistency of thick syrup.

Growth hormone   Hormone that promotes cell division; in adults, it is implicated in the repair and regeneration of tissue.

Guarding   Contraction of muscles in a splinting action, surrounding an injured area.

Hacking   Type of tapotement/percussion that alternately strikes the surface of the body with quick, snapping movements.

Half-life   Amount of time required for half of a hormone to be eliminated from the bloodstream.

Hardening   Method of teaching the body to deal more effectively with stress; sometimes called toughening.

Hardiness   The physical and mental ability to withstand external stressors.

Healing   The restoration of well-being.

Health   Condition of homeostasis that results in a state of physical, emotional, social, and spiritual well-being. Optimum functioning with freedom from disease or abnormal processes.

Heart   The pump of the cardiovascular system; the heart is hollow, cone shaped, and about the size of a fist, and it is located in the mediastinum of the thoracic cavity. The myocardium is the heart muscle itself, the endocardium is the thin inner lining, and the epicardium is the outer membrane.

Heart rate   The number of cardiac cycles in 1 minute. In the average healthy person, the rate works out to be 60–70 cycles or beats per minute.

Heart sounds   The two main sounds that result from closure of the valves. Murmurs are extra sounds, such as those produced by faulty valves.

Heart valves   Four sets of valves that keep the blood flowing in the correct direction through the heart.

Heavy pressure   Compressive force that extends to the bone under the tissue.

Hemoglobin   Oxygen-carrying, red molecule in the blood.

Hemorrhage   The passage of blood outside of the cardiovascular system.

Hepatitis   A viral inflammatory process and infection of the liver.

Hernia   Weakness in a muscle or structure that allows protrusion of a muscle, organ, or structure through the resultant opening.

Herpes simplex   DNA virus that causes painful blisters and small ulcers in and around the mouth and on the genital area.

High-energy bonds   Covalent bonds created in specific organic substrates in the presence of enzymes.

Hinge joint   Joint that allows flexion and extension in one direction, while changing the angle of the bones at the joint, like a door hinge.

Histamine   A chemical produced by the body that dilates the blood vessels. A neurotransmitter that is considered a stimulant. Histamine is released by the mast cells as part of the inflammatory process and can cause itching.

History   Information from the client about past and present medical conditions and patterns of symptoms.

Homeostasis   Dynamic equilibrium of the internal environment of the body achieved through processes of feedback and regulation; the relatively constant state of the internal environment of the body that is maintained by adaptive responses. Specific control and feedback mechanisms are responsible for adjusting body systems to maintain this state.

Horizontal abduction   Movement of the humerus in the horizontal plane away from the midline of the body. Also known as horizontal extension or transverse abduction.

Horizontal adduction   Movement of the humerus in the horizontal plane toward the midline of the body. Also known as horizontal flexion or transverse adduction.

Hormone   A messenger chemical in the bloodstream.

Human immunodeficiency virus   Virus that appears to be responsible for acquired immunodeficiency syndrome. Abbreviated HIV.

Hyaline cartilage   Thin covering of articular connective tissue on the ends of the bones in freely movable joints in the adult skeleton. Hyaline cartilage forms a smooth, resilient, low-friction surface for the articulation of one bone with another, distributes forces, and helps to absorb some of the pressure imposed on joint surfaces.

Hydrotherapy   The use of various types of water applications and temperatures for therapy.

Hygiene   Practices and conditions that promote health and prevent disease.

Hyperalgesia   Increased sensitivity to pain.

Hyperextension   Movement that takes the body part farther in the direction of extension and farther out of anatomic position.

Hypermobility   Range of motion of a joint that is greater than would be permitted normally by the structure. Hypermobility results in instability.

Hyperplasia   Uncontrolled increase in the number of cells in a body part.

Hypersecretion   Excessive release of a hormone.

Hyperstimulation analgesia   Technique that diminishes the perception of a sensation by stimulating large-diameter nerve fibers. Methods used include application of ice or heat, counterirritation, acupressure, acupuncture, rocking, music, and repetitive massage strokes.

Hypertension   An increase in systolic and diastolic pressures.

Hypertrophy   An increase in the size of a cell, which results in an increase in the size of a body part or organ.

Hyperventilation   Abnormally deep or rapid breathing, in excess of physical demands.

Hypomobility   Range of motion of a joint that is less than what would be permitted normally by the structure.

Hyposecretion   Insufficient release of a hormone.

Hypotension   Decrease in systolic and diastolic pressures. Hypotension is an important manifestation of shock, which causes inadequate blood supply to vital organs.

Hypothesis   The starting point of research; it is based on the statement, "If this happens, then that will happen."

Immunity   Resistance to disease provided by the body through specific or nonspecific immunity. The immune system is a functional system rather than an organ system in the anatomic sense. The most important immune cells are lymphocytes and macrophages. The key to immunity is the ability of the body to distinguish self from nonself.

Impermeable   The quality of not permitting entry of a substance.

Impingement syndromes   Conditions that involve pathologic pressure on nerves and vessels; the two types of impingement are compression and entrapment.

Implicit bias   Unconscious attitudes and stereotypes that can influence relationships and understanding of individuals.

Incontinence   The inability to control urination or defecation, most often because of weak pelvic floor muscles or nerve damage.

Indication   A therapeutic application that promotes health or assists in a healing process.

Inertia   The reluctance of matter to change its state of motion.

Inflammation   Protective response of the tissues to irritation or injury that may be chronic or acute. The four primary signs are redness, heat, swelling, and pain.

Inflammatory response   Sequence of events that involves chemical and cellular activation that destroys pathogens and aids in repairing tissues.

Informed consent   Client authorization for any service received from a professional based on adequate information provided by the professional. Obtaining informed consent is a consumer protection process that requires that clients have knowledge of what will occur, that their participation is voluntary, and that they are competent to give consent. Informed consent is an educational procedure that allows clients to make knowledgeable decisions about whether they want to receive a massage.

Ingestion   Taking food into the mouth.

Inhibition   A decrease in or cessation of a response or function.

Initial treatment plan   Plan that states therapeutic goals, the duration of treatment sessions, the number of appointments necessary to meet agreed-upon goals, costs, the general classifications of interventions to be used, and the objective progress measurement that will be used to confirm the attainment of goals.

Inorganic compounds   Chemical structures that do not consist of carbon and hydrogen atoms as the primary structure.

Insertion   The distal attachment of a muscle; the part of a muscle that attaches farthest from the midline, or center, of the body. The muscle attachment point that is closest to the moving joint.

Integrated approaches   Combined methods of various forms of massage and bodywork styles.

Integration   Process of remembering an event while one is able to remain in the present moment, with an awareness of the difference between then and now, to bring some sort of resolution to the event.

Integument   The skin and its appendages: hair, sebaceous and sweat glands, nails, and breasts.

Intercompetition massage   Massage provided during an athletic event.

Internal respiration   The exchange of gases between tissues and blood.

Internal rotation   Medial rotary movement of a bone. Also known as rotation medially, inward rotation, and medial rotation.

Interphase   Period during which a cell grows and carries out its activities.

Intimacy   A tender, familiar, and understanding experience between beings.

Intractable pain   The continuation of chronic pain without the presence of active disease, or the persistence of chronic pain even with treatment.

Intuition   Knowledge of something attained by using subconscious information.

Inversion   Movement of the sole of the foot inward toward the midline.

Ion pumps   Carriers that transport substances into or out of a cell with the use of energy.

Ischemia   Temporary deficiency or decreased supply of blood to a tissue.

Isometric contraction   Action of the prime mover that occurs when tension develops within the muscle but no appreciable change occurs in the joint angle or in the length of the muscle. Movement does not occur.

Isotonic contraction   Contraction in which the effort of the target muscle or group of muscles is matched in part by counterpressure, allowing a degree of resisted movement; the action of the prime mover that occurs when tension develops in the muscle while it is shortening or lengthening.

Job   A regular activity performed for payment.

Joint capsule   Connective tissue structure that indirectly connects the bony components of a joint.

Joint end feel   Sensation that is felt when a normal joint is taken to its physiologic limit. (*See* End feel.)

Joint kinesthetic receptors   Receptors in the capsules of joints that respond to pressure and to acceleration and deceleration of joint movement. The two main types of joint kinesthetic receptors are type II cutaneous mechanoreceptors and Pacinian (lamellated) corpuscles.

Joint movement   Movement of the joint through its normal range of motion.

Joint play   The inherent laxity that is present in a joint; involuntary movement that occurs between articular surfaces that is separate from the range of motion of a joint produced by muscles. Joint play, which is an essential component of joint motion, must occur for normal functioning of the joint.

Keratin   Fibrous protein produced in the epidermis that protects our skin and makes it waterproof.

Kinematics   Branch of mechanics that involves the time, space, and mass aspects of a moving system.

Kinesiology   The study of movement that combines the fields of anatomy, physiology, physics, and geometry and relates them to human movement.

Kinetic chain   An integrated functional unit. The kinetic chain is made up of the myofascial system (muscle, ligament, tendon, and fascia), the articular (joint) system, and the nervous system. Each of these systems works interdependently to allow structural and functional efficiency in all three planes of motion: sagittal, frontal, and transverse. The process by which each individual joint movement pattern is part of an interconnected aspect of the neurologic coordination pattern of muscle movement.

Kinetics   Those forces that cause movement in a system.

Kyphosis   Condition of exaggeration of the thoracic curve.

Lateral flexion (side bending) Movement of the head or trunk laterally away from the midline; abduction of the spine.

Lateral recumbency (side-lying) Lying horizontally on the right or left side.

Law Scientific statement that is uniformly true for a whole class of natural occurrences.

Lengthening Process in which the muscle assumes a normal resting length by means of the neuromuscular mechanism.

Leukocytes White blood cells that protect the body from pathogens and that remove dead cells and substances.

Lever A solid mass, such as a crowbar or a person's arm, that rotates around a fixed point called the fulcrum. The rotation is produced by a force applied to a lever at some distance from the fulcrum.

Leverage Leaning with the body weight to provide pressure.

License Type of credential required by law; licenses are used to regulate the practice of a profession to protect the public health, safety, and welfare.

Ligaments Dense bundles of parallel connective tissue fibers, primarily collagen, that connect bones and strengthen and stabilize the joint.

Lipids Fats and oils; organic compounds that are made up of carbon, hydrogen, and oxygen atoms but in a different proportion than that of carbohydrates.

List A lateral tilt of the spine.

Locomotion Moving from one place to another; walking.

Longitudinal stretching A stretch applied along the fiber direction of connective tissues and muscles.

Loose-packed position Position of a synovial joint in which the joint capsule is most lax. Joints tend to assume this position when inflammation occurs, to accommodate the increased volume of synovial fluid.

Lordosis Exaggeration of the normal lumbar curve.

Lower respiratory tract The larynx, trachea, bronchi, and alveoli.

Lubricant Substance that reduces friction on the skin during massage movements.

Lungs The primary organs of respiration, the lungs are soft, spongy, highly vascular structures that are separated into left and right lungs by the mediastinum. Each lung is separated into lobes. The right lung consists of three lobes: an upper, middle, and lower; the left consists of two lobes: an upper and lower.

Lymph Clear interstitial tissue fluid that bathes the cell is considered lymph when it moves into the lymph vessels. Lymph contains lymphocytes, which provide immune response. It returns plasma proteins that have leaked out through capillary walls, and it transports fats from the gastrointestinal system to the bloodstream.

Lymph nodes Small, round structures distributed along the network of lymph vessels that provide a filtering system for removing waste products and transferring them to the bloodstream for removal to the spleen, intestines, and kidneys for detoxification. Lymph nodes are centers for lymphocyte production. Their main function is to prevent bacteria and viruses from gaining access to the bloodstream. Generally clustered at the joints for assistance in pumping when the joint moves, they are especially numerous in the axillae, groin, and neck and along certain blood vessels of the pelvic, abdominal, and thoracic cavities.

Lymph system Specialized component of the circulatory system that is responsible for waste disposal and immune response.

Lymphatic drainage Specific type of massage that enhances movement of interstitial fluid into lymph vessels.

Lysosome Cell organelle that is part of the intracellular digestive system.

Malignant Type of tumor (cancer) that tends to spread to other regions of the body.

Manipulation Skillful use of the hands in a therapeutic manner. Massage manipulations focus on the soft tissues of the body and are not to be confused with joint manipulation in which a high-velocity thrust is used.

Manual lymph drainage Methods of bodywork that influence lymphatic movement.

Marketing Advertising and other promotional activities required to sell a product or service.

Massage The scientific art and system of assessment and manual application of certain techniques to the superficial soft tissue of skin, muscles, tendons, ligaments, and fasciae and structures that lie within the superficial tissue. The hand, foot, knee, arm, elbow, and forearm are used for the systematic external application of touch, stroking (effleurage), friction, vibration, percussion, kneading (pétrissage), stretching, compression, or passive and active joint movements within the normal physiologic range of motion. Massage methods introduce mechanical forces into the soft tissue. Massage therapy can include adjunctive external applications of water, heat, and cold for the purposes of establishing and maintaining good physical condition and health by normalizing and improving muscle tone, promoting relaxation, stimulating circulation, and producing therapeutic effects on the respiratory and nervous systems and subtle interactions among all body systems. These intended effects are accomplished through physiologic energetic and mind/body connections in a safe, nonsexual environment that respects the client's self-determined outcome for the session.

Massage chair Specially designed chair that allows the client to sit comfortably during the massage.

Massage environment Area or location where a massage is given.

Massage equipment Tables, mats, chairs, and other incidental supplies and implements used during the massage.

Massage mat Cushioned surface that is placed on the floor.

Massage routine Step-by-step protocol and sequence used to give a massage.

Massage table Specially designed table that allows massage to be done with the client lying down.

Matrix Basic substance between the cells of a tissue. Matrix is composed of amorphous ground substance consisting of molecules that expand when water molecules and electrolytes bind to them. Up to 90% of connective tissue is ground substance. Fibers make up the other component of matrix.

Maximum stimulus Point at which all motor units of a muscle have been recruited and the muscle is unable to increase in strength.

Mechanical methods Techniques that directly affect the soft tissue by normalizing the connective tissue or moving body fluids and intestinal contents.

Mechanical receptors Sensory receptors that detect changes in pressure, movement, temperature, or other mechanical forces.

Mechanical response Response that is based on a structural change in the tissue. The tissue change is caused directly by application of the technique.

Mechanical touch Touch applied with the intent of achieving a specific anatomic or physiologic outcome.

Mechanics Branch of physics that deals with the study of forces and the motion produced by their actions.

Medications Substances prescribed to stimulate or inhibit a body process or replace a chemical in the body.

Meiosis Type of cell division in which each daughter cell divides again. In the second division, each daughter cell receives half the normal number of chromosomes, forming two reproductive cells (a total of four reproductive cells from one meiotic cycle).

Melanin Pigment that colors our skin and works as a natural sunscreen to protect us from ultraviolet rays by darkening our skin.

Membrane Thin, sheetlike layer of tissue that covers a cell, an organ, or some other structure; that lines a tube or a cavity; or that divides or separates one part from another.

Mental impairment Any mental or psychological disorder, such as mental retardation, developmental disabilities, organic brain syndrome, emotional or mental illness, and specific learning disabilities.

Mentoring Career support provided by someone who is more experienced.

Metabolism Chemical processes in the body that convert food and oxygen into energy to support growth, distribution of nutrients, and elimination of waste.

Metabolites Molecules synthesized or broken down inside the body by chemical reactions.

Metastasis Migration of cancer cells.

Microorganisms Small life forms that may be damaging to the body or that may interfere with its function.

Microvilli Small projections of the cell membrane that increase the surface area of the cell.

Micturition Clinical term for urination or voiding.

Mitochondria Cell organelles of rod or oval shape.

Mitosis Cell division in which the cell duplicates its DNA and divides into two identical daughter cells.

Mixed nerves Nerves that contain sensory and motor axons.

Moderate pressure Compressive pressure that extends to the muscle layer but does not press the tissue against the underlying bone.

Mole Also known as a nevus, a mole is a benign pigmented skin growth formed of melanocytes.

Molecule The combination of two or more atoms. A molecule is the smallest portion of a substance that can exist separately without losing the physical and chemical properties of that substance.

Monoplegia Paralysis of a single limb or a single group of muscles.

Motivation The internal drive that provides the energy to do what is necessary to accomplish a goal.

Motor point Location at which the motor neuron enters the muscle and a visible contraction can be elicited with a minimum amount of stimulation. Motor points most often are located in the belly of the muscle.

Motor unit A motor neuron and all of the muscle fibers it controls.

Movement cure Term used in the 19th and early 20th centuries for a system of exercise and massage manipulations that are focused on treating a variety of ailments.

Multiple isotonic contractions Movement of the joint and associated muscles by the client through a full range of motion against partial resistance applied by the massage therapist.

Muscle energy techniques Neuromuscular facilitation; specific use of active contraction in individual muscles or groups of muscles to increase tolerance to stretch.

Muscle spindles Structures located primarily in the belly of the muscle that respond to sudden and prolonged stretches.

Muscle testing procedure Assessment process that uses muscle contraction. Strength testing is done to determine whether a muscle responds with sufficient strength to perform the required body functions. Neurologic muscle testing is designed to determine whether the neurologic interaction of muscles is working smoothly.

Muscle tissue Specialized form of tissue that contracts and shortens to provide movement, maintain posture, and produce heat.

Musculotendinous junction Point at which muscle fibers end and the connective tissue continues to form the tendon; a major site of injury.

Myasthenia gravis Disorder that usually affects muscles in the face, lips, tongue, neck, and throat, which are innervated by the cranial nerves, but that can affect any muscle group.

Myelin A white, fatty, insulating substance formed by the Schwann cells that surrounds some axons; also produced in the central nervous system by oligodendrocytes.

Myofascial approaches Styles of bodywork that affect the connective tissues; often called deep tissue massage, soft-tissue manipulation, or myofascial release.

Myofascial release System of bodywork that affects the connective tissue of the body through various methods that elongate and alter the plastic component and the ground matrix of connective tissue.

Myotome A skeletal muscle or group of skeletal muscles that receives motor axons from a particular spinal nerve.

Negative feedback system Control mechanism that provides a stimulus to decrease a function, such as a fire alarm, which causes a series of reactions that work to reduce the fire.

Neoplasm Abnormal growth of new tissue. Also called a tumor, a neoplasm may be benign or malignant.

Nerve   A bundle of axons or dendrites or both.

Nerve impingement   Pressure against a nerve exerted by skin, fascia, muscles, ligaments, or joints.

Nervous tissue   Specialized tissue that coordinates and regulates body activity and that can develop more excitability and conductivity than other types of tissue.

Neurilemma   The outer cell membrane of a Schwann cell that is essential in the regeneration of injured axons. The thin membrane spirally wraps the myelin layers of certain fibers, especially of peripheral nerves, or the axons of certain unmyelinated nerve fibers. Also called Schwann's membrane, sheath of Schwann, and endoneural membrane.

Neuroglia   Specialized connective tissue cells that support, protect, and hold neurons together.

Neurologic muscle testing   Testing designed to determine whether the neurologic interaction of muscles is proceeding smoothly.

Neuromuscular   Term that describes the interaction between nervous system control of muscles and the response of muscles to nerve signals.

Neuromuscular approaches   Methods of bodywork that influence the reflexive responses of the nervous system and its connection to muscular function.

Neuromuscular mechanism   The interplay and reflex connection between sensory and motor neurons and muscle function.

Neurons   Nerve cells that conduct impulses.

Neurotransmitters   Chemical compounds that generate action potentials when released in the synapses from presynaptic cells.

Nociceptors   Sensory receptors that detect painful or intense stimuli.

Norepinephrine   Catecholamine that is primarily involved in emotional responses. Norepinephrine is found in the central nervous system and the sympathetic division of the autonomic nervous system and causes constriction of blood vessels within skeletal muscles.

Norepinephrine/noradrenaline   Neurochemical that functions in a manner similar to that of epinephrine but that is more concentrated in the brain.

Nucleic acids   The two types of nucleic acid are deoxyribonucleic acid (DNA) and ribonucleic acid (RNA).

Nutrients   Essential elements and molecules obtained through the diet that the body requires for normal body function.

Nutrition   The use of food for growth and maintenance of the body.

Occupation   Productive or creative activity that serves as a regular source of livelihood.

Oil   Type of liquid lubricant.

Open kinematic chain   Position in which the ends of the limbs or the parts of the body are free to move without causing motion at another joint.

Open-ended question   A question that cannot be answered with a simple, one-word response.

Opportunistic invasion   Potentially pathogenic organisms that are found on the skin and mucous membranes of nearly everyone but that do not cause disease until they have the opportunity to do so, as in depressed immunity.

Opportunistic pathogens   Organisms that cause disease only when immunity is low in a host.

Opposition   Movement of the thumb across the palmar aspect to make contact with the fingers.

Organelles   The basic components of a cell that perform specific functions within the cell.

Organic compounds   Substances that include carbon and hydrogen as part of their basic structure.

Origin   The attachment point of a muscle at the fixed point during movement. The proximal attachment of a muscle; the part that attaches closest to the midline (center) of the body; the least movable part of a muscle.

Osmosis   Diffusion of water from a region of lower concentration of solution to a region of higher concentration of solution across the semipermeable membrane of a cell.

Osteokinematic movements   The movements of flexion, extension, abduction, adduction, and rotation; also known as physiologic movements.

Osteokinematics   The movement of bones as opposed to the movement of articular surfaces; also known as range of motion.

Osteoporosis   Disorder of the bones in which a lack of calcium and other minerals and a decrease in bone protein leave the bones soft, fragile, and likely to break.

Overload principle   Stress on an organism is greater than the stress that is regularly encountered during everyday life.

Oxygen debt   The extra amount of oxygen that must be taken in to convert lactic acid to glucose or glycogen.

Oxytocin   Hormone that is implicated in pair or couple bonding, parental bonding, feelings of attachment, and caretaking, along with its more commonly known functions in pregnancy, delivery, and lactation.

Pain   An unpleasant sensation. Pain is a complex, private experience with physiologic, psychological, and social aspects. Because pain is subjective, it is often difficult to explain or describe.

Pain and fatigue syndromes   Multicausal, often chronic, nonproductive patterns that interfere with well-being, activities of living, and productivity.

Pain neuroscience education   Information describing the neurobiology and neurophysiology of pain and pain processing by the nervous system. The intention is to help clients better understand acute and chronic pain supporting a reduction in fear avoidance behaviors.

Pain–spasm–pain cycle   Steady contraction of muscles, which causes ischemia and stimulates pain receptors in muscles. The pain, in turn, initiates additional spasms.

Palliative care   Care intended to relieve or reduce the intensity of uncomfortable symptoms but that cannot effect a cure.

Palpation   Assessment through touch.

Panic   Intense, sudden, and overwhelming fear or feeling of anxiety that produces terror and immediate physiologic change, resulting in immobility or senseless, hysterical behavior.

Paraplegia Paralysis of the lower portion of the body and of both legs.

Parasympathetic autonomic nervous system The restorative part of the autonomic nervous system. The parasympathetic response often is called the relaxation response.

Parasympathetic nervous system The energy conservation and restorative system associated with what commonly is called the relaxation response.

Passive joint movement Movement of a joint by the massage practitioner without the assistance of the client.

Passive range of motion Movement of a joint in which the therapist, not the client, effects the motion.

Passive transport Transportation of a substance across the cell membrane without the use of energy.

Pathogenesis The development of a disease.

Pathogenic animals Large, multicellular organisms, sometimes called metazoa. Most metazoa are worms that feed off human tissue or cause other disease processes.

Pathogenicity The ability of an infectious agent to cause disease.

Pathogens Microorganisms that are capable of producing disease.

Pathologic barrier Adaptation of the physiologic barrier that allows the protective function to limit rather than support optimum functioning.

Pathologic range of motion Amount of motion at a joint that fails to reach the normal physiologic range or that exceeds the normal anatomic limits of motion of that joint.

Pathology The study of disease as observed in the structure and function of the body.

Peer support Interaction among those involved in the same pursuit. Regular interaction with other massage practitioners creates an environment in which technical information and dilemmas and interpersonal dilemmas can be sorted out.

Pericardium Double-membranous, serous sac that surrounds the heart. The pericardium secretes a lubricating fluid to prevent friction caused by movement of the heart.

Periosteum Thin membrane of connective tissue that covers bones, except at articulations.

Peripheral nervous system System of somatic and autonomic neurons outside the central nervous system. The peripheral nervous system comprises the afferent (sensory) division and the efferent (motor) division.

Peristalsis Rhythmic contraction of smooth muscles that propels products of digestion along the tract from the esophagus to the anus.

Peritoneum Mucous membrane that lines the abdominal cavity to prevent friction produced by the organs.

Person-to-person contact Pathogens often can be carried in the air from one person to another.

Personal protective equipment Commonly referred to as "PPE," is equipment worn to minimize exposure to hazards that cause serious workplace injuries and illnesses. Common types include masks, gloves, and gowns.

Pétrissage Kneading; rhythmic rolling, lifting, squeezing, and wringing of soft tissue.

Phagocytosis Process of endocytosis followed by digestion of vesicle contents by enzymes present in the cytoplasm.

Phantom pain A form of pain or other sensation experienced at the site of the missing extremity after a limb amputation.

Pharynx The throat.

Phasic muscles Muscles that move the body.

Phospholipid bilayer Cell membrane made up of lipids, carbohydrates, and proteins.

Physical assessment Evaluation of body balance, efficient function, basic symmetry, range of motion, and ability to function.

Physical disability Any physiologic disorder, condition, cosmetic disfigurement, or anatomic loss that affects one or more of the following body systems: neurologic, musculoskeletal, special sense organ, respiratory (including speech organs), cardiovascular, reproductive, digestive, genitourinary, hemic and lymphatic, skin, and endocrine. Extremes in size and extensive burns also may be considered physical impairments.

Physiologic barriers The result of limits in range of motion imposed by protective nervous and sensory functions to support optimal performance.

Physiologic range of motion Amount of motion available to a joint as determined by the nervous system from information provided by joint sensory receptors. This information usually prevents a joint from being positioned so that injury could occur.

Physiology The study of the processes and functions of the body involved in supporting life.

Piezoelectric Quality of bones that allows them to deform slightly and vibrate when electrical currents pass through them. Bone formation patterns follow lines of stress load directed by piezoelectric currents.

Piezoelectricity Production of an electrical current by application of pressure to certain crystals such as mica, quartz, Rochelle salt, and connective tissue.

Pivot joint The bony projection from one bone fits into a "ring" formed by another bone and ligament structure to allow rotation around its own axis.

Placebo Treatment for an illness that influences the course of the disease, even if the treatment has not been validated specifically.

Plantar flexion Extension movement of the ankle that results in moving the foot and toes away from the body.

Plasma Thick, straw-colored fluid that makes up about 55% of the blood.

Plastic range Range of movement of connective tissue that is taken beyond the elastic limits. In this range, the tissue permanently deforms and cannot return to its original state.

Plexus Network of intertwining nerves that innervates a particular region of the body.

Polarity Holistic health practice that encompasses some of the theory base of Asian medicine and Ayurveda. Polarity is an eclectic, multifaceted system.

Polio (or poliomyelitis) Viral infection that affects the nerves that control skeletal muscle movement.

Positional release   Method of moving the body into the direction of ease (the way the body wants to move out of the position that causes the pain); proprioception is taken into a state of safety and may stop signaling for protective spasm.

Postevent massage   Massage provided after an athletic event.

Postisometric relaxation   State that occurs after isometric contraction of a muscle; it results from the activity of minute neural reporting stations called the Golgi tendon bodies.

Posttraumatic stress disorder   Disorder characterized by episodes of flashback memory, state-dependent memory, somatization, anxiety, irritability, sleep disturbance, concentration difficulties, times of melancholy or depression, grief, fear, worry, anger, and avoidance behavior.

Posterior pelvic rotation   Posterior movement of the upper pelvis; the iliac crest tilts backward in a sagittal plane.

Postural muscles   Muscles that support the body against gravity.

Powder   Type of lubricant that consists of a finely ground substance.

Prefix   Word element added to the beginning of a root to change the meaning of the word.

Premassage activity   Any activity that is involved in preparation for a massage, including setting up the massage room, obtaining supplies, and determining the temperature of the room.

Pressure   Compressive force; the amount of force on a specific area.

PRICE first aid   Protection, rest, ice, compression, elevation.

Prime movers   The muscles responsible for movement.

Principle   Basic truth or rule of conduct.

Process   Any prominent bony growth that projects out from the bone.

Profession   An occupation that requires training and specialized study.

Professional   A person who practices a profession.

Professional touch   Skilled touch delivered to achieve a specific outcome; the recipient in some way reimburses the professional for services rendered.

Professionalism   Adherence to professional status, methods, standards, and character.

Pronation   Internal rotary movement of the radius on the ulna that results in movement of the hand from the palm-up to the palm-down position.

Prone   Lying horizontal with the face down.

Proprioceptive neuromuscular facilitation   Specific application of muscle energy techniques that use strong contraction combined with stretching and muscular pattern retraining.

Proprioceptors   Sensory receptors that provide the body with information about position, movement, muscle tension, joint activity, and equilibrium.

Proteins   Substances formed from amino acids.

Protozoa   One-celled organisms that are larger than bacteria and that can infest human fluids, causing disease by parasitizing (living off) or directly destroying cells.

Protraction   Forward movement while one remains in a horizontal plane.

Psoriasis   A common, chronic skin disease characterized by reddened skin covered by dry, silvery scales. Psoriasis most often is found on the scalp, elbows, knees, back, or buttocks.

Pulmonary trunk   Large artery that carries blood to the lungs to release carbon dioxide and take in oxygen.

Pulmonary veins   The four veins from the lungs that bring oxygen-rich blood to the left atrium.

Pulsed muscle energy   Procedures that involve engaging the barrier and using minute, resisted contractions (usually 20 in 10 seconds); introduces mechanical pumping as well as postisometric relaxation or reciprocal inhibition.

Qi   Also known as chi, Qi refers to the life force.

Quadriplegia   Paralysis or loss of movement in all four limbs.

Qualified   Criteria that indicate when the goal is achieved.

Quantified   Goals measured in terms of objective criteria, such as time, frequency, a 1-to-10 scale, a measurable increase or decrease in the ability to perform an activity, or a measurable increase or decrease in sensation, such as relaxation or pain.

Quiet expiration   Movement of air out of the body through passive action. This occurs through relaxation of the external intercostals and elastic recoil of the thoracic wall and tissue of the lungs and bronchi, with gravity pulling the rib cage down from its elevated position.

Quiet inspiration   Movement of air into the body while resting or sitting quietly. The diaphragm and external intercostals are the prime movers.

Range of motion   Movement of joints.

Rapport   Development of a relationship based on mutual trust and harmony.

Reciprocal inhibition   Effect that occurs when a muscle contracts, obliging its antagonist to relax in order to allow normal movement to take place.

Reciprocal innervation   The circuitry of neurons that allows reciprocal inhibition to take place. One can use reciprocal innervation therapeutically to assist in muscle relaxation.

Reciprocity   Exchange of privileges between governing bodies.

Recovery massage   Massage that is structured primarily for the uninjured athlete who wants to recover from a strenuous workout or competition.

Reduction   Return of the spinal column to the anatomic position from lateral flexion; adduction of the spine.

Reenactment   Reliving an event as though it were happening at the moment.

Referral   Sending a client to a healthcare professional for specific diagnosis and treatment of a disease.

Referred pain   Pain felt in a surface area far from the stimulated organ.

Reflex   Involuntary response to a stimulus. Reflexes are specific, predictable, adaptive, and purposeful. Reflexive methods work by stimulating the nervous system (sensory neurons), and tissue changes occur in response to the body's adaptation to neural stimulation.

Reflex arc   Pathway that a nerve impulse follows in a reflex action.

Reflexive methods   Massage techniques that stimulate the nervous system, the endocrine system, and the chemicals of the body.

Reflexology   Massage system directed primarily toward the feet and hands.

Refractory period   Period after a muscle contraction during which the muscle is unable to contract again.

Regional anatomy   The study of the structures of a particular area of the body.

Regional contraindications   Contraindications that relate to a specific area of the body.

Rehabilitation massage   Massage used for severe injury or as part of intervention after surgery.

Remedial massage   Massage used for minor to moderate injuries.

Remission   Reversal of signs and symptoms in chronic disease that can be temporary or permanent.

Resourceful compensation   Adjustments made by the body to manage a permanent or chronic dysfunction.

Respiration   Movement of air into and out of the lungs, the exchange of oxygen and carbon dioxide between the lungs and blood, and the exchange of oxygen and carbon dioxide between blood and body tissues.

Respiratory rate   The number of breaths taken in 1 minute.

Resting position   The first stroke of the massage; the simple laying on of hands. Also called holding.

Reticular fibers   Delicate connective tissue fibers that occur in networks and support small structures, such as capillaries, nerve fibers, and the basement membrane. Reticular fibers are made of a specialized type of collagen called reticulin.

Retraction   Backward movement in a horizontal plane.

Rhythm   The regularity of application of a technique. If the method is applied at regular intervals, it is considered even or rhythmic. If the method is choppy or irregular, it is considered uneven or not rhythmic.

Ribonucleic acid   Nucleic acid that transfers genetic information and controls cellular chemical activities. Abbreviated RNA.

Right of refusal   The entitlement of the client and the professional to stop the session.

Rocking   Rhythmic movement of the body.

Root word   The part of a word that provides the fundamental meaning.

Rotation   Partial turning or pivoting in an arc around a central axis.

Rupture   Tearing or disruption of connective tissue fibers that takes place when they exceed the limits of the plastic range.

Saddle joint   Joint that is convex in one plane and concave in the other, with the surfaces fitting together like a rider on a saddle.

Safe touch   Secure, respectful, considerate, sensitive, responsive, sympathetic, understanding, supportive, and empathetic contact.

Sanitation   The formulation and application of measures to promote and establish conditions favorable to health, specifically public health.

Schwann cell   Specialized cell that forms myelin.

Science   Intellectual process of understanding through observation, measurement, accumulation of data, and analysis of findings.

Scoliosis   Lateral curvature of the spine.

Scope of practice   The knowledge base and practice parameters of a profession.

Sebaceous glands   Oil glands found in the skin.

Sebum   Oily substance secreted by sebaceous glands that prevents dehydration, softens skin and hair, and slows the growth of bacteria.

Self-employment   To work for oneself rather than another.

Serotonin   A neurotransmitter that works primarily as an inhibitor in the central nervous system and is synthesized into melatonin and affects our sleep and moods. The neurochemical that regulates mood in terms of appropriate emotions, attention to thoughts, and calming, quieting, and comforting effects; it also subdues irritability and regulates drive states.

Service   Action performed for another person that results in a specific outcome.

Sesamoid bones   Round bones that often are embedded in tendons and joint capsules.

Seven Emotions   The Asian concept that joy, anger, fear, fright, sadness, worry, and grief are emotional responses that may trigger disharmony in the body, mind, or spirit under certain conditions.

Sexual misconduct   Any behavior that is sexually oriented in the professional setting.

Shaking   Technique in which the body area is grasped and shaken in a quick, loose movement; sometimes classified as rhythmic mobilization.

Shiatsu   Acupressure- and meridian-focused bodywork system from Japan.

Shock   Inadequate blood supply to vital organs, causing reduced function in these organs.

Side-lying   Position in which the client is lying on his or her side.

Signs   Objective changes that someone other than the client or patient can observe and measure.

Sinus   Four groups of air-filled spaces that open into the internal nose. They are located in the frontal, ethmoid, sphenoid, and maxillary bones of the skull. Sinuses are lined with mucosa and function to lighten the weight of the skull, making it easier to hold the head up and help in the production of sound.

Six Pernicious Influences   The Asian concept that heat, cold, wind, dampness, dryness, and summer heat, which are natural climate changes, may induce disease under certain conditions.

Skeletal muscle fibers   Large, cross-striated cells that are connected to the skeleton and are under voluntary control of the nervous system.

Skin rolling   Form of massage that lifts the skin.

Slapping   Form of percussion/tapotement that uses a flat hand.

Smooth muscle fibers   Muscle fibers that are neither striated nor voluntary. These muscle cells help regulate blood flow through the cardiovascular system, propel food through the gut, and squeeze secretions from glands.

SOAP charting Problem-oriented method of medical record keeping; the acronym SOAP stands for subjective, objective, assessment (analysis), and plan.

SOAP notes Acronym that refers to subjective, objective, analysis or assessment, and plan—the four parts of the written account of record keeping.

Soft tissue The skin, fasciae, muscles, tendons, joint capsules, and ligaments of the body.

Somatic Pertaining to the body.

Somatic nervous system System of nerves that keeps the body in balance with its external environment by transmitting impulses between the central nervous system, skeletal muscles, and skin.

Somatic pain Pain that arises from the body as opposed to the viscera. Superficial somatic pain results from the stimulation of receptors in the skin, whereas deep somatic pain arises from stimulation of receptors in skeletal muscles, joints, tendons, and fasciae.

Spa treatments Various hydrotherapies, applications of preparations to the body, and massage applications found in the spa setting.

Spastic Term used to describe a muscle with excessive tone.

Speed Rate of application (i.e., fast, slow, or varied).

Spinal cord Portion of the central nervous system that exits the skull into the vertebral column. The two major functions of the spinal cord are to conduct nerve impulses and to serve as a center for spinal reflexes.

Spinal nerves Thirty-one pairs of mixed nerves, originating in the spinal cord and emerging from the vertebral column, that make sensation and movement possible.

Spindle cells Sensory receptors in the belly of the muscle that detect stretch.

Spongy (cancellous) bone The lighter-weight portion of bone made up of trabeculae.

Stabilization Holding the body in a fixed position during joint movement, lengthening, and stretching.

Stabilizer A force or an object that helps maintain a position. Stabilization is essential to the accurate assessment of movement patterns.

Standard Precautions Safety measures established by the Centers for Disease Control and Prevention. These precautions were instituted to prevent the spread of bacterial and viral infections by setting up specific methods of dealing with human fluids and waste products. Standard Precautions protect client and practitioner from pathogens.

Standards of practice Principles that serve as specific guidelines to direct professional ethical practice and quality care, including a structure for evaluating the quality of care. Standards of practice represent an attempt to define the parameters of quality care.

Start-up costs Initial expenses involved in starting a business.

State-dependent memory Encoding and storing of a memory based on the effects of the autonomic nervous system and resultant chemical levels in the body. The memory is retrievable only during a similar physiologic experience in the body.

Static force Force applied to an object in such a way that it does not produce movement.

Sterilization Process by which all microorganisms are destroyed.

Stimulation Excitation that activates the sensory nerves.

Strain–counterstrain Use of tender points to guide the positioning of the body into a space where the muscle tension can be released on its own.

Strength testing Testing intended to determine whether a muscle is responding with sufficient strength to perform required body functions. Strength testing determines the force of contraction of a muscle.

Stress Any external or internal stimulus that requires a change or response to prevent an imbalance in the internal environment of the body, mind, or emotions. Stress may characterize any activity that makes demands on mental and emotional resources. Some responses to stress may stimulate neurons of the hypothalamus to release corticotropin-releasing hormone.

Stressors Any internal perceptions or external stimuli that demand a change in the body.

Stretching Mechanical tension applied to lengthen the myofascial unit (muscles and fasciae); two types are longitudinal and cross-directional stretching.

Stroke Technique of therapeutic massage that is applied with movement on the surface of the body, whether superficial or deep.

Structural and postural integration approaches Methods of bodywork derived from biomechanics, postural alignment, and the importance of connective tissue structures.

Subacute Diseases that manifest with characteristics between those of acute and chronic conditions.

Subtle energies Weak electrical fields that surround and run through the body.

Suffering Overall impairment of a person's quality of life.

Suffix A word element that is added to the end of a root to change the meaning of the word.

Superficial fascia Subcutaneous tissue that composes the third layer of skin, consists of loose connective tissue, and contains fat or adipose tissue.

Superficial pressure Pressure that remains on the skin.

Supervision Support from more experienced professionals.

Supination External rotary movement of the radius on the ulna that results in movement of the hand from the palm-down to the palm-up position.

Supine Lying horizontal with the face up.

Surface anatomy The study of internal organs and structures as they can be recognized and related to external features.

Suture Synarthrotic joint in which two bony components are united by a thin layer of dense fibrous tissue.

Sweat glands Sudoriferous glands in the skin; they are classified as apocrine or eccrine on the basis of their location and structure.

Symmetrical stance Position in which body weight is distributed equally between the feet.

Sympathetic autonomic nervous system Energy-using part of the autonomic nervous system, the division in which the fight-or-flight response is activated.

Sympathetic nervous system The portion of the autonomic nervous system that provides for most of the active function of the body; when the body is under stress, the sympathetic nervous system predominates with fight-or-flight responses.

Symphysis Cartilaginous joint in which the two bony components are joined directly by fibrocartilage in the form of a disk or plate.

Symptoms Subjective changes noticed or felt only by the client or patient.

Synapse Space between neurons or between a neuron and an effector organ.

Synarthrosis A limited-movement, nonsynovial joint.

Synchondrosis Joint in which the material used to connect the two components is hyaline growth cartilage.

Syndesmosis Fibrous joint in which two bony components are joined directly by a ligament, cord, or aponeurotic membrane.

Syndrome A group of different signs and symptoms that identify a pathologic condition, especially when they have a common cause.

Synergist A muscle that aids or assists the action of the agonist but is not primarily responsible for the action; also known as a guiding muscle.

Synergistic The interaction of medication and massage to stimulate the same process or effects.

Synovial fluid Thick, colorless lubricating fluid secreted by the joint cavity membrane.

Synovial joint A freely moving joint that allows motion in one or more planes.

System A group of interacting elements that function as a complex whole.

Systemic anatomy The study of the structure of a particular body system.

Systemic massage Massage that is structured to affect one body system primarily. This approach usually is used for lymphatic and circulation enhancement massage.

Tao An ancient philosophic concept that represents the whole and its parts as one and the same.

Tapotement Springy blows to the body delivered at a fast rate to create rhythmic compression of the tissue; also called percussion.

Tapping Type of tapotement that uses the fingertips.

Target muscle The muscle or groups of muscles on which the response of the methods is focused specifically.

Techniques Methods of therapeutic massage that provide sensory stimulation or mechanical changes to the soft tissue of the body.

Tendon organs Structures found in the tendon and the musculotendinous junction that respond to tension at the tendon. Articular (joint) ligaments contain receptors that are similar to tendon organs and that adjust reflex inhibition of the adjacent muscle when excessive strain is placed on the joints.

Tendonitis Inflammation of a tendon.

Tenosynovitis Inflammation of a tendon sheath.

Tensegrity Architectural principle developed in 1948 by R. Buckminster Fuller. The tensegrity principle underlies geodesic domes. A tensegrity system is characterized by a continuous tensional network (tendons, ligaments, and fascial structures) connected by a discontinuous set of compressive elements, or struts (bones).

Therapeutic applications Healing or curative powers.

Therapeutic change Beneficial change produced by a bodywork process that results in modification of physical form or function that can affect a client's physical, mental, or spiritual state.

Therapeutic relationship The interpersonal structure and professional boundaries between professionals and the clients they serve.

Thermal receptors Sensory receptors that detect changes in temperature.

Thorax Also known as the chest cavity, the thorax is the upper region of the torso that is enclosed by the sternum, ribs, and thoracic vertebrae and contains the lungs, heart, and great vessels.

Threshold stimulus Stimulus at which the first observable muscle contraction occurs.

Tissue A group of similar cells that combine to perform a common function.

Tone State of tension in resting muscles.

Tonic vibration reflex Reflex that tones a muscle via stimulation through vibration methods at the tendon.

Touch Contact with no movement.

Touch technique Technique that serves as the basis for soft-tissue forms of bodywork methods.

Toughening/hardening Reaction to repeated exposure to stimuli that elicit arousal responses.

Trabecula Irregular meshing of small, bony plates that makes up spongy bone; its spaces are filled with red marrow.

Traction Gentle pull on the joint capsule to increase the joint space.

Tracts Collections of nerve fibers in the brain and spinal cord that have a common function.

Training stimulus threshold Stimulus that elicits a training response.

Transference Personalization of the professional relationship by the client.

Trauma Physical injury caused by violent or disruptive action, toxic substances, or psychic injury resulting from a severe long- or short-term emotional shock.

Trigger point Area of local nerve facilitation; pressure on the trigger point results in hypertonicity of a muscle bundle and referred pain patterns; a hyperirritable area within a taut band of skeletal muscle, located in the muscular tissue or its associated fascia. The spot is painful on compression and can cause characteristic referred pain and autonomic phenomena.

Trochanter One of two large bony processes found only on the femur.

Tropic (or trophic) hormones Hormones produced by the endocrine glands that affect other endocrine glands.

Tubercle A small rounded process on a bone.

Tuberculosis Infection caused by bacteria that usually affects the lungs but may invade other body systems.

Tuberosity A large rounded protuberance on a bone.

Tumor Also referred to as a neoplasm, a tumor results from growth of new tissues that may be benign (nonthreatening or noncancerous) or malignant (cancerous).

Ulcer Round, open sore of the skin or mucous membrane.

Upper respiratory tract The nasal cavity and all its structures and the pharynx.

Upward rotation Scapular motion that turns the glenoid fossa upward and that moves the inferior angle superiorly and laterally away from the spinal column.

Vector The direction of force.

Veins Blood vessels that collect blood from the capillaries and transport it back to the heart. Seventy-five percent of the blood in the body is found in the venous system. Larger veins often contain a set of valves that ensure that blood flows in the correct direction to the heart and also prevent backflow.

Vena cava One of two large arteries that return poorly oxygenated blood to the right atrium of the heart.

Ventral root One of two roots that attach a spinal nerve to the spinal cord.

Ventricles The two large, lower chambers of the heart; they are thick-walled and are separated by a thick interventricular septum.

Venules The smallest veins.

Vibration Fine or coarse tremulous movement that creates reflexive responses.

Virulent Quality of organisms that readily causes disease.

Viruses Microorganisms that invade cells and insert their genetic code into the genetic code of the host cell. Viruses use host cell nutrients and organelles to produce additional virus particles.

Visceral pain Pain that results from the stimulation of receptors or from an abnormal condition in the viscera (internal organs).

Viscoelasticity The combination of resistance offered by a fluid to a change in form and the ability of material to return to its original state after deformation. This term is used to describe connective tissue.

Wellness The efficient balance of body, mind, and spirit, with all working in a harmonious way to enhance quality of life.

Whiplash Injury to the soft tissues of the neck caused by sudden hyperextension or flexion of the neck.

Word elements The parts of a word; the prefix, root, and suffix.

Yang The portion of the whole realm of function of the body, mind, and spirit in Eastern thought that corresponds with sympathetic autonomic nervous system functions.

Yellow elastic cartilage Cartilage that is more opaque, flexible, and elastic than hyaline cartilage and that is distinguished further by its yellow color. The ground substance is penetrated in all directions by frequently branching fibers that produce all of the reactions for elastin.

Yin The portion of the whole realm of function of the body, mind, and spirit in Eastern thought that corresponds with parasympathetic autonomic nervous system functions.

Yin/yang Yin and yang are terms that are used to describe polar relationships. Yin/yang refers to the dynamic balance between opposing forces and the continual process of creation and destruction. Yin/yang reflects the natural order and duality of the whole universe and everything in it, including the individual.

Answer Key

ANSWERS TO PART II

Answers and Rationales

CHAPTER 4:
Anatomy and Physiology

Answer Key for Labeling Exercise 1
Mitochondrion
Secretory vesicle
Nuclear membrane
Nucleolus
Centrioles
Cytoplasm
Cell membrane
Cilia
Rough endoplasmic reticulum
Ribosomes
Lysosome
Chromatin
Microtubules
Nucleus
Golgi apparatus
Smooth endoplasmic reticulum

Answer Key for Labeling Exercise 2
Cervical lordotic curve
Thoracic kyphotic curve
Lumbar lordotic curve
Sacral kyphotic curve
First cervical vertebra (atlas)
Second cervical vertebra (axis)

Seventh cervical vertebra
First thoracic vertebra
Intervertebral disk
Intervertebral foramina
First lumbar vertebra
Body
Transverse process
Spinous process

Answer Key for Labeling Exercise 3, Part A
Clavicle
Scapula
Humerus
Radius
Ulna
Carpals
Metacarpals
Phalanges
Skull (cranium)
Mandible
Cervical vertebrae
Sternum
Rib cage
Thoracic vertebrae
Lumbar vertebrae
Sacrum
Pelvic bone
Femur
Patella
Tibia

Fibula
Tarsals
Metatarsals
Phalanges

Answer Key for Labeling Exercise 3, Part B
Phalanges
Metacarpals
Carpals
Radius
Ulna
Humerus
Scapula
Clavicle
Skull (cranium)
Mandible
Cervical vertebrae
Thoracic vertebrae
Rib cage
Lumbar vertebrae
Sacrum
Pelvic bone
Coccyx
Femur
Fibula
Tibia
Tarsals
Metatarsals
Phalanges

Answer Key for Labeling Exercise 4
Jugular notch
Clavicle
True ribs
False ribs
Costal cartilage
Seventh cervical vertebra
First thoracic vertebra
Sternum
Manubrium
Sternal angle
Body
Xiphoid process
Floating ribs
Sternal end
Body
Head
Articular facets for body of vertebrae
Neck
Articular facet for transverse process of vertebra
Tubercle
Angle
Xiphoid process
Body
Sternal angle
Manubrium
Clavicular notch

Jugular notch
Facets for attachment of costal cartilages 1 to 7

Answer Key for Labeling Exercise 5
Sternal end
Body
Acromial end

Answer Key for Labeling Exercise 6
Superior angle
Supraspinous fossa
Scapular spine
Infraspinous fossa
Inferior angle
Suprascapular notch
Acromion
Glenoid fossa
Infraglenoid tubercle
Lateral border
Coracoid process
Supraglenoid tubercle
Medial border
Scapular spine
Coracoid fossa
Glenoid fossa

Answer Key for Labeling Exercise 7
Greater tubercle
Lesser tubercle
Deltoid tuberosity
Radial fossa
Lateral epicondyle
Capitulum
Trochlea
Medial epicondyle
Coronoid fossa
Head
Greater tubercle
Surgical neck
Olecranon fossa

Answer Key for Labeling Exercise 8
Radial head
Radial tuberosity
Radius
Radial styloid
Olecranon process of ulna
Trochlear notch
Coronoid process
Interosseous membrane
Ulna
Ulnar styloid

Answer Key for Labeling Exercise 9
Phalanges
Metacarpus
Carpal bones

Capitate
Hook of hamate
Hamate
Pisiform
Triquetrum
Lunate
Ulna
Distal
Middle
Proximal
Distal
Proximal
Carpal bones
Trapezoid
Tubercle of trapezium
Trapezium
Tubercle of scaphoid
Scaphoid
Wrist joint
Radius
Pisiform
Triquetrum
Hamate
Tubercle
Trapezium
Trapezoid
Capitate

Answer Key for Labeling Exercise 10
Sacroiliac joint
Sacral promontory
Anterior superior iliac spine
Obturator foramen
Ilium
Pubis
Ischium
Symphysis pubis
Posterior superior iliac spine
Posterior inferior iliac spine
Greater sciatic notch
Ischial spine
Lesser sciatic notch
Obturator foramen
Ischial tuberosity
Iliac crest
Ilium
Anterior superior iliac spine
Anterior inferior iliac spine
Lunate surface
Acetabulum
Inferior pubic ramus
Acetabular notch
Ischial ramus
Iliac crest
Ilium
Iliac fossa
Anterior superior iliac spine

Anterior inferior iliac spine
Iliopectineal line
Superior pubic ramus
Pubic crest
Symphysis pubis
Obturator foramen
Articular surface
Posterior superior iliac spine
Posterior inferior iliac spine
Greater sciatic notch
Body of ischium
Ischial spine
Lesser sciatic notch
Ischial ramus
Inferior pubic ramus

Answer Key for Labeling Exercise 11
Greater trochanter
Lateral and medial supracondylar ridges
Patellar groove
Lateral epicondyle
Lateral condyle
Fovea capitis
Head of femur
Neck
Intertrochanteric fossa
Lesser trochanter
Intertrochanteric line
Intertrochanteric crest
Pectineal line
Linea aspera
Medial and lateral supracondylar lines
Adductor tubercle
Medial epicondyle
Medial condyle
Greater trochanter
Gluteal tuberosity
Intercondylar fossa

Answer Key for Labeling Exercise 12
Intercondylar eminence
Lateral condyle
Head
Neck of fibula
Fibula
Lateral malleolus
Medial malleolus
Tibia
Tibial tuberosity
Medial condyle

Answer Key for Labeling Exercise 13
Tarsals
Cuboid
Lateral cuneiform
Metatarsals
Phalanges

Proximal phalanx
Middle phalanx
Distal phalanx
Tarsals
Calcaneus
Talus
Navicular
Intermediate cuneiform
Medial cuneiform
Proximal phalanx of great toe
Distal phalanx of great toe
Tibia
Talus
Navicular
Cuneiforms
Phalanges
Metatarsals
Tarsals
Cuboid
Calcaneus
Talus
Fibula

Answer Key for Labeling Exercise 14
Coronal suture
Sagittal suture
Frontal bone
Parietal bone
Occipital bone

Answer Key for Labeling Exercise 15
Temporal bone, squamous part
Lateral temporomandibular ligament
External auditory meatus
Stylomandibular ligament

Answer Key for Labeling Exercise 16
Coracoclavicular ligament
Conoid ligament
Trapezoid ligament
Acromioclavicular ligament
Transverse humeral ligament
Long head of biceps muscle
Humerus
Clavicle
Transverse scapular ligament
Suprascapular notch
Glenohumeral ligament
Scapula
Acromioclavicular ligament
Scapular spine and acromion

Answer Key for Labeling Exercise 17
Synovial chondrosternal joint
Sternoclavicular joint
Articular disk
Manubrium of sternum

Sternoclavicular ligament
Clavicle
First rib
Costoclavicular ligament
Second rib
Costal cartilages
Body of sternum

Answer Key for Labeling Exercise 18
Sternum
Clavicle
Coracoclavicular ligament
Acromioclavicular ligament
Acromioclavicular joint
Acromion
Scapular spine
Supraspinous fossa

Answer Key for Labeling Exercise 19
Lateral epicondyle
Radial collateral ligament
Annular ligament of radius
Radius
Ulna
Ulnar collateral ligament
Elbow joint capsule
Medial epicondyle
Annular ligament
Radial tuberosity
Radius
Ulna
Olecranon of ulna
Medial (ulnar) collateral ligament
Anterior band
Transverse band
Posterior band
Anterior elbow capsule

Answer Key for Labeling Exercise 20
Interphalangeal joint (DIP)
Metacarpophalangeal joint (MCP)
Distal interphalangeal joint (DIP)
Proximal interphalangeal joint (PIP)
Metacarpophalangeal joint (MCP)

Answer Key for Labeling Exercise 21
Iliolumbar ligament
Sacroiliac ligament
Sacrospinous ligament
Sacrotuberous ligament
Pectineal line
Pubic tubercle
Pubic symphysis
Ischium
Coccyx
Acetabulum
Lesser sciatic foramen

Inguinal ligament
Arcuate line
Greater sciatic foramen
Sacroiliac joint

Answer Key for Labeling Exercise 22
Ilium
Iliofemoral ligament
Greater trochanter
Lesser trochanter
Pubofemoral ligament
Inferior pubic ramus
Ischial tuberosity
Lesser trochanter
Greater trochanter
Ischiofemoral ligament

Answer Key for Labeling Exercise 23
Anterior cruciate ligament
Fibular (lateral) collateral ligament
Tendon of popliteus muscle
Lateral meniscus
Transverse ligament
Fibular head
Patellar tendon
Anterior cruciate ligament
Posterior cruciate ligament
Medial condyle
Tibial (medial) collateral ligament
Medial meniscus
Semimembranous tendon
Patellar ligament
Patella
Popliteus muscle
Tibia
Posterior meniscus femoral ligament
Fibular (lateral) collateral ligament
Lateral condyle
Lateral meniscus
Popliteus tendon
Oblique popliteal ligament
Fibular head

Answer Key for Labeling Exercise 24
Medial malleolus
Medial cuneiform
Navicular
Calcaneus
Deltoid ligament
Anterior tibiotalar
Tibionavicular
Tibiocalcaneal
Posterior tibiotalar

Answer Key for Labeling Exercise 25
Femur
Fibrous capsule

Synovial membrane
Articular cartilage
Menisci
Tibia
Quadriceps femoris muscle
Synovial membrane
Suprapatellar bursa
Patella
Prepatellar bursa
Subpatellar fat
Subcutaneous infrapatellar bursa
Infrapatellar bursa

Answer Key for Labeling Exercise 26
Muscle
Epimysium
Perimysium
Endomysium
Axon of motor neuron
Blood vessel
Fascicle
Muscle fiber (muscle cell)
Nucleus
Sarcolemma
Sarcoplasmic reticulum
Muscle fiber (muscle cell)
Thick filaments
Thin filaments
Myofibril
Bone
Tendon
Fascia
Fascicle
Perimysium
Endomysium

Answer Key for Labeling Exercise 27
Facial muscles
Deltoid
Biceps brachii
Linea alba
Aponeurosis of the biceps
Extensors of the wrist and fingers
Adductors of thigh
Flexor retinaculum
Sartorius
Vastus medialis
Patellar tendon
Gastrocnemius
Soleus
Superior extensor retinaculum
Extensor hallucis longus tendon
Peroneus brevis fibularis
Peroneus longus fibularis
Extensor digitorum longus
Tibialis anterior
Patella

Rectus femoris
Vastus lateralis
Tensor fasciae latae
External obliques
Flexors of wrist and fingers
Rectus abdominis
Serratus anterior
Pectoralis major
Trapezius
Sternocleidomastoid
Cranial muscles

Answer Key for Labeling Exercise 28
Sternocleidomastoideus
Seventh cervical vertebra
Deltoid
Teres minor
Teres major
Triceps
Latissimus dorsi
Extensors of the wrist and fingers
Semitendinosus
Biceps femoris
Semimembranosus
Gastrocnemius
Peroneus longus fibularis
Peroneus brevis fibularis
Superior peroneal retinaculum
Soleus
Gastrocnemius tendon (Achilles tendon)
Plantaris
Iliotibial tract
Gracilis
Adductor magnus
Gluteus maximus
External obliques
Portion of rhomboid
Infraspinatus
Trapezius
Splenius capitis

Answer Key for Labeling Exercise 29
Superior auricular
Anterior auricular
Frontal belly of occipitofrontalis
Orbicularis oculi
Procerus
Nasalis
Levator labii superioris alaeque nasi
Levator labii superioris
Zygomatic minor
Zygomatic major
Orbicularis oris
Depressor labii inferioris
Mentalis
Depressor anguli oris
Risorius

Buccinator muscle
Platysma
Posterior auricular
Occipital belly of occipitofrontalis

Answer Key for Labeling Exercise 30
Semispinalis capitis muscle
Levator scapulae muscle
Rhomboid minor muscle
Rhomboid major muscle
Latissimus dorsi muscle
Trapezius muscle
Splenius capitis muscle

Answer Key for Labeling Exercise 31, Part A
Acromion
Deltoid
Supraspinatus tendon
Fibrous membrane
Glenoid cavity
Synovial membrane
Infraspinatus
Glenoid labrum
Teres minor
Subscapularis
Teres major
Latissimus dorsi
Long head of triceps brachii
Short head of biceps brachii and coracobrachialis
Pectoralis major
Subscapular bursae
Coracoid process
Coracoacromial ligament
Long head of biceps brachii tendon
Subacromial bursa (subdeltoid)

Answer Key for Labeling Exercise 31, Part B
Transverse humeral ligament
Long head of biceps brachii muscle
Short head of biceps brachii muscle
Radial tuberosity
Tuberosity of ulna
Bicipital aponeurosis (cut)
Brachialis muscle
Coracobrachialis muscle

Answer Key for Labeling Exercise 32
Supinator (superficial head)
Extensor carpi ulnaris
Extensor digitorum
Extensor pollicis longus
Supinator (deep head)
Interosseous membrane
Extensor pollicis longus
Extensor indicis
Extensor carpi radialis longus
Extensor carpi radialis brevis

Abductor pollicis longus
Extensor pollicis brevis
Supinator (superficial head)
Abductor pollicis longus
Extensor pollicis brevis

Answer Key for Labeling Exercise 33
Longitudinal fibers of palmar aponeurosis
Transverse fibers of palmar aponeurosis
Palmar brevis muscle

Answer Key for Labeling Exercise 34
Tensor fasciae latae
Rectus femoris
Pectineus
Vastus intermedius
Adductor longus
Vastus medialis
Fibularis longus
Tibialis anterior
Extensor digitorum longus
Sartorius
Gluteus maximus
Adductor magnus
Vastus lateralis
Semitendinosus
Biceps femoris
Semimembranosus
Plantaris
Soleus
Gastrocnemius
Calcaneal (Achilles) tendon

Answer Key for Labeling Exercise 35
Spinal cord
Dorsal root ganglion
Epineurium
Perineurium
Endoneurium
Axon
Motor end plate
Skin
Ventral root
Blood vessels
Nerve bundles (fasciculus)
Node of Ranvier
Myelin sheath
Muscle
Pain receptors

Answer Key for Labeling Exercise 36
C2
C3
C4
C5
T2
T1

C6
C7
C8
L1
S1
Posterior femoral cutaneous (S1 to S3)
Dorsal rami (S1 to S3)
Lateral femoral cutaneous (L2, L3)
Dorsal rami (L1 to L3)
Medial antebrachial cutaneous (C8, T1)
Posterior brachial cutaneous (radial C5 to C8)
Medial brachial cutaneous (C8, T1) and intercostobrachial (T2)
Dorsal rami (C3 to C5)
Lesser occipital (C2)
Greater occipital (C2, C3)

Answer Key for Labeling Exercise 37
Superficial temporal artery
Common carotid artery
Axillary artery
Dorsalis pedis artery
Popliteal (posterior to patella) artery
Femoral artery
Radial artery
Brachial artery
Facial artery

Answer Key for Labeling Exercise 38
Facial nodes
Deep cervical nodes
Right lymphatic duct
Subclavicular node
Axillary nodes
Mammary plexus
Cubital nodes
Superficial inguinal nodes
Palmar plexus
Thoracic duct
Superficial cervical nodes
Occipital nodes
Parotid nodes
Popliteal nodes
Plantar plexus

Answer Key for Labeling Exercise 39
Upper respiratory tract
Lower respiratory tract
Nasal cavity
Pharynx
Nasopharynx
Oropharynx
Laryngopharynx
Larynx
Trachea
Left and right primary bronchi
Bronchioles

Alveolar duct
Alveolar sac
Alveoli
Capillary

Answer Key for Labeling Exercise 40
Rectum
Seminal vesicle
Levator ani muscle
Ejaculatory duct
Anus
Bulbocavernosus muscle
Epididymis
Testis
Penis
Urinary bladder
Symphysis pubis
Prostate gland
Corpus cavernosum
Corpus spongiosum
Urethra
Glans

Answer Key for Labeling Exercise 41
Sacral promontory
Ureter
Sacrouterine ligament
Posterior cul-de-sac
Cervix
Levator ani muscle
Fornix of vagina
External anal sphincter
Anus
Urogenital diaphragm
Vagina
Labium majus
Labium minus
Urethra
Crus of clitoris
Symphysis pubis
Bladder
Anterior cul-de-sac
Fundus of uterus
Round ligament
Corpus of uterus
Ovarian ligament
External iliac vessels
Fallopian tube

ANSWER KEY FOR CHAPTERS 5 AND 6 COMPREHENSION ACTIVITY

Scenario 1

1. a
2. d

3. c
4. b
5. a
6. a
7. a
8. c
9. a
10. b
11. d
12. b
13. d
14. a
15. a
16. b
17. c
18. c
19. c

Scenario 2

1. c
2. a.
3. d
4. b
5. a
6. b
7. a
8. c
9. a
10. c
11. d
12. b
13. a
14. c
15. a
16. d
17. c
18. c
19. b
20. c
21. d
22. b
23. d
24. a

Scenario 3

1. b
2. c
3. a
4. c
5. c
6. b
7. d
8. c

9. a
10. b
11. a
12. c
13. a
14. c
15. c
16. a
17. b
18. b
19. d
20. a
21. b
22. a

Scenario 4

1. a
2. c
3. c
4. a
5. b
6. a

7. c
8. b
9. b
10. c
11. a
12. a
13. b
14. d
15. b
16. a
17. d
18. c
19. d
20. b
21. c
22. b
23. b
24. c
25. a
26. a
27. a
28. d
29. c
30. b

ANSWERS TO PART IV

Answers and Rationales

CHAPTER 7:
Therapeutic Massage

FOUNDATIONS OF THERAPEUTIC APPLICATIONS OF TOUCH

Answers and Rationales to Factual Recall Questions

1. d
   Factual recall
   Rationale: The correct answer is the definition of professionalism.
2. b
   Factual recall
   Rationale: The correct answer is the definition of culture.
3. b
   Factual recall
   Rationale: Being able to define the various forms of touch is necessary to identify touch technique and mechanical touch.

4. a
   Factual recall
   Rationale: Biopsychosocial (BPS) Model is a comprehensive model that includes biological, psychological, and social components to understand the possible causes of an illness.
5. a
   Factual recall
   Rationale: While the practitioner's education and the influence of the practice setting are important the best answer is the relationship between the practitioner and client called the therapeutic alliance.
6. c
   Factual recall
   Rationale: Shiatsu is a form of bodywork from Japan where compression over clothing is part of the application.
7. a
   Factual recall
   Rationale: Myofascial release is a type of method that targets superficial fascia, a type of connective tissue.

8. b
Factual recall
Rationale: The Swedish form of massage uses the terms effleurage, petrissage, and tapotement.

9. a
Factual recall
Rationale: Neuromuscular therapy is a modern form of bodywork.

10. b
Factual recall
Rationale: The question is the definition of reflexology.

Answer/Rationale to Application and Concept Identification Question

1. b
Application and concept identification
Rationale: The question addresses the issue of how an individual can experience touch interaction.

2. c
Application and concept identification
Rationale: Age differences can be an issue in the therapeutic setting.

PROFESSIONALISM AND LEGAL ISSUES

Answers and Rationales to Factual Recall Questions

1. a
Factual recall
Rationale: The question is the definition of scope of practice.

2. c
Factual recall
Rationale: The question provides an example of the scope of practice involved in working with those with complex situations but who are not ill.

3. d
Factual recall
Rationale: The question describes the ethical principle of client autonomy and self-determination.

4. a
Factual recall
Rationale: The question is the definition of a needs assessment.

5. b
Factual recall
Rationale: The question lists all the components of a policy statement except fee structure. The wrong answers are part of a treatment plan or a clinical reasoning process.

6. a
Factual recall
Rationale: Locking the door could be considered entrapment.

7. b
Factual recall
Rationale: The question gives examples of listening difficulties.

8. c
Factual recall
Rationale: The next step in dealing with unethical peer behavior is to talk with those involved. Direct communication to get all the facts is the most appropriate approach.

9. d
Factual recall
Rationale: This question is about zoning; the other answers are not about zoning.

10. c
Factual recall
Rationale: This is the definition of conflict.

11. a
Factual recall
Rationale: The supervisor has the authority to use power, regardless of whether or not this is the best method.

12. d
Factual recall
Rationale: The Health Insurance Portability and Accountability Act encompasses three primary areas and involves privacy standards, patient rights, and administrative requirements.

Answers and Rationales to Application and Concept Identification Questions

1. d
Application and concept identification
Rationale: The question gives an example of countertransference. The answer is determined by comparing the behavior of the massage professional described in the question to the definition of countertransference.

2. b
Application and concept identification
Rationale: The question provides an example of a breach in a standard of practice. The answer is determined by comparing the behavior of the massage professional described in the question to the standards of practice for massage therapy.

3. c
Application and concept identification
Rationale: The question addresses various approaches to massage and bodywork. A description of the population and the indication for application of a variety of methods indicate that this professional uses an integrated approach.

4. b
Application and concept identification
Rationale: The question provides an example of a breach in scope of practice. The answer is determined by comparing the behavior of the massage professional described in the question to the scope of practice for massage therapy.

5. d

Application and concept identification

Rationale: This situation is not a dual role, transference, or even a technical breach in the scope of practice for massage. However, the massage professional's personal scope of practice is most likely affected because perhaps the massage professional did not receive enough training to address this complex disease condition.

6. c

Application and concept identification

Rationale: The correct answer would indicate that confidentiality has been breached. The three wrong answers are examples of maintaining confidentiality.

7. a

Application and concept identification

Rationale: Only information that would directly affect the massage interaction is to be disclosed. The three wrong answers are examples of inappropriate conversation with a client.

8. c

Application and concept identification

Rationale: The question asks for a rationale for the right of refusal. The only answer that is logical based on the facts in the question is answer *c*.

9. a

Application and concept identification

Rationale: The question gives an example of the power differential but in a different context than the examples in the textbook. The other terms, once defined, would not be logical in relation to the facts of the question.

10. b

Application and concept identification

Rationale: The answer is determined by comparing the definition of transference to the behavior of the massage professional described in each of the possible answers.

11. c

Application and concept identification

Rationale: The question indicates that the client is confused about the sensations and indicates no intentional acts by either party.

12. c

Concept identification

Rationale: The nature of the conflict is "not enough to go around." This is a conflict of interest.

13. d

Clinical reasoning

Rationale: The question provides an example of a situation in which peer support is helpful in ethical decision-making. The three wrong answers indicate that the professional has decided what the problem is, but the question indicates otherwise. Peer support and ethical decision-making are helpful in identifying the area of concern and in developing plans to rectify the situation.

BUSINESS CONSIDERATIONS FOR A CAREER IN THERAPEUTIC MASSAGE

Answers and Rationales to Factual Recall Questions

1. b

Factual recall

Rationale: A standard comparison of the two types of positions indicates that stable income is considered an advantage.

2. d

Factual recall

Rationale: The question is the definition of start-up costs.

3. a

Factual recall

Rationale: The question provides an example of marketing.

4. c

Factual recall

Rationale: By comparing the common elements included in a brochure with the list provided in the question, the missing element can be identified as fees.

5. d

Factual recall

Rationale: The question provides an example of management.

6. a

Factual recall

Rationale: The government department that deals with zoning would determine whether the business was located in the proper district.

7. c

Factual recall

Rationale: The question is the definition of net income.

8. b

Factual recall

Rationale: The question defines premise liability insurance.

9. a

Factual recall

Rationale: All the components of a business plan have been identified in the question except for retirement investment.

10 a

Factual recall

Rationale: Employees are eligible for unemployment.

11. a

Factual recall

Rationale: Those who are self-employed pay self-employment taxes.

12. c

Factual recall

Rationale: Workers' compensation is an insurance employers pay to cover employees injured on the job.

13. b

Factual recall

Rationale: Home office deductions for tax purposes require regular and exclusive use as a principal place of business.

14. a

Factual recall

Rationale: The question defines the National Provider Identification (NPI) number.

Answer and Rationale to Application and Concept Identification Questions

1. c

Application and concept identification

Rationale: When all the information provided in the question is considered, burnout is the most likely answer.

MEDICAL TERMINOLOGY

Answers and Rationales to Factual Recall Questions

1. c

Factual recall

Rationale: The answer describes record-keeping responsibilities.

2. d

Factual recall

Rationale: The correct answer is the definition of charting.

3. b

Factual recall

Rationale: The correct answer is the definition of a quantifiable goal.

4. a

Factual recall

Rationale: The question is the definition of abscess.

5. a

Factual recall

Rationale: -algesia means capacity to feel pain.

6. d

Factual recall

Rationale: The correct answer describes the reason for assessment.

7. c

Factual recall

Rationale: The correct answer describes the proper reason for data analysis.

8. b

Factual recall

Rationale: A treatment plan is a guide for a series of sessions.

9. b

Factual recall

Rationale: The answer describes data recorded as part of the plan.

10. c

Factual recall

Rationale: "-plasty" means surgical repair.

11. c

Factual recall

Rationale: Myalgia means muscle pain.

12. a

Factual recall

Rationale: Vasodilation refers to enlargement of the lumen of blood vessels; blood vessels are a component of the cardiovascular system.

13. b

Factual recall

Rationale: The information in the question is objective.

Answers and Rationales to Application/Concept Identification and Clinical Reasoning/Synthesis Questions

1. a

Application and concept identification

Rationale: The answer is determined by comparing the definition of quantified outcome goal to the activities described in each of the possible answers. Two of the wrong answers are examples of qualified goals.

2. c

Application and concept identification

Rationale: A type of objective data is information collected from assessment, as described in the correct answer. Answers *a* and *b* are subjective data, and answer *d* is information related to the treatment plan.

3. c

Application and concept identification

Rationale: The decision-making process is being described in the question, and this happens during the analysis.

4. a

Application and concept identification

Rationale: Clinical reasoning is a process of thinking. The wrong answers are reasons for record-keeping.

5. b

Application and concept identification

Rationale: The question asks for components of analysis. Required are a preassessment and a postassessment analysis to determine results.

6. d

Application and concept identification

Rationale: Neuritis is nerve inflammation.

RESEARCH LITERACY AND EVIDENCE-BASED PRACTICE

Answers and Rationales to Factual Recall Questions

1. c
   Factual recall
   Rationale: The correct answer is a definition of science.
2. b
   Factual recall
   Rationale: The correct answer is a definition of centering.
3. b
   Factual recall
   Rationale: Research objectively validates massage.
4. b
   Factual recall
   Rationale: Only rubbing provides manual stimulation.
5. a
   Factual recall
   Rationale: The effects of massage are explained by reflexive/neuro and mechanical methods.
6. c
   Factual recall
   Rationale: Mechanical methods directly stimulate the nervous system.
7. a
   Factual recall
   Rationale: Anxiety is a mood disorder. None of the other answers are problems in behavior, mood, or perception of stress and pain.
8. c
   Factual recall
   Rationale: Dopamine coordinates fine motor movement, and research shows that dopamine availability increases with massage.
9. b
   Factual recall
   Rationale: Serotonin is involved in satiety, and its availability is increased by massage.
10. c
    Factual recall
    Rationale: The three stages in the stress response are alarm, resistance, and exhaustion.
11. a
    Factual recall
    Rationale: Alarm is used to describe the initial activation of the sympathetic nervous system.
12. b
    Factual recall
    Rationale: The correct answer describes parasympathetic functions.
13. c
    Factual recall
    Rationale: The third type of proprioceptor is joint kinesthetic receptors.
14. a
    Factual recall
    Rationale: The stretch reflex can cause cramping when tissues are elongated too quickly. There is no such thing as Hooke's reflex, but Hooke's neurologic law does exist.
15. d
    Factual recall
    Rationale: The crossed extensor reflex is involved in maintaining balance.
16. d
    Factual recall
    Rationale: The correct answer defines gate control.
17. d
    Factual recall
    Rationale: The question is the definition of experiment replication.
18. b
    Factual recall
    Rationale: All research begins with a question to be answered.
19. a
    Factual recall
    Rationale: The discovery phase is when the researcher identifies what exists.
20. d
    Factual recall
    Rationale: This is the definition of theory.
21. b
    Factual recall
    Rationale: Factors that have an effect on the experiment are called variables.
22. c
    Factual recall
    Rationale: The purpose of an experiment is to test the hypothesis.
23. d
    Factual recall
    Rationale: The methods part describes how the experiment was designed.
24. b
    Factual recall
    Rationale: A researcher who influences the research findings but objectively reports on outcomes of the research makes the research biased.

Answers and Rationales to Application/Concept Identification and Clinical Reasoning/Synthesis Questions

1. b
   Application and concept identification
   Rationale: The question asks for a correlation between relaxation, the sympathetic symptoms displayed, and a massage outcome.

2. b

Application and concept identification

Rationale: Answers *a* and *c* indicate an adrenaline response. The symptoms provided in the question indicate the resistance response and the result of long-term exposure to cortisol. Answer *d* is a parasympathetic response pattern.

3. b

Application and concept identification

Rationale: The question asks for the reason for a physiologic response to massage related to normal flow in the arteries.

4. c

Application and concept identification

Rationale: The aspect of research where the variable that is manipulated is the independent variable.

5. c

Application and concept identification

Rationale: The correct answer requires the least amount of adaption and is most relaxing for an exhausted client. The facts provided in the question involve long-term stress and a breakdown in adaptive capacity (exhaustion). There would also be long-term cortisol effects, indications, and contraindications. Because the body is overstressed, care must be taken that the massage does not add excessive stress to the system. The wrong answers strain the system or do not provide for a long enough intervention.

INDICATIONS AND CONTRAINDICATIONS FOR THERAPEUTIC MASSAGE

Answers and Rationales to Factual Recall Questions

1. a

Factual recall

Rationale: The three wrong answers are correct examples of types of contraindications.

2. c

Factual recall

Rationale: In this question, massage does everything but inhibits homeostasis.

3. c

Factual recall

Rationale: The correct answer is the definition of chronic pain.

4. c

Factual recall

Rationale: All of the answers describe pain, but it is important to differentiate between types of pain to identify indications and contraindications for massage.

5. d

Factual recall

Rationale: The correct answer is the definition of somatic pain. *Soma* means body and is used to describe the soft tissue, including skin, muscles, joints, tendons, and fasciae.

6. b

Factual recall

Rationale: The question is the definition of referred pain.

7. d

Factual recall

Rationale: The liver and gallbladder refer pain to the right side of the neck.

8. a

Factual recall

Rationale: Lung and diaphragm pain may be referred to the left side of the neck.

9. d

Factual recall

Rationale: Impingement of the cervical plexus would have symptoms that extend into the head and neck area.

10. a

Factual recall

Rationale: Sacral plexus nerve impingement is indicated by pain into the leg and gluteal area.

11. d

Factual recall

Rationale: The correct answer defines health. The other three answers indicate that the mechanisms of health are breaking down.

12. c

Factual recall

Rationale: The correct answer defines pathology.

13. b

Factual recall

Rationale: The correct answer defines a sign in relation to information presented in the question. Signs describe objective and observable information. The wrong answers are examples of subjective data.

14. c

Factual recall

Rationale: The correct answer is the definition of homeostasis.

15. b

Factual recall

Rationale: The general adaptation syndrome has three stages: alarm, resistance, and exhaustion.

16. c

Factual recall

Rationale: A sign of the inflammatory response is heat.

17. d

Factual recall

Rationale: *Regeneration* is the term for new cells that are similar to those they replace.

18. d

Factual recall

Rationale: The correct answer is the definition of regional contraindication.

19 c

Factual recall

Rationale: The difference between benign tumors and malignant tumors is that benign tumors remain localized; malignant tumors tend to spread.

20. c

Factual recall

Rationale: The similarity between medication effect and massage benefit is seen in these three basic interactions: replace, stimulate, and inhibit.

21. b

Factual recall

Rationale: When massage and medication perform a similar function, the relationship is synergistic.

22. c

Factual recall

Rationale: The answer is the definition of intractable pain.

23. d

Factual recall

Rationale: The question defines risk factors.

24. c

Factual recall

Rationale: The question defines signs.

25 a

Factual recall

Rationale: The question defines connective tissue.

Answers and Rationales to Application/ Concept Identification and Clinical Reasoning/Synthesis Questions

1. d

Application and concept identification

Rationale: Endangerment sites are areas of the body that are susceptible to pressure damage.

2. a

Application and concept identification

Rationale: The treatment plan approach of condition management is defined in the question. The correct answer conforms to this definition. Answers b and c describe therapeutic change, and answer d may indicate a breach in scope of practice.

3. b

Application and concept identification

Rationale: Referral in this situation seems overly cautious because there is a reason for the discomfort and it fits the criteria of stage 1, which is easily reversible. Reversible conditions respond to therapeutic change.

4. c

Application and concept identification

Rationale: Palliative care reduces suffering and would be most appropriate for the man with terminal cancer. This does not mean that the other three conditions would not respond to palliation, but condition management would be more appropriate.

5. b

Application and concept identification

Rationale: Creation of therapeutic inflammation would be appropriate when fibrotic connective tissue causes dysfunction. Answers a, c, and d are contraindicated for this approach.

6. b

Application and concept identification

Rationale: Because massage most specifically addresses soft tissue nerve entrapment by increasing the resting length of muscles, answer b is the best method of those listed.

7. c

Application and concept identification

Rationale: Acute pain is most effectively managed with an intervention that is less invasive and supports the current healing process.

8. b

Application and concept identification

Rationale: An anticoagulant prevents or reduces blood clotting, so friction may cause bruising.

9. a

Application and concept identification

Rationale: Lymph nodes are endangerment sites and so are contraindicated for deep sustained compression. Answers b, c, and d do not indicate aspects of endangerment sites.

10. c

Clinical reasoning and synthesis

Rationale: Answer a provides facts about edema, the severity of the condition, and a logical explanation. No referral would be necessary. Answer b does not represent a condition in relation to massage. Answer c is the correct answer because no explanation is provided for the condition, and bruising can be a sign of a serious pathologic condition. Answer d does not represent a contraindication unless something is contraindicated with use of the medication.

HYGIENE, SANITATION, AND SAFETY

Answers and Rationales to Factual Recall Questions

1. c

Factual recall

Rationale: The correct answer provides examples of pathogenic organisms.

2. b

Factual recall

Rationale: The question defines fungi.

3. a

Factual recall

Rationale: Opportunistic invasion is a route by which pathogens are spread. The three wrong answers name methods that prevent the spread of disease.

4. d

Factual recall

Rationale: The three primary ways that pathogens are spread are person-to-person contact, opportunistic invasion, and environmental contact. The three wrong answers name methods that prevent the spread of disease.

5. b

Factual recall

Rationale: The question provides an example of sterilization.

6. a

Factual recall

Rationale: Proper hand washing is essential to the practice of sanitary massage therapy.

7. a

Factual recall

Rationale: The correct answer is an example of disinfection.

8. c

Factual recall

Rationale: The correct answer is the definition of acquired immunodeficiency syndrome.

9. b

Factual recall

Rationale: An open flame is a safety hazard.

10. b

Factual recall

Rationale: Standard Precautions are a specific protocol of sanitary procedures developed by the Centers for Disease Control and Prevention.

11. b

Factual recall

Rationale: Severe acute respiratory syndrome is a very contagious disease.

Answer and Rationale to Clinical Reasoning and Synthesis Question

1. c

Rationale: This type of question asks for a decision. The correct answer is the one that best conforms to standards of sanitary practice. All of the answers are correct, but the safety of the client always is a priority.

2. a.

Clinical reasoning and synthesis

Rationale: Zero tolerance is the appropriate action for sexual solicitation.

BODY MECHANICS

Answers and Rationales to Factual Recall Questions

1. b

Factual recall

Rationale: The relaxed standing position conserves muscle energy while maintaining balance with the gastrocnemius and soleus muscles.

2. c

Factual recall

Rationale: The incorrect answers are fatiguing.

3. c

Factual recall

Rationale: Two directional forces are used with massage: compressive force down with a forward momentum.

4. a

Factual recall

Rationale: The correct answer describes proper weight distribution.

5. b

Factual recall

Rationale: The center of gravity changes, resulting in increased pressure if the weight-bearing foot is moved farther away from the table but not to the point that one stands on the toes.

Answers and Rationales to Application and Concept Identification Questions

1. d

Application and concept identification

Rationale: If the massage practitioner shifts the weight to the front foot at the end of the stroke, the focus of the pressure is smaller and would be uncomfortable.

2. a

Application and concept identification

Rationale: The question provides information about correct body mechanics except in one area: excessive trunk flexion.

3. c

Application and concept identification

Rationale: This massage outcome would be accomplished most efficiently by using the method described in the correct answer.

4. a

Application and concept identification

Rationale: One of the most important aspects of perpendicularity and weight transfer is core stability.

5. a

Clinical reasoning and synthesis

Rationale: Facts in the question suggest that something is incorrect with delivery of the massage. The incorrect answers describe appropriate body mechanics, whereas the correct answer provides a logical explanation for the strain in the arms and shoulders.

6. b

Clinical reasoning and synthesis

Rationale: The facts in the question describe low back pain that is getting worse and full-time massage practice. Answer *a* likely would make the condition worse and add knee strain. Answers *c* and *d* describe actions that would increase the strain.

7. c

Clinical reasoning and synthesis

Rationale: The question indicates that something is wrong with the body mechanics, resulting in pain. All three of the incorrect answers would increase the pain.

8. c

Clinical reasoning and synthesis

Rationale: The question asks for a decision on the cause of knee pain. After each answer is analyzed, the only one that is logical describes flexed and static knees.

PREPARATION FOR MASSAGE: EQUIPMENT, SUPPLIES, PROFESSIONAL ENVIRONMENT, POSITIONING, AND DRAPING

Answers and Rationales to Factual Recall Questions

1. b

Factual recall

Rationale: The cable support is the structural design component for stability, and the center hinge is the weak point.

2. c

Factual recall

Rationale: Draping material provides warmth and modesty, so the material must be opaque.

3. a

Factual recall

Rationale: Sanitation is a priority, and disinfection is appropriate for linens.

4. d

Factual recall

Rationale: The most common reason for an allergic reaction to a lubricant is the volatile oils that are used to scent the product.

5. b

Factual recall

Rationale: The only reason for using a lubricant is to reduce skin drag when gliding or kneading massage methods are used. All other reasons, such as medicinal or cosmetic ones, may indicate a breach in the scope of practice.

6. c

Factual recall

Rationale: Of the four answers provided, going to a client's home presents the most difficult boundary issues.

Answers and Rationales to Application/Concept Identification and Clinical Reasoning/Synthesis Questions

1. a

Application and concept identification

Rationale: The mat would allow work to be done on the floor, where falling would not be an issue.

2. d

Clinical reasoning and synthesis

Rationale: Answer *a* is not recommended because scents may cause an allergic reaction in sensitive individuals, and personal preference varies. A lock on the massage door can be considered entrapment, so this is inappropriate. Because the file cabinet is locked, confidentiality is maintained. It is recommended that the plants be removed, again because many persons are allergic to them.

3. b

Clinical reasoning and synthesis

Rationale: A summary of the facts provided in the question indicates that boundary issues have been breached and conversation with the client was inappropriate.

4. a

Application and concept identification

Rationale: The question reflects a comprehensive, first-client orientation process. Explaining massage flow to clients is an important factor in making them more comfortable with the process. The incorrect answers describe a boundary violation or are not part of the orientation process.

5. a

Application and concept identification

Rationale: Prone and supine positions tend to aggravate low back pain. Even a seated position can be tiring to the low back. Therefore, the side-lying position is the best choice.

6. c

Clinical reasoning and synthesis

Rationale: The question presents a common massage practice situation. In this situation, the wrong answers do not provide enough body coverage to accommodate this client.

7. c

Application and concept identification

Rationale: When the client conditions as presented are considered, the elderly woman with blood pressure concerns is correct because she could be dizzy after the massage.

8. d

Clinical reasoning and synthesis

Rationale: Massage can be done without asking the client to remove clothing. Methods can be modified to adjust to the situation, or the client can wear clothing that is easy to work around. Attempts to change the client's beliefs by demonstrating draping or providing an educational session are not necessary when having the client wear shorts and a loose shirt solves the problem.

9. a

Clinical reasoning and synthesis

Rationale: In this question, a client does not leave after the session, which makes it difficult for the professional to maintain a work schedule. Usually, this occurs because the policies and client rules were not enforced from the beginning, as described in the correct answer. Wrong answers *b* and *c* would predispose to future problems, and answer *d* indicates incorrect word usage.

MASSAGE MANIPULATIONS AND TECHNIQUES

Answers and Rationales to Factual Recall Questions

1. a

Factual recall

Rationale: The correct answer is the definition of massage manipulations.

2. c

Factual recall

Rationale: Osteokinematic movement is produced voluntarily.

3. b

Factual recall

Rationale: The question defines pétrissage/kneading.

4. d

Factual recall

Rationale: Only gliding requires the use of lubricant.

5. a

Factual recall

Rationale: The incorrect answers may increase the tickle sensation.

6. d

Factual recall

Rationale: Only rocking does not require that the client actively contracts muscle groups.

7. b

Factual recall

Rationale: The question describes postisometric relaxation.

8. d

Factual recall

Rationale: The veins in the legs are more susceptible to blood clot development.

9. c

Factual recall

Rationale: The question describes a common application of effleurage/gliding.

10. a

Factual recall

Rationale: Pathogen transmission through the mucous membranes in the face is a matter of concern.

11. c

Factual recall

Rationale: The chest area should be draped carefully to protect breast tissue.

12. d

Factual recall

Rationale: The back is often massaged longer than is effective.

13. b

Factual recall

Rationale: Gliding effectively creates tension force.

14. b

Factual recall

Rationale: Twisting creates torsion force.

15. d

Factual recall

Rationale: This is the definition of friction.

16. c

Factual recall

Rationale: Kneading/pétrissage results in bending and torsion forces.

Answers and Rationales to Application/ Concept Identification and Clinical Reasoning/Synthesis Questions

1. d

Application and concept identification

Rationale: This type of massage application would stimulate the body, increasing alertness.

2. c

Application and concept identification

Rationale: The rhythm of the massage was not appropriate to the client's needs.

3. a

Application and concept identification

Rationale: In this particular situation, gliding is the best choice.

4. c

Application and concept identification

Rationale: Only tapping is appropriate for the face.

5. a

Application and concept identification

Rationale: Passive joint movement is the best choice for assessing range of motion because all the other methods involve a muscle contraction.

6. a

Application and concept identification

Rationale: Only if proper stabilization is used can joint movement isolate its effects.

7. c

Application and concept identification

Rationale: Postisometric relaxation methods first cause the target muscle to contract. In this instance, the contraction is causing cramping.

8. a

Application and concept identification

Rationale: Only the correct answer lists methods that do not stimulate a sympathetic response.

9. d

Application and concept identification

Rationale: Any of the possible answers would allow the neck to be massaged, but the side-lying position provides the best mechanical advantage for the massage therapist to use efficient body mechanics.

10. d

Application and concept identification

Rationale: Compression on the lymphatic plexuses located in the hands and feet would provide the best outcome among the methods listed as possible answers.

11. a

Application and concept identification

Rationale: Of those listed, skin rolling is the best method by which to affect the connective tissue.

12. c

Application and concept identification

Rationale: Compression does not require lubricant.

13. b

Clinical reasoning and synthesis

Rationale: Increased range of motion can be achieved through mechanical methods. An analysis of the incorrect answers indicates that the information is flawed or is not presented in context with the question.

14. b

Clinical reasoning and synthesis

Rationale: All methods listed may provide benefit, but focused stretching is used most specifically to increase range of motion by creating more pliable tissue.

15. b

Clinical reasoning and synthesis

Rationale: The connective tissue method would most enhance mobility in the lumbar and hip region. Lymphatic drainage is not focused on the goal. Answers *c* and *d* present other types of muscle energy methods.

16. a

Clinical reasoning and synthesis

Rationale: Usually, back tension is caused by shortening of the soft tissue structures of the chest.

17. b

Clinical reasoning and synthesis

Rationale: The key to the correct answer is sensitivity to pressure. Only the correct answer provides a method that can be applied lightly, although the side-lying position allows the client to see more of what is happening, thus making the client more comfortable.

18. b

Clinical reasoning and synthesis

Rationale: The problem presented by the question involves which body areas should be massaged in a

limited time to achieve the strongest relaxation effect. Face, hands, and feet have the largest nervous system distribution.

ASSESSMENT PROCEDURES FOR DEVELOPING A CARE PLAN

Answers and Rationales to Factual Recall Questions

1. a

Factual recall

Rationale: The question is providing an example of a breakdown in rapport.

2. d

Factual recall

Rationale: The sequence of assessment places interpretation of the data after data collection.

3. d

Factual recall

Rationale: The question provides an example of assessment by observation.

4. a

Factual recall

Rationale: The question provides an example of an open-ended question.

5. c

Factual recall

Rationale: The therapist needs to confirm the information received during subjective assessment with the client, to ensure that the therapist understands it.

6. c

Factual recall

Rationale: Single-session massage applications do not require an extensive assessment process, but the therapist does need to identify possible contraindications.

7. b

Factual recall

Rationale: Symmetry means the same on both sides, as is reflected in the correct answer.

8. a

Factual recall

Rationale: Arms swinging freely opposite the leg swing is part of a normal gait pattern.

9. c

Factual recall

Rationale: The question gives an example of palpation.

10. b

Factual recall

Rationale: The only answer that focuses palpation to the skin surface is light fingertip stroking to assess for areas of dampness or drag.

11. a

Factual recall

Rationale: End feel is identified by passive joint movement as an assessment method.

12. d
Factual recall
Rationale: Pulses assess arterial circulation.

13. c
Factual recall
Rationale: Grooves in fascial sheaths are where the massage practitioner would focus palpation assessment for the status of acupuncture meridians.

14. b
Factual recall
Rationale: Flexors are typically stronger than extensors.

15. a
Factual recall
Rationale: Only measuring skinfold by lifting the tissue would identify connective tissue shortening.

Answers and Rationales to Application/Concept Identification and Clinical Reasoning/Synthesis Questions

1. b
Application and concept identification
Rationale: Immediate application of an intervention method changed the condition before there was a chance to gather more information to understand the rest of the pattern.

2. b
Application and concept identification
Rationale: Synergistic or fixator muscles should not be recruited. If this happens, the pressure is excessive.

3. d
Application and concept identification
Rationale: The client is gesturing. Pulling on tissue usually indicates connective tissue shortening.

4. c
Application and concept identification
Rationale: The question presents an example of a clinical reasoning process. Brainstorming generates options.

5. d
Application and concept identification
Rationale: The client has resourceful compensation that was disturbed by the massage intervention.

6. d
Application and concept identification
Rationale: Evaluation of a treatment plan is an analytic process that involves the use of the clinical reasoning model. One area that is considered is the feelings of the persons involved, and this is the area that the question targets. Answers a and b pertain to fact gathering, and answer c involves brainstorming. Only answer d indicates the feelings of the persons involved because compliance is all about feelings.

7. b
Application and concept identification
Rationale: This is an example of the gait aspect of kinetic chain reflex interactions.

8. a
Clinical reasoning and synthesis
Rationale: The correct answer describes a repetitive movement pattern that, over time, could affect shoulder girdle position.

9. d
Clinical reasoning and synthesis
Rationale: The correct answer describes a common compensation pattern.

10. a
Clinical reasoning and synthesis
Rationale: The area described is the thorax. The facts of the question report the dysfunction as a pulling, which typically results from contracted muscles or shortened connective tissue, and often from both. The shortened tissues described in the wrong answers would not result in the postural change.

11. b
Clinical reasoning and synthesis
Rationale: If internal rotation is increased, the muscles that produce this movement are overly tense with inhibited external rotators, or the connective tissue of the area is shortened, thus pulling the shoulder into internal rotation. If the condition is recent, it is probably neuromuscular; if it is chronic, a myofascial shortening aspect to the dysfunction is likely. Local intervention to the area is best achieved by combining muscle energy methods to restore a normal resting length with stretching to enhance the pliability of connective tissue in the area. Answers a and d would increase the weakness of the external rotators. Answer c would enhance the contraction of the internal rotator.

12. d
Clinical reasoning synthesis
Rationale: The shoulder should not have a hard end feel. Typically, a hard end feel indicates joint dysfunction.

COMPLEMENTARY BODYWORK SYSTEMS

Answers and Rationales to Factual Recall Questions

1. a
Factual recall
Rationale: Eastern and Asian bodywork methods focus on meridians and points.

2. d
Factual recall
Rationale: Cold applications of hydrotherapy to reduce swelling are called antiedemic.

3. b
Factual recall
Rationale: The question describes an effect of cold after the primary effect, which is increased localized circulation.

4. c

Factual recall

Rationale: A neutral bath is 92—98°F.

5. d

Factual recall

Rationale: A pack is a folded towel soaked in water of the desired temperature and placed on a large area of skin.

6. c

Factual recall

Rationale: The base of the large toe is the area on the foot that would affect the neck.

7. a

Factual recall

Rationale: The correct answer provides a scientific explanation for the benefits of foot massage.

8. d

Factual recall

Rationale: Myofascial methods are focused most specifically on change in the ground substance.

9. b

Factual recall

Rationale: The correct answer describes the physiologic effects of deep transverse friction-controlled inflammation.

10. a

Factual recall

Rationale: Muscles that contain trigger points must be lengthened to restore normal resting length. No more than 15 minutes of this type of intervention is recommended.

11. d

Factual recall

Rationale: Trigger points refer pain.

12. b

Factual recall

Rationale: Lavender is a safe and commonly used essential oil. Clove is not. Spirulina is a seaweed that is used in thalassotherapy baths, and paraffin is a heat application.

13. b

Factual recall

Rationale: Dry brush is specific for circulation. Answers *a* and *c* relate to exfoliation, and Mylar is a material that is used for wraps.

Answers and Rationales to Application/Concept Identification and Clinical Reasoning/Synthesis Questions

1. c

Application and concept identification

Rationale: The approach that is the most appropriate self-help method is hydrotherapy.

2. b

Application and concept identification

Rationale: Deep transverse friction is too aggressive. Compression and lymphatic drain are likely to be less effective than the correct answer, which is superficial myofascial release.

3. c

Application and concept identification

Rationale: Changes that occur when a condition such as trigger points becomes chronic instead of acute involve fibrotic changes.

4. b

Application and concept identification

Rationale: The recommendation for treatment of trigger points is to use least invasive measures first. The wrong answers are too aggressive (answers *a* and *c*) or provide misinformation (answer *d*).

5. d

Application and concept identification

Rationale: Various levels of pressure are used, and direction can vary as well. Fluid movement in the lymphatic system is slow, and the massage mimics a pump.

6. d

Application and concept identification

Rationale: Weight loss is a healthcare intervention that commonly involves medical expertise.

7. c

Application and concept identification

Rationale: Although spas are innovative and creative, a common theme involves various applications of hydrotherapy.

8. a

Clinical reasoning and synthesis

Rationale: The facts presented in the question offer a logical explanation for mild edema. The correct answer describes the combination of methods recommended to support normal lymphatic function. The incorrect answers present misinformation or less effective applications of methods.

9. b

Clinical reasoning and synthesis

Rationale: The main focus is on increasing arterial blood flow without interfering with performance. Any massage longer than 30 minutes would be fatiguing, which eliminates answers *a* and *c*. Any work that would substantially change muscle tone or create pain is contraindicated before an athletic performance, so the only logical answer is answer *b*.

10. b

Clinical reasoning and synthesis

Rationale: The only clear indication for lymphatic drainage is the condition described in the correct answer. The other scenarios are risky unless physician support is provided.

ADAPTIVE MASSAGE

Answers and Rationales to Factual Recall Questions

1. b
   Factual recall
   Rationale: Massage methods do not change, but because everyone is unique and certain populations need adaptations, special situations require additional study.

2. a
   Factual recall
   Rationale: For many, massage is the professional structure for human contact.

3. d
   Factual recall
   Rationale: Pleasurable and secure touch supports bonding.

4. c
   Factual recall
   Rationale: Working with special populations in a health-care setting requires special attention to record-keeping.

5. a
   Factual recall
   Rationale: The most common accommodation for those with physical disability is barrier-free access to the facility.

6. d
   Factual recall
   Rationale: In this population, a common factor that can be managed with massage is breathing in excess of demand, which triggers a sympathetic nervous system dominance pattern that contributes to anxiety symptoms.

7. c
   Factual recall
   Rationale: Deep abdominal massage is contraindicated for a client in the first trimester of pregnancy.

8. b
   Factual recall
   Rationale: Palliative care is indicated for a client with a terminal illness.

9. b
   Factual recall
   Rationale: Nausea, capsulitis, and heat cramp are not medical emergencies, but heatstroke is life-threatening.

Answers and Rationales to Application/Concept Identification and Clinical Reasoning/Synthesis Questions

1. c
   Application and concept identification
   Rationale: The question describes dissociation and provides a logical explanation for why the client might respond in such a way.

2. c
   Application and concept identification
   Rationale: Rehabilitation massage is being performed to help with the athlete's healing process.

3. c
   Application and concept identification
   Rationale: Ethical concerns relate to breast massage for the female client. Scar tissue massage is the most relevant form of massage to the breast area.

4. b
   Application and concept identification
   Rationale: Dealing with those with chronic pain can frustrate the massage professional.

5. b
   Application and concept identification
   Rationale: With mental health issues, the ability of the client to make an informed decision is a priority.

6. a
   Clinical reasoning and synthesis
   Rationale: Answers b, c, and d describe conditions that are more complex than growing pains.

7. c
   Application and concept identification
   Rationale: Laceration is a wound type. Muscle guarding and cramp is a neurologic issue, but delayed-onset muscle soreness is a fluid and inflammation issue.

8. c
   Application and concept identification
   Rationale: Breast changes and constipation are common in the first trimester. Positioning is provided for comfort, but preeclampsia is a medical emergency.

9. d
   Clinical reasoning and synthesis
   Rationale: Grade 3 strain is a regional contraindication in the acute phase. Answers b and c do not respond to massage as a primary treatment, but massage can be used to address the tight and rubbing structures involved in tendonitis.

WELLNESS EDUCATION

Answers and Rationales to Factual Recall Questions

1. b
   Factual recall
   Rationale: The question provides an example of mind issues.

2. b
   Factual recall
   Rationale: The question provides an example of defensive measures.

3. c
   Factual recall
   Rationale: The reduction in demand means letting go of something to lighten the stress load.

4. d
   Factual recall
   Rationale: The correct answer describes correct breathing when relaxed.

5. d
   Factual recall
   Rationale: The three wrong answers can interfere with sleep.
6. a
   Factual recall
   Rationale: The question defines effective coping.

Answers and Rationales to Application and Concept Identification Questions

1. a
   Application and concept identification
   Rationale: The correct answer states a logical connection. All three of the wrong answers present incorrect information.
2. c
   Application and concept identification
   Rationale: Although massage can support various lifestyle changes, it can influence breathing function directly.
3. a
   Application and concept identification
   Rationale: The client has not exercised extensively and likely is deconditioned.
4. b
   Application and concept identification
   Rationale: A walking program would stimulate aerobic function and is continuous.

CHAPTER 8: Anatomy, Physiology, and Pathology

THE BODY AS A WHOLE

Answers and Rationales to Factual Recall Questions

1. c
   Factual recall
   Rationale: Adenosine triphosphate is a compound that stores energy in muscle. This energy is released during the chemical process of catabolism.
2. a
   Factual recall
   Rationale: The question is the definition of matrix.
3. d
   Factual recall
   Rationale: The question is a definition of metabolism.
4. c
   Factual recall
   Rationale: The question describes a function of electrons.
5. d
   Factual recall
   Rationale: The question is the definition of a chemical reaction.
6. a
   Factual recall
   Rationale: The question is a definition of metabolism.
7. a
   Factual recall
   Rationale: The question is the definition of anabolism.
8. d
   Factual recall
   Rationale: The question describes an organelle function. Ribosomes manufacture proteins.
9. a
   Factual recall
   Rationale: Of the four listed components that make up cells, water is the most abundant.
10. b
    Factual recall
    Rationale: Mitosis is the reproductive process of cells.
11. c
    Factual recall
    Rationale: The question is the definition of differentiation.
12. d
    Factual recall
    Rationale: The question describes a function of basement membrane.
13. a
    Factual recall
    Rationale: Skin is the largest cutaneous membrane.
14. c
    Factual recall
    Rationale: The question is the definition of serous membranes.
15. b
    Factual recall
    Rationale: Of the four tissue types, connective tissue is the most abundant in the body.
16. a
    Factual recall
    Rationale: Support is a major function of connective tissue.
17. c
    Factual recall
    Rationale: Areolar connective tissue has a high vascularity, in contrast to the other types mentioned, which have limited blood flow.
18. a
    Factual recall
    Rationale: The question describes the location of dense regular connective tissue.
19. c
    Factual recall
    Rationale: The question is the definition of an osteoblast.
20. b
    Factual recall

Rationale: Deforming collagen creates a piezoelectric current.

21. b

Factual recall

Rationale: The thigh is a regional location. Physiology relates to function, not location. Systems anatomy describes body systems such as the digestive system and muscular system. Collagenous fibers are made of connective tissue; they do not represent a body location.

22. a

Factual recall

Rationale: Basement membrane relates to epithelial tissue, and reticular fibers relate to connective tissue.

Answers and Rationales to Application and Concept Identification Questions

1. c

Application and concept identification

Rationale: The question asks for an application of the study of physiology to massage and bodywork. Most benefits derived from massage are the result of physiologic changes. The potential of these changes helps in determining the outcomes of the massage.

2. a

Application and concept identification

Rationale: The question is asking for the relationship between two concepts that define life. Although anatomy can be studied on cadavers, physiology is apparent when life is manifested.

3. a

Application and concept identification

Rationale: The question asks for an understanding of homeostasis and its relationship to the development of disease. The chemical level of the organizational structure of the body is often where homeostasis begins to break down and disease begins.

4. a

Application and concept identification

Rationale: Massage generates a stimulus to chemical reactions.

5. b

Application and concept identification

Rationale: Many massage treatment benefits are derived from chemical reactions.

6. a

Application and concept identification

Rationale: The only answer provided that correctly describes connective tissue is related to the properties of cells and the composition of the matrix.

7. a

Application and concept identification

Rationale: Hyaline cartilage is found at the ends of bones in synovial joints such as the hip and knee and is subject to damage caused by repetitive movement.

8. d

Application and concept identification

Rationale: Massage methods applied to connective tissue affect its thixotropic properties by agitating ground substance and encouraging a softer, more pliable texture.

9. c

Application and concept identification

Rationale: The question describes changes in body function, or physiology. Organizational physiology targets how the organs all function together. Function is physiology, not anatomy, and characteristics of life are not relevant to the question.

10. c

Application and concept identification

Rationale: The term *lipid* relates to fat. Answer *a* is wrong because it indicates a diet high in fat. Answer *b* is incorrect because amino acids are related to protein. Carbohydrates are sugars and starches, not fats.

MECHANISMS OF HEALTH AND DISEASE

Answers and Rationales to Factual Recall Questions

1. c

Factual recall

Rationale: The question is a definition of stress.

2. d

Factual recall

Rationale: The question lists the parts of a feedback loop.

3. b

Factual recall

Rationale: The question gives a definition of negative feedback.

4. a

Factual recall

Rationale: Circadian patterns keep body rhythms organized.

5. a

Factual recall

Rationale: The question gives a definition of health.

6. b

Factual recall

Rationale: The question gives a definition of pathology.

7. d

Factual recall

Rationale: The question gives a definition of a syndrome.

8. c

Factual recall

Rationale: The question gives a definition of chronic.

9. a

Factual recall

Rationale: "Parasites" is the only answer that fits the criterion of being pathogenic organisms.

10. c

Factual recall

Rationale: A neoplasm is abnormal tissue growth, hyperplasia is an uncontrolled increase in cell number, and the definition of benign includes growths that are contained and encapsulated as opposed to malignant, which is a nonencapsulated mass.

11. d
    Factual recall
    Rationale: The question gives a definition of anaplasia.
12. d
    Factual recall
    Rationale: The question gives a definition of inflammation.
13. b
    Factual recall
    Rationale: The question asks for the function of exudates, which is to dilute irritants that cause inflammation.
14. a
    Factual recall
    Rationale: Histamine is a vasodilator.
15. b
    Factual recall
    Rationale: The correct answer describes the function of increased fluid volume during inflammation.
16. b
    Factual recall
    Rationale: Tissue repair that results in a scar is replacement.
17. d
    Factual recall
    Rationale: Collagen is the major component of scar tissue.
18. b
    Factual recall
    Rationale: The correct answer describes risk factors appropriately, whereas the incorrect answers are not correlated to the information in the question.
19. d
    Factual recall
    Rationale: Pain is the chief complaint over the other three listed.
20. a
    Factual recall
    Rationale: The question describes a function of pain.
21. d
    Factual recall
    Rationale: The question is the definition of deep pain.
22. c
    Factual recall
    Rationale: Organ pain is perceived as an aching. Differentiation of the types of pain is important so that appropriate referral can be made to the physician.
23. c
    Factual recall
    Rationale: The soma relates to the soft tissue elements described in the question.
24. a
    Factual recall
    Rationale: The question is a definition of counterirritation.
25. d
    Factual recall
    Rationale: The question is a definition of referred pain.

26. c
    Factual recall
    Rationale: Aspirin has an effect on pain perception through its effects on prostaglandins.
27. d
    Factual recall
    Rationale: The question is a definition of the general adaptation syndrome.
28. a
    Factual recall
    Rationale: The only term listed in the answer that is related to breathing is *hyperventilation syndrome*, which is a common functional disturbance of the stress response.
29. c
    Factual recall
    Rationale: The very young and the old are not as capable of maintaining homeostasis, whereas young adults and those in the middle of life are most able to stay healthy.

Answers and Rationales to Application/Concept Identification and Clinical Reasoning/Synthesis Questions

1. c
   Application and concept identification
   Rationale: If massage caused a decrease in blood pressure, this would be a negative feedback response.
2. b
   Application and concept identification
   Rationale: Entrainment concerns body rhythms, general adaptation syndrome relates to the stress response, and threshold and tolerance describe aspects of pain. Only feedback loop addresses the information in the question.
3. a
   Application and concept identification
   Rationale: Specifically, hypnosis and medication are not within the scope of practice of massage, and none of the terms is a risk factor. These methods are not specific for treating inflammation.
4. d
   Application and concept identification
   Rationale: The listed terms are symptoms. They do not necessarily involve inflammation, and they are not necessarily genetic.
5. c
   Application and concept identification
   Rationale: Information exchange is necessary for a feedback loop, and feedback loops support homeostasis.
6. d
   Application and concept identification
   Rationale: The question is asking about a connection between massage and feedback loops. Massage and bodywork methods initially are processed as a stress stimulus.

7. a

Application and concept identification

Rationale: The correct answer identifies how massage begins a feedback process.

8. d

Application and concept identification

Rationale: Three concepts are correlated: biologic rhythms, entrainment, and autonomic nervous system functions. All three must be connected correctly. Only answer *d* is correct.

9. c

Application and concept identification

Rationale: The question asks about the physiologic outcomes of certain massage methods when used to resolve a type of chronic inflammation. This is done by creating a controlled therapeutic inflammation, and friction, stretching, and pulling of tissue are the best methods to accomplish this goal.

10. b

Application and concept identification

Rationale: The question asks for a correlation between symptoms and referred pain patterns. The kidney most often refers pain to the lumbar area.

11. a

Application and concept identification

Rationale: Massage therapy is a stimulus, and analgesia relates to pain.

12. b

Application and concept identification

Rationale: The hypothalamus is the first responder to the perception of threat; then the hypothalamus releases corticotropin-releasing hormones.

13. d

Clinical reasoning and synthesis

Rationale: The facts of the question describe the referred pain pattern of the gallbladder.

14. c

Clinical reasoning and synthesis

Rationale: The question is asking for an explanation for a client behavior—in this instance, high pain tolerance. The other answers describe a massage outcome or a response that is contradictory (i.e., if endorphin levels drop, then the client would be more aware of pain, not less aware of pain).

15. b

Clinical reasoning and synthesis

Rationale: Answer *a* is incorrect because there is no such thing as stress threshold straining, and cortisol is usually an immune suppressant. Answer *c* is incorrect because the client's adaptive capacity is inadequate, and the client's stress levels, including age, decrease adaptive capacity.

MEDICAL TERMINOLOGY

Answers and Rationales to Factual Recall Questions

1. c

Factual recall

Rationale: A prefix, root, or suffix is based on Latin or Greek word elements.

2. a

Factual recall

Rationale: The prefix *auto-* means "self."

3. c

Factual recall

Rationale: The prefix meaning "against" or "opposite" is *contra-*.

4. d

Factual recall

Rationale: The prefix *mal-* means "illness" or "disease."

5. c

Factual recall

Rationale: The prefix for "hard" is *scler(o)-*.

6. b

Factual recall

Rationale: The root word *pneum(o)-* means "lung" or "gas."

7. a

Factual recall

Rationale: The root word for "kidney" is *nephr(o)-*.

8. c

Factual recall

Rationale: The suffix for "pain" is *-algia*.

9. a

Factual recall

Rationale: The suffix *-pnea* means "to breathe."

10. d

Factual recall

Rationale: The question is a definition of clinical reasoning.

11. a

Factual recall

Rationale: The question is a definition of subjective data.

12. b

Factual recall

Rationale: The question is a definition of functional assessment.

13. b

Factual recall

Rationale: The question is a definition of objective data.

14. c

Factual recall

Rationale: The question is a definition of analysis.

15. c

Factual recall

Rationale: The question is representative of information in a plan.

16. c

Factual recall

Rationale: The question is a list of structures in the axial area.

17. d

Factual recall

Rationale: The bladder is located in the hypogastric region of the abdomen.

18. a

Factual recall

Rationale: The liver is located in the right upper quadrant.

19. a

Factual recall

Rationale: Flexion decreases the angle of a joint.

20. c

Factual recall

Rationale: The term meaning "on the same side" is *ipsilateral.*

21. d

Factual recall

Rationale: The term meaning "closer to the trunk or point of origin" is *proximal.*

22. c

Factual recall

Rationale: The question is representative of information that correlates Eastern theory with Western science. Many different systems have developed a point theory, and the location of these points consistently falls over nerves and sensory receptors.

23. b

Factual recall

Rationale: They are prefixes.

24. c

Factual recall

Rationale: The occipital area is where the head joins the neck.

Answers and Rationales to Application/ Concept Identification and Clinical Reasoning/Synthesis Questions

1. b

Application and concept identification

Rationale: Twisted would be a rotation, and rotation occurs in the transverse plane. Abduction does not occur in the sagittal plane, and flexion and extension are sagittal plane movements.

2. c

Application and concept identification

Rationale: Whenever nonstandard abbreviations are used, a deciphering key is necessary.

3. b

Application and concept identification

Rationale: Accumulated experience provided the base for consistent patterns observed by ancient healers.

NERVOUS SYSTEM BASICS AND THE CENTRAL NERVOUS SYSTEM

Answers and Rationales to Factual Recall Questions

1. d

Factual recall

Rationale: The correct answer is a primary function of this specialized connective tissue. The three wrong answers describe other nervous system functions.

2. a

Factual recall

Rationale: Myelin, dendrites, and axons do not form or secrete any substance. Only Schwann cells form myelin and its outer covering, which is called the neurilemma.

3. a

Factual recall

Rationale: The question is a definition of sensory neurons.

4. b

Factual recall

Rationale: The question is the definition of membrane potential when the nerve is at rest.

5. c

Factual recall

Rationale: The question describes a function of neurilemma.

6. a

Factual recall

Rationale: The question describes a function of neurotransmitters.

7. b

Factual recall

Rationale: The question describes a function of acetylcholine.

8. c

Factual recall

Rationale: The question describes a function of the cerebrum.

9. c

Factual recall

Rationale: The question describes the location of the corpus callosum.

10. b

Factual recall

Rationale: The question describes a function of the parietal lobe.

11. a

Factual recall

Rationale: The question describes integrative functions of the cortex.

12. b

Factual recall

Rationale: The question describes a function of the reticular activating system.

13. d

Factual recall

Rationale: The question describes a function of parietal lobes in the brain.

14. c
Factual recall
Rationale: The question describes a function of the limbic system.

15. c
Factual recall
Rationale: The question describes substances that affect the central nervous system.

16. d
Factual recall
Rationale: The question describes a function of the medulla oblongata.

17. a
Factual recall
Rationale: The question describes a function of the thalamus.

18. a
Factual recall
Rationale: The question describes a function of the cerebellum.

19. d
Factual recall
Rationale: The question describes the location of the pia mater.

20. b
Factual recall
Rationale: Substance P enhances pain transmission.

Answers and Rationales to Application/Concept Identification and Clinical Reasoning/Synthesis Questions

1. d
Application and concept identification
Rationale: The physiology of these two systems is involved in the control of body function.

2. c
Application and concept identification
Rationale: The question asks how massage causes the neuron to transmit a signal. A stimulus such as the pressure of massage causes a change in the charge of one segment of a neuron. This is depolarization.

3. b
Application and concept identification
Rationale: The refractory period occurs after nerve transmission. During this time, the nerve does not readily respond to stimuli, which allows the muscle that it controls to be lengthened.

4. d
Application and concept identification
Rationale: The question describes a function of dopamine in relationship to behavior.

5. b
Application and concept identification

Rationale: The question provides half of a balancing pair of neurotransmitters. Enkephalin inhibits pain signals, and substance P transmits pain signals.

6. a
Application and concept identification
Rationale: The question describes a function of histamine in relationship to behavior. You must define all terms in the question and in the answers before you can answer the question correctly.

7. c
Application and concept identification
Rationale: The question describes a function of serotonin in relationship to behavior and in response to massage.

8. a
Application and concept identification
Rationale: The question describes functions of serotonin and endorphin in relationship to massage applications.

9. a
Application and concept identification
Rationale: The question asks for an application of central nervous system functions. Only the correct answer is reasonable in relation to the concept of higher consciousness.

10. c
Application and concept identification
Rationale: The question asks for an application of central nervous system function and an interpretation of sensory perception that is based on sensory and motor distribution in these areas of the brain. Only the correct answer explains why self-massage is less than successful.

11. a
Application and concept identification
Rationale: The question is asking for an understanding of how sensory signals of massage are processed.

12. b
Application and concept identification
Rationale: The question is asking for an understanding of how massage may be indicated for pathologic conditions of the central nervous system. Lower motor neuron injury results in flaccid muscles, and the pumping action of muscles in assisting fluid movement is lost.

13. c
Application and concept identification
Rationale: Depression may respond to an increase in the availability of neurotransmitters described in the question. Schizophrenia may temporarily worsen. The other two are not linked directly to neurotransmitters.

14. b
Application and concept identification
Rationale: Essential tremor is not affected by massage.

15. a
Application and concept identification
Rationale: Because only one limb is effective in monoplegia, walking may be possible. Answers *b, c,* and *d* would limit the ability to walk.

16. d

Application and concept identification

Rationale: An aneurysm is a bulging artery. A contusion is a bruise that the client may have, but the symptoms indicate a concussion. Answer *c* is a stroke.

17. d

Application and concept identification

Rationale: Epinephrine is a central nervous system stimulant. Therefore, sleep would be disturbed, the skeletal system would be tense, and serotonin would be decreased. Dopamine is also a stimulant.

PERIPHERAL NERVOUS SYSTEM

Answers and Rationales to Factual Recall Questions

1. c

Factual recall

Rationale: The question is a definition of somatic nerves.

2. b

Factual recall

Rationale: The question is a definition of nerves.

3. c

Factual recall

Rationale: The connective tissue covering that surrounds the fasciculus is called perineurium.

4. a

Factual recall

Rationale: The vagus nerve affects visceral function.

5. a

Factual recall

Rationale: The dorsal root ganglion contains cell bodies of sensory neurons.

6. a

Factual recall

Rationale: The phrenic nerve is part of the cervical plexus.

7. c

Factual recall

Rationale: The obturator nerve is found in the lumbar plexus.

8. c

Factual recall

Rationale: Blood pressure is monitored by visceroreceptors that detect changes in the internal body environment.

9. d

Factual recall

Rationale: Most reflexes do not make their way past the brainstem, so the spinal cord is the correct answer.

10. c

Factual recall

Rationale: The question is the definition of a proprioceptor.

11. a

Factual recall

Rationale: The question describes a function of the parasympathetic system.

12. a

Factual recall

Rationale: The question describes the locations of sympathetic nerves and ganglia near the spine.

13. b

Factual recall

Rationale: The term *adrenergic* is used to describe sympathetic stimulation, and epinephrine is one of the neurotransmitters involved.

14. a

Factual recall

Rationale: The main neurotransmitter of the parasympathetic system is acetylcholine.

15. b

Factual recall

Rationale: The terms in the answers are related to the ear, but only the term *ossicles* describes the bones.

16. a

Factual recall

Rationale: The question asks for a specific visual interpretation, which is processed in the frontal lobes.

17. b

Factual recall

Rationale: The only logical answer is answer *b*.

18. a

Factual recall

Rationale: The only logical answer is answer *a*.

19. c

Factual recall

Rationale: Only the turbinate is located in the nose.

20. d

Factual recall

Rationale: Only the proprioceptors are specific for detecting movement.

21. d

Factual recall

Rationale: Of the offered combinations, only answer *d* includes both conditions that have a viral cause.

Answers and Rationales to Application/ Concept Identification and Clinical Reasoning/Synthesis Questions

1. c

Application and concept identification

Rationale: The femoral nerve is not part of the sacral plexus, the thoracodorsal nerve innervates the latissimus dorsi muscle, and the brachial plexus supplies the arm. By elimination, the lumbar plexus would contain the nerve that would explain these symptoms.

2. a

Application and concept identification

Rationale: Parasympathetic influence on the eye involves constriction of the pupil. This is an autonomic function, and the accessory nerve is a cranial nerve that influences speaking and movement of the head.

3. b

Application and concept identification

Rationale: Smell can be emotional because of the connection to emotional brain centers in the limbic system.

4. c

Application and concept identification

Rationale: Symptoms indicate that the lumbar plexus is involved.

5. b

Application and concept identification

Rationale: Symptoms indicate that the brachial plexus is involved.

6. a

Application and concept identification

Rationale: Symptoms described in the question result from inappropriate pressure on the greater auricular nerve.

7. d

Application and concept identification

Rationale: Symptoms indicate that a range in dermatome distribution between L1 and L3 is likely. Answer *d* is the only answer that represents this area.

8. b

Application and concept identification

Rationale: *Mono* means "one," and *poly* means "many." Many reflex actions are required before one can regain balance.

9. b

Application and concept identification

Rationale: The question describes sensations that indicate that the client is not getting used to the draping material. The ability of the nervous system to adapt to sensation is what allows the body to tolerate ongoing sensation.

10. d

Application and concept identification

Rationale: The question is asking for a connection between massage methods that create deep compressive forces and the sensory receptor affected. Ruffini end organs would respond to compressive force. The other mechanical sensory receptors listed respond more to light touch.

11. a

Application and concept identification

Rationale: The question is asking for a connection between massage methods that create deep compressive forces and the sensory receptor affected. Meissner's corpuscles adapt quickly.

12. c

Application and concept identification

Rationale: The question is asking for a connection between massage methods that create deep compressive forces and the sensory receptor affected and the location of that receptor. Muscle spindles are located

primarily in the belly of the muscle and are active when a muscle cramps.

13. d

Application and concept identification

Rationale: The question is asking for a connection between massage methods and reflex responses. Because the question describes a pattern involving opposite sides of the body, the contralateral reflex is the correct answer.

14. c

Application and concept identification

Rationale: The question is asking for a connection between massage methods and changes in the autonomic nervous system. Because the question describes a pattern of parasympathetic dominance, massage would have to be designed to inhibit sympathetic activation.

15. d

Application and concept identification

Rationale: The question is asking for a connection between the vestibule mechanism and massage application. Rocking of the head in particular affects this system.

16. c

Application and concept identification

Rationale: The question is asking for a connection between the vestibule mechanism, a pathologic condition, and massage application. Rocking of the head in particular can result in motion sickness.

17. a

Clinical reasoning and synthesis

Rationale: Coordination is disrupted, which is described as timing being off. Knowledge of the types of reflexes is necessary to select the best answer. Golf is something that is learned, so the conditioned reflex is the best answer.

18. b

Clinical reasoning and synthesis

Rationale: The symptoms include headache brought on by bright light, recent onset, and increased job stress. Increased workload is likely to stimulate sympathetic dominance. An effect of this is pupil dilation, which would increase light sensitivity. The incorrect answers do not describe the correct functions of the autonomic nervous system.

19. b

Clinical reasoning and synthesis

Rationale: The question is asking for identification of symptoms to support a referral. The facts of the question indicate brachial plexus involvement.

20. d

Clinical reasoning and synthesis

Rationale: The question is representative of a decision that is based on a pathologic condition. The question is asking for identification of symptoms to support an appropriate massage intervention. The facts of the question include a current outbreak of herpes zoster and pain. Each of the answers is a possible approach that would have to be analyzed before the best answer could be determined. Outcomes would include increased tolerance to pain and reduced pain perception. These outcomes are best achieved with parasympathetic dominance and an increase in serotonin and endorphins. In addition, appropriate sanitation is a factor. The client also is immune-compromised because an active infection is present. Only answer *d* addresses all of these issues.

21. c

Clinical reasoning and synthesis

Rationale: The question is asking for the development of realistic outcomes for massage intervention. The only fact is a diagnosis of neuralgia, which would have to be researched. Neuralgia is a noninflammatory disorder of the nerve that results in pain. Nerve pain is difficult to manage. The only logical answer is *c*.

22. c

Clinical reasoning and synthesis

Rationale: The question is representative of a decision that is based on a pathologic condition. The question is asking for identification of symptoms to support an appropriate massage intervention. The facts of the question include recent sleep disturbance, feeling of agitation, work stress, and a diagnosis of exogenous anxiety. Information about exogenous anxiety becomes part of the factual information and indicates that the client is reacting to changes in the environment. For this type of reactive anxiety, short-term therapy and medication use usually are successful. Massage would have to support these interventions. The only logical treatment plan is given in answer *c*.

ENDOCRINE SYSTEM

Answers and Rationales to Factual Recall Questions

1. c

Factual recall

Rationale: The question is a portion of the definition of a hormone.

2. a

Factual recall

Rationale: The correct answer describes a function of a hormone. The three incorrect answers are flawed and do not state true information in relationship to the question.

3. d

Factual recall

Rationale: *Hyper* means "too much."

4. c

Factual recall

Rationale: The question describes a function of the hypothalamus.

5. a

Factual recall

Rationale: The pituitary is the main source of tropic hormones.

6. a

Factual recall

Rationale: Epinephrine extends the fight-or-flight response produced by the sympathetic autonomic nervous system.

7. d

Factual recall

Rationale: Androgens are gonadocorticoids that are produced by the gonads and the adrenal glands.

8. c

Factual recall

Rationale: The pineal gland is responsive to light and dark cycles.

9. a

Factual recall

Rationale: Only prostaglandin is a tissue hormone.

Answers and Rationales to Application/Concept Identification and Clinical Reasoning/Synthesis Questions

1. c

Application and concept identification

Rationale: The primary influence on the endocrine system achieved by massage is a secondary effect that results from a shift in autonomic nervous system dominance. Lymphatic is more about fluids, and stimulation of mechanoreceptors has many different influences on the body, but most are directed to the somatic nervous system.

2. a

Application and concept identification

Rationale: Touch stimulates the hypothalamus, which in turn regulates the endocrine responses. The other responses have not been shown to result from massage application or are flawed in terminology.

3. d

Application and concept identification

Rationale: These are hypothyroid symptoms.

4. a

Application and concept identification

Rationale: The key is that prostaglandins are involved in inflammation and are influenced by aspirin.

5. a

Application and concept identification

Rationale: The nervous system responds quickly but sustained responses involve the endocrine system.

6. c

Application and concept identification

Rationale: The question is asking for a connection between hydrotherapy applications and pituitary hormones. The three incorrect answers involve anterior pituitary hormones that have not been shown to be influenced by cold applications.

7. c

Application and concept identification

Rationale: The pancreatic pathology of type 2 diabetes is defined in the correct answer. The three incorrect answers provide misinformation.

8. b

Application and concept identification

Rationale: Cortisol exerts a long-term effect on the body and therefore is more involved with resistance to stress.

9. a

Application and concept identification

Rationale: The question asks for a connection between long-term stress and the development of diabetes. Only answer a makes the correct correlation.

10. a

Application and concept identification

Rationale: An effect of androgen is increased facial hair and acne.

11. b

Clinical reasoning and synthesis

Rationale: The facts presented by the question include an elderly client, slow tissue healing, gradual weight loss, and improvement in all areas after 3 months of weekly massage. The question asks for justification of this outcome. Research has shown that touch stimulates the hypothalamus. A function of the hypothalamus is to stimulate the pituitary to produce and release growth hormone, which would account for the benefits observed.

12. b

Clinical reasoning and synthesis

Rationale: The facts presented by the question include a middle-aged woman, hypothyroid symptoms, increased stress and reduced ability to cope, and no blood work done during the physical. Hypothyroidism is the condition with these symptoms.

13. b

Clinical reasoning and synthesis

Rationale: The facts provided in the question include the client is a runner, has an inflamed knee, received a steroid injection at the site, and asks for deep massage to the area. Only answer b is a logical response. The other three answers present incorrect information. Massage at the site of a recent injection is contraindicated. Deep massage would tend to increase inflammation in the area. Corticosteroids would decrease tissue repair processes.

14. d

Clinical reasoning and synthesis

Rationale: Three types of information are presented in the question and in the possible answers: the behavior change and result, what primary endocrine function is disrupted, and what massage intervention would

support a return to homeostasis. All three areas must connect logically for a correct answer. Only in the correct answer does this occur.

15. b

Clinical reasoning and synthesis

Rationale: Oxytocin is influenced by touch and bonding and by parasympathetic dominance. Antidiuretic hormone influences water balance, and luteinizing hormone influences ovulation, progesterone, and testosterone. Cortisol would be most influenced by sleep. The adrenal hormone is specific, and during deep restorative sleep, it would be least active.

SKELETAL SYSTEM

Answers and Rationales to Factual Recall Questions

1. c
Factual recall
Rationale: Generating heat is a function of muscle, not of bone.

2. a
Factual recall
Rationale: The question is the definition of a sesamoid bone.

3. b
Factual recall
Rationale: The question asks for the elastic component of bone provided by the organic material.

4. d
Factual recall
Rationale: The question asks for the piezo material of bone, which is collagen.

5. c
Factual recall
Rationale: Periosteum is the external connective tissue covering of bone.

6. a
Factual recall
Rationale: The bone function that is described as a change in the bone in response to demand is remodeling.

7. b
Factual recall
Rationale: Cancellous bone contains trabeculae.

8. c
Factual recall
Rationale: Long bones contain a diaphysis.

9. b
Factual recall
Rationale: A depression on a bone is a fossa.

10. b
Factual recall
Rationale: The clavicle is located in the appendicular skeleton.

11. c
   Factual recall
   Rationale: The lambdoidal suture joins the parietal bones and the occipital bone.
12. a
   Factual recall
   Rationale: The vomer forms the structure of the nose.
13. c
   Factual recall
   Rationale: The thoracic vertebra has a superior articular facet.
14. d
   Factual recall
   Rationale: The olecranon fossa is located on the humerus.
15. a
   Factual recall
   Rationale: The coracoid process is located on the scapula.
16. c
   Factual recall
   Rationale: The nuchal ligament is palpated in the posterior cervical area.
17. d
   Factual recall
   Rationale: The costal angle is located on the rib.
18. b
   Factual recall
   Rationale: The foot contains 26 bones.
19. b
   Factual recall
   Rationale: Epicondyle, sulcus, and fissure refer to bony landmarks.
20. a
   Factual recall
   Rationale: Coccyx, occipital, and sternum are axial skeleton bones.
21. c
   Factual recall
   Rationale: Olecranon fossa and lesser tubercle are bony landmarks of the humerus.
22. b
   Factual recall
   Rationale: The lamina is located in the vertebral column.
23. d
   Factual recall
   Rationale: The acetabulum is part of the pelvis.
24. b
   Factual recall
   Rationale: When the area over the vertebral column is palpated, the structure most prominently felt is the spinous process.

Answers and Rationales to Application/Concept Identification and Clinical Reasoning/Synthesis Questions

1. d
   Application and concept identification
   Rationale: Scoliosis is characterized by curves in both areas. Scurvy and whiplash are not spinal deformities.
2. b
   Application and concept identification
   Rationale: This question asks about the connection between a structure that is connected with bone and an injury. If the trunk were placed in exaggerated extension, the anterior longitudinal ligament could be overstretched.
3. a
   Application and concept identification
   Rationale: The question is asking about the connection between hormone effects on bone and symptoms of aching. Answer *a* explains why this could be happening. The other three answers present incorrect information. Estrogen and testosterone produce long bone growth, but increasing estrogen levels, primarily in females, stop the growth. Because a male is described in the question, *a* is the correct answer.
4. a
   Application and concept identification
   Rationale: The question is asking what happens if the disk ruptures. The correct answer is narrowed disk space caused by leakage of the nucleus pulposus.
5. c
   Application and concept identification
   Rationale: The question asks for the name of an excessive lumbar curve that may be responsible for low back pain, which is lordosis.
6. d
   Clinical reasoning and synthesis
   Rationale: The facts in the question identify the predisposition to the pathologic condition osteoporosis. The question also indicates that caution should be used during the massage because osteoporosis predisposes one to bone fracture.
7. a
   Clinical reasoning and synthesis
   Rationale: The facts in the question include pain in the tibia and endurance running the day before. The most logical answer is a stress fracture, given the history provided by the question.

JOINTS

Answers and Rationales to Factual Recall Questions

1. c
   Factual recall
   Rationale: The function of simple joint design is stability and that of complex joint design is mobility.

2. d
   Factual recall
   Rationale: Many joints serve dual functions of stability and mobility.

3. b
   Factual recall
   Rationale: Hyaline cartilage is found at the ends of bone in synovial joints.

4. a
   Factual recall
   Rationale: A major component of ground substance is water.

5. c
   Factual recall
   Rationale: The question is the definition of creep.

6. a
   Factual recall
   Rationale: Amphiarthrosis is the type of joint that has the most limited mobility.

7. b
   Factual recall
   Rationale: Bones separated by fibrocartilage is *not* a characteristic of a synovial joint.

8. c
   Factual recall
   Rationale: Stratum fibrosum is highly innervated and serves as a source of sensory data related to movement and position of a joint.

9. b
   Factual recall
   Rationale: The question is the definition of arthrokinematics.

10. d
    Factual recall
    Rationale: The correct answer defines the close-packed position of a joint.

11. b
    Factual recall
    Rationale: The question is the definition of physiologic range of motion.

12. d
    Factual recall
    Rationale: The anatomic limits of motion of the knee are provided primarily by soft tissue, such as the joint capsule and ligaments, instead of by bone, as found in the elbow and hip. The ankle is similar to the knee but is held more stable by the bone structure.

13. c
    Factual recall
    Rationale: Eversion is a movement of the foot.

14. b
    Factual recall
    Rationale: Scapular retraction is movement toward the spine.

15. d
    Factual recall
    Rationale: A ball-and-socket joint is a multiaxial joint.

16. c
    Factual recall
    Rationale: The question is the definition of kinematic chains.

17. a
    Factual recall
    Rationale: The question describes the outcomes of functional change in closed kinematic chains.

18. c
    Factual recall
    Rationale: The two articulating bones of the temporomandibular joint are the mandible and temporal.

19. a
    Factual recall
    Rationale: The glenohumeral joint exhibits extensive mobility because it has range-of-motion limits provided primarily by soft tissue.

20. b
    Factual recall
    Rationale: Rotation is allowed at the sternoclavicular joint.

21. d
    Factual recall
    Rationale: The coracoclavicular ligament indirectly assists in stabilizing the acromioclavicular joint.

22. b
    Factual recall
    Rationale: The radioulnar joint allows for pronation and supination.

23. a
    Factual recall
    Rationale: Wrist movement is greatest in flexion and extension because the joint capsule is loose in superior and inferior directions.

24. c
    Factual recall
    Rationale: The joint at which the fingers join the body of the hand is called the metacarpophalangeal.

25. b
    Factual recall
    Rationale: The articulating bones of the sacroiliac joint are the sacrum and ilium.

26. d
    Factual recall
    Rationale: The sacroiliac joint is responsible for helping the vertebral column to remain relatively still during walking.

27. d
    Factual recall
    Rationale: The question describes the function of a meniscus.

28. c
    Factual recall
    Rationale: The most stable position is full dorsiflexion.
29. b
    Factual recall
    Rationale: The atlantoaxial joint allows rotation as a motion pattern.
30. d
    Factual recall
    Rationale: The costovertebral and costochondral joints are most active during breathing.
31. b
    Factual recall
    Rationale: The ribs are raised during inspiration.
32. a
    Factual recall
    Rationale: Plantar flexion occurs in the ankle, and pronation occurs in the wrist; c and d are similar actions.

Answers and Rationales to Application/Concept Identification and Clinical Reasoning/Synthesis Questions

1. c
   Application and concept identification
   Rationale: Only synovial joints are freely movable. The remaining terms indicate structures with limited movement.
2. d
   Application and concept identification
   Rationale: A convexity is characteristic of a bend strain to the ligament and a tension-based injury. The hit on the lateral side would cause a concavity. Shear force consists of concavities and convexities but does not fit the description of the injury.
3. d
   Application and concept identification
   Rationale: Inspiration is inhalation, and the ribs move up and out.
4. b
   Application and concept identification
   Rationale: The function of joints is based on stability and mobility. Bones, landmarks, articulations, diarthroses, and synovial fluid do not describe function.
5. a
   Application and concept identification
   Rationale: The question asks what happens when lax ligaments reduce stability, and the answer is that joint play increases. The concepts presented in the question include stability and laxity; in the answers, concepts include joint play, hypomobility, and muscle relaxation. The term *plasma membrane* refers to cellular structure.
6. c
   Application and concept identification
   Rationale: The question asks why the least-packed position is the most comfortable when a joint is injured.

7. d
   Application and concept identification
   Rationale: The question asks about the connection between a massage method (passive range of motion) and the way the method would be implemented. Only answer d correctly describes circumduction.
8. c
   Application and concept identification
   Rationale: The action described by the correct answer must result in external rotation of the hip. Only answer c is correct.
9. c
   Application and concept identification
   Rationale: The question is asking about the relationship between two joints: the sternoclavicular joint and the scapula.
10. b
    Application and concept identification
    Rationale: The question asks for an explanation as to why the heel would increase the potential for sprained ankle. The heel puts the ankle into plantar flexion, which is a less stable position for the ankle, predisposing one to ankle sprains.
11. a
    Application and concept identification
    Rationale: The connection between the location of the anterior longitudinal ligament and its function in relation to the vertebral joints means that this ligament stabilizes against trunk extension.
12. a
    Application and concept identification
    Rationale: The loose-packed position of the hip joint consists of flexion, abduction, and lateral rotation.
13. b
    Application and concept identification
    Rationale: If the leg is fixed and the pelvis moves forward into anteversion, the result is increased lordosis.
14. c
    Application and concept identification
    Rationale: The most stable position of the knee joint is in locked extension.
15. b
    Application and concept identification
    Rationale: In this situation, the medial ligament would be pushed into extension, causing damage.
16. c
    Application and concept identification
    Rationale: Only answer c is correct. Dislocation is contraindicated. Rheumatoid arthritis has a limited response to massage and requires caution. Kyphosis is structural.
17. b
    Clinical reasoning and synthesis
    Rationale: The facts presented in the question include a 1-year stretching program that was initially beneficial and increased the intensity of the program over the previous 3 months, resulting in joint pain. The question asks why

this is the outcome, given the changes in connective tissue structure. Only answer *b* presents correct information in relation to the facts of the question; it provides a logical explanation for decreased joint stability and the development of joint pain.

18. a

Clinical reasoning and synthesis

Rationale: The case study format presents the following facts: sensation of shortening in the lumbosacral area, confirmed by assessment revealing decreased mobility of the tissue in the area. Next, limits are put on the type of intervention allowed. Only answer *a* presents a treatment plan that is cautious yet effective. The three incorrect answers are not logical and would require cautions with their use.

19. d

Clinical reasoning and synthesis

Rationale: The facts presented by the question are limited to information about a hypermobile knee joint. Safe application of massage methods is always a priority. Answer *d* describes the most logical approach because protective and compensatory muscle contraction is not eliminated but instead is managed. The three wrong answers would further increase hypermobility.

20. c

Clinical reasoning and synthesis

Rationale: The facts presented in the question include information about multiple dislocations of a shoulder joint that now has reduced mobility and muscle spasms. Answer *c* describes the most logical approach because protective and compensatory muscle contraction is not eliminated but instead is managed. The three wrong answers would further increase underlying hypermobility.

21. a

Clinical reasoning and synthesis

Rationale: The facts include a broken wrist, an extended period of joint immobility while in a cast, and current limited range of motion of the wrist. The only probable outcome is that described in answer *a*. The condition described is hypomobility, so answer *c* can be eliminated. Muscles atrophy when immobile, so answer *b* can be eliminated. Answer *d* states the opposite of what is stated in the question.

22. c

Clinical reasoning and synthesis

Rationale: The facts presented in the question indicate that the disk bulged posteriorly, which would be the result of a flexion injury. The most common location in the lower back is at the lumbosacral junction.

23. d

Clinical reasoning and synthesis

Rationale: The question provides the following fact: the client has degenerative joint disease. The question also places cautions on treatment, indicating the need for conservative measures. The correct treatment plan would have to address the condition and the cautions.

Answer *d* presents the best plan. Bed rest is not indicated, nor is cortisone injection used for conservative treatment. Intense exercise and connective tissue massage are too aggressive.

24. a

Clinical reasoning and synthesis

Rationale: The facts from the question include repetitive strain injury, long-term decreased mobility, and reduced range of motion. Of possible reasons for the reduced range of motion, massage would best reverse muscle and connective tissue abnormality.

25. b

Clinical reasoning and synthesis

Rationale: Zero degrees is the anatomic position. The question is measuring a limit in flexion, so answer *b* is correct, and *a* and *c* should be eliminated. Answer *d* would indicate an increase in range of motion, not a decrease.

26. c

Clinical reasoning and synthesis

Rationale: An anterior tilt means that the ischial tuberosity is up and the iliac crest is moving forward. This would suggest that the hips need to flex.

MUSCLES

Answers and Rationales to Factual Recall Questions

1. b

Factual recall

Rationale: Adenosine triphosphate produces mechanical energy to exert force.

2. b

Factual recall

Rationale: Contractility is the ability of muscle tissue to shorten.

3. c

Factual recall

Rationale: The structural units of contraction in skeletal muscle fibers are called sarcomeres.

4. a

Factual recall

Rationale: The attachment of myosin to cross-bridges on actin requires calcium.

5. d

Factual recall

Rationale: The questions and the possible answers describe a physiologic process in terms of muscle contractile ability and control based on the number of muscle fibers per motor unit. The fewer the fibers, the more precise is the movement.

6. c

Factual recall

Rationale: A strong correlation has been noted among the locations of motor points, acupuncture points, and trigger points.

7. b
   Factual recall
   Rationale: The question is a definition of tone.
8. b
   Factual recall
   Rationale: The structure of capillaries is long and winding to accommodate the changes in muscle shape.
9. d
   Factual recall
   Rationale: The connective tissue is continuous with muscle fibers. The three incorrect answers describe functions of muscles.
10. a
   Factual recall
   Rationale: Intermuscular septa are formed primarily from deep fascia.
11. b
   Factual recall
   Rationale: The long head of biceps brachii is an example of an insertion also called the distal attachment.
12. b
   Factual recall
   Rationale: The question defines a function of pennate muscle shape.
13. c
   Factual recall
   Rationale: The question provides a function of smooth muscle.
14. d
   Factual recall
   Rationale: Before this question can be answered, a factual basis regarding attachments, innervation, function, myotatic unit, common trigger points, and referred pain patterns of the individual muscles is needed. The question asks about a referred pain pattern.
15. b
   Factual recall
   Rationale: Lateral pterygoid is a muscle of mastication.
16. a
   Factual recall
   Rationale: The muscles of the anterior triangle of the neck as defined by the sternocleidomastoid have a primary function of assisting in swallowing.
17. c
   Factual recall
   Rationale: Compression by the scalene group against the brachial nerve plexus often refers pain to the pectoralis, to the rhomboid area, and into the arm and hand.
18. b
   Factual recall
   Rationale: The question asks about myotatic unit interaction. The abdominal and psoas muscles are the major antagonists for longissimus thoracis.
19. d
   Factual recall
   Rationale: External intercostals may be involved because they lift the ribs.

20. a
   Factual recall
   Rationale: The question asks about a referred pain pattern. The muscle likely to be involved is quadratus lumborum.
21. c
   Factual recall
   Rationale: The question asks about origin and insertion. Rectus abdominis has the attachments described in the question.
22. a
   Factual recall
   Rationale: The question asks about nerve supply. Levator ani is innervated by the perineal division of the pudendal nerve.
23. b
   Factual recall
   Rationale: Trapezius has three distinct parts with distinct functions, allowing the muscle to be an antagonist to itself.
24. c
   Factual recall
   Rationale: Pectoralis minor and serratus anterior are likely to be tense and shortened if the scapular area is rounded forward and protracted.
25. d
   Factual recall
   Rationale: The question asks about the myotatic unit, particularly the antagonist to the subscapularis.
26. c
   Factual recall
   Rationale: The question asks about impaired function of an antagonist pattern. Latissimus dorsi is likely to be tight and short if a client is having difficulty raising the arm to comb the hair.
27. d
   Factual recall
   Rationale: Brachialis is attached to the distal half of the anterior surface of the humerus, medial and lateral intermuscular septa, and coronoid process and tuberosity of the ulna.
28. c
   Factual recall
   Rationale: The question asks about the myotatic unit. Anconeus is synergistic to triceps brachii.
29. a
   Factual recall
   Rationale: The question provides a definition of myotatic units.
30. b
   Factual recall
   Rationale: The question provides a definition of the flexor reflex.
31. b
   Factual recall
   Rationale: Opponens pollicis is located in the thenar eminence.

32. c

Factual recall

Rationale: Gluteus maximus extends, laterally rotates the hip joint with lower fibers, assists in adduction of the hip with the femur fixed, and assists in extension of the trunk.

33. d

Factual recall

Rationale: Piriformis is the deepest layer.

34. a

Factual recall

Rationale: Gemellus superior may be tense and shortened in a leg that is externally (laterally) rotated.

35. a

Factual recall

Rationale: The question asks about the myotatic unit. Biceps femoris and gluteus maximus are synergistic with each other.

36. c

Factual recall

Rationale: Sartorius is a flexor of the hip that assists in flexion of the torso to the thigh if the legs are fixed.

37. d

Factual recall

Rationale: The question asks about the myotatic unit. The hamstring group is likely to be tense and short if a client has difficulty extending the knee.

38. c

Factual recall

Rationale: Popliteus is likely to be involved in the situation described in the question.

39. a

Factual recall

Rationale: Anterior leg muscles are most responsible for dorsiflexion.

40. b

Factual recall

Rationale: Soleus may be inhibited if it is difficult to sustain movement that requires being up on the toes because soleus performs plantarflexion.

41. d

Factual recall

Rationale: Plantaris plantarflexes the ankle and assists with knee flexion.

42. b

Factual recall

Rationale: The question asks about the myotatic unit. Tibialis anterior is likely to be inhibited if gastrocnemius is tight and short.

43. c

Factual recall

Rationale: Flexor halluces brevis has its attachment on the great toe.

44. d

Factual recall

Rationale: The question asks about identification of antiinflammatory medication. Tendonitis is an inflammatory condition.

45. a

Factual recall

Rationale: An analgesic is a painkiller. Therefore, feedback mechanisms for pain will be altered.

46. b

Factual recall

Rationale: Only myositis ossificans has a regional contraindication. The three wrong answers indicate general contraindications.

47. a

Factual recall

Rationale: Stabilization, but not movement, is produced in this contraction.

Answers and Rationales to Application/Concept Identification and Clinical Reasoning/Synthesis Questions

1. c

Application and concept identification

Rationale: Typically, the eccentric function of any muscle is to restrain and decelerate the opposite action.

2. a

Application and concept identification

Rationale: A synergist assists movement, and an antagonist produces the opposite movement. For answers c and d, the muscles are in the wrong location, as is the fibularis.

3. b

Application and concept identification

Rationale: The muscles are located in the leg, not in the thigh; do not cross the knee; and share function at the ankle.

4. c

Application and concept identification

Rationale: Because of reverse actions of muscles wherein stabilizing and moving attachments can change according to action, the terms *origin* and *insertion* are being phased out in favor of *proximal* and *distal*. Proximal attachments would be *from*, and the distal attachment would be *to*.

5. a

Application and concept identification

Rationale: The question asks for the connection between an action (pushing a car), the result (fatigue and muscle soreness), and the best description for the action. Generating static force expends energy with no result in movement.

6. d

Application and concept identification

Rationale: Assessment identifies hypermobile joints. The correct answer explains the role of muscles in joint stability.

7. c

Application and concept identification

Rationale: The question identifies the genetic tendency for fast-twitch and slow-twitch fiber types in muscles. The wrong answers are not logical in relation to the facts in the question or there is a misuse of terminology in relation to other terms in the sentence.

8. a

Application and concept identification

Rationale: Postural muscles are fatigue resistant and usually are made of a higher percentage of slow-twitch red fibers. To affect these muscles, a sustained force must be applied at the threshold stimulus.

9. b

Application and concept identification

Rationale: Slow stretching affects the viscous aspect of the connective tissue to a greater extent than does the neurologic or chemical action of muscle fibers. Slow stretching has a minimum effect on blood flow. Answer *c* is incorrect because slow stretching would increase, not decrease, water binding.

10. d

Application and concept identification

Rationale: Only answer *d* correctly describes the reason for increased tenderness on palpation. The wrong answers use all the right words in the wrong context. This is a common strategy for writing wrong answers.

11. c

Application and concept identification

Rationale: The question describes a myotatic unit. The answers listed are components of myotatic units, and you need to define these terms. The agonist for abduction requires that the antagonist (the adductor) must relax to allow movement. If this is not happening, then the antagonist is the likely cause.

12. b

Application and concept identification

Rationale: The action described in the question stimulated the protective action of the tendon reflex. The question asks about a correlation of reflex physiology to an actual situation.

13. b

Application and concept identification

Rationale: The question is describing the pain—spasm—pain cycle.

14. c

Application and concept identification

Rationale: Muscle tension headache commonly responds well to general massage, which generates a parasympathetic effect. The three wrong answers present contraindications or complex conditions that require specific intervention.

15. c

Clinical reasoning and synthesis

Rationale: Client A has near normal function, whereas client B has dysfunction. You need to decide why this occurred on the basis of correct information. Only answer *c* has correct information about tissue healing. Limiting exercise and wrapping the area would result in less mobility, and client A had near-normal function. Satellite cell activity results in replacement during healing, not increased scar development. Increased circulation and decreased adhesions result in mobility, not rigidity.

16. a

Clinical reasoning and synthesis

Rationale: The facts presented in the question include extended contraction of the muscles used to grip (the flexor group of the forearm and the intrinsic muscles of the palm) and inhibition of the wrist extensors. The possible answers provide a reason for this condition.

17. d

Clinical reasoning and synthesis

Rationale: Fibromyalgia, or muscle pain syndrome, responds best to general massage provided to support sleep and relieve pain symptoms. Any type of massage that creates inflammation or that excessively strains the system is contraindicated.

BIOMECHANICS

Answers and Rationales to Factual Recall Questions

1. d

Factual recall

Rationale: The question is the definition of an isotonic eccentric contraction.

2. a

Factual recall

Rationale: The question is a definition of pressure.

3. b

Factual recall

Rationale: The question describes dynamic balance.

4. b

Factual recall

Rationale: The center of gravity outside the base of support would have the least amount of balance.

5. c

Factual recall

Rationale: A third-class lever provides the greatest speed. There is no combined lever type.

6. a

Factual recall

Rationale: When the foot is on the floor, this is the stance phase. No double swing is noted during gait.

7. c

Factual recall

Rationale: Plantar flexors move the foot onto the toes; therefore, toe-off preswing is the correct answer.

8. d

Factual recall

Rationale: The question is the definition of functional block.

9. d
   Factual recall
   Rationale: The question defines stabilization.
10. b
    Factual recall
    Rationale: Range of motion beyond normal is considered hypermobility.
11. a
    Factual recall
    Rationale: The typical range of motion in extension for the lumbar spine is 25 degrees.
12. b
    Factual recall
    Rationale: Only sternocleidomastoid is a cervical flexor.
13. b
    Factual recall
    Rationale: Restricted mobility on the left should indicate shortened and contracted muscles on the right.
14. d
    Factual recall
    Rationale: Only the pectoralis major exerts influence on the sternoclavicular joint.
15. b
    Factual recall
    Rationale: The primary function of the shoulder girdle muscles that have attachments at the axial skeleton, the scapula, and the clavicle is stability of the scapula.
16. c
    Factual recall
    Rationale: Normal elbow flexion is 150 degrees, so the joint is hypomobile.
17. b
    Factual recall
    Rationale: The wrist is flexed and resistance is applied against the palm of the hand when a muscle test for normal function of the wrist flexors is performed.
18. c
    Factual recall
    Rationale: The question describes a function of the iliopsoas.
19. d
    Factual recall
    Rationale: The question asks about which muscle is testing weak for hip extension. Semimembranosus is the only listed muscle involved in hip extension.
20. c
    Factual recall
    Rationale: The loose-packed position of the knee is at about 30 degrees of flexion, allowing for the movements of internal and external rotation.
21. c
    Factual recall
    Rationale: This is the definition of a firing pattern.
22. d
    Factual recall

Rationale: Upper crossed syndrome is indicated because the muscles listed are not found in the lower body, nor are they actively involved in gait. Muscle testing typically does not assess myofascial dysfunction.
23. b
    Factual recall
    Rationale: Only the shoulder complex has 80 degrees of internal rotation. All other areas exhibit less rotational movement.
24. a
    Factual recall
    Rationale: When a joint is moved so that the joint angle is decreased, prime movers and the synergist concentrically contract. The antagonist eccentrically functions while lengthening to allow movement.

Answers and Rationales to Application/Concept Identification and Clinical Reasoning/Synthesis Questions

1. a
   Application and concept identification
   Rationale: Edema usually would not cause joint dysfunction, and loading of a joint more likely would cause the damage. Closed kinematic chain and optimal firing pattern are the names of types of function, not dysfunction.
2. d
   Application and concept identification
   Rationale: Transversus abdominis is the answer. Core muscles stabilize the trunk, which eliminates answers *b* and *c*. Inner unit muscles attach intrinsically, which eliminate answer *a*.
3. d
   Application and concept identification
   Rationale: A fulcrum is a fixed point around which a lever rotates. Only the joint can be a fulcrum; bones are levers, and muscles provide force.
4. b
   Application and concept identification
   Rationale: The question describes an action and asks for muscle function. Muscles exert a force to generate effort to overcome resistance.
5. a
   Application and concept identification
   Rationale: Visual input during gait requires that the eyes remain forward and be kept level.
6. a
   Application and concept identification
   Rationale: Because of recent onset in response to slight trauma, answer *a* is the most logical.
7. c
   Application and concept identification
   Rationale: Resistance is applied to the distal end of the lever.

8. c

Application and concept identification

Rationale: The question asks about a condition of a muscle group in response to repetitive strain to the scalene muscles caused by an inappropriate breathing pattern.

9. c

Application and concept identification

Rationale: Information from the question indicates the latissimus dorsi.

10. a

Application and concept identification

Rationale: The entire shoulder complex moves as a unit.

11. c

Application and concept identification

Rationale: A joint function is provided to identify a biomechanical principle. Information about the glenohumeral joint design is necessary before the question can be answered. Because this joint is one that exhibits the greatest mobility, answer c is the most logical.

12. a

Application and concept identification

Rationale: The action limited is supination.

13. b

Application and concept identification

Rationale: The question is asking about the relationship between observed internal rotation and outcomes of muscle testing. Answer a reverses the information. The two muscles in answers c and d are not involved in the movement described.

14. d

Application and concept identification

Rationale: The concentrically contracting group of muscles in the knee that is being held in extension is the quadriceps.

15. a

Application and concept identification

Rationale: The fibularis longus is the only muscle that would be overstretched by this action.

16. b

Clinical reasoning and synthesis

Rationale: This question requires analysis of normal gait patterns against the disrupted gait described in the question. The arms counterbalance the legs, with the right arm counterbalancing the left leg, and vice versa. This means that when the shoulder flexors contract on the right, the thigh flexors on the left also are contracting. If the tension in the left biceps brachii has increased, this would inhibit the thigh flexors on the left, and the thigh flexors on the right would increase in tone.

17. d

Clinical reasoning and synthesis

Rationale: Answer d describes a change in compensation patterns and is the most logical reason for the pain. Because the condition changed from reduced range of motion without pain to increased range of motion with onset of pain, a shift from a second-degree to a first-degree dysfunction would not be logical. With mobility increasing, stability would decrease around the area.

18. b

Clinical reasoning and synthesis

Rationale: Facts presented in the question include knee joint pain with hypermobility and pain with passive movement. The knee is moving beyond 150 degrees of flexion and 135 degrees of extension. Pain on passive movement often suggests joint dysfunction or nerve entrapment. Answer b provides massage but refers the client for specific work on the knee because joint or nerve involvement is indicated by the assessment. Answer a would increase hypermobility. Answer c is too conservative, and answer d is too aggressive.

19. d

Clinical reasoning and synthesis

Rationale: Facts presented in the question include right shoulder pain on external rotation with a slow onset. Range of motion is 40 degrees and normal is 90 degrees. Infraspinatus, posterior deltoid, and teres minor are inhibited by the subscapularis, pectoralis major, latissimus dorsi, teres major, and anterior deltoid. Only answer d addresses the muscle listed as causal and applies proper methods to normalize the condition.

INTEGUMENTARY, CARDIOVASCULAR, LYMPHATIC, AND IMMUNE SYSTEMS

Answers and Rationales to Factual Recall Questions

1. a

Factual recall

Rationale: The epidermis is the outer layer of the skin.

2. d

Factual recall

Rationale: Melanocytes produce dark pigment in the skin.

3. b

Factual recall

Rationale: The erector pili muscles are located at the hair root.

4. c

Factual recall

Rationale: Sebum is produced by sebaceous glands.

5. b

Factual recall

Rationale: Apocrine glands produce sweat with the strongest odor.

6. b

Factual recall

Rationale: The right atrium receives blood from the superior and inferior venae cavae.

7. d
   Factual recall
   Rationale: Systole and diastole are part of the cardiac cycle, with diastole being the portion during which the ventricles relax.

8. a
   Factual recall
   Rationale: Impetigo is a contagious skin disease.

9. b
   Factual recall
   Rationale: A mole has the greatest potential for becoming malignant.

10. d
    Factual recall
    Rationale: Fibrocystic disease is a pathologic concern with lumps in the axillary area.

11. b
    Factual recall
    Rationale: The heart muscle is myocardium.

12. d
    Factual recall
    Rationale: The semilunar valve controls flow of blood from the left ventricle into the aorta.

13. c
    Factual recall
    Rationale: The pulmonary trunk carries blood to the lungs.

14. d
    Factual recall
    Rationale: The dorsalis pedis pulse is located in the ankle.

15. c
    Factual recall
    Rationale: A normal blood pressure is somewhere around 120/80 mm Hg. The blood pressure described in the question is low, indicating hypotension.

16. b
    Factual recall
    Rationale: The only artery listed that is in the neck is the carotid.

17. c
    Factual recall
    Rationale: The popliteal artery is located behind the knee.

18. a
    Factual recall
    Rationale: The basilic vein is located in the arm.

19. d
    Factual recall
    Rationale: The saphenous vein is commonly removed during surgery for varicose veins.

20. c
    Factual recall
    Rationale: Stem cells are involved in blood cell development.

21. d
    Factual recall
    Rationale: Ischemia results from a temporary deficiency or diminished supply of blood to a tissue.

22. a
    Factual recall
    Rationale: An embolism often begins as a thrombus.

23. b
    Factual recall
    Rationale: Lymph is clear interstitial tissue fluid that has moved into open-ended capillaries.

24. b
    Factual recall
    Rationale: Both lymphatic ducts empty lymph into the subclavian veins.

25. d
    Factual recall
    Rationale: The question describes a function of the spleen.

26. b
    Factual recall
    Rationale: Mononucleosis is contagious.

27. c
    Factual recall
    Rationale: The question is an example of specific immunity.

28. b
    Factual recall
    Rationale: The question describes a function of antibodies.

29. a
    Factual recall
    Rationale: The correct answer describes the nonspecific immune defense of mucus.

30. c
    Factual recall
    Rationale: The correct answer is a definition of allergy.

31. a
    Factual recall
    Rationale: This function of the urinary system supports nonspecific immunity.

32. d
    Factual recall
    Rationale: Sanitary measures support the immune system by isolating and destroying pathogens. Extreme heat kills most pathogens.

33. b
    Factual recall
    Rationale: These two diseases are transmitted in body fluids.

34. a
    Factual recall
    Rationale: Edema is a result of congestive heart failure.

35. c
    Factual recall
    Rationale: A ventricle is a part of the heart.

36. d
    Factual recall
    Rationale: Rheumatoid arthritis is an autoimmune disorder. Answers *a*, *b*, and *c* usually occur as the result of overuse or trauma.

Answers and Rationales to Application/ Concept Identification and Clinical Reasoning/Synthesis Questions

1. b
   Application and concept identification
   Rationale: Breathing and muscle contraction are aspects of the venous pump. Capillaries, arteries, and pulses are not involved directly in the venous pump. Answer *d* indicates pathologic conditions of the heart.

2. b
   Application and concept identification
   Rationale: Plexuses and nodes respond best to compression and deep lymphatic circulation through muscle action and respiration.

3. c
   Application and concept identification
   Rationale: Sanitary practices support the protective barrier of the skin.

4. d
   Application and concept identification
   Rationale: Color changes in the skin can indicate a pathologic condition. A yellow cast may indicate jaundice.

5. a
   Application and concept identification
   Rationale: The question provides information about the locations of vessels by stating that the client had a heart attack with reduced blood flow to the heart. The coronary arteries supply blood to the heart.

6. c
   Application and concept identification
   Rationale: The client has a reduced return of blood in the veins, and the correct answer explains why. The three wrong answers would increase blood flow within the veins. Only standing still for long periods would reduce blood flow.

7. a
   Application and concept identification
   Rationale: A normal pulse is between 50 and 70 beats per minute. Although 85 beats per minute is below what is considered tachycardia, it is faster than what usually is considered normal.

8. a
   Application and concept identification
   Rationale: Care must be taken so that clients do not have low blood pressure after a massage. The three wrong answers would indicate an increase in blood pressure, and pressure on the baroreceptors can lower it.

9. c
   Application and concept identification
   Rationale: There is a lymphatic plexus on the bottom of the foot, and compression to the area stimulates lymphatic fluid movement.

10. c
    Application and concept identification

Rationale: The question is asking for a correlation with immune suppression and stress levels. Only answer *c* is correct because stress tends to suppress the entire immune function through an increase in cortisol levels.

11. d
    Clinical reasoning and synthesis
    Rationale: The facts in the question indicate that the immune system is unable to fight pathogens. Precautions must be taken to protect the client. No methods should be used to increase the stress response or strain the adaptive capacity of the client. Therefore, the correct answer is to support nonspecific homeostatic regulation and restorative sleep.

RESPIRATORY, DIGESTIVE, URINARY, AND REPRODUCTIVE SYSTEMS

Answers and Rationales to Factual Recall Questions

1. a
   Factual recall
   Rationale: The question is the definition of breathing.

2. d
   Factual recall
   Rationale: The question describes the location of the septum.

3. d
   Factual recall
   Rationale: The question defines alveoli.

4. a
   Factual recall
   Rationale: The bronchioles bronchodilate under sympathetic nervous system dominance.

5. b
   Factual recall
   Rationale: Because the phrenic nerve allows the diaphragm to function and the injury is below this area, breathing without assistance is possible.

6. c
   Factual recall
   Rationale: The question is about muscle function that results in rib movement up and out, which creates the vacuum that draws air into the lungs.

7. a
   Factual recall
   Rationale: Tuberculosis is contagious.

8. b
   Factual recall
   Rationale: Addictive behavior is related to stimulation of pleasure sensations.

9. a
   Factual recall
   Rationale: The question describes the peritoneum.

10. d
Factual recall
Rationale: Amylase digests carbohydrates.

11. b
Factual recall
Rationale: The question describes the rugae.

12. c
Factual recall
Rationale: The question describes the duodenum.

13. c
Factual recall
Rationale: The question describes the liver.

14. a
Factual recall
Rationale: A major function of the large intestine is to absorb water.

15. b
Factual recall
Rationale: The question describes the appendix.

16. a
Factual recall
Rationale: The question describes protein.

17. c
Factual recall
Rationale: The question describes cirrhosis.

18. b
Factual recall
Rationale: The question describes hepatitis.

19. d
Factual recall
Rationale: The question describes a strangulated hernia.

20. a
Factual recall
Rationale: Micturition is parasympathetic action to void urine.

21. d
Factual recall
Rationale: The detrusor muscle contracts to empty the bladder.

22. c
Factual recall
Rationale: *Cyst* means "bladder"; cystitis is a bladder infection.

23. a
Factual recall
Rationale: The correct answer explains the physiology of erectile tissue.

24. b
Factual recall
Rationale: The Bartholin gland secretes a lubricating fluid in the female external genitalia.

25. d
Factual recall
Rationale: Ovulation is the last to occur as the female sexually matures.

26. b
Factual recall

Rationale: The alkaline role of semen is to counteract the acidic nature of vaginal fluid.

27. c
Factual recall
Rationale: Gonorrhea is bacterial in origin.

28. d
Factual recall
Rationale: Benign prostatic hyperplasia is the most likely diagnosis.

29. b
Factual recall
Rationale: Total metabolic rate is the amount of energy expended by the body at any given time. The citric acid cycle is the way that food becomes energy. Digestion breaks food down, and the basal metabolic rate is related to energy usage while one is awake.

30. c
Factual recall
Rationale: Combined fluid inside the cells accounts for most of the body fluid.

31. a
Factual recall
Rationale: Force exerted by water is called hydrostatic pressure.

32. c
Factual recall
Rationale: Prelabor is normal, as is lactation. Vaginitis is an infection that needs to be treated, but an ectopic pregnancy could cause the fallopian tube to burst.

Answers and Rationales to Application/Concept Identification and Clinical Reasoning/Synthesis Questions

1. b
Application and concept identification
Rationale: The key words are "directly and mechanically influence," which is possible with constipation.

2. b
Application and concept identification
Rationale: Swell bodies in the nose are unable to function properly, so normal movement during sleep is disrupted. This leads to low back stiffness.

3. d
Application and concept identification
Rationale: Tachypnea is fast breathing, which would increase oxygen levels, drop carbon dioxide levels, and trigger sympathetic dominance. This is a cause of hyperventilation syndrome.

4. c
Application and concept identification
Rationale: Massage methods that modulate the breathing rhythm also interact with the autonomic nervous system. The three wrong answers present information contrary to the identified effects of massage.

5. b

Application and concept identification

Rationale: A diet with severely limited fat can lead to difficulty with hormone production because many hormones are lipid based.

6. b

Application and concept identification

Rationale: Stimulation of movement of fecal material through the large intestine may be assisted by massage that simulates the peristaltic action of the large intestine and the fecal flows along the same anatomic route.

7. b

Application and concept identification

Rationale: Renal insufficiency would make it difficult for the kidneys to handle increased blood volume.

8. b

Application and concept identification

Rationale: The correct answer explains the physiology of the male erection in response to parasympathetic dominance.

9. b

Application and concept identification

Rationale: An understanding of the stages of pregnancy, positioning of the client, and indications and contraindications for massage is required before the question can be answered.

10. a

Application and concept identification

Rationale: Massage stimulates the release of oxytocin, a hormone involved in lactation.

11. b

Clinical reasoning and synthesis

Rationale: The problem is bronchoconstriction, so answer *b* is correct. Answer *a* is incorrect. Answers *c* and *d* would worsen the problem.

12. c

Clinical reasoning and synthesis

Rationale: Sympathetic dominance tends to aggravate digestive problems. Answer *b* is not a safe practice. Answer *d* includes supporting upper chest breathing, indicating sympathetic dominance, so the content in the answer is flawed.

13. b

Clinical reasoning and synthesis

Rationale: Given the symptoms described in the question, the most logical cause is disrupted breathing function, which creates sympathetic dominance. The treatment described in answer *b* would address this situation best.

14. c

Clinical reasoning and synthesis

Rationale: The correct answer would provide correct justification for how massage may help some types of infertility conditions that are related to stress. Adrenaline does not promote a decreased stress response. Massage has not been shown to affect follicle-stimulating hormone. Massage has not been shown to affect the hormones listed, and these same hormones may inhibit ovulation.

15. a

Clinical reasoning and synthesis

Rationale: Answer *a* is the most logical. Massage done correctly should not be excessively fatiguing. Massage promotes entrainment. Answer *d* is not logical.

Where are the questions to this part.

ANSWER KEY FOR CHAPTER 9 PRACTICE TESTS IN THE BOOK

Practice Test 1

Mock Exam Modeling the MBLEx—100 Questions

1. Correct answer and rational C

Decreased arterial pressure occurs when parasympathetic activation occurs and stress is decreased.

Incorrect answers rationales

Increased blood pressure and vasoconstriction are more related to sympathetic ANS function.

2. Correct answer and rational B

Meridians are channels that direct the flow of energy through specific pathways of the body.

Incorrect answers rationales

Nerves are described in traditional anatomy and self-care is a variety of activities to support health.

3. Correct answer and rational A

The cerebellum is responsible for smooth, coordinated voluntary movements.

Incorrect answers rationales

The thalamus is the relay center of the brain. It receives afferent impulses from sensory receptors located throughout the body and processes the information for distribution to the appropriate cortical area. The medulla oblongata is at the bottom of the brain stem, where the spinal cord meets the foramen magnum of the skull. It is responsible for autonomic functions.

4. Correct answer and rationale A

Regional anatomy: The study of all the structures of a particular area would be the answer that best fits the intent of the question-massage/bodywork of an area.

Incorrect answers rationales

Developmental anatomy: How anatomy changes over the life cycle. Gross anatomy: The study of body structures large enough to be visible to the naked eye.

5. Correct answer and rational B

The hypogastric region (below the stomach) contains the organs of the reproductive system, such as the uterus and ovaries. The menstrual cycle involves shedding of the lining of the uterus if fertilization does not occur.

Incorrect answers rationales

The thorax consists of a bony framework that is held together by 12 thoracic vertebrae posteriorly and ribs that encircle the lateral and anterior thoracic cavity. Upper left quadrant is the area of the abdomen that is on the left side region of the navel and extends up to the left rib cage.

6. Correct answer and rationale B

The cell membrane acts to structure the cell and filter movement of particles in and out of the cell.

Incorrect answers rationales

Cytoplasm is contained within the cell and lysosome is an organelle.

7. Correct answer and rational A

The secretion of hydrochloric acid by the stomach plays an important role in protecting the body against pathogens ingested with food or water.

Incorrect answers rationales

Suppression of mucus production would not support immunity since mucus forms a protective barrier which helps trap foreign bodies or flushes them out of the body. While antibodies are components of immunity, the stomach is not specifically involved in production. Antibodies are produced by a type of white blood cell called a B cell (B lymphocyte). B cells develop from stem cells in bone marrow.

8. Correct answer and rationale C

The sinoatrial node initiates the impulse in the heart and is referred to as the pacemaker.

Incorrect answers rationales

The atrioventricular (AV) node is a key part of the heart's electrical system, controlling the transmission of the heart's electrical impulse from the atria to the ventricles.

9. Correct answer and rational A

The peritoneum is the serous membrane forming the lining of the abdominal cavity.

Incorrect answers rationales

Pericardium relates to the heart and visceral relates to the internal organs of the body, specifically those within the chest or abdomen.

10. Correct answer and rational B

The adrenal glands secrete androgens and are located in the trunk.

Incorrect answers rationales

The cranium is not located in the trunk and the pleura is not hormone producing.

11. Correct answer and rational B

The muscle spindles are proprioceptors detecting muscle length. A stretch reflex occurs if muscle is stretched quickly.

Incorrect answers rationales

The muscle spindle's associated muscle is primarily stimulated when rapidly stretched, not when slowly lengthened or shortened.

12. Correct answer and rational C

Interstitial fluid around the cells moves into the open-ended lymphatic capillaries.

Incorrect answers rationales

Ventricles are in the heart and lymph nodes filter fluid after it has entered the lymph vessels.

13. Correct answer and rational C

The application of counter force resists the movement.

Incorrect answers rationales

Assisted and passive movement does not resist the movement produced by the client.

14. Correct answer and rational A

Diarthrosis type joints are able to be actively moved.

Incorrect answers rationales

Cartilaginous joints have little if any mobility and syndesmoses is an immovable joint in which bones are joined by connective tissue.

15. Correct answer and rational C

In isometric exercise and contraction, the muscle length does not change, but the tension does.

Incorrect answers rationales

In an isotonic exercise, the muscle length changes during tension increase. An eccentric action is the lengthening of a muscle fiber.

16. Correct answer and rational B

Self-Employment Tax (SE tax) is a social security and Medicare tax primarily for individuals who work for themselves.

Incorrect answers and rationales

Income tax is paid on income and workers' compensation is paid by an employer.

17. Correct answer and rational A

The adductors of the hip would need to shorten, producing a concentric contraction and returning the area to anatomical position.

Incorrect answers rationales

The adductor group would already be lengthened when the hip is in the abducted position. Stabilizing would be involved, but the question is asking for what is happening during a movement.

18. Correct answer and rational C

The ischial tuberosity is the posterior portion of the ramus of the ischium. The hamstrings attach to the ischial tuberosity at the proximal end.

Incorrect answers rationales

Quadriceps and sartorius are located on the anterior thigh.

19. Correct answer and rational B

All healthcare providers who are considered covered entities under HIPAA, and those who file claims electronically or use a clearinghouse to bill insurance, are required to apply for an NPI. All other healthcare providers are eligible to receive an NPI if they desire.

Incorrect answers and rationales

Employer Identification Number (EIN) and Taxpayer Identification Number (TIN) are two names for the same thing—federal tax identification numbers.

20. Correct answer and rational C
    Business gross per year needs to be $65,000 and the number of sessions per year is 1000. Thus, services must be $65 per hour.
    Incorrect answers and rationales
    $50 is too low to generate enough gross business income. $90 would generate a surplus, but the question is asking for the breakeven point.

21. Correct answer and rational C
    Abduction means to move away from the midline.
    Incorrect answers and rationales
    Adduction means to add to the midline or bring it closer as indicated in arms moving toward trunk or over abdomen.

22. Correct answer and rational A
    In flexion of the lumbar spine, the back flattens, leading to a decrease in lordosis.
    Incorrect answers and rationales
    Extension increases lordosis and kyphosis is the curve of the thoracic spine.

23. Correct answer and rational C
    Nut and nut product allergic reactions can result in the medical emergency anaphylaxis.
    Incorrect answers and rationales
    Water and alcohol are unlikely to cause an allergic reaction.

24. Correct answer and rational A
    Isopropyl alcohol is an antiseptic.
    Incorrect answers and rationales
    Sodium hypochlorite and quaternary ammonium are disinfectants.

25. Correct answer and rational A
    Both latissimus dorsi and teres major are adductors of the glenohumeral joint.
    Incorrect answers and rationales
    Gluteus medius and adductor magnus are antagonist. Supraspinatus acts on the glenohumeral joint and pectoralis minor acts on the scapula.

26. Correct answer and rational B
    Professional communication about confidentiality helps set boundaries related to interaction with the clients who are also friends.
    Incorrect answers and rationales
    The incorrect response about the practitioner being nervous is more of a personal response than a professional communication. Regardless of the relationship between clients the practitioner needs to maintain confidentiality.

27. Correct answer and rational C
    Sexual harassment is behavior characterized by the making of unwelcome and inappropriate sexual remarks or physical advances in a workplace or other professional or social situation.
    Incorrect answers and rationales
    A practitioner explaining sexual boundaries is ethical and professional communication. Gossip is both unethical and unprofessional.

28. Correct answer and rational B
    Spinalis cervicis: extends and hyperextends the cervical (neck), moving the head into extension.
    Incorrect answers and rationales
    The longus capitis and longus colli muscles are located at the anterior aspect of the cervical vertebrae and produce flexion of the head.

29. Correct answer and rational C
    Signs are observable and symptoms are an experience of a disease.
    Incorrect answers and rationales
    Subjective feelings of discomfort can be a symptom, but disease typically is described by signs and symptoms. An acute episode of a chronic illness can occur but is not specifically related to the manifestation of a disease.

30. Correct answer and rational A
    An aneurysm is an abnormal bulge or ballooning in the wall of a blood vessel.
    Incorrect answers and rationales
    Cerebrovascular accident (CVA) is a stroke, and edema is increased swelling related to excess fluid accumulation in the body tissues.

31. Correct answer and rational B
    Synarthrosis is a term that classifies a joint as an immovable fixed joint between bones connected by fibrous tissue.
    Incorrect answers and rationales
    The symphysis refers to a specific joint, not a classification. Synovial joints are types of freely moveable joints which are functionally classified as diarthroses.

32. Correct answer and rational B
    Latissimus dorsi would internally rotate the arm to the point that the palms are facing the lateral aspect of the upper thigh.
    Incorrect answers and rationales
    Triceps functions at the elbow and shoulder but does not produce rotation. Anterior serratus acts on the scapula.

33. Correct answer and rational C
    When a massage practitioner talks about personal issues during the massage session, they fail to respect professional boundaries.
    Incorrect answers and rationales
    Dual relationships involve the practitioner interacting with the client in multiple professional capacities. Confidentiality respects the client's privacy.

34. Correct answer and rational A
    The activity described is an ethics violation and sexual misconduct.
    Incorrect answers and rationales
    A therapeutic alliance is based on respect. Values conflict is associated with contrasting belief systems.

35. Correct answer and rational B
    Atrophy is gradual loss of muscle usually because of disease or lack of use.
    Incorrect answers and rationales

Hypertrophy is the enlargement of an organ or tissue from the increase in size of its cells.

Regeneration is the process of replacing or restoring damaged or missing cells and tissues.

36. Correct answer and rational A

Hepatitis is a viral disease.

Incorrect answers and rationales

MRSA is methicillin-resistant *Staphylococcus aureus*, a bacterial infection, and thrush is a contagious fungal/yeast condition.

37. Correct answer and rational B

A hiatal hernia occurs when the upper part of the stomach bulges through the diaphragm muscle.

Incorrect answers and rationales

The other types of hernias occur in other locations—umbilical relates to navel and inguinal the groin.

38. Correct answer and rational B

A person acts with autonomy, making one's own choices, free from any controlling interference from others and is self-determination.

Incorrect answers and rationales

Ability to pay for services and right to medical insurance are different issues than autonomy.

39. Correct answer and rational C

The axillary nerve lies near the humerus and can be injured during anterior shoulder dislocation or fracture of the humeral neck.

Incorrect answers and rationales

The median and radial nerves while located in the arm are less likely to be injured in shoulder dislocation.

40. Correct answer and rational B

To avoid or minimize possible harm to the client is the essence of nonmaleficence.

Incorrect answers and rationales

Proportionality relates to benefits being more than burden of treatment. Justice denotes acting in a fair and impartial manner.

41. Correct answer and rational A

Orthostatic hypotension is a decrease in cardiac output and lowering of arterial pressure decreasing blood pressure.

Incorrect answers and rationales

Myocardial ischemia occurs when blood flow to the heart is reduced, preventing the heart muscle from receiving enough oxygen. Vasodilation is the widening of blood vessels as a result of relaxation of the blood vessel's muscular walls.

42. Correct answer and rational B

The healing phase of ligaments is divided into the following categories: inflammatory phase/acute (first few days after injury), proliferative phase/subacute (1–6 weeks after injury), and remodeling phase/chronic (begins 7 weeks after injury).

Incorrect answers and rationales

2–6 weeks after injury is the proliferative phase of healing.

43. Correct answer and rational A

Kneading is the correct answer.

Incorrect answers and rationales

Vibration is a rigorous shake or rocking of specific muscles or body segments. Gliding is a method that moves horizontally.

44. Correct answer and rational C

Along with tremor and rigidity, people with Parkinson's disease show bradykinesia, impaired balance, and poor postural control. There is also usually a masklike expression in the face.

Incorrect answers and rationales

Alzheimer's disease involves cognition impairments in the disease process. Multiple sclerosis is a disease that affects the central nervous system. The immune system attacks the myelin, the protective layer around nerve fibers, and causes inflammation and lesions, making it difficult for the brain to send signals to rest of the body.

45. Correct answer and rational A

The anterior triangle of the neck defined by the sternocleidomastoid muscles and the inferior border of the mandible contain structures sensitive to pressure including the common carotid, external carotid, and internal carotid arteries; the thyroid gland; and the anterior and internal jugular veins and nerves including the vagus nerve.

Incorrect answers and rationales

The foot and thigh do not have as many structures vulnerable to pressure.

46. Correct answer and rational B

Improved mobility best targets efficient performance of daily living such as dressing and cleaning.

Incorrect answers and rationales

Stress management is helpful but would not specifically support increase physical function. A facility that is peaceful and soothing is also helpful but does not specifically target goals and outcomes related to mobility.

47. Correct answer and rational C

Post assessment is used to evaluate response to previous treatment.

Incorrect answers and rationales

Identifying contraindications is part of the initial pre-assessment process. Pre, not post, assessment would determine if treatment is within scope of practice.

48. Correct answer and rational C

Myofascial release (MFR) is a form of manual therapy that involves the application of a low load, long duration stretch to the myofascial complex, intended to restore optimal length, decrease pain, and improve function.

Incorrect answers and rationales

Polarity therapy targets proposed energy fields, and lymphatic drainage targets fluid movement.

49. Correct answer and rational A

The biopsychosocial model indicates that biological, psychological, and social factors all play a significant role in human functioning in the context of disease or illness and health is best understood in terms of these combined factors rather than purely in biological terms.

Incorrect answers and rationales

Approaches to care based on fixed outcomes such as increased mobility or adaptions for those with similar issues as found in population specialization may or may not consider whole person care.

50. Correct answer and rational B

The holding/resting position targets the skin for stimulation of the cutaneous (skin) sensory receptors.

Incorrect answers and rationales

Kneading and shaking methods involve more pressure.

51. Correct answer and rational C

Research indicates that responses of the nervous system have shown to be valid.

Incorrect answers and rationales

Research results related to fluid exchange and postural changes have not been validated by research.

52. Correct answer and rational B

Tension headache is commonly caused by changes in soft tissue structures that can be safely addressed by massage therapy application.

Incorrect answers and rationales

Pancreatitis is an inflammation (swelling) of the pancreas. When the pancreas is inflamed, the powerful digestive enzymes it makes can damage its tissue. The inflamed pancreas can cause release of inflammatory cells and toxins that may harm other body organs.

Pulmonary edema is a condition where fluid accumulates in lung tissues causing shortness of breath, wheezing, and coughing up blood.

53. Correct answer and rational C

Valid research supports massage as a method to reduce pain and anxiety in those with a cancer diagnosis.

Incorrect answers and rationales

Research does not support claims of massage therapy directly increasing the action of chemotherapy or detoxing the body of cancer cells.

54. Correct answer and rational A

Improved mobility outcomes involve more targeted assessment with appropriate intervention.

Incorrect answers and rationales

Outcomes based on relaxation and stress management have fewer focused interventions.

Pain management outcome does not mean short frequent sessions are needed.

55. Correct answer and rational C

Rheumatoid arthritis is an autoimmune condition affecting joints, and caution is indicated specifically to reduce potential for increasing inflammatory response.

Incorrect answers and rationales

Diverticulosis is a condition where small pouches called diverticula develop in the large intestine. Diverticulitis means the small pouches are inflamed.

Plantar fasciitis is a chronic local inflammation of the ligament stretching underneath the sole that attaches at the heel.

56. Correct answer and rational A

Selective serotonin reuptake inhibitors (SSRIs) are a class of medications most commonly prescribed to treat depression. They are often used as first-line pharmacotherapy for depression and numerous other psychiatric disorders due to their safety, efficacy, and tolerability.

Incorrect answers and rationales

Hypertension is high blood pressure. Classes of blood pressure medications include diuretics, beta-blockers, and ACE inhibitors.

Diabetes is treated with medication that lowers the amount of glucose the liver makes and helps the body use insulin better.

57. Correct answer and rational B

Friction is an intervention intended to target local areas.

Incorrect answers and rationales

Joint movement and gliding address larger areas.

58. Correct answer and rational C

Mechanisms of action for massage therapy benefit are elusive but research consistently shows ANS affects.

Incorrect answers and rationales

Research of blood flow is inconsistent and massage sensory stimulation is processed through reflex mechanisms related to neuroendocrine mechanisms.

59. Correct answer and rational B

Immersion in warm water is the use of both approaches.

Incorrect answers and rationales

Hot stones may be warmed in water but it is not a combined application.

Counterirritation ointment usually containing some sort of menthol will feel cold.

60. Correct answer and rational A

It is important to understand how the condition is being treated to determine contraindications.

Incorrect answers and rationales

Referral is not necessarily indicated nor is posture and gait assessment required.

61. Correct answer and rational B

Compression provides pressure and gliding elongates tissue when using enough drag.

Incorrect answers and rationales

Friction, vibration, kneading, and shaking are not specifically focused on general massage pressure or a sense of tissue stretching.

62. Correct answer and rational C

Massage may promote sliding in the fascial layers.

Incorrect answers and rationales

It is unlikely manual therapy changes the length of collagen fibers or breaks down adhesions.

63. Correct answer and rational B
Twisting is a combined force application resulting in torsion.
Incorrect answers and rationales
Shear stress is created when the mechanical force application causes tissues to slide against adjacent tissues.
Compression stress is created by a push/pull force application.

64. Correct answer and rational C
Vessels constrict in response to cold.
Incorrect answers and rationales
Histamine causes the surrounding blood vessels to dilate.
Heat causes vasodilation.

65. Correct answer and rational B
Visual assessment is providing the information in the questions.
Incorrect answers and rationales
Orthopedic tests and muscle strength assessments tend to be regional or tissue specific.

66. Correct answer and rational C
Visual assessment is used as the practitioner watches the client perform the movements.
Incorrect answers and rationales
Postural assessment does not typically involve movements and history taking is most often based on client conversation.

67. Correct answer and rational A
Shiatsu is performed over clothing—preferably a thin garment made from natural fibers—and disrobing is not required. Pressure is often applied using the thumbs, though various other parts of the body may be employed, including fingertips, palms, knuckles, elbows, and knees—some therapists even use their feet.
Incorrect answers and rationales
Swedish and manual lymph drain use gliding on skin.

68. Correct answer and rational A
Compression can be applied via static pressure.
Incorrect answers and rationales
Drag is a method modifier associated with the amount of lubricant used.
Friction involves movement.

69. Correct answer and rational A
Palpation involves physical contact.
Incorrect answers and rationales
Assessing activities of daily living and taking an accurate history involve observation and interviewing.

70. Correct answer and rational B
Postural assessment involves comparison of left and right sides of the body.
Incorrect answers and rationales
Treatment planning and documentation occur after assessments are performed.

71. Correct answer and rational C
Foremost for safety it is necessary to identify possible contraindications before decisions are made related to treatment plan and referral.
Incorrect answers and rationales
Referral and session timing occurs after health history discussion.

72. Correct answer and rational B
While legislation mandates and requirements for client files are important, the client is asking for reasons related to the session.
Incorrect answers and rationales
Legislation mandates and requirements for client files are important but less relate to how information is used for the specific session.

73. Correct answer and rational C
First the practitioner needs to determine if the area is contraindicated. If more of a caution then methods would be adapted. Avoiding the area may not be necessary.
Incorrect answers and rationales
Explaining that the area is a local contraindication and determining adaptations comes after evaluating the rash.

74. Correct answer and rational A
The client is participating in daily living activities, has been diagnosed, and has treatment scheduled. Stress management is a logical outcome and the session could be helpful so long as the client is comfortable, the session is general, and the abdominal area is avoided.
Incorrect answers and rationales
It is not necessary to postpone treatment or obtain a doctor's permission to work with this client.

75. Correct answer and rational B
Head trauma is a medical emergency.
Incorrect answers and rationales
Providing the session then calling emergency contact and performing a balance assessment are not indicated since head trauma is a medical emergency.

76. Correct answer and rational C
Client requested outcomes may or may not be congruent with realistic treatment goals. Evidence informed practice uses the best available research to guide valid expectations in session outcomes.
Incorrect answers and rationales
While it is valid to explain research supporting valid expectations for session outcomes when there is a conflict related to unrealistic client expectations, the question does not indicate that conflict exists nor is there evidence of boundary issues in the therapeutic relationship.

77. Correct answer and rational A
A more general approach with a focus on wellbeing is logical for the initial session focusing on the clients ability to enjoy the session.

Incorrect answers and rationales

Pain relief and increased mobility as goals would involve intervention-based methods which would be a more complex care approach than warranted for a client during the first session.

78. Correct answer and rational A

Supine with lower legs elevated would support normal lymphatic flow.

Incorrect answers and rationales

Supine with knees bent and heels on the table and prone with lower legs flat on the table do not help passively move fluid using gravity.

79. Correct answer and rational B

The practitioner is using critical thinking to develop a treatment strategy.

Incorrect answers and rationales

Performing an intake assessment and determining outcome goals have been completed. The question indicates stress management and functional mobility as outcomes. The practitioner needs to strategize how to work with this client and not use the prone position.

80. Correct answer and rational C

The practitioner is developing an application strategy for this client.

Incorrect answers and rationales

Using primarily compression methods is too limited and focusing on head, hands, and feet may not address client outcomes.

81. Correct answer and rational A

Countertransference is a therapist's reactions and feelings toward a client.

Incorrect answers and rationales

Transference is the client's feelings about a practitioner and a dual relationship occurs when a professional assumes a second role with a client and unsettles the power differential in the therapeutic relationship.

82. Correct answer and rational C

A dual relationship arises when a client is a friend, family member, or business associate. These relationships make it difficult to maintain professional boundaries.

Incorrect answers and rationales

Transference is a phenomenon in which one seems to direct feelings or desires related to an important figure in one's life—such as a parent—toward someone who is not that person.

Power differential means the basic inequality inherent in the professional relationship.

83. Correct answer and rational A

Scope of practice includes everything that the practitioner is trained to do under the specific certificate/license with which they are currently working. Scope of practice for massage excludes diagnosis and prescribing.

Incorrect answers and rationales

A dual relationship can confuse the professional boundaries.

Emotional boundaries include transference, countertransference, and the power differential.

84. Correct answer and rational C

Interest conflict arises when what is in a person's best interest is not in the best interest of another person.

Incorrect answers and rationales

Differing credentials are not indicated as an issue or as a reason for the difference in fees.

Confidentiality as the protection of information is not an issue since both fees are disclosed.

85. Correct answer and rational A

Respect for others means to equally express and practice dignity, autonomy, privacy, rights, and interests for all.

Incorrect answers and rationales

The principle of beneficence is a moral obligation to act for the benefit of others.

The principle of justice obliges us to equitably distribute benefits, risks, costs, and resources.

86. Correct answer and rational B

Manipulation of joints, including the spine, is out of scope of practice for massage therapy.

Incorrect answer and rationales

Including methods with spinal adjustment potential and inferring that spinal adjustment naturally occurs is providing misleading information.

87. Correct answer and rational B

Jurisdiction is the power, right, or authority to interpret and apply the law. Completing all requirements to practice legally is necessary. Following state licensing mandates and local government requirement is necessary.

Incorrect answers and rationales

Investigating forms of business structures and developing marketing for the target market primarily apply to self-employment and are not legally required.

88. Correct answer and rational C

While stretching within the normal functional range is typically part of massage therapy scope of practice as determined by licensure, when working with a higher credentialed professional such as a physical therapist and when the condition is related to a pathology, the referral is made to that professional. The professional then either provides the intervention or gives guidance to the massage therapist on how to proceed with the intervention.

Incorrect answers and rationales

In this scenario, it would be the PT's responsibility to perform more specific assessment, and the massage therapist would need authorization by the PT to include stretching as requested.

89. Correct answer and rational A

Permits for home occupations are available. Cities and towns have laws that govern most aspects of daily life. The locations of businesses are severely restricted in most developed countries, as well as the conditions under which they can operate.

Incorrect answers and rationales

Limited liability corporation business structure is not necessary and a health department inspection may or may not be required by the local government.

90. Correct answer and rational A

Respect must be shown for clients, other professionals, and oneself. This includes following safe and modest draping practices.

Incorrect answer and rationales

Client autonomy and self-determination is the freedom to decide and the right to sufficient information to make decisions, while veracity is the right to the objective truth.

91. Correct answer and rational B

Disinfectants are primarily applied to non-living surfaces. Do not put disinfectants in or on your body. They can kill you. When using disinfectants, follow the label directions.

Incorrect answers and rationales

Antiseptics are applied to living tissues, often to the skin in the form of hand rubs or washes.

Air purifiers allow for clean, circulated air. Air filters should be cleaned/replaced regularly.

92. Correct answer and rational B

For safety the parking area needs to have outdoor lighting.

Incorrect answers and rationales

Access to designated smoking areas and having multiple trash receptacles are not as essential as proper lighting for safety.

93. Correct answer and rational C

The structure of the hand consists of many small bones, joints, and intrinsic muscles supporting fine movement instead of gross impact movements involved with massage application.

Incorrect answers and rationales

The hinge joints in the fingers are able to be stabilized.

Intrinsic hand muscles have attachments only in the hand, not at the elbow.

94. Correct answer and rational A

National Institute for Occupational Safety and Health (NIOSH) guidelines indicate the shoulder joint should not exceed 45% of flexion to stay within safe ranges.

Incorrect answers and rationales

Trunk flexion should not exceed 20 degrees and occurs at the hip joint.

Supination/pronation should be limited but is not directly related to excursion/stroke length.

95. Correct answer and rational B

The trunk should be maintained at no more than 20 degrees flexion.

Incorrect answers and rationales

The feet position about shoulder width apart and in asymmetrical stance is considered appropriate while standing on balls of the feet would indicate table is too high.

96. Correct answer and rational C

A mask limits transmission of droplet and aerosol spread pathogens.

Incorrect answers and rationales

A face shield does not limit transmission since it is open at the bottom and edges.

A smock protects the practitioner's clothing.

97. Correct answer and rational A

Sole proprietor is able to use social security number for tax identification.

Incorrect answers and rationales

Employer Identification Number (EIN), also known as a Federal Tax Identification Number (TIN), is used to identify a business entity of partnership and corporations.

98. Correct answer and rational A

The franchise structure uses brand recognition as a marketing strategy.

Incorrect answers and rationales

Fees for service are not often adapted and a lead therapist is not always on staff.

99. Correct answer and rational C

A W-2 is a report of income and tax withholdings at the end of the year.

Incorrect answers and rationales

W-4 forms serve as a set of instructions for how an employer should withhold taxes from an employee's paycheck.

1099 forms report various types of income to the IRS. 1099-NEC is the form to report nonemployee compensation—sometimes referred to as self-employment income.

100. Correct answer and rational A

Each session is individually documented and kept on file either by paper or electronically.

Incorrect answers and rationales

Treatment plan is created once then updated, while informed consent is completed during the initial intake and updated as needed.

Practice Test 2

Just Anatomy and Physiology—150 Questions

1. Correct answer and rational B

Frontal is the correct answer.

Incorrect answers and rationales

Transverse plane divides the upper trunk from the lower body horizontally. Midsagittal plane is center of the body as the division line.

2. Correct answer and rational A

Medical Definition of pedal: of or relating to the foot.

Incorrect answers and rationales

Cervical relates to neck and femoral the thigh.

3. Correct answer and rational A
    Lateral: the further from the midline toward the side of body, the more lateral.
    Incorrect answers and rationales
    Caudal refers to a body part toward the tail. Dorsal refers to the back of the body.

4. Correct answer and rationale B
    Regional anatomy: The study of all the structures of a particular area would be the answer that best fits the intent of the question-massage/bodywork of an area.
    Incorrect answers and rationales
    Developmental anatomy: How anatomy changes over the life cycle. Gross anatomy: The study of body structures large enough to be visible to the naked eye.

5. Correct answer and rationale A
    Pathophysiology: The study of disease and changes in body function during illness.
    Incorrect answers and rationales
    Systemic physiology is the study of body systems not the diseases. Metabolism describes all the physiological processes that take place in our bodies.

6. Correct answer and rationale B
    Epithelial tissues cover and protect the surface of the body. Light pressure touches skin surface.
    Incorrect answers and rationales
    While all massage/bodywork methods access the skin, an epithelial tissue, as well as connective and muscle tissue, the concept of light pressure best describes skin surface contact.

7. Correct answer and rationale A
    Fascia is classified as connective tissue.
    Incorrect answers and rationales
    Epithelial and muscle tissue have fascial components, but fascia is classified as a connective tissue.

8. Correct answer and rationale C
    Cardiovascular and lymphatic systems are considered systems that move fluid. Therefore methods that target fluid movement would target these systems.
    Incorrect answers and rationales
    While integumentary, exocrine, renal, and digestive structures have aspects of fluid exchange, these systems are not specifically targeted for supporting fluid movement.

9. Correct answer and rationale C
    Hyaline cartilage is found at the ends of bones in most synovial joints.
    Incorrect answers and rationales
    Adipose cells and collagen fibers are components of connective tissue.

10. Correct answer and rationale C
    Skeletal muscle tissue makes up muscles connected to the skeleton.
    Incorrect answers and rationales
    Cardiac muscle tissue is found in the heart and smooth muscle tissue is found in organs and viscera.

11. Correct answer and rationale B
    Organism level: Composed of the unity of all structural levels (simple to complex) that can carry out the various processes of life.
    Incorrect answers and rationales
    The system and organ levels do not reflect a whole in body organization. System level: Composed of groups of organs that combine to perform more complex body functions. Organ level: Composed of groups of two or more kinds of tissue that combine to perform a special function.

12. Correct answer and rationale A
    The question is the definition of catabolism
    Incorrect answers and rationales
    Causation: An event that is the result of the occurrence of another event—also referred to as cause and effect. Anabolism: Chemical processes in the body that join simple compounds to form more complex compounds of carbohydrates, lipids, proteins, and nucleic acids.

13. Correct answer and rationale B
    Physiology: the study of the processes and functions of the body involved in supporting life. Homeostasis: the relatively constant state of the internal environment of the body that is maintained by adaptive responses. Specific control and feedback mechanisms are responsible for adjusting body systems to maintain this state.
    Incorrect answers and rationales
    Correlation: A relationship between two or more events that appear to be related but are not. Collagen: A protein substance composed of small fibrils that combine to create the connective tissue of fasciae, tendons, and ligaments.

14. Correct answer and rationale A
    The cell membrane gives structure to the cell and filters movement of particles in and out of the cell.
    Incorrect answers and rationales
    Cytoplasm is contained within the cell and lysosome is an organelle.

15. Correct answer and rational C
    Cytoplasm: the gelatinous liquid that fills the inside of a cell
    Incorrect answers and rationales
    Endoplasmic reticulum: a network of membranes inside a cell through which proteins and other molecules move. Cell membrane: separates the interior of the cell from the outside environment. The cell membrane consists of a lipid bilayer that is semipermeable.

16. Correct answer and rational A
    The atrioventricular (AV) node is a key part of the heart's electrical system, controlling the transmission of the heart's electrical impulse from the atria to the ventricles.

Incorrect answers and rationales

The sinoatrial node initiates the impulse in the heart and is referred to as the pacemaker. The atria are the upper chambers of the heart.

17. Correct answer and rational B

Coronary arteries provide blood to the heart.

Incorrect answers and rationales

Carotid artery is located in the neck. Vena Cava is a large vein in the middle of the body.

18. Correct answer and rational A

The right ventricle pumps the blood to the lungs where it becomes oxygenated.

Incorrect answers and rationales

The oxygenated blood from the lungs is brought back to the heart by the pulmonary veins which enter the left atrium. Left ventricular contraction forces oxygenated blood through the aortic valve to be distributed to the entire body.

19. Correct answer and rational C

The oxygenated blood from the lungs is brought back to the heart by the pulmonary veins which enter the left atrium.

Incorrect answers and rationales

The main difference between the aorta and vena cava is that the aorta is an artery that carries oxygenated blood whereas the vena cava is a vein which carries deoxygenated blood.

20. Correct answer and rational C

The right atrium receives oxygen-poor blood from the body and pumps it to the right ventricle through the tricuspid valve. The right ventricle pumps the oxygen-poor blood to the lungs through the pulmonary valve.

Incorrect answers and rationales

The left atrium receives oxygen-rich blood from the lungs and pumps it to the left ventricle through the mitral valve. The left ventricle pumps the oxygen-rich blood through the aortic valve out to the rest of the body.

21. Correct answer and rational B

The mediastinum is the area in the chest between the lungs that contains the heart.

Incorrect answers and rationales

The myocardium is the muscular layer of the heart made up of cardiac muscle whereas the pericardium is the fibrous encase of the heart made up of connective tissue.

22. Correct answer and rational C

The heart is anchored on top of the diaphragm in order to keep it in place. The diaphragm also reduces friction to the outer membranes of the heart.

Incorrect answers and rationales

Diaphragmic movement would not have a direct effect on mitral valve function. The heart position stabilizes the diaphragm

23. Correct answer and rational A

Anterior medial thigh distal to the groin is the location of the femoral artery.

Incorrect answers and rationales

There are no major arteries in the plantar aspect of the foot or between the scapula from C7 to T5.

24. Correct answer and rational C

The vena cava is the largest vein in the body that delivers oxygen-poor or deoxygenated blood to the right atrium of the heart.

Incorrect answers and rationales

Arterial blood flows in arteries not veins. The left and right brachiocephalic veins are major veins in the upper chest.

25. Correct answer and rational A

Hematopoiesis is the production of all the cellular components of blood and blood plasma.

Incorrect answers and rationales

Phagocytosis is the process by which a cell engulfs a particle and digests it. Thrombophlebitis is inflammation of a vein related to a blood clot.

26. Correct answer and rational A

Parasympathetic stimulation also relaxes the smooth musculature of the peripheral blood vessels, which results in vasodilation.

Incorrect answers and rationales

Increased blood pressure and vasoconstriction are sympathetic autonomic nervous system responses.

27. Correct answer and rational B

Ghrelin and leptin play a role in appetite.

Incorrect answers and rationales

Menstruation and bone healing are not directly affected by ghrelin and leptin.

28. Correct answer and rational A

The liver is an accessory organ of the digestive system that assists with digestive processes. The liver assists the digestive system by secreting bile and bile salts to help emulsify fats and aid in their digestion in the small intestine.

Incorrect answers and rationales

The lymphatic system returns lymph fluid via vessels to the cardiovascular system for eventual elimination of toxic byproducts by end organs, such as the kidney, liver, colon, skin, and lungs, but the liver is classified as part of the digestive system. Respiratory system main organs are the lungs.

29. Correct answer and rational B

The gastrointestinal tract is another name for the alimentary canal. The alimentary canal is a continuous passage starting from the mouth and ending at the anus, which carries food through different parts of the digestive system and allows waste to exit the body.

Incorrect answers and rationales

The omentum and mesentery are two supporting tissues present in the abdominal cavity, surrounding the gastrointestinal organs.

30. Correct answer and rational C

The peritoneum is a continuous transparent membrane which lines the abdominal cavity and covers the abdominal organs (or viscera). It acts to support the viscera while also providing a pathway for blood vessels and lymph.

Incorrect answers and rationale

The pericardium is the membrane enclosing the heart. Viscera are the internal organs, especially those in the abdominal cavity.

31. Correct answer and rational A

The duodenum is the first part of the small intestine which connects to the stomach.

Incorrect answers and rationale

The jejunum and ileum are also parts of the small intestine but do not directly connect to the stomach. The jejunum lies between the duodenum and the ileum. On its distal end, the ileum is the last segment of the small intestine which connects to the large intestine.

32. Correct answer and rational B

The liver is a large vascular organ that can be susceptible to damage from focused pressure.

Incorrect answers and rationale

The cecum is a small pouch at the beginning of the large intestine. The pylorus is the opening from the stomach into the duodenum. Neither are as susceptible to pressure as the liver.

33. Correct answer and rational C

Hydrochloric acid is a natural component of gastric juices produced by cells in the stomach.

Incorrect answers and rationales

Sulfuric acid can cause severe burns and tissue damage when it comes into contact with the skin or mucous membranes. Nitric acid is corrosive and poisonous.

34. Correct answer and rational A

Bile is produced in your liver and stored in your gallbladder.

Incorrect answers and rationales

The gallbladder holds bile but does not make it. The pancreas makes pancreatic juices, which contain enzymes that aid in digestion, and it produces several hormones, including insulin.

35. Correct answer and rational A

The secretion of hydrochloric acid by the stomach plays an important role in protecting the body against pathogens ingested with food or water.

Incorrect answers and rationales

Suppression of mucus production would interfere with immune function. Antibodies are proteins that your immune system makes to help fight infection.

36. Correct answer and rational C

The human microbiota consists of bacteria, viruses, fungi, and other single-celled animals that live in the body.

Incorrect answers and rationales

Gastric juices are released from the lining the stomach and mucus is a slimy substance secreted by mucous membranes and glands.

37. Correct answer and rational C

Adrenaline is a hormone secreted by the adrenal glands, especially related to stress.

Incorrect answers and rationales

GABA is a non-protein amino acid that functions as an inhibitory neurotransmitter throughout the central nervous system. Oxytocin is a hormone that acts as a neurotransmitter and plays an important role in reproduction. It's also linked to a host of relationship-enhancing effects. These chemicals would be more active once adrenaline decreases.

38. Correct answer and rational A

The thyroid gland is located in the neck.

Incorrect answers and rationale

The pancreas is in the thorax. The pineal gland is in the cranial cavity.

39. Correct answer and rational B

The adrenal glands secrete androgens and are located in the trunk.

Incorrect answers and rationale

The cranium is the skull. The pleura is a serous membrane that lines each half of the thorax and folds back over the surface of the lung.

40. Correct answer and rational C

The thymus is an organ that is part of the lymphatic system, in which T lymphocytes grow and multiply. The thymus is in the chest behind the breastbone.

Incorrect answers and rationale

The hypothalamus and pituitary are located in the diencephalon of the brain.

41. Correct answer and rational B

The key components of the "stress system" are the hypothalamic-pituitary-adrenal (HPA) axis and the sympathetic nervous system (SNS).

Incorrect answers and rationale

Hypothalamic—pituitary—gonadal axis is a hormone-regulating mechanism containing three different component structures that operate in a coordinated fashion and which are involved in the regulation of several reproductive and developmental processes. Hypothalamic-pituitary-thyroid axis controls energy expenditure and whole body metabolism.

42. Correct answer and rational A

Exocrine glands release secretions onto an epithelial surface via a duct.

Incorrect answers and rationale

All tissues have blood vessels. Islets of Langerhans are pancreatic cells secreting insulin and glucagon.

43. Correct answer and rational C

PRH (prolactin-releasing hormone) induces prolactin production. Prolactin induces REM sleep, modulates the immune system, and milk production. Prolactin is suppressed by the hypothalamus' production of dopamine.

Incorrect answers and rationales

Cortisol and thyroxin are indirectly affected by the hypothalamus which secretes releasing hormones, which are transported via the blood to the pituitary gland. There, the releasing hormones induce the production and secretion of pituitary hormones, which in turn are transported by the blood to their target glands.

44. Correct answer and rational A

Endocrine glands secrete hormones.

Incorrect answers and rationales

Exocrine glands secrete saliva and mucus.

45. Correct answer and rational B

The hypothalamus links the nervous system to the endocrine system via the pituitary gland.

Incorrect answers and rationales

Circadian rhythms are physical, mental, and behavioral changes that follow a 24-hour cycle. The pineal gland produces the hormone melatonin. Melatonin influences sexual development and sleep-wake cycles.

46. Correct answer and rational A

Dermis is the answer. The order from superficial to deep: dermis, hypodermis, stratum germinativum.

Incorrect answers and rationale

Epidermis is a superficial layer of stratified epithelium. The stratum germinativum is the deepest layer of the epidermis. It is also referred to as the basal layer of the skin.

47. Correct answer and rational B

The stratum corneum is the outermost epidermal layer of the skin, which consists of dead cells called corneocytes.

Incorrect answers and rationale

The dermis is a connective tissue layer sandwiched between the epidermis and subcutaneous tissue. The interstitium is a supporting material or connective tissue that lies between the principal cells of an organ or between structures in the body.

48. Correct answer and rational B

A sebaceous gland is a microscopic exocrine gland in the skin that opens into a hair follicle to secrete an oily or waxy matter, called sebum.

Incorrect answers and rationale

Sebaceous glands are not located on soles of the feet or the palms of the hands.

49. Correct answer and rational C

Apocrine sweat glands refer to a gland, especially a sweat gland, that secretes a viscous fluid into a hair follicle.

Incorrect answers and rationale

Endocrine organs are located inside the body. Proprioceptors are in muscles, tendons, ligaments etc.

50. Correct answer and rational A

The interstitium is a network of collagen fibers and fluid-filled spaces that underlies the skin and surrounds the gut, muscles, and blood vessels.

Incorrect answers and rationale

Chyme is the semifluid mass of partly digested food expelled by the stomach into the duodenum. Alveoli are tiny, thin-walled, capillary-rich sacks in the lungs where the exchange of oxygen and carbon dioxide takes place.

51. Correct answer and rational C

Pressure applied to the skin is the primary stimulus for touch sensations.

Incorrect answers and rationales

Muscle tone is the amount of tension a muscle has at rest and is regulated by the local spinal cord reflexes at the segmental level which innervate that muscle. Visceral pain originates from the internal organs.

52. Correct answer and rational B

The integumentary system functions to guard the body, providing a barrier to infection.

Incorrect answers and rationales

The skin does synthesize Vitamin D. It excretes waste products into the sweat but these functions are not directly related to the immune function.

53. Correct answer and rational A

Pacinian corpuscles are rapidly adapting (phasic) receptors that detect gross pressure changes and vibrations in the skin. Pacinian corpuscles have been found mainly in the deep portions of the skin tissue.

Incorrect answers and rationales

Merkel's Disks are located superficially in the dermis of skin at the base of the epidermis and lie adjacent to Meissner's corpuscles and sweat glands. These receptors respond to indentation of the skin. They adapt slowly to pressure, and therefore record the sustained presence of pressure on the skin. Ruffini Endings (or Corpuscles) are found in the superficial dermis of both hairy and the thick hairless skin that is located on the soles of our feet and the palms of the hands, detecting low-frequency vibration or pressure.

54. Correct answer and rational C

The tongue, lips, and fingertips are the most touch-sensitive parts of the body.

Incorrect answers and rationales

Back and abdomen contain fewer sensory receptors than the hands.

55. Correct answer and rational A

The tonsils are part of the lymphatic system, which help to fight infections.

Incorrect answers and rationale

Integumentary system is most related to skin. Digestive system includes organs such as stomach, liver, etc.

56. Correct answer and rational B

The spleen is part of the lymphatic system.

Incorrect answers and rationales

The appendix is a small pouch attached at the other end to the cecum. The pancreas makes pancreatic juices, which contain enzymes that aid in digestion, and produces several hormones, including insulin.

57. Correct answer and rational C
    When pressure is greater in the interstitial fluid around the cells interstitial fluid enters the lymphatic capillary.
    Incorrect answers and rationales
    Ventricles are located in the heart and lymph nodes filter lymph.

58. Correct answer and rational A
    Interstitial fluid slips through spaces between the overlapping endothelial cells that compose the lymphatic capillary. Once the fluid is in the lymphatic capillary it is called lymph.
    Incorrect answers and rationales
    Lymph is not located in the spaces between the cells. That fluid is interstitial fluid. Lacteals transfer chyle to lymph vessels in the walls of the small intestine.

59. Correct answer and rational C
    Plasma flows through arteries, smaller arteriole blood vessels, and capillaries. Most plasma is returned by way of veins but some seeps through the capillaries and into interstitial spaces. The lymphatic system collects this excess fluid.
    Incorrect answers and rationales
    Lymphocytes are a type of immune cell that is made in the bone marrow and is found in the blood and in lymph tissue. Enzymes are proteins that act as biological catalysts.

60. Correct answer and rational B
    The rhythmic contraction and relaxation of breathing acts as a pump for the lymphatic system.
    Incorrect answers and rationales
    Smooth muscle peristalsis is a series of wave-like muscle contractions that move food through the digestive tract. The period of time that begins with contraction of the atria and ends with ventricular relaxation is known as the cardiac cycle controlled by the cardiac conducting system which is regulated by the medulla via the autonomic nervous system.

61. Correct answer and rational A
    Popliteal nodes are in the area of the knee.
    Incorrect answers and rationales
    Superficial cubital nodes are in the elbow area. Inguinal notes are in the groin area.

62. Correct answer and rational B
    Plasma moves into the spaces around cells and is called interstitial fluid. Lymph capillaries collect interstitial fluid into the lymph vessels where it is then called lymph.
    Incorrect answers and rationales
    Urine is a waste fluid from the kidneys. Cytoplasm is found inside cells.

63. Correct answer and rational B
    Lymphocytes are immune cells made in bone marrow and found in blood and lymph tissue.
    Incorrect answers and rationales
    Erythrocytes are red blood cells. Platelets are part of the blood clotting process.

64. Correct answer and rational C
    The left subclavian vein plays a key role in the absorption of lipids, by allowing products that have been carried by lymph in the thoracic duct to enter the bloodstream.
    Incorrect answers and rationales
    Lymphatic fluid is returned to the bloodstream in veins not arteries. Hepatic relates to the liver.

65. Correct answer and rational A
    Lacteals are special lymphatic vessels in the small intestine that absorb and transport fat. The smallest of the lacteals are the lacteal capillaries, running down the center of a villus, in the mucous membrane lining the small intestine.
    Incorrect answers and rationales
    The esophagus and stomach do not contain lacteals.

66. Correct answer and rational C
    Gliding moves the skin and superficial facia in a horizontal manner that opens lymph capillaries which take in interstitial fluid from tissue spaces.
    Incorrect answers and rationales
    Percussion and friction would not be as effective in opening the lymphatic capillaries since there is much less horizontal direction focus during the application of the method.

67. Correct answer and rational B
    Muscle fibers in a pennate muscle can only pull at an angle, and as a result, contracting pennate muscles do not move their tendons very far. However, because a pennate muscle generally can hold more muscle fibers within it, it can produce relatively more tension for its size.
    Incorrect answers and rationales
    A convergent muscle arises from a broad area and converges to form a single tendon with the ability to move in multiple directions but not with as much force. Parallel muscles have a long excursion (% of shortening), but they are only moderately strong in terms of the whole muscle force they can generate.

68. Correct answer and rational A
    A motor unit refers to one motor neuron, located in the spinal cord, and the population of muscle fibers that it innervates.
    Incorrect answers and rationales
    A nerve plexus is a system of connected nerve fibers that link spinal nerves with specific areas of the body. A sarcomere is the basic contractile unit of muscle fiber.

69. Correct answer and rational C
    The term *myotatic unit* describes synergistic and antagonistic muscles controlling a joint.
    Incorrect answers and rationales
    The crossed extensor reflex is a contralateral reflex that allows the body to compensate on one side for a stimulus on the other. The threshold stimulus a stimulus that is just strong enough to elicit a response.

70. Correct answer and rational B

Peristalsis is the involuntary constriction and relaxation of the smooth muscles of the intestine or another canal, creating wave-like movements that push the contents of the canal forward.

Incorrect answers and rationales

Skeletal muscle relates to joint movement and cardiac muscle to heart pumping.

71. Correct answer and rational C

The neuromuscular junction is a type of synapse where neuronal signals from the brain or spinal cord interact with skeletal muscle fibers, causing them to contract. The activation of many muscle fibers together causes muscles to contract.

Incorrect answers and rationales

Sliding of the filaments is produced by the action of numerous cross bridges that extend out from the myosin toward the actin after the neuro input.

72. Correct answer and rational A

An isometric contraction is a muscle contraction without motion.

Incorrect answers and rationales

Concentric action happens when the muscle contracts and produces movement. Eccentric action happens when the muscle lengthens.

73. Correct answer and rational A

The nervous system is involved in receiving information about the environment around us (sensation) and generating responses to that information.

Incorrect answers and rationales

The cardiovascular system moves blood through the body. The immune system protects against disease.

74. Correct answer and rational C

Accessory nerves are the 11th pair of cranial nerves, consisting of motor fibers from the spinal cord that innervate the pharyngeal, trapezius, and sternocleidomastoid.

Incorrect answers and rationales

The suprascapular nerves main function is to provide motor supply for two of five muscles of the rotator cuff. Quadratus lumborum is innervated by the subcostal nerve (T12)

75. Correct answer and rational B

Neurons are the fundamental units of the brain and nervous system.

Incorrect answers and rationales

Neuroglia are cells whose primary function is to protect and maintain the optimum functioning of your nervous system. A nerve is a bundle of fibers which uses electrical and chemical signals to transmit sensory and motor information from one body part to another.

76. Correct answer and rational C

Mixed nerves are composed of both motor and sensory fibers, transmitting messages in both directions.

Incorrect answers and rationales

Neurons are the fundamental units of the brain and nervous system. A ganglion is a collection of neuronal bodies found in the peripheral nervous system.

77. Correct answer and rational A

The medulla oblongata is a portion of the hindbrain that controls autonomic functions such as breathing, digestion, heart and blood vessel function, swallowing, etc.

Incorrect answers and rationales

The cerebrum is a major part of the brain. Its upper layer, called the cerebral cortex, is responsible for a range of complex functions and the source of intellect and personality.

The cerebellum is the brain region that coordinates sensory input with muscular responses.

78. Correct answer and rational C

The thalamus is the part of the brain where sensory information from all over the body converges and is then sent to various areas of the cortex.

Incorrect answers and rationales

Cerebellum is the brain region that coordinates sensory input with muscular responses, contributing to balance. The limbic system involves functions including emotion, behavior, long-term memory, and is the sensation of smell.

79. Correct answer and rational A

The pituitary gland is a pea-sized organ. It's the "master gland" because it tells other glands to release hormones.

Incorrect answers and rationales

The cerebellum contributes to sense of balance and coordination. The thalamus where sensory information from all over the body converges and is sent to various areas of the cortex.

80. Correct answer and rational B

The cerebellum is the brain region that coordinates sensory input with muscular responses.

Incorrect answers and rationales

The medulla oblongata is a portion of the hindbrain that controls autonomic functions such as breathing, digestion, heart and blood vessel function, swallowing, etc. The limbic system involves functions including emotion, behavior, long-term memory, and the sensation of smell.

81. Correct answer and rational B

The limbic system involves functions including emotion, behavior, long-term memory, and is the sensation of smell.

Incorrect answers and rationales

The pituitary is involved in releasing hormones and regulating endocrine glands. The hippocampus functions in storage of new information in memory.

82. Correct answer and rational A

Broca's area is a region in the frontal lobe of the dominant hemisphere, usually the left, of the brain with functions linked to speech production.

Incorrect answers and rationales

The hippocampus functions in storage of new information in memory and is part of the limbic system. Injury to the Wernicke's Area of the brain would interfere with comprehension of speech.

83. Correct answer and rational C

The hippocampus functions in storage of new information in memory and is part of the limbic system.

Incorrect answers and rationales

Broca's area is a region in the frontal lobe of the dominant hemisphere linked to the ability to talk. Speech comprehension involves the Wernicke's area of the brain.

84. Correct answer and rational B

The five terminal branches of the brachial plexus are the musculocutaneous, median, ulnar, axillary, and radial nerves. This plexus arises from the anterior rami of spinal nerves C5-T1.

Incorrect answers and rationales

The brachial plexus is not located in the leg. Cervicogenic headache occurs when pain is referred from a specific source in the neck up to the head. Cervicogenic headache is felt to be referred from the first three spinal nerves—known as C1-C3 of the upper cervical spine.

85. Correct answer and rational C

There are 31 pairs of spinal nerves.

Incorrect answers and rationales

There are 31 pairs of spinal nerves not 12 or 18.

86. Correct answer and rational A

The axillary nerve provides function to three muscles: the deltoid, the teres minor, and the long head of the triceps muscle.

Incorrect answers and rationales

The musculocutaneous nerve travels along the front of the humerus and provides function to the coracobrachialis, biceps, and brachialis muscles. The ulnar nerve innervates the majority of the intrinsic hand muscles.

87. Correct answer and rational A

The vertebral column, also known as the spinal column, is a flexible column that encloses the spinal cord.

Incorrect answers and rationales

The skull protects the brain. The ribcage protects the heart and lungs.

88. Correct answer and rational B

The tibial nerve branches off from the sciatic nerve. It provides innervation to the muscles of the lower leg and foot.

Incorrect answers and rationales

The radial nerve is in the arm. The latissimus dorsi muscle is innervated by the thoracodorsal nerve.

89. Correct answer and rational A

The fibular (peroneal) nerve can cause knee pain. This nerve starts in the back part of the knee and controls some of the muscles in the leg and the foot.

Incorrect answers and rationales

The median nerve crosses the elbow anteriorly, controlling flexion movement muscles of the forearm and hand. The pudendal nerve innervates the perineum and external genitalia.

90. Correct answer and rational B

The saphenous nerve is the largest and terminal branch of the femoral nerve and passes under the inguinal ligament laterally following the femoral artery.

Incorrect answers and rationales

The obturator nerve descends through the fibers of the psoas major and emerges from its medial border. The accessory nerve is a cranial nerve.

91. Correct answer and rational C

Ascending tracts refer to the neural pathways by which sensory information from the peripheral nerves are transmitted to the cerebral cortex.

Incorrect answers and rationales

Neurolemma is the thin sheath around a nerve axon. Descending tracts are the pathways by which motor signals are sent from the brain to lower motor neurons.

92. Correct answer and rational A

A synapse is the junction between two nerve cells, consisting of a minute gap across which impulses pass by diffusion of a neurotransmitter.

Incorrect answers and rationales

A dendrite is a structure that extends away from the cell body to receive messages from other neurons. Glial cells are also known as neuroglia or simply glia and are essentially any of several kinds of cells that principally focus on supporting nerve cells.

93. Correct answer and rational B

Myelinated nerve fibers allow for fast transmission of the nerve impulse as depolarization occurs only at the nodes of Ranvier.

Incorrect answers and rationales

C group nerve fibers are unmyelinated and have a small diameter and low conduction velocity. Neuroglia are any of several kinds of cells that principally support nerve cells.

94. Correct answer and rational A

Stimulus-sensory neuron-motor neuron-action is the correct sequence of events in a reflex.

Incorrect answers and rationales

Stimulus-motor neuron-sensory neuron-action is incorrect because a stimulus travels on a sensory neuron. Action-sensory neuron-motor neuron-stimulus is incorrect since a reflex begins with a stimulus.

95. Correct answer and rational C

Massage and bodywork application of touch are sensory stimuli.

Incorrect answers and rationales

A motor response is the output from the cortex to control the musculature through motor neurons. The reticular activating system coordinates both the sleep-wake cycle and wakefulness.

96. Correct answer and rational B

The medulla oblongata is continuous with the spinal cord.

Incorrect answers and rationales

The frontal cortex and corpus callosum are part of the brain but do not directly attach to the spinal cord.

97. Correct answer and rational C

The myelin sheath covers the axon in myelinated nerves.

Incorrect answers and rationales

Dendrites are projections from the nerve cell body. A synapse is where a signal moves from one neuron to another.

98. Correct answer and rational A

The prostate is part of the male reproductive system.

Incorrect answers and rationales

The prostate is not part of the female reproductive system or digestive system.

99. Correct answer and rational B

Estrogen is one of two main female sex hormones. The other is progesterone. Estrogen is responsible for female physical features and reproduction. Men have estrogen but in smaller amounts.

Incorrect answers and rationales

In men, the testicles primarily make testosterone. Women's ovaries also make testosterone, though in much smaller amounts. Thyroxine is the primary hormone secreted by the thyroid gland.

100. Correct answer and rational A

The uterus is located in the hypogastric region.

Incorrect answers and rationales

The organs found in the left upper quadrant are the left sections of the liver and kidney, adrenal gland, spleen, stomach, pancreas, colon's splenic flexure and lower portion of the colon. The anterior thorax includes the chest.

101. Correct answer and rational C

Female organs are primarily located inside the body while male testes are outside of the body cavity.

Incorrect answers and rationales

Both male and females have gonads. Gonads are the primary reproductive glands that produce reproductive cells (gametes). In males the gonads are called testes; the gonads in females are called ovaries. Both males and females make testosterone.

102. Correct answer and rational B

The reproductive systems involve hormones.

Incorrect answers and rationales

Neurotransmitters are chemicals in the nervous system. The corpus callosum is a brain structure.

103. Correct answer and rational A

Ovulation is the release of eggs from the ovaries.

Incorrect answers and rationales

Menopause refers cessation of the menstrual cycle. Menstruation is the process of shedding blood and other materials from the lining of the uterus if pregnancy does not occur.

104. Correct answer and rational C

Positive feedback is a process in which the end products of an action cause more of that action to occur in a feedback loop. This amplifies the original action.

Incorrect answers and rationales

An action potential begins when the cell's membrane potential reaches threshold. Once initiated the action potential has a consistent structure and is an all-or-nothing event. Negative feedback is when the end results of an action inhibit that action from continuing to occur.

105. Correct answer and rational C

The mediastinum is the area in the chest between the lungs.

Incorrect answers and rationales

The mediastinum is the anatomic region located between the lungs that contains all the principal tissues and organs of the chest including the heart but not the lungs. The kidneys are located on either side of the spine, with the top of each kidney beginning around the 11th or 12th rib space closer to the back side of the abdomen.

106. Correct answer and rational A

Intercostal means pertaining to muscles, parts, or intervals between the ribs.

Incorrect answers and rationales

Costovertebral relates to the ribs and the thoracic vertebrae where ribs articulate. The metacarpals are long bones of the hand that are connected to the carpals, or wrist bones, and to the phalanges, or finger bones.

107. Correct answer and rational B

Pleura are serous membranes lining the thorax and enveloping the lungs.

Incorrect answers and rationales

Mucus is a normal, slippery, and stringy fluid substance produced by many lining tissues in the body. Serous fluid is a clear to pale yellow watery fluid that is found in the body, especially in the spaces between organs and the membranes which line or enclose them.

108. Correct answer and rational A

At its bottom end the trachea divides into left and right air tubes called bronchi connected to the lungs.

Incorrect answers and rationales

The trachea divides into left and right air tubes called bronchi at the distal end not proximal end. The larynx is connected to the top of the trachea.

109. Correct answer and rational B

The lungs are enclosed in the rib cage.

Incorrect answers and rationales

The dorsal cavity contains the skull, brain, and spinal cavity. Organs located in the right lower quadrant include the ascending colon, the cecum, the right ovary and fallopian tube, the right ureter, and the appendix.

110. Correct answer and rational B

Trachea, bronchi, bronchioles is the correct branching order into the lungs.

Incorrect answers and rationales

111. Correct answer and rational C
Carbon dioxide is the byproduct of respiration.
Incorrect answers and rationales
Hydrogen and methane are mostly produced in the large intestine.

112. Correct answer and rational A
Expiration moves carbon dioxide out of the body.
Incorrect answers and rationales
Inspiration brings air is. Peristalsis is smooth muscle contraction.
The incorrect answers are in the wrong order.

113. Correct answer and rational C
Anaerobic respiration is the type of respiration through which cells can break down sugars to generate energy in the absence of oxygen.
Incorrect answers and rationales
Carbon dioxide is a waste product of respiration. Aerobic respiration occurs with oxygen.

114. Correct answer and rational A
Alveoli are air sacs in the lungs.
Incorrect answers and rationales
The lungs are surrounded by two membranes called the pleurae. Two hollow tubes leading into the lungs are called bronchi.

115. Correct answer and rational B
Anaerobic metabolism produces lactic acid.
Incorrect answers and rationales
Nitric oxide is produced within skeletal muscle fibers and has various functions in skeletal muscle supporting glucose uptake during contraction/exercise. Aside from glucose produced by your liver, food is the main source of plasma glucose. Glucose is used by all cells and is a common fuel for the body.

116. Correct answer and rational B
The primary inspiratory muscles are the diaphragm and external intercostals.
Incorrect answers and rationales
Micturition is a process where urine is expelled from the body. Peristalsis is the involuntary constriction and relaxation of the muscles of the intestine or another canal, creating wave-like movements that push the contents of the canal forward.

117. Correct answer and rational C
The alveolar surface is moist to aid the diffusion of gases. Alveoli are located in the alveolar sacs of the lungs, allowing for the exchange of oxygen and carbon dioxide during breathing.
Incorrect answers and rationales

118. Correct answer and rational A
When arm and shoulder are in a fixed and stable position, the serratus anterior helps to elevate ribs. This occurs during normal breathing therefore the serratus anterior muscles are considered secondary/accessory muscles of respiration.
Incorrect answers and rationales
The primary inspiratory muscles are the diaphragm and external intercostals. The obturator internus muscle is located in the obturator fossa of the pelvis and not considered a respiratory muscle.
Alveoli do not aid swallowing or blood flow in the intestines.

119. Correct answer and rational C
Hemoglobin in red blood cells binds with oxygen.
Incorrect answers and rationales
Fibrin together with platelets form plugs over damaged areas of blood vessels

120. Correct answer and rational B
The mucus in the trachea helps capture microorganisms such as viruses and harmful bacteria before they enter the lungs.
Incorrect answers and rationales
Mucus does not aid in gas diffusion or increased blood flow.

121. Correct answer and rational A
The scalene muscles act as accessory muscles of respiration and perform flexion at the neck.
Incorrect answers and rationales
The main accessory muscles of expiration are the abdominal wall muscles. Vomiting is the involuntary, forceful expulsion of the contents of one's stomach through the mouth and sometimes the nose.

122. Correct answer and rational C
An increase in carbon dioxide concentration leads to a decrease in the pH of blood due to the production of H^+ ions from carbonic acid. In response to a decrease in blood pH, the respiratory center in the medulla sends nervous impulses to the external intercostal muscles and the diaphragm, to increase the breathing rate and the volume of the lungs during inhalation.
Incorrect answers and rationales
The cough reflex is a protective mechanism that allows the body to expel inhaled particles. Carbon monoxide poisoning occurs when carbon monoxide builds up in your bloodstream. When too much carbon monoxide is in the air, your body replaces the oxygen in your red blood cells with carbon monoxide.

123. Correct answer and rational C
During expiration, the elastic recoil of the lungs and chest wall causes intra-pleural pressure to decrease.
Incorrect answers and rationales
Inspiration expands the chest wall including the ribs and pressure in the lungs increases.

124. Correct answer and rational A
Oxygen debt occurs when the body reaches a state of anaerobic respiration during intense exercise.
Incorrect answers and rationales
Aerobic exercise is when oxygen is used during exercise and is also called endurance exercise.

125. Correct answer and rational B
Breathing is both voluntary/somatic and automatic/autonomic in regulation.
Incorrect answers and rationales

Chewing and jumping are voluntary/somatic.
126. Correct answer and rational A

Hyperventilation is breathing that is deeper and more rapid than normal. It causes a decrease in the amount of a gas in the blood (called carbon dioxide, or CO_2). This decrease typically causes light-headedness, numbness or tingling in hands or feet, a rapid heartbeat, and shortness of breath. It also can lead to anxiety, fainting, and sore chest muscles.

Incorrect answers and rationales

Tachycardia is the medical term for a heart rate over 100 beats per minute. Bradypnea is an abnormally slow breathing rate.

127. Correct answer and rational C

The tibia is in the leg which is part of the appendicular skeleton.

Incorrect answers and rationales

The pelvic girdle does not contain the tibia. The axial skeleton is the ribcage, spine, and skull.

128. Correct answer and rational A

Breastbone is the sternum.

Incorrect answers and rationales

Collarbone is the clavicle. Shoulder blade is the scapula.

129. Correct answer and rational C

Periosteum is a dense layer of vascular connective tissue enveloping the bones except at the surfaces of the joints.

Incorrect answers and rationales

Diaphysis is the long shaft of a bone. Endosteum is the thin layer of connective tissue which makes up the medullary cavity.

130. Correct answer and rational B

Pedicle is a short bony process lying on either side of a vertebra that projects posteriorly from the vertebral body.

Incorrect answers and rationales

An epicondyle is a protuberance above or on the condyle of a long bone, especially either of the two at the elbow end of the humerus or knee end of the femur. A malleolus is a rounded prominence on either side of the ankle joint.

131. Correct answer and rational A

Articulation is the correct answer. It is where two bones meet to form a joint.

Incorrect answers and rationales

A ligament is connective tissue that attaches bone to bone. Bursa is the fluid filled sac found between bones/tissues at the joint to counter friction.

132. Correct answer and rational C

The tibial tuberosity is the bony protrusion at the top of the tibia bone in the lower leg. It is located just underneath the patella.

Incorrect answers and rationales

A malleolus is a rounded prominence on either side of the ankle joint. The fibula is a small bone that runs along the outside of the lower leg.

133. Correct answer and rational A

Sesamoid is a small independent bone or bony nodule developed in a tendon where it passes over an angular structure, typically in the hands and feet. The kneecap is a particularly large sesamoid bone.

Incorrect answers and rationales

Flat bones are generally flat and broad providing protection and more space for muscle attachment. Irregular bones are the bones whose shape serves a very specific purpose.

134. Correct answer and rational A

The bone marrow is generally collected from the Ilium in the pelvic girdle.

Incorrect answers and rationales

The calcaneus is in the foot. The clavicle is part of the shoulder girdle.

135. Correct answer and rational B

In adults, hematopoiesis of red blood cells and platelets occurs primarily in the bone marrow.

Incorrect answers and rationales

Bone marrow fills the cavities of the bones and therefore is not a point of tendon attachment or protection of the brain.

136. Correct answer and rational C

The bony framework of the chest is a called the thoracic cage and protects vital organs such as the heart and lungs.

Incorrect answers and rationales

The shoulder girdle is the set of bones in the appendicular skeleton which connects to the arm on each side and the upper limb to the torso. The xiphoid process is a small projection off the sternum.

137. Correct answer and rational B

The Vestibulo-Ocular Reflex produces compensatory eye movements in response to head movement.

Incorrect answers and rationales

The mitral valve is in the heart. The nares are the openings of the nose and nasal cavity.

138. Correct answer and rational A

The semicircular canals are organs that are part of the vestibular system in the inner ear.

Incorrect answers and rationales

The semicircular canals are not located in the eyes or nose.

139. Correct answer and rational C

The vestibular system is the sensory apparatus of the inner ear that helps the body maintain its postural equilibrium. The information furnished by the vestibular system is also essential for coordinating the position of the head and the movement of the eyes.

Incorrect answers and rationales

Swallowing and nociceptors are not specifically part of vestibular function.

140. Correct answer and rational B

An odor is caused by one or more volatilized chemical compounds that stimulate the chemoreceptors in the nose.

Incorrect answers and rationales

Mechanoreceptors detect external stimuli usually in the form of touch, pressure, stretching. Proprioceptors are sensory receptors which receive stimuli from within the body and respond to position and movement.

141. Correct answer and rational A

Depth perception is the ability to see things in three dimensions including length, width, and depth.

Incorrect answers and rationales

Ears and nose are not directly involved in depth perception.

142. Correct answer and rational C

The vestibular system apparatus of the inner ear is involved in balance.

Incorrect answers and rationales

The tongue involves sense of taste. Olfactory nerves involve smell.

143. Correct answer and rational C

The kidneys maintain blood pressure through regulation of blood volume in the body. When electrolyte levels are high, the body retains more water, increasing the volume of blood.

Incorrect answers and rationales

The liver and the spleen are the major site of red blood cell elimination and iron recycling. The kidneys filter and eliminate liquid waste and make red blood cells.

144. Correct answer and rational A

Bladder is the organ that holds urine until it is ready to be released and then helps to expel it from the body.

Incorrect answers and rationales

Ureters bring urine to the bladder from the kidneys. The urethra is the tube that allows urine to pass out of the body.

145. Correct answer and rational B

The urinary system, also known as the renal system or urinary tract, consists of the kidneys, ureters, bladder, and the urethra. The purpose of the urinary system is to eliminate liquid waste from the body, regulate blood volume and blood pressure, control levels of electrolytes and metabolites, and regulate blood pH.

Incorrect answers and rationales

The lymphatic system helps maintain fluid balance in the body by collecting excess fluid and particulate matter from tissues but does not eliminate waste. The endocrine system is involved in homeostasis regulation using hormones.

146. Correct answer and rational A

The kidneys are located on either side of the spine, with the top of each kidney beginning around the 11th or 12th rib space.

Incorrect answers and rationales

Above and behind the pubic bone or anterior to the ilium are not kidney locations.

147. Correct answer and rational C

Kidneys are part of the urinary system.

Incorrect answers and rationales

The adrenal gland is part of the endocrine system. The spleen is part of the lymphatic system.

148. Correct answer and rational B

The urinary bladder is a muscular sac in the pelvis, just above and behind the pubic bone.

Incorrect answers and rationales

The stomach is located between the esophagus and the small intestine. The gallbladder is located below the liver.

149. Correct answer and rational A

The detrusor muscle is the muscle in the bladder that controls the emptying of the bladder.

Incorrect answers and rationales

The uterus and prostrate are part of the reproductive system.

150. Correct answer and rational B

In the kidneys and bladder, parasympathetic function stimulates peristalsis of ureters, contraction of the detrusor muscle, and relaxation of the internal urethral sphincter aiding in the flow and excretion of urine.

Incorrect answers and rationales

The enteric nervous system is found within the walls of the entire gastrointestinal tract. When the sympathetic nervous system is active, it causes the bladder to increase in capacity and stimulates the internal urinary sphincter to remain tightly closed.

Practice Test 3

Just Kinesiology—100 Questions

1. Correct answer and rational C

Muscles located in the transverse plan are typically internal or external rotators; also called medial and lateral rotation.

Incorrect answers and rationales

Muscles that function in the frontal (coronal) plane are adductors and abductors. Muscles located in the sagittal plane are primarily flexors and extensors.

2. Correct answer and rational C

Flexion and extension occur in the sagittal plane.

Incorrect answers and rationales

Muscles functioning in the transverse plan are typically internal or external rotators. Muscles that function in the frontal (coronal) plane are adductors and abductors.

3. Correct answer and rational A

In isometric exercise and contraction, the muscle length does not change, but the tension does.

Incorrect answers and rationales

In an isotonic exercise, the muscle length changes. An eccentric action is the lengthening of a muscle fiber.

4. Correct answer and rational B

Synergist muscles act around a moveable joint to produce motion similar to or in concert with agonist muscles.

Incorrect answers and rationales

An antagonist muscle acts to oppose the action of another muscle (the agonist). A fixator muscle holds a body part in a certain position or restricts its movement, usually so that other muscles may operate effectively.

5. Correct answer and rational A

Muscles functioning in the sagittal plane are primarily flexors and extensors.

Incorrect answers and rationales

Muscles functioning in the transverse plan are typically internal or external rotators. Muscles that function in the frontal (coronal) plane are adductors and abductors.

6. Correct answer and rational B

Muscles that function in the frontal (coronal) plane are adductors and abductors.

Incorrect answers and rationales

Muscles functioning in the transverse plan are typically internal or external rotators. Muscles functioning in the sagittal plane are primarily flexors and extensors.

7. Correct answer and rational A

When a joint is moved out of anatomical position the muscles producing the movement are acting concentrically shortening. To reverse the action and move back to anatomical position the muscles that were functioning eccentrically now need to shift to concentric movement shortening to reverse the position.

Incorrect answers and rationales

Lengthening relates to eccentric function. Stabilizing immobilizes or assists movement.

8. Correct answer and rational A

The fixator functions as a synergist but also provides stability.

Incorrect answers and rationales

Synergists help the prime mover. Antagonists resist agonists.

9. Correct answer and rational B

Concentric movement happens when muscles shorten. Eccentric movement occurs when muscles lengthen. Eccentric action controls motion by resisting shortening.

Incorrect answers and rationales

Isometric movement involves muscle contraction without movement. Pennate is a muscle shape.

10. Correct answer and rational C

An agonist, also called the prime mover would be shortening when contracting. This is a concentric function.

11. Correct answer and rational B

Joint kinesthetic receptors consist of different types of receptors located in the capsules of synovial joints, providing information about joint position. Ligaments structurally blend into the joint capsule.

Incorrect answers and rationales

Neuromuscular spindles are stretch receptor organs that regulate muscle tone via the spinal stretch reflex. Lamellar corpuscles are "rapidly adapting" mechanoreceptors that are particularly specialized in receiving vibrational, touch, and pressure stimuli

Incorrect answers and rationales

Antagonists function eccentrically in relationship to agonists.

12. Correct answer and rational A

Proprioceptors are sensory receptors which receives stimuli from within the body, especially related to position and movement.

Incorrect answers and rationales

Nociceptors are sensory receptors for painful stimuli. Tactile receptors are sensory receptors which respond to touch.

13. Correct answer and rational C

Muscle contains muscle spindles, sensory receptors that inform the central nervous system about changes in the length of individual muscles and the speed of stretching. The responses of muscle spindles to changes in length also play an important role in regulating the contraction of muscles, by activating motor neurons via the stretch reflex to resist muscle stretch.

Incorrect answers and rationales

The function of the Golgi tendon receptors can be considered opposite of muscle spindles causing associated muscles to relax by interrupting contraction. Free nerve endings trigger signals associated with the perception of pain and respond to a number of different substances that are released by damaged tissue.

14. Correct answer and rational A

The muscle spindles are proprioceptors detecting muscle length. A stretch reflex occurs if muscle is stretched quickly.

Incorrect answers and rationales

When muscles contract they produce tension at the point where the muscle is connected to the tendon, where the Golgi tendon organ is located. The Golgi tendon organ records the change in tension, and the rate of change of the tension, and sends signals to the CNS. When this tension exceeds a certain threshold, it triggers the lengthening reaction which inhibits the muscles from contracting and causes them to relax.

15. Correct answer and rational A

The ischial tuberosity is the posterior portion of the ramus of the ischium, where body weight is supported when seated. The hamstrings attach to the ischial tuberosity at the proximal end.

Incorrect answers and rationales

The quadriceps and sartorius would not be directly compressed when seated.

16. Correct answer and rational B

The flexor digiti minimi brevis flexes the little toe.

Incorrect answers and rationales

The extensor hallucis brevis and flexor hallucis brevis move the great toe.

17. Correct answer and rational C
Both latissimus dorsi and teres major are adductors of the glenohumeral joint.
Incorrect answers and rationales
Gluteus Medius and adductor magnus are antagonists. Supraspinatus acts on the glenohumeral joint and Pectoralis Minor acts on the scapula.

18. Correct answer and rational A
Biceps femoris short head flexes the knee. Vastus lateralis extends of the knee.
Incorrect answers and rationales
Gracilis action is adduction and medial rotation. Rectus femoris is part of quadriceps muscles that extend the knee.

19. Correct answer and rational A
The triceps brachii proximal attachment is at the infraglenoid tubercle of the scapula. The triceps brachii muscle is the primary extensor of the elbow.
Incorrect answers and rationales
The brachioradialis and the trapezius muscles are not located at the lateral aspect of the scapula, inferior to the glenoid cavity.

20. Correct answer and rational B
The radial styloid process is found on the lateral surface of the distal radius bone. The tendon of the brachioradialis attaches at its base.
Incorrect answers and rationales
The lateral supracondylar ridge is a narrow ridge running proximally from the lateral epicondyle of the humerus and is the proximal attachment site of the brachioradialis. The fifth metacarpal is the bone of the little finger.

21. Correct answer and rational C
The olecranon process of the ulna is the most proximal part of the ulna. The triceps brachii is the primary extensor of the elbow, attaching from the ulna to the humerus and scapula.
Incorrect answers and rationales
The infraglenoid tubercle is the part of the scapula from which the long head of the triceps brachii muscle originates. Biceps brachii muscle inserts on the radial tuberosity and bicipital aponeurosis into deep fascia on the medial part of the forearm.

22. Correct answer and rational B
The function of the anterior and mid fibers of the temporalis muscle is to elevate the mandible. The posterior fibers of the temporalis muscle function to retract the mandible.
Incorrect answers and rationales
The mentalis muscle elevates, everts, and protrudes the lower lip. Medial Rectus muscle located on the side of the eyeball closer to the nose is responsible for moving eyes toward the nose.

23. Correct answer and rational C

The main function of the levator scapulae muscle is to elevate and retract the shoulder girdle at the scapulothoracic joint.
Incorrect answers and rationales
The occipitals draw the scalp backward. The major muscle that laterally flexes and rotates the head is the sternocleidomastoid.

24. Correct answer and rational C
The upper trapezius can elevate the shoulder girdle.
Incorrect answers and rationales
The middle trapezius retracts the scapula toward the spine. The lower trapezius depresses the shoulder girdle.

25. Correct answer and rational A
The rectus capitis lateralis, trapezius, splenius capitis, and sternocleidomastoid all act on the atlanto-occipital joint, but the rectus capitis lateralis is the deepest muscle in the area.
Incorrect answers and rationales
The splenius capitis is located on the posterior neck, below the most superficial muscles and on top of the sub occipital muscles. The sternocleidomastoid muscle is more superficial.

26. Correct answer and rational C
The sub-occipital muscles are located in the posterior neck at the base of the skull under many other structures.
Incorrect answers and rationales
Muscles of mastication that are located on the surface and easy to access are the masseter and temporalis. The pterygoids are more difficult to access. The plantar group consists of all the other intrinsic muscles of the foot.

27. Correct answer and rational B
The Splenius Capitis acts as an extensor and lateral flexor of the neck, while assisting rotation.
Incorrect answers and rationales
Zygomaticus major elevates and draws the angle of the mouth laterally. The sternocleidomastoid muscles flex the neck and assist movement of the head.

28. Correct answer and rational A
The scalenes function as elevators of the first and second ribs during inspiration. The anterior and medial scalenes elevate the first rib and the posterior scalene elevates the second rib.
Incorrect answers and rationales
External intercostal muscles and posterior scalenes are synergists since both contract during inspiration and lift the ribs. The antagonist would be the internal intercostal muscles that move the ribcage inward and downward. The xiphoid process is the most distal edge of the sternum.

29. Correct answer and rational B
Abductor muscles are the muscles that pull body parts outwards away from the midline.
Incorrect answers and rationales

The adductor muscles are the muscles that pull body parts towards the midline/midsagittal/median plane of the body. Flexion is a movement in the sagittal plane.

30. Correct answer and rational A

Muscles functioning to extend the head would have attachments on the occipital bone.

Incorrect answers and rationales

The sternum in located on the anterior torso. The mandible is the jaw bone.

31. Correct answer and rational C

The main actions for rectus abdominis are flexion of the trunk by drawing the pubic symphysis and sternum toward each other.

Incorrect answers and rationales

Extensor muscles are attached to the back of the spine, including the erector spinae which help hold up the spine. The gluteal muscles and deep lateral hip rotators are involved in hip rotation.

32. Correct answer and rational B

The adductors are layered muscles of the medial thigh that fan out from the small area of attachment on the pubic bone toward the femur to insert into the linea aspera of the femur.

Incorrect answers and rationales

Abductor muscles of hip would be found on the lateral side of the hip. Hip flexors are located on the anterior aspect of the femur.

33. Correct answer and rational C

Quadratus femoris externally rotates the thigh which is a transverse plane movement.

Incorrect answers and rationales

The quadratus lumborum contributes to the stabilization and movement of the spine and the pelvis. A bilateral contraction causes extension of the lumbar area, a sagittal plane movement. The quadratus plantae muscle flexes the second to fifth toes, a sagittal plane movement.

34. Correct answer and rational C

The triceps muscle is a pennate muscle with three heads: long, lateral, and medial which produce elbow extension.

Incorrect answers and rationales

The brachialis muscle is a flexor of the forearm at the elbow joint. It is fusiform in shape. The interossei muscles are intrinsic muscles of the hand or foot.

35. Correct answer and rational A

The knee flexors include the gastrocnemius which has proximal attachments on the medial and lateral condyles of the femur located on the distal posterior femur.

Incorrect answers and rationales

Hip extension involves the gluteal muscle group which is attached to the proximal femur, while the hamstrings distal attachments are on the medial tibia and fibular head. The shoulder adduction muscles are latissimus dorsi and pectoralis major.

36. Correct answer and rational B

The lesser tubercle of the humerus is the insertion of the subscapularis muscle.

Incorrect answers and rationales

The ligamentum nuchae is a midline or median structure found in the posterior aspect of the neck. The clavicle joins the scapula and sternum.

37. Correct answer and rational A

Latissimus dorsi would internally rotate the arm to the point that the palms are facing the lateral aspect of the upper thigh.

Incorrect answers and rationales

Triceps function at the elbow and scapula. Anterior serratus protracts the scapula.

38. Correct answer and rational C

The pelvic diaphragm is composed of the levator ani and coccygeus muscles. This pelvic diaphragm assists in forced expiration, coughing, sneezing, vomiting, urinating, defecating.

Incorrect answers and rationales

Gluteus maximus, gluteus medius, gemelli superior, and gemelli inferior function at the hip.

39. Correct answer and rational B

The spinalis cervicis muscles extend and hyperextend the cervical portion of the vertebral column when acting together.

Incorrect answers and rationales

The longus capitis and longus colli muscles are located anterior to the cervical vertebrae and produce flexion of the head.

40. Correct answer and rational A

The movement of the sole towards the median plane is inversion.

Incorrect answers and rationales

Rotation is a pivotal movement, a revolving around a single axis. Abduction is a movement away from the midline.

41. Correct answer and rational B

Hyaline cartilage coats the ends of the bone surfaces, reducing friction in the joints.

Incorrect answers and rationales

Fibrocartilage is normally found on tendon and ligament insertions. Elastic cartilage is found either in the trachea or earlobe.

42. Correct answer and rational C

Abduction means to move away from the midline.

Incorrect answers and rationales

Adduction means to add to the midline or bring it closer.

43. Correct answer and rational C

In flexion of the lumbar spine, the back flattens, leading to a decrease in lordosis.

Incorrect answers and rationales

Extension increases lordosis. Kyphosis is a normal outward curve of the spine in the thorax. Hyper-kyphosis, or an enlarged outward curve, is an abnormal curving of the spine.

44. Correct answer and rational A

Elevation is the upward movement of a body structures i.e. cranial towards the skull.

Incorrect answers and rationales

Extension refers to movement where the angle between two bones increases, otherwise known as straightening. Eversion is the movement of the foot causing the sole of the foot to face outward.

45. Correct answer and rational B

In anatomic position, the body is erect with the head and torso upright. Arms are at the sides of the torso with the shoulders in neutral rotation. Elbows are extended with palms facing forward. The lower extremities are straight and parallel, with the second toe facing straight forward. For measuring joint movement this is the 0 position.

Incorrect answers and rationales

Ideal alignment is a standard, theoretical position in which all joints of the body are centered and balanced. In anatomy, the sagittal plane, or longitudinal plane, is an anatomical plane which divides the body into right and left parts.

46. Correct answer and rational A

Caudal describes how close something is to the tail bone. Depression of the shoulder in is the direction of the tailbone/coccyx.

Incorrect answers and rationales

Contraction is to tighten or shorten. Abduction is movement away from the midline.

47. Correct answer and rational B

Osteokinematics is the gross movement that happens between two bones which can be done voluntarily such as flexion, extension, rotation, adduction, and abduction.

Incorrect answers and rationales

Arthrokinematics represents the small movements happening at the joint surface such a spin, roll, and glide. Equilibrium is a state of body balance, either stationary or moving.

48. Correct answer and rational C

Active range of motion refers to the ability of the client to voluntarily move the limb through an arc of movement.

Incorrect answers and rationales

Passive range of motion refers to the amount of movement that a joint obtains by the practitioner moving the segment without resistance or assistance from the client. Manual muscle testing is used to identify muscle strength or weakness.

49. Correct answer and rational A

Accessory motion is the ability of the joint surfaces to glide, roll, and spin on each other which is described as arthrokinematics.

Incorrect answers and rationales

Oscillatory motion is a repeating motion in which an object continuously repeats in the same motion again and again. Linear motions are one-dimensional on a straight line.

50. Correct answer and rational B

Synovial joint movement is under somatic nervous system control.

Incorrect answers and rationales

The vagus nerve is one of the most important nerves of the autonomic nervous system. Synovial joint movement is primarily voluntary.

51. Correct answer and rational B

The main movements in the knee joint are flexion and extension but also limited medial rotation in a flexed position and in the last stage of extension, as well as lateral rotation when "unlocking" and flexing the knee.

Incorrect answers and rationales

Adduction occurs when a joint moves a part of the body toward the midline in one plane. Nutation and counternutation are movements that happen at the sacroiliac joint.

52. Correct answer and rational C

The sacroiliac joints are the joints where the sacrum (part of the axial skeleton) connects to the pelvis (part of the appendicular skeleton).

Incorrect answers and rationales

The atlanto-axial joint is a joint between the first and second cervical vertebrae; the atlas and axis. The glenohumeral joint articulates the scapula with the humerus, both of which are part of the appendicular skeleton.

53. Correct answer and rational C

The medial collateral ligaments of the ankle joint are collectively called the deltoid ligament.

Incorrect answers and rationales

The elbow or hip are not the location of the deltoid ligament.

54. Correct answer and rational A

Circumduction is the movement of the limb, hand, or fingers in a circular pattern, using the sequential combination of flexion, adduction, extension, and abduction motions. This motion can occur at a ball and socket joint or a saddle joint.

Incorrect answers and rationales

Hinge and gliding joint types do not allow circumduction.

55. Correct answer and rational A

Adduction/abduction are frontal/coronal plane movements.

Incorrect answers and rationales

Flexion/extension occurs in the sagittal plane. Medial/lateral rotation occurs in the transverse plane.

56. Correct answer and rational A

Range of motion is commonly abbreviated as ROM.

Incorrect answers and rationales

Repair of muscles and restriction of movement are not abbreviated as ROM.

57. Correct answer and rational B

The ligament on the inside of the elbow is the ulnar collateral ligament. The thumb also has an ulnar collateral ligament. Both are in the upper limb.

Incorrect answers and rationales

Lower limb and thorax are not locations for the ulnar collateral ligament.

58. Correct answer and rational C

Synovial fluid is contained by synovial membranes, located in cavities between bones of joints. Articular cartilage contains chondrocytes which produce the thick liquid part of synovial fluid.

Incorrect answers and rationales

Lymph fluid is in the lymph vessels. Plasma fluid carries blood components throughout the body.

59. Correct answer and rational B

The multifidus muscle starts at the sacral bone at the base of the spine and extends up to the axis. The muscle attaches at multiple points along the spine, specifically into the spinous process of each vertebra.

Incorrect answers and rationales

Carpal joints are in the wrist. Acromioclavicular joints include the scapula and clavicle.

60. Correct answer and rational C

A uniaxial joint only allows for a motion in a single plane around a single axis. The elbow joint, which only allows for bending or straightening, is an example of a uniaxial joint.

Incorrect answers and rationales

A biaxial joint allows for motions within two planes. The shoulder and hip joints are multiaxial joints. The temporomandibular joint (TMJ) or jaw joint is a bi-arthroidal hinge joint that allows for complex movements.

61. Correct answer and rational B

A suture is a type of fibrous joint.

Incorrect answers and rationales

A diarthrosis is a freely moveable joint. Ellipsoid joints allow back and forth and side to side movement and are found between the metacarpals and phalanges.

62. Correct answer and rational A

The hip joint, also known as the acetabulofemoral joint, is a synovial joint that allows flexion, extension, abduction, adduction, rotation, and circumduction.

Incorrect answers and rationales

The superior tibiofibular joint is a plane synovial joint, while the inferior one is a syndesmosis (fibrous joint). These joints allow no active movements except a small range of gliding to accommodate the movements of the ankle joint. The knee joint, also known as the tibiofemoral joint, is a synovial biaxial modified hinge joint.

63. Correct answer and rational C

A diarthrosis is a freely moveable joint.

Incorrect answers and rationales

Syndesmoses are slightly movable fibrous joints held together by ligaments. A cartilaginous joint is also called an amphiarthrosis where two bones are linked by cartilage. The two types of cartilaginous joints are synchondroses and symphyses.

64. Correct answer and rational C

The functional classification of joints is determined by the amount of mobility found between the adjacent bones. Joints are thus functionally classified as a synarthrosis or immobile joint, an amphiarthrosis or slightly moveable joint, or as a diarthrosis, which is a freely moveable joint

Incorrect answers and rationales

Synovial and *symphyses* are not terms related to function. Joint classification based on structure relates to the presence/absence of a joint cavity as well as what types of tissue bind the bones together: fibrous joint, cartilaginous joint, synovial joint.

65. Correct answer and rational A

The sternoclavicular joint has three planes of movement: superior and inferior elevation/depression, anterior and posterior protraction/retraction, and rotation.

Incorrect answers and rationales

Sternochondral joints (aka chondrosternal or sternocostal joints) are synovial plane joints that attach the sternum with the costal cartilages. Plane joints permit gliding or sliding movements in the plane of the articular surface. The tibiofibular joints are the articulations between the tibia and fibula which allows very little movement.

66. Correct answer and rational B

Zygapophyseal joints (aka facet joints or apophyseal joints) are a set of synovial, plane joints between the articular processes of two adjacent vertebrae.

Incorrect answers and rationales

A saddle joint is a type of biaxial joint that allows movements on two planes: flexion or extension, and abduction or adduction. A pivot joint, also known as a rotary joint, is a type of synovial joint in which a circular bone rotates upon the axis of another bone.

67. Correct answer and rational A

Joints of the fingers and toes are classified as synovial hinge joints capable of flexing and extending.

Incorrect answers and rationales

Syndesmosis: a fibrous joint held together by ligaments. Synarthrosis: an immovable fixed joint between bones connected by fibrous tissue.

68. Correct answer and rational A

Range of motion assessed by moving the joint.

Incorrect answers and rationales

Palpation and pain scale would not determine joint range of motion.

69. Correct answer and rational B

Joint range of motion is described as the amount of motion available at a specific joint.

Incorrect answers and rationales

Range of motion assesses the mobility of a joint, not soft tissue. Tissue flexibility influences ROM. Shortened soft tissue intervention may include stretching.

70. Correct answer and rational C

The amount of movement through a normal range of motion is commonly measured in degrees.

Incorrect answers and rationales

Weight or pounds are not joint range of motion measures.

71. Correct answer and rational A

Generally accepted values for normal range of motion for the elbow moving away from anatomical position is 0 to 150 degrees.

Incorrect answers and rationales

0 to 45 degrees would be hypomobile movement for the elbow. 80 to 0 degrees indicates moving back to the anatomical position.

72. Correct answer and rational A

Normal backward/hyper extension of the hip joint is 0 to 30 degrees.

Incorrect answers and rationales

0 to 5 degrees would indicate hypo mobility. 0 to 110 degrees likely more relates to hip flexion.

73. Correct answer and rational B

This movement is occurring at the atlanto-occipital and atlantoaxial joints. Generally accepted values for normal range of motion at these joints is 0 to 15 degrees.

Incorrect answers and rationales

45 to 0 degrees indicates moving back to the anatomical position. 0 to 5 degrees would be hypomobile.

74. Correct answer and rational C

The first 30 degrees of abduction of the glenohumeral joint occurs solely in the shoulder joint. Abduction from 30 to 180 degrees requires combined movement of the glenohumeral joint and scapula.

Incorrect answers and rationales

180 to 0 degrees would indicate movement back to anatomical position. 90 to 5 degrees would indicate movement back to anatomical position 0 with additional hyper movement of 5 degrees beyond 0.

75. Correct answer and rational B

The hip joint would have a range of motion of adduction 45 to 0 degrees indicating the starting point of 45 degrees of abduction and returning to anatomical position.

Incorrect answers and rationales

Wrist adduction (ulnar deviation) is 30 degrees and wrist abduction (radial deviation) 20 degrees. The knee does not allow adduction or abduction.

76. Correct answer and rational B

Resistant joint movement occurs when the massage practitioner attempts to prevent the client's active joint movement.

Incorrect answers and rationales

Passive joint movement occurs when the massage practitioner provides the movement. Assisted joint movement occurs when together the client and the practitioner move the joint.

77. Correct answer and rational C

Active joint movement occurs when the client provides the movement.

Incorrect answers and rationales

Passive joint movement occurs when the massage practitioner provides the movement. Assisted joint movement occurs when together the client and the practitioner move the joint.

78. Correct answer and rational A

Passive joint movement occurs when the massage practitioner provides the movement.

Incorrect answers and rationales

Assisted joint movement occurs when together the client and the practitioner move the joint. Resistant joint movement occurs when the massage practitioner attempts to prevent the client's active joint movement.

79. Correct answer and rational C

Assisted joint movement occurs when together the client and the practitioner move the joint.

Incorrect answers and rationales

Resistant joint movement occurs when the massage practitioner attempts to prevent the client's active joint movement. Isometric joint movement is not a term related to joint movement.

80. Correct answer and rational B

Gastrocnemius stabilizes the knee and ankle joints and is involved in maintaining balance in static standing when functioning isometrically.

Incorrect answers and rationales

Pectoralis major and middle trapezius act on the upper limb.

81. Correct answer and rational C

Joint kinesthetic receptors are proprioceptors located in the joints where bones connect.

Incorrect answers and rationales

Cervical/lumbar plexuses consist of the networks of branching nerves. Spinal nerves are peripheral nerves that transmit messages between the spinal cord and the rest of the body.

82. Correct answer and rational A

The gripping action for extended periods could alter normal responses between agonists and antagonists.

Incorrect answers and rationales

If wrist extensors were facilitated the muscles would be strong not weak. Muscles located in the same muscle grouping are synergists.

83. Correct answer and rational C

Muscle spindles are stretch receptors within the body of a skeletal muscle that primarily detect changes in the length of the muscle.

Incorrect answers and rationales

Joint kinesthetic receptors and Golgi tendons organs are not located in the muscle belly.

84. Correct answer and rational C
Latissimus dorsi acts at the low back and at the arm.
Incorrect answers and rationales
Psoas major and rectus abdominis do not attach to the upper limb.

85. Correct answer and rational A
Full range of motion at the shoulder requires the scapula to move.
Incorrect answers and rationales
Glenohumeral joint rotation and flexion are not as involved in combined scapular movement for full range of motion.

86. Correct answer and rational B
Extensor muscle groups are generally smaller and produce less force than flexor muscle groups. If the muscles assess equal in strength their function will be non-optimal.
Incorrect answers and rationales
Gait patterns are not relevant to the questions. Extensors are not stronger than adductors.

87. Correct answer and rational C
Osteokinematic movement is visible movement of a bone as it moves about the axis of a joint.
Incorrect answers and rationales
Arthrokinematics refers to the movement of joint surfaces. Joint play is the intrinsic space between bones in the joint capsule that allows arthrokinematic movement.

88. Correct answer and rational B
If the shoulder in internally rotated the internal rotators are short so muscle energy methods and elongation of the internal rotators would reverse the condition.
Incorrect answers and rationales
Friction and traction to the external rotators would have a tendency to inhibit external rotators which are already long. Tapotement to internal rotators would likely increase tone, adding to shortness.

89. Correct answer and rational C
Antagonists are any muscles that opposes the action of another. If the antagonist will not lengthen then the agonist will have limited ability to produce movement.
Incorrect answers and rationales
Agonists and synergists perform similar actions. In the question the hip abductors are agonists and synergists.

90. Correct answer and rational A
The external intercostals are the more surface-level muscles between the ribs which serve to elevate the rib cage and assist the lungs in expanding to take in air.
Incorrect answers and rationales
Contraction of the internal intercostal muscles depresses the ribs and pulls them closer together,

facilitating exhalation. The diaphragm is involved in respiration but flattens during inhalation. During inhalation the diaphragm contracts (tightens) and moves downward, allowing the lungs to expand.

91. Correct answer and rational A
Joint play is an involuntary movement related to space in the joint capsule. If ligaments are loose the space increases.
Incorrect answers and rationales
Joint laxity would create hypermobility and resultant muscle contraction to support stability.

92. Correct answer and rational C
The clavicle connects the sternum and scapula.
Incorrect answers and rationales
Radius and olecranon are not located in the area described.

93. Correct answer and rational C
The least packed position of the bones in a joint allows the most space in the joint capsule.
Incorrect answers and rationales
The closed packed position would not allow for normal swelling. Movement would be limited in an injured joint.

94. Correct answer and rational C
When the toes turn out from the midline the hip will externally rotate.
Incorrect answers and rationales
Crossing the ankles and pointing toes toward each other would be internal rotation.

95. Correct answer and rational A
Muscles on the anterior torso that function in the sagittal plane would be flexors and the extensors would be located on the posterior torso.
Incorrect answers and rationales
Muscles of the lateral thigh and upper limb are not in specific agonist/antagonist functional groups with the torso muscles.

96. Correct answer and rational A
Opponens pollicis and flexor pollicis brevis are synergists. Opponens pollicis is a short intrinsic muscle of the hand. It belongs to a group called thenar muscles, along with adductor pollicis, abductor pollicis, and flexor pollicis brevis.
Incorrect answers and rationales
Opponens digiti minimi and flexor digitorum profundus function on the little finger.

97. Correct answer and rational B
Rectus femoris flexes the hip and extends the knee.
Incorrect answers and rationales
Vastus lateralis and soleus only act on one joint.

98. Correct answer and rational C
Hip extension involves concentric contraction of the gluteus maximus which attaches to the IT band.
Incorrect answers and rationales
Trunk flexion and plantar flexion do not directly involve muscles that act on the IT band

99. Correct answer and rational B
The serratus anterior protracts and stabilizes the scapula and lifts the ribcage and supports breathing.
Incorrect answers and rationales
Adductor magnus is the largest muscle of the medial thigh. Psoas runs from the lumbar spine through the groin on either side and, with the iliacus, flex the hip.

100. Correct answer and rational A
The question describes the location of the temporalis muscles.
Incorrect answers and rationales
Masseter and pterygoid muscles are more involved with TMJ issues.

Practice Test 4

Pathology, Contraindications, Areas of Caution, Special Populations—175 Questions

1. Correct answer and rational A
Proper hand washing is the single most effective deterrent to the spread of disease.
Incorrect answers and rationales
Linen sterilization and sanitizing equipment are important but do not supersede handwashing in infection control.

2. Correct answer and rational B
Signs and symptoms are the observed or detectable signs and experienced symptoms of an illness, injury, or condition.
Incorrect answers and rationales
Feelings of discomfort would be a symptom since a sign is a phenomenon that can be detected by someone other than the individual. An acute episode of a chronic illness would be described by signs and symptoms.

3. Correct answer and rational A
Fever is a systemic (body wide) sign of a disease.
Incorrect answers and rationales
Swelling of the knee and rash on face are local signs.

4. Correct answer and rational C
An aneurysm is dilatation in the wall of an artery supplying blood to a specific area.
Incorrect answers and rationales
Cerebrovascular accident (CVA) is the medical term for a stroke. A stroke is when blood flow to a part of your brain is stopped either by a blockage or the rupture of a blood vessel. Edema is swelling as a result of fluid retention.

5. Correct answer and rational B
A chronic condition is a human health condition or disease that is persistent/continuous.
Incorrect answers and rationales
Temporary means short term. Acute conditions resolve during the normal course of healing.

6. Correct answer and rational C
Atrophy is the term used to describe the wasting away or reduction in size of a body part.
Incorrect answers and rationales
Hypertrophy is an increase in the size of a tissue or organ caused by enlargement of the individual cells. Regeneration is the process in which a lost body part regrows.

7. Correct answer and rational A
Thoracic outlet syndrome describes a condition caused by nerve compression in the upper body, specifically the nerves in the neck, chest, shoulders, and arms.
Incorrect answers and rationales
Lumbar spine and posterior knee are not specially related to thoracic outlet syndrome

8. Correct answer and rational B
Homeostatic imbalance may lead to a state of disease.
Incorrect answers and rationales
Stages in tissue healing relate to healing an injury. Acquired immune response is pathogen specific and occurs when the body first encounters a pathogen it produces a response that is remembered by the immune system to protect against future infection.

9. Correct answer and rational A
Hyperplasia is the enlargement of an organ or tissue caused by an increase in the reproduction rate of its cells, often as an initial stage in the development of cancer.
Incorrect answers and rationales
Paresthesia is a burning, tingling, or numb feeling that generally affects the hands, arms, legs, or feet. Hyperalgesia is an abnormally increased sensitivity to pain.

10. Correct answer and rational B
Resilience is the ability to become strong, healthy, or successful again after something bad happens.
Incorrect answers and rationales
Allodynia is when things that don't usually cause pain suddenly seem to be painful. Stress can be defined as any type of change that causes physical, emotional, or psychological strain.

11. Correct answer and rational C
Bacteria cause infections as do viruses, fungi, or parasites.
Incorrect answers and rationales
Allergies occur when the immune system reacts to a foreign substance that doesn't cause a reaction in most people. A contusion is an injury that causes bleeding and tissue damage underneath the skin, usually without breaking the skin.

12. Correct answer and rational C
Hyperalgesia is an abnormally increased sensitivity to pain.
Incorrect answers and rationales

Salutogenesis is a stress resource—orientated concept, which focuses on assets, strengths, and motivation as a way to maintain and improve the movement toward health. An ultradian rhythm is a rhythm that plays out in 80—120 minute cycles.

13. Correct answer and rational A

Visceral pain: pain originating from the internal organs which may refer to the body surface.

Incorrect answers and rationales

Joint pain is regional to a jointed area. Connective tissue pain can take many forms and does not necessarily have specific referral patterns like visceral pain.

14. Correct answer and rational B

Adaptive capacity is the ability to respond and adapt with minimum loss of function.

Incorrect answers and rationales

Decreased immune response and resilience decline would indicate decreased adaptive capacity.

15. Correct answer and rational C

Restorative care is based on optimizing and maintaining functional abilities. Thus the client would be generally healthy.

Incorrect answers and rationales

If a client is exhibiting stress symptoms or prone to infection the ability to maintain homeostasis is strained.

16. Correct answer and rational C

The variety of upper respiratory infections are common.

Incorrect answers and rationales

Bone cancer and phantom pain are not common conditions.

17. Correct answer and rational A

Adaptive capacity is the ability to respond and adapt with minimum loss of function. An autoimmune condition would stain adaptive capacity.

Incorrect answers and rationales

A chronic illness would interfere with homeostasis and normal biological rhythms.

18. Correct answer and rational B

Stress is the ability to respond to adaptive demand.

Incorrect answers and rationales

Ongoing stress would decrease the overall health. A congenital disease is present at birth.

19. Correct answer and rational A

Nonproductive inflammation is a common underlying cause of chronic disease.

Incorrect answers and rationales

Resilience is the ability to adapt. Restorative sleep is part of a healing process.

20. Correct answer and rational C

The injection site for insulin is considered a local contraindication.

Incorrect answers and rationales

Cervical spine is not an injection site. A medical port is not typically indicated for insulin use.

21. Correct answer and rational B

Inflammation is productive in the acute and subacute heal stages.

Incorrect answers and rationales

Inflammation is nonproductive in autoimmune conditions such as multiple sclerosis. Available evidence strongly suggests that type 2 diabetes is an inflammatory disease and that inflammation is a primary cause of obesity-linked insulin resistance.

22. Correct answer and rational A

Rheumatoid arthritis is an autoimmune inflammatory condition that can be aggravated with aggressive pressure.

Incorrect answers and rationales

Diverticulosis is a condition in which there are small pouches or pockets in the wall or lining of any portion of the digestive tract. Plantar fasciopathy is an acute or chronic painful disorder of the plantar fascia which spans between the medial calcaneal tubercle and the proximal phalanges of the toes. Thickening and degenerative tissue findings are more common than inflammatory changes, so the term *plantar fasciopathy* should better define the disorder known as *plantar fasciitis*.

23. Correct answer and rational B

Psoriasis is an autoimmune condition and not contagious.

Incorrect answers and rationales

Herpes simplex and hepatitis are both contagious. Hepatitis is a liver disease.

24. Correct answer and rational B

Osteoarthrosis is a common disorder of synovial joints, seen most often in older clients.

Incorrect answers and rationales

Pancreatitis is a condition characterized by inflammation of the pancreas. Meningitis is a disease caused by inflammation of the meninges, the membranes that surround the brain and spinal cord, usually caused by a virus.

25. Correct answer and rational C

Changes in mental status and challenged breathing are considered medical emergencies.

Incorrect answers and rationales

An overwhelming emotional response is of concern and would indicate a referral but is not a medical emergency. Negative feedback is a type of regulation in biological systems in which the end product of a process reduces the stimulus of that same process.

26. Correct answer and rational A

Having obesity increases the development of diabetes, the condition of having too much glucose circulating in the bloodstream. Obesity also causes diabetes to worsen faster.

Incorrect answers and rationales

Depression and cancer are not specifically comorbid with diabetes.

27. Correct answer and rational C

A sign is objective evidence of a disease that another person can detect, whereas only the individual in question will be able to recognize a symptom. A rash is observable therefore a sign.

Incorrect answers and rationales

Only the individual in question will be able to recognize a symptom. Nausea and anxiety are symptoms.

28. Correct answer and rational A

Myocardial infarction follows the occlusion/blockage of a coronary artery by a thrombus generated over a ruptured atherosclerotic plaque.

Incorrect answers and rationales

Peripheral neuropathy is dysfunction of the nerves outside of the brain and the spinal cord. Parkinson's disease is a neurological movement disorder associated with dopamine.

29. Correct answer and rational B

Spondylolisthesis is a condition involving spine instability, which means the vertebrae move more than they should.

Incorrect answers and rationales

Preeclampsia is a condition that occurs only during pregnancy. Cystic fibrosis is an inherited disease characterized by an abnormality in the glands that produce sweat and mucus.

30. Correct answer and rational B

Tuberculosis is a contagious infection caused by bacteria that mainly affects the lungs but can also affect other organs including bone and the brain.

Incorrect answers and rationales

Scabies is a contagious itchy skin condition caused by a tiny burrowing mite called Sarcoptes scabiei. Infectious mononucleosis is an infection usually caused by the Epstein—Barr virus (EBV).

31. Correct answer and rational C

One of the most common causes of yellowing skin is jaundice, a liver condition.

Incorrect answers and rationales

Cyanosis is a bluish hue to the skin, gums, fingernails, or mucous membranes due to a lack of oxygen in the blood. Vitiligo is a skin condition characterized by patches of the skin losing their pigment.

32. Correct answer and rational A

Hepatitis is inflammation of the liver tissue that can be a viral condition.

Incorrect answers and rationales

Methicillin-resistant *Staphylococcus aureus* (MRSA) is a cause of staph infection that is difficult to treat because of resistance to some antibiotics. Thrush is a fungal infection.

33. Correct answer and rational C

Droplet transmission occurs when bacteria or viruses travel on relatively large respiratory droplets that people sneeze, cough, drip, or exhale.

Incorrect answers and rationales

Vectors are living organisms that can transmit infectious pathogens between humans, or from animals to humans. Direct contact transmission occurs through direct body contact with the tissues or fluids of an infected individual.

34. Correct answer and rational A

The suffix "-algesia" pertains to a condition in which the client is either very sensitive to pain (hyperalgesia) or has a difficulty perceiving pain (hypoalgesia).

Incorrect answers and rationales

The prefix "-asthenia" pertains to a lack of strength. The prefix "-itis" indicates inflammation.

35. Correct answer and rational C

A hiatal hernia occurs when the upper part of the stomach bulges through the diaphragm muscle.

Incorrect answers and rationales

The other types of hernias occur in other locations— umbilical relates to navel and inguinal the groin.

36. Correct answer and rational B

Olecranon bursitis is an inflammation of the bursa at the olecranon process of the ulna which is part of the elbow joint.

Incorrect answers and rationales

The boney landmark called the olecranon process is not located at the ankle or hip.

37. Correct answer and rational A

Stress involves altered ANS regulation especially increasing sympathetic output which in turn increases vigilance which often disturbs sleep.

Incorrect answers and rationales

While lumbar pain and joint stiffness may occur, these issues do not specifically relate to stress.

38. Correct answer and rational B

Lice is the answer.

Incorrect answers and rationales

Bad breath is halitosis. Athlete's foot is tinea pedis.

39. Correct answer and rational C

Grade II muscle strains involve incomplete muscle tearing with some strength loss.

Incorrect answers and rationales

Tearing of a few muscle fibers without strength loss refers to a grade I strain. Complete tearing of the muscle with complete strength loss is a grade III strain.

40. Correct answer and rational B

The most common area for strain or tear of any muscle is the musculotendinous junction.

Incorrect answers and rationales

It is uncommon for muscle strains to occur in the muscle belly. The biceps brachii does not attach to the spine of the scapula.

41. Correct answer and rational A

Torticollis involves the contracted state of the sternocleidomastoid muscle, producing head tilt to the affected side with rotation of the chin to the opposite side.

Incorrect answers and rationales

Torticollis is specific to the neck, not the pelvis or shoulder.

42. Correct answer and rational C

An avulsion fracture is when a sudden muscular contraction occurs and the ligament pulls away from the bone.

Incorrect answers and rationales

Impaction fracture is when one fragment of the bone is driven into another. A stress fracture is caused by repeated low-force trauma.

43. Correct answer and rational C

The axillary nerve is near the humerus and most likely to be injured during anterior shoulder dislocation or fracture of the humeral neck.

Incorrect answers and rationales

The median and radial nerves are in the forearm.

44. Correct answer and rational A

Bursitis is inflammation of the bursae, which are the fluid-filled sacs located throughout the body situated in places in tissues where friction can occur.

Incorrect answers and rationales

Nerve entrapment develops when nerves become compressed (or entrapped) and restricted. Tendinopathy, also called tendinosis, refers to the degeneration of collagen in a tendon.

45. Correct answer and rational A

The saphenous nerve lies just anterior to the medial malleolus and runs parallel the great saphenous vein.

Incorrect answers and rationales

The axillary nerve is in the upper body. The intermediate dorsal cutaneous nerve innervates the top outside part of the foot.

46. Correct answer and rational C

Bradypnea is defined as less than 10 breaths/minute in a resting adult.

Incorrect answers and rationales

Tachypnea is defined as more than 20 breaths/minute in an adult. Hypoventilation occurs when ventilation is inadequate to perform needed gas exchange.

47. Correct answer and rational B

When ligaments are overstretched, their fibers can tear and cause pain and instability of the joint, resulting in a sprain.

Incorrect answers and rationales

An injury to a tendon or muscle would be a strain.

48. Correct answer and rational B

Tachycardia is defined as a pulse above 100 beats/minute.

Incorrect answers and rationales

Bradycardia is defined as a heart rate of less than 60 beats/minute at rest. Tachypnea is a rapid shallow respiratory rate.

49. Correct answer and rational A

Orthostatic hypotension is a decrease in cardiac output and lowering of arterial pressure which decreases blood pressure resulting in feeling dizzy or lightheaded. This could cause a client to faint.

Incorrect answers and rationales

Myocardial ischemia occurs when blood flow to the heart is reduced, preventing the heart muscle from receiving enough oxygen. Vasodilation is the widening of blood vessels as a result of the relaxation of blood vessel muscular walls.

50. Correct answer and rational B

White blood cell count increase suggests infection or other inflammatory responses.

Incorrect answers and rationales

Red blood cells are responsible for carrying oxygen from the lungs to other cells in the body. Blood platelets are responsible for helping blood clot and stop bleeding.

51. Correct answer and rational C

The myocardium of the heart receives its blood supply from two major vessels: the right and upper coronary arteries. A blockage prevents oxygen supply to the heart.

Incorrect answers and rationales

Purkinje fibers are a part of the relaying system of electrical signals in the heart. Pulmonary veins are a group of blood vessels that drain oxygenated blood from the lungs and return it to the heart.

52. Correct answer and rational A

Lymphedema is swelling that occurs when protein-rich lymph fluid accumulates in the interstitial tissue.

Incorrect answers and rationales

Accumulation of lymphocytes in the blood and tissues would be more a sign of chronic lymphocytic leukemia. A bruise, or contusion, is caused when blood vessels are damaged or broken as the result of a blow to the skin and blood leaks into the tissues.

53. Correct answer and rational B

Inguinal hernias occur in the abdominal wall.

Incorrect answers and rationales

A femoral hernia is a protrusion of loop of intestine into the femoral canal. Umbilical hernia occurs through a congenital defect in the abdominal muscle at the umbilical ring.

54. Correct answer and rational B

Vertebral compression fractures are the most common osteoporosis-related spinal fractures.

Incorrect answers and rationales

Rib fractures and metacarpal fractures can occur but are not as common as fractures in the vertebral column.

55. Correct answer and rational C

Herpes simplex virus type 1 lesions typically occur around the mouth and lips.

Incorrect answers and rationales

Herpes does not occur on an area such as the foot. Herpes simplex virus type 2 is most often seen in the genitals.

56. Correct answer and rational A

A Baker's cyst is a subtype of ganglion that often communicates within a joint space. A Baker's cyst is most often palpated behind the knee in older adults with osteoarthritis.

Incorrect answers and rationales

A lipoma is a lump of fatty tissue that grows just under the skin. A nevus is a congenital (present at birth) or acquired growth or pigmented blemish on the skin; birthmarks/moles.

57. Correct answer and rational C

A stress fracture is caused by the bones' inability to withstand stress applied in a rhythmic, repeated fashion.

Incorrect answers and rationales

A compound fracture is bone break with perforation of the skin. A greenstick fracture is a crack or break on one side of a long bone in the arm or leg that does not extend all the way through the bone. Children are more likely to have greenstick fractures because their bones are softer and less brittle.

58. Correct answer and rational B

Inflammatory phase/acute occurs during the first few days after injury.

59. Correct answer and rational A

Osgood-Schlatter syndrome results from the patella tendon pulling small bits of immature bone from the tibial tuberosity. It is most commonly seen in active adolescent boys 10—15 years of age but also can affect girls 8—13 years of age.

Incorrect answers and rationales

Toddlers and infants are not prone to this condition.

Incorrect answers and rationales

Proliferative phase/subacute is 1—6 weeks after injury. Remodeling phase/chronic begins 7 weeks after injury.

60. Correct answer and rational C

The stretch or pressure on the meninges caused by meningitis will cause a severe headache.

Incorrect answers and rationales

Tinnitus is ringing in the ears, even though no external sound is present. Confusion occurs when a person has difficulty understanding a situation or has disordered or unclear thoughts.

61. Correct answer and rational A

Alzheimer's disease is the most common cause of dementia overall. It is one of the principal causes of disability and decreased quality of life among older adults.

Incorrect answers and rationales

Lewy body dementia is second most common. Frontotemporal dementia is less common.

62. Correct answer and rational B

Tremor is the most common initial manifestation of Parkinson's disease.

Incorrect answers and rationales

Neuropathy and edema can occur with Parkinson's disease, but tremor is most common.

63. Correct answer and rational C

The practitioner should have the client sit down because there is an increased risk for falls. Nystagmus is a condition that causes involuntary, rapid movement of one or both eyes. It often occurs with vision problems, including blurriness, and could increase dizziness.

Incorrect answers and rationales

Walking slowly with the client could increase potential for falls. Returning client to the supine position could increase symptoms.

64. Correct answer and rational B

Examples of primary headaches are migraine headaches, tension headaches, and cluster headaches.

Incorrect answers and rationales

Secondary headaches are caused by associated disease such as fever and irregularities in blood pressure.

65. Correct answer and rational A

Along with tremor and rigidity, people with Parkinson's disease show bradykinesia, impaired balance, and poor postural control. There is also usually a masklike expression in the face.

Incorrect answers and rationales

Alzheimer's disease involves cognition impairments early in the disease process. Multiple sclerosis is a disease that affects the central nervous system—the immune system attacks the myelin, the protective layer around nerve fibers and causes inflammation and lesions. This makes it difficult for the brain to send signals to rest of the body.

66. Correct answer and rational C

A painful neuroma in the space between the third and the fourth metatarsal heads is called Morton's neuroma.

Incorrect answers and rationales

Second and third, fourth and fifth metatarsal heads are not the location for Morton's neuroma.

67. Correct answer and rational A

Edema is a condition of swelling due to excess fluid accumulation in the body tissues.

Incorrect answers and rationales

Dilatation means being stretched beyond normal dimensions. *Emesis* is the medical term for vomiting.

68. Correct answer and rational B

Neuralgia is nerve pain and also called neuropathy, neuropathic pain, or neurogenic pain.

Incorrect answers and rationales

Neuroplasticity refers to the brain's ability to adapt. Neuroglia is the delicate connective tissue which supports and binds together the nervous elements of the central nervous system.

69. Correct answer and rational B

Hyperthermia occurs when body temperature is greatly elevated due to retention of body.

Incorrect answers and rationales

Orthopnea is a shortness of breath some people experience when lying down. Hypothermia occurs when your body loses heat faster than it produces it. The most common causes of hypothermia are exposure to cold-weather conditions or cold water.

70. Correct answer and rational C

An adhesion is a band of scar tissue that binds two parts of tissue or organs together. Adhesions may appear as thin sheets of tissue similar to plastic wrap or as thick fibrous bands.

Incorrect answers and rationales

Anaphylaxis is a serious life-threatening allergic reaction which usually occurs within seconds or minutes of exposure to allergic substances. Diaphoresis causes sudden, all-over sweating for no apparent reason.

71. Correct answer and rational C

Cyanosis is a pathologic condition that is characterized by a bluish discoloration of the skin or mucous membranes.

Incorrect answers and rationales

Erythrocytosis is an increase in RBCs relative to the volume of blood. Xanthosis is an abnormal yellow discoloration of the skin.

72. Correct answer and rational A

Gastric ulcers are a break in the mucosa of the stomach lining.

Incorrect answers and rationales

A hiatal hernia occurs when a portion of the stomach protrudes into the upper chest area. Gastroesophageal reflux disease (GERD) is a chronic gastrointestinal disorder characterized by the regurgitation of gastric contents into the esophagus

73. Correct answer and rational A

Narcolepsy is a chronic sleep disorder characterized by overwhelming daytime drowsiness and sudden attacks of sleep.

Incorrect answers and rationales

Epilepsy is a neurological disorder that causes seizures or unusual sensations and behaviors. Polydipsia is a medical name for the feeling of extreme thirstiness.

74. Correct answer and rational B

A cerebrovascular accident is also called a CVA, brain attack, or stroke. It occurs when blood flow to a part of the brain is suddenly stopped and oxygen cannot get to that area.

Incorrect answers and rationales

A myocardial infarction, also called a heart attack, is caused by a lack of blood flow to the heart muscle.

Angina is a type of chest pain caused by reduced blood flow to the heart.

75. Correct answer and rational C

Angina pectoris is the medical term for chest pain or discomfort due to coronary heart disease. It occurs when the heart muscle doesn't get as much blood as it needs.

Incorrect answers and rationales

Aortic stenosis occurs when the heart's aortic valve narrows. Mitral valve prolapse is a common cause of a heart murmur.

76. Correct answer and rational B

Cirrhosis is a slowly developing disease in which healthy liver tissue is replaced with scar tissue.

Incorrect answers and rationales

Cholecystitis is the most common type of gallbladder disease. It presents itself as either an acute or chronic inflammation of the gallbladder. Colon conditions include inflammatory bowel disease, diverticular disease, polyps, and cancer.

77. Correct answer and rational C

An abrasion is a minor injury that occurs when the skin is rubbed or torn off. It is a shallow wound, typically a wearing away of the top layer of skin.

Incorrect answers and rationales

A contusion is an injury that causes bleeding and tissue damage underneath the skin, usually without breaking the skin. An incision is a surgical cut made in skin or flesh.

78. Correct answer and rational A

Shingles is a viral infection that causes a painful rash. Although shingles can occur anywhere on the body, it most often appears as a single stripe of blisters that wraps around either the left or the right side of the torso.

Incorrect answers and rationales

Diuresis occurs when the kidneys filter too much bodily fluid with increased urine production. Myelitis is inflammation of the spinal cord.

79. Correct answer and rational A

An abscess is a pocket of pus that accumulates when a bacterial infection breaks down tissue.

Incorrect answers and rationales

Cellulitis is a serious bacterial infection of the skin usually affecting the leg causing swelling, redness, and pain. Acne is a common skin condition caused by inflammation of the hair follicles and oil-producing (sebaceous) glands of the skin.

80. Correct answer and rational A

Initial inflammation should start 48–72 hours following the injury and then move into the proliferation stage.

Incorrect answers and rationales

Wound remodeling usually starts at week 2 or 3 and can last up to a year. Inflammation at this time would be non productive.

81. Correct answer and rational B
Proliferation involves angiogenesis (forming of new blood vessels).
Incorrect answers and rationales
Inflammation is the first stage of healing and begins to resolve during proliferation. Remodeling occurs over time after the proliferation stage of healing.

82. Correct answer and rational C
Initial blood loss is decreased by the immediate vaso-constriction of the vessels. This vasoconstrictive response may last 5—10 minutes.
Incorrect answers and rationales
Vasodilation would increase potential blood loss and capillary density refers to the number of capillaries present at a certain site in the body.

83. Correct answer and rational A
Specific contraction at the wound site occurs during the proliferative phase because fibroblasts, particularly myofibroblasts, have contractile capability.
Incorrect answers and rationales
The inflammatory phase begins immediately after injury and last 3—6 days and involves deposition of fibrin, and the formation of blood clots in the area. The macrophages clear cellular debris by the process known as phagocytosis. Maturation phase, also called the remodeling stage of wound healing, is when collagen is remodeled. When collagen is laid down during the proliferative phase, it is disorganized and the wound is thick. During the maturation phase, collagen is aligned along tension lines.

84. Correct answer and rational B
The remodeling stage of healing should not involve pain.
Incorrect answers and rationales
The acute healing stage involves acute pain. The sub-acute stage involves pain but should be reduced compared to acute pain.

85. Correct answer and rational C
In 6 weeks the subacute healing stage would be completing and entering the remodeling stage resulting in reduced pain and more confident movement.
Incorrect answers and rationales
6 weeks post injury would typically be too soon to fully resume preinjury activity levels. Localized aching and edema post activity typically occurs during the subacute healing stage.

86. Correct answer and rational A
Endangerment sites are places on the body where caution or avoidance is required since massage could cause damage.
Incorrect answers and rationales
Referred pain is visceral pain that is felt in another area of the body and occurs when organs share a common nerve pathway. The tooth is made of several layers of varying density and hardness: the enamel, dentin, cementum, and pulp.

87. Correct answer and rational B
Epilepsy is neurological disorder that causes seizures or unusual sensations and behaviors often treated by a neurologist.
Incorrect answers and rationales
Primary aldosteronism is a hormonal disorder that leads to high blood pressure. It occurs when adrenal glands produce too much of a hormone called aldosterone, typically treated by an endocrinologist. Emphysema is a lung disease which results in shortness of breath due to destruction and dilatation of the alveoli, treated by a pulmonologist.

88. Correct answer and rational C
A tension headache is the most common type of headache. It is pain or discomfort in the head, scalp, or neck, and is often associated with muscle tight-ness in these areas.
Incorrect answers and rationales
Pancreatitis occurs when digestive enzymes become activated while still in the pancreas, irritating the cells of the pancreas and causing inflammation. Pulmonary edema is condition where fluid accu-mulates in lung tissues and can cause shortness of breath, wheezing, and coughing up blood. Both conditions are organ related, involve medical treat-ment, and less likely to be affected by massage methods.

89. Correct answer and rational B
The contents of the anterior triangle include muscles, nerves, arteries, veins, and lymph nodes which can be damaged when compressed.
Incorrect answers and rationales
The plantar aspect of the foot (sole) and the anterior thigh have nerves, arteries, veins better protected by muscles and connective tissue than the anterior neck

90. Correct answer and rational C
The external iliac artery, femoral artery, and femoral nerve are located in the inguinal triangle.
Incorrect answers and rationales
The popliteal fossa is the main conduit for neuro-vascular structures entering and leaving the leg. Its contents are the popliteal artery and vein and tibial nerve. The carotid artery, jugular vein, and vagus nerve are located in the carotid triangle.

91. Correct answer and rational A
At the medial epicondyle of the humerus the ulnar nerve and radial and ulnar arteries pass around its posterior aspect to enter the forearm and can easily be compressed or damaged.
Incorrect answers and rationales
The inguinal triangle contains the external iliac artery, femoral artery, and femoral nerve. Posterior triangle of the neck contains many important vascular and neural structures but not the ulnar nerve or the radial and ulnar arteries.

92. Correct answer and rational C
The 12th rib is in the general location of the kidneys.

Incorrect answers and rationales

The brachial plexus is in the cervical and axillary area. The saphenous vein is in the lower limb.

93. Correct answer and rational A

Lymph nodes are located in the cervical, axilla, and inguinal areas.

Incorrect answers and rationales

Carotid arteries are in the cervical area only. A styloid process is a small, pointed bony prominence extending from a bone that acts as an anchoring site for muscles and ligaments.

94. Correct answer and rational B

The median nerve begins in the axillary region and runs between the biceps and triceps muscles.

Incorrect answers and rationales

The popliteal fossa is at the knee. The femoral artery is in the lower limb.

95. Correct answer and rational B

The umbilicus area of the abdomen is the location of the descending aorta. Pressure should not be directly applied to this structure.

Incorrect answers and rationales

The axilla area is commonly known as the arm pit. The bump on the outer side of the elbow is called the lateral epicondyle.

96. Correct answer and rational C

Stop the session, explain why and urgently refer to client their physician or emergency room. Venous thromboembolism (VTE) is the third most common cause of vascular mortality worldwide and comprises deep-vein thrombosis (DVT) and pulmonary embolism (PE). Swelling, redness, and pain are some of the signs and symptoms of deep vein thrombosis. A pulmonary embolism can cause sudden chest pain and shortness of breath.

Incorrect answers and rationales

While serious, the condition is not quite a medical emergency unless breathing symptoms are involved, so an ambulance should not be required. However, this condition can progress quickly and should be evaluated by a physician, so the session should stop.

97. Correct answer and rational A

Potential stroke is a life-threatening medical emergency.

Incorrect answers and rationales

Potential concussion and symptoms of rhabdomyolysis are serious. Urgent referral to physical or emergency care is indicated but not to the same extent as a stroke.

98. Correct answer and rational B

Posttraumatic stress disorder can be a result of persistent trauma-related mental and emotional stress involving disturbance of sleep and constant vivid recall of the experience, with dulled responses to others and to the outside world.

Incorrect answers and rationales

Biological rhythms are cyclic variations in the intensity and character of biological processes and

phenomena supporting adaption to cyclic changes in the environment. Stress and coping involve mental, emotional, or physical response/adaptation to real or perceived changes/challenges.

99. Correct answer and rational A

Stress management as a goal has clinically shown improvements for anxiety and accompanying sleep disorder likely due to generalized relaxation responses.

Incorrect answers and rationales

Inflammation reduction research related to massage is in early stages and relates more to healing stages than anxiety and sleep. Functional mobility is also a common outcome for massage application and can have a secondary rather than primary influence on anxiety and sleep disorders.

100. Correct answer and rational A

Pneumonia is an infection that inflames the air sacs of the lungs. A variety of organisms, including bacteria, viruses, and fungi can cause pneumonia.

Incorrect answers and rationales

Raynaud's disease is a disorder of the blood vessels, usually in the fingers and toes, causing the blood vessels to narrow when the person is cold or feeling stressed. Sickle cell disease is a group of inherited red blood cell disorders where the red blood cells become hard and sticky and look like a C-shaped farm tool called a "sickle."

101. Correct answer and rational C

The etiology of pain and fatigue syndromes involves various components of the central nervous system including the hypothalamic pituitary axes, pain-processing pathways, and autonomic nervous system. These central nervous system changes lead to corresponding changes in immune function.

Incorrect answers and rationales

The neuromatrix theory of pain describes a multidimensional experience produced by patterns of nerve impulses generated by a widely distributed neural network in the brain. These neurosignature patterns may be triggered by sensory inputs, but they may also be generated independently. Central sensitization is defined as an increased responsiveness of nociceptors in the central nervous system to either normal or subthreshold afferent input pain sensation. Peripheral sensitization refers to reduced threshold and augmented responses of the sensory nerve fibers in the peripheral to external stimulus experienced as enhanced stimulus-dependent pain called primary hyperalgesia. Both may contribute to pain and fatigue syndromes.

102. Correct answer and rational A

Tinea corporis is commonly called ringworm and is a fungal infection that spreads on the top layer of the skin which can be transmitted by direct skin-to-skin contact.

Incorrect answers and rationales

An angioma is a benign non-contagious growth that consists of small blood vessels. Seborrheic keratosis is a benign skin tumor that originates from cells in the outer layer of the skin and occurs more often as people age.

103. Correct answer and rational C

A contusion is a caused by a direct trauma to the muscle.

Incorrect answers and rationales

Cellulitis is a common, potentially serious bacterial skin infection. Spina bifida is a birth defect that occurs when the spine and spinal cord don't form properly.

104. Correct answer and rational B

The difference between injury and illness is that injury is damage to the body and illness is a disease. A concussion is an injury.

Incorrect answers and rationales

Atherosclerosis and prostatitis are considered illnesses.

105. Correct answer and rational C

Stomach ulcers are open sores that develop when the lining of the stomach has become damaged. Stomach ulcers are also called gastric ulcers.

Incorrect answers and rationales

Duodenal ulcers occur on the inside of the upper portion of the small intestine called the duodenum. The cecum is a small sac-like structure at the beginning of the large intestine.

106. Correct answer and rational A

Diverticula are small, bulging pouches that can form in the lining of your digestive system. They are found most often in the lower part of the large intestine.

Incorrect answers and rationales

Pancreatitis is inflammation of the pancreas. Appendicitis occurs when the appendix becomes inflamed or infected.

107. Correct answer and rational A

Stress fractures result from recurrent and repetitive loading of bone. The stress fracture differs from other types of fractures in that in most cases, no acute traumatic event precedes the symptoms.

Incorrect answers and rationales

Spiral fractures happen when the bone gets twisted to the point of breaking and can be detected by Xray. Compound fractures puncture through the skin.

108. Correct answer and rational B

A hiatal hernia is a condition in which the upper part of the stomach bulges through an opening in the diaphragm.

Incorrect answers and rationales

The duodenum is a short portion of the small intestine connecting it to the stomach. The transverse colon is the portion of the large intestine that crosses the upper abdomen from right to left.

109. Correct answer and rational B

Sebaceous glands in the skin secrete a lubricating oily matter called sebum into the hair follicles to lubricate the skin and hair. Sebaceous glands can become overactive, leading to an excess amount of oil being created. This can then cause dead skin cells to stick together instead of shed off, clogging the pore and resulting in a blackhead.

Incorrect answers and rationales

Sudoriferous glands (aka sweat glands) are exocrine glands in the human body responsible for producing perspiration/sweat. Ceruminous glands are modified sweat glands of the ear which produce earwax.

110. Correct answer and rational C

Brachial plexus injuries cut off all or some parts of communication between the spinal cord and the arm, wrist, and hand. This may mean impaired use of the arm or hand. Often, brachial plexus injuries also result in total loss of sensation in the area.

Incorrect answers and rationales

The pharyngeal plexus originates from cranial nerve IX through XI and innervates muscles and skin of the front of the neck and aids in the swallowing mechanism. The sacral plexus has extensive functions throughout the pelvis and legs.

111. Correct answer and rational A

Osteoporosis is a disease that causes bones to become weak and brittle over time. Osteoporosis is a "silent" disease because symptoms may not present until a fracture occurs.

Incorrect answers and rationales

Osteomyelitis is infection in the bone caused by bacteria or fungi usually affecting the long bones of arms or legs in children and the spine, feet, or hips among adults. Osteogenesis imperfecta is a genetic bone disease. People born with the condition have bones that break easily.

112. Correct answer and rational B

A person with scoliosis has a sideways curve to their spine. The curve is often S-shaped or C-shaped.

Incorrect answers and rationales

Lordosis occurs when the spine of a person curves significantly inward at the lower back. Kyphosis is characterized by an abnormally rounded upper back (more than 50 degrees of curvature).

113. Correct answer and rational A

A first-degree burn is the least severe of burn types. First-degree burns affect only the epidermis, causing pain and reddening.

Incorrect answers and rationales

A second-degree burn is classified as a burn that affects both the epidermis and the dermis, or the second layer of skin. Second-degree burns look red and often create burn blisters. Third-degree burn injuries penetrate deeper than the dermis to the underlying layer of fat with white, black, deep red, or charred skin.

114. Correct answer and rational C

Edema is swelling caused by excess fluid trapped in body tissues.

Incorrect answers and rationales

An aneurysm is an abnormal bulge or ballooning in the wall of a blood vessel. Infarction is the death of tissue resulting from a failure of blood supply, commonly due to obstruction of a blood vessel by a blood clot or narrowing of the blood-vessel channel.

115. Correct answer and rational B

Bone to bone (bony) end feel occurs when one would not expect to find a hard, unyielding end feel when joint assessment occurs, and is a sign of pathology that needs to be identified.

Incorrect answers and rationales

Soft tissue approximation occurs when range of motion is restricted by the normal muscular bulk and is painless. The anatomical barrier is the end of available motion without causing tissue damage.

116. Correct answer and rational A

An ulcer is an area of destroyed mucous membrane causing an open sore or lesion

Incorrect answers and rationales

A laceration is a wound that occurs when skin, tissue, and/or muscle is torn or cut open. A hiatal hernia is a protrusion of the stomach into the diaphragm.

117. Correct answer and rational B

Rotator cuff tendinitis is a condition of the shoulder joint which is a synovial joint.

Incorrect answers and rationales

Fibrous joints are immovable and cartilaginous joints are partially moveable. Tendinitis typically occurs in mobile synovial joints.

118. Correct answer and rational C

Phlebitis is inflammation of veins causing pain, discomfort, and swelling. It commonly occurs in the legs but can occur elsewhere in the body.

Incorrect answers and rationales

Varicose veins are swollen, twisted blood vessels that bulge just under the skin's surface. Vasodilation refers to a widening of the blood vessels within the body.

119. Correct answer and rational C

Tic douloureux, also called trigeminal neuralgia. is a shock like pain in the face.

Incorrect answers and rationales

Olfactory nerve relates to the sense of smell. Optic nerve relates to vision.

120. Correct answer and rational A

Quality research indicates that those undergoing cancer treatment have less pain and anxiety after a massage session.

Incorrect answers and rationales

Increasing the action of chemotherapy and detoxing the body of cancer cells are not indicated benefits of massage.

121. Correct answer and rational B

Athletes may experience a variety of conditions but are prone to joint injury.

Incorrect answers and rationales

Endocrine disorders and autoimmune conditions can occur in athletes however joint injury is more common.

122. Correct answer and rational C

Effects of sport specific training can alter joint movement. Athletes depend on the effects of training and the resulting neurological responses for precise functioning. Because they use their bodies in specific ways to achieve performance, athletes create functional alterations in their bodies.

Incorrect answers and rationales

Travel schedules can be stressful but don't relate specifically to joint function. The type of counterirritant ointment used would not specifically relate to joint hyper/hypomobility.

123. Correct answer and rational C

Numerous mechanical stresses and strains can adversely affect the skin's integrity, such as friction (rubbing), scraping, compression (pressure), tearing, cutting, and penetration. Abrasions commonly arise from conditions in which the skin is scraped against a rough surface.

Incorrect answers and rationales

A puncture would be a penetrating injury. A contusion is a bruise.

124. Correct answer and rational A

Use of nonsteroidal anti-inflammatory medications available over the counter is common.

Incorrect answers and rationales

Muscle relaxers and diuretics are not readily available without prescription.

125. Correct answer and rational B

Trauma is a physical injury or wound sustained in a sport produced by external or internal force.

Incorrect answers and rationales

Illness and depression can occur but don't specifically relate to physical demand.

126. Correct answer and rational A

A contusion or skin bruise occurs when a blow compresses or crushes the skin surface and causes bleeding under the skin.

Incorrect answers and rationales

Puncture injuries are rare. Blisters may occur if equipment is rubbing against the skin.

127. Correct answer and rational B

Localized injury such as bruising, abrasions, sprains, etc. are treated as regional contraindications.

Incorrect answers and rationales

Direct work over an injury is contraindicated until healing has progressed to the subacute/remodeling stage. Most injuries are not general contraindications, meaning total avoidance of massage application.

128. Correct answer and rational C

Overtraining and over exertion is reflected by muscle soreness, decreased joint flexibility, and general fatigue 24 hours after activity. Four specific indicators of possible overexertion are acute muscle soreness, delayed-onset muscle soreness, muscle stiffness, and muscle cramps/spasms.

Incorrect answers and rationales

New equipment might cause some symptoms related to adaptation. An ankle sprain would be tender and cause guarding with reduced movement but generally not fatigue.

129. Correct answer and rational A

A sprain is the most common ankle injury.

Incorrect answers and rationales

The event described in the question is more likely to cause a sprain than a fracture or dislocation.

130. Correct answer and rational C

A strain is a stretch, tear, or rip in the muscle or adjacent tissue.

Incorrect answers and rationales

Avulsion occurs when tissue is pulled away from other structures. A sprain occurs in ligaments.

131. Correct answer and rational B

Muscle strain usually causes muscle guarding. The body's normal response is to cause the muscles around the injured area to tighten up and guard the injured area as a protective mechanism to limit mobility. The guarding should not be reduced because it protects the area from further injury.

Incorrect answers and rationales

The other possible answers are related to grade 3 injury. Grade 1 (mild) strain: Local pain, which is increased by tension of the muscle, and minor loss of strength; mild swelling and local tenderness. Grade 2 (moderate) strain: Similar to a mild strain but with moderate signs and symptoms and impaired muscle function. Grade 3 (severe) strain: Severe signs and symptoms, with loss of muscle function and commonly a palpable defect in the muscle.

132. Correct answer and rational A

Tenosynovitis is inflammation of the synovial sheath surrounding a tendon. The cause of the inflammation may be unknown, or it may result from diseases that cause inflammation, infection, injury, overuse, strain, or a combination.

Incorrect answers and rationales

Tendinitis is marked by a gradual onset, degenerative changes, and diffuse tenderness caused by repeated microtrauma. Obvious signs of tendinitis are swelling and pain. Tendinosis occurs when an inflamed or irritated tendon (tendonitis) fails to heal, and the tendon degenerates.

133. Correct answer and rational B

Heatstroke is a life-threatening emergency.

Incorrect answers and rationales

Heat exhaustion is more severe than heat cramps and results from a loss of water and salt in the body. Both are heat-related illnesses and are serious, but heatstroke is the most serious.

134. Correct answer and rational C

Most pregnant individuals clot blood more readily than normal and are predisposed to deep-vein thrombosis or other clot-related conditions.

Incorrect answers and rationales

Gestational diabetes mellitus (GDM) is a condition in which a hormone made by the placenta prevents the body from using insulin effectively. Fatigue is common during pregnancy.

135. Correct answer and rational B

Diastasis recti is a separation of the abdominal wall where the connective tissue that runs directly down the center of the linea alba is stretched and weak.

Incorrect answers and rationales

Pelvic organ prolapse is defined as the descent of one or more compartments of the vagina. A hernia is a protrusion or bulge of an organ or part of an organ through the body wall.

136. Correct answer and rational A

Most pregnant individuals clot blood more readily than normal and are predisposed to deep-vein thrombosis or other clot-related conditions.

Incorrect answers and rationales

Gestational diabetes mellitus (GDM) is a condition in which a hormone made by the placenta prevents the body from using insulin effectively. Preeclampsia is a pregnancy complication characterized by high blood pressure and signs of damage to another organ system, most often the liver and kidneys.

137. Correct answer and rational B

Typically, the side lying position is necessary to adapted to the growing baby.

Incorrect answers and rationales

In a normal pregnancy it is not necessary to avoiding work on the legs, but the pressure and aggressiveness of massage application should be reduced as the pregnancy progresses. Increasing the duration of the session is not recommended.

138. Correct answer and rational C

The period after the birth is post-partum.

Incorrect answers and rationales

Trimester is a stage of pregnancy. Transition is a stage of labor.

139. Correct answer and rational A

Depression is common postpartum.

Incorrect answers and rationales

Preeclampsia is a pregnancy complication characterized by high blood pressure and signs of damage to another organ system, most often the liver and kidneys. Menopause is when menstrual periods stop permanently.

140. Correct answer and rational C

Minors and those unable to provide consent require permission from a parent, spouse, or guardian.

Incorrect answers and rationales

It is the capacity to provide consent, not the condition (i.e., illness or disability) that influences the need for permission to provide massage services.

141. Correct answer and rational A

To adapt appropriately for this population it is necessary to learn about the effects of aging.

Incorrect answers and rationales

There are no specific methods or required education.

142. Correct answer and rational C

Considered an acute wound the surgical site is vulnerable to infection.

Incorrect answers and rationales

Since this was a minor procedure pain management would not be a primary concern. Scar tissue development is a part of wound healing.

143. Correct answer and rational B

Acute illness is generally contraindicated in most situations until the acute phase passes.

Incorrect answers and rationales

Acute injury would present local contraindication. Chronic illness would fall into the caution category with adaptation.

144. Correct answer and rational A

In the acute phase of an illness or injury pain management is a primary goal.

Incorrect answers and rationales

Improved mobility and faster wound healing are important outcomes, but pain management is the first goal in acute care.

145. Correct answer and rational B

Acute mean active, a sudden onset or of a short duration.

Incorrect answers and rationales

An assumption cannot be made about if the person is under the care of a physician or has a diagnosis. Referral is often indicated.

146. Correct answer and rational C

The hemostasis phase starts immediately after an injury and overlaps with the inflammatory phase of healing. The inflammatory phase should only last a few days.

Incorrect answers and rationales

The proliferation phase is the actual construction phase of the tissue. Cautious massage application near the area would support pliable scar formation. Wound remodeling is the last phase and would be treated as non-injured tissue.

147. Correct answer and rational B

Regional contraindication, sometimes called local contraindication, is where a condition exists indicating massage application is avoided in a specific location.

Incorrect answers and rationales

Absolute contraindication and systemic contraindication refer to a situation where the condition is such that massage should be entirely avoided.

148. Correct answer and rational A

An absolute contraindication means no bodywork is performed.

Incorrect answers and rationales

Localized avoidance and method adaptation indicate caution but not complete avoidance of treatment.

149. Correct answer and rational C

Osteoporosis causes bones to become weak and brittle, potentially so brittle that a fall or even mild stresses such as bending over or coughing can cause fracture.

Incorrect answers and rationales

Fibrotic tendons and necrotic joint surfaces are not typical signs of osteoporosis.

150. Correct answer and rational A

Phlebitis is the inflammation of a vein. It can occur in veins on the surface of the skin (also called superficial phlebitis), in varicose veins, and in deeper veins, typically in the legs.

Incorrect answers and rationales

An embolus is a particle that moves either in the veins or arteries. Most emboli are composed of clotted blood cells. A blood clot is called a thrombus and a moving blood clot is called a thromboembolus. An embolus can occur with phlebitis but not always. A hematoma is a collection of blood outside of a blood vessel.

151. Correct answer and rational B

Edema is swelling as a result of fluid retention. There are many different kinds and causes of edema and can be a symptom of serious illnesses.

Incorrect answers and rationales

A hematoma is a collection of blood outside of a blood vessel. An aneurysm is an abnormal ballooning in the wall of a blood vessel. If an aneurysm bursts, it often leads to death.

152. Correct answer and rational B

The axilla or arm pit contains nerves and vessels that should not be compressed.

Incorrect answers and rationales

The nerves/vessels in the plantar surface of foot and forearm are better protected by soft tissue.

153. Correct answer and rational C

Dermatitis is a general term for conditions that cause inflammation of the skin. Examples include atopic dermatitis (eczema), contact dermatitis, and seborrheic dermatitis (dandruff). These conditions cause red rashes, dry skin, and itchiness among other symptoms. The condition is not contagious.

Incorrect answers and rationales

Nerves and joints are not involved in dermatitis

154. Correct answer and rational A

Pushing in gently on the swollen area for at least 5 seconds and then removing your finger will leave a dimple in the skin when edema is present.

Incorrect answers and rationales

Skin springing back or red flushing would not specifically be a sign of edema.

155. Correct answer and rational C
The upper right quadrant of the abdomen contains the liver.
Incorrect answers and rationales
The ulnar nerve in is the upper limb. The aorta is the large artery in the posterior abdominal area located along the anterior aspect of the spinal column.

156. Correct answer and rational B
Botulinum toxin paralyzes muscles by inhibiting the release of acetylcholine at the neuromuscular junction. If spasticity is reduced, often range of motion and function will increase in children with cerebral palsy.
Incorrect answers and rationales
Fibrosis and circulation are not specifically affected by botulinum toxin injections.

157. Correct answer and rational A
Diuretic drugs increase urine output by the kidneys.
Incorrect answers and rationales
Diuresis is an increase in the production of urine by the kidneys, which typically results in a corresponding increase in urine expelled by the body. The glomerulus is a collection of capillaries inside the nephron which allow the kidney to perform the filtration process.

158. Correct answer and rational C
Warfarin sodium has been proved to be significantly more effective than aspirin in the prevention of stroke in individuals with atrial fibrillation.
Incorrect answers and rationales
Aspirin is the most commonly used oral antiplatelet drug. Atorvastatin/Lipitor targets cholesterol.

159. Correct answer and rational A
Selective serotonin reuptake inhibitors (SSRIs) are the most commonly prescribed antidepressants.
Incorrect answers and rationales
Hypertension and diabetes are not typically treated with SSRI medications.

160. Correct answer and rational B
Anticoagulants are medicines that help prevent blood clots.
Incorrect answers and rationales
Antihistamines are a class of drugs commonly used to treat symptoms of allergies. These drugs help treat conditions caused by too much histamine. Diuretics are a common treatment for high blood pressure.

161. Correct answer and rational A
A beta agonist stimulates cardiac beta receptors, leading to an increase in heart rate and blood pressure.
Incorrect answers and rationales
Side effects of a beta agonist are not a decrease in blood pressure or incoordination.

162. Correct answer and rational B
Nitrates relax blood vessels, allowing more blood to flow to the heart and thereby decreasing pain.
Incorrect answers and rationales

Proton pump inhibitors are medicines that work by reducing the amount of stomach acid made by glands in the lining of the stomach. Bronchodilators are a type of medication that make breathing easier by relaxing the muscles in the lungs and widening the airways (bronchi).

163. Correct answer and rational C
Pain medication can interfere with the client's ability to provide feedback related to pressure and intensity increasing risk of tissue injury.
Incorrect answers and rationales
Relaxation massage and reflexology have less potential for tissue injury.

164. Correct answer and rational C
Opioids are a class of drugs that cause pain relief by binding to opioid receptors.
Incorrect answers and rationales
Ibuprofen is a nonsteroidal anti-inflammatory medication. Acetaminophen is a pain reliever and a fever reducer.

165. Correct answer and rational A
Diuretics are used to treat hypertension.
Incorrect answers and rationales
Antiarrhythmics and beta-blockers are used to control heart rate.

166. Correct answer and rational B
The oral route is the most frequently used route for drug administration.
Incorrect answers and rationales
Medication administration using the topical or injection route is less common.

167. Correct answer and rational A
Brand/trade name is chosen by the company that makes it. Several companies may make the same generic medicine, each with their own brand name. Tylenol is the trade name for acetaminophen.
Incorrect answers and rationales
Each medicine has an approved name called the generic name. A group of medicines that have similar actions often have similar-sounding generic names. Acetaminophen and metformin are generic.

168. Correct answer and rational A
Antihypertensive medications treat high blood pressure.
Incorrect answers and rationales
Steroid medication is for inflammation. Antibiotics treat bacterial infection.

169. Correct answer and rational B
Analgesics treat pain.
Incorrect answers and rationales
Antitussives treat coughs. Anti-parkinsonism medications treat Parkinson's disease.

170. Correct answer and rational A
Bronchodilators are used to treat respiratory conditions.
Incorrect answers and rationales
Anticonvulsants are used to treat seizures. Antidepressants are prescribed for depression.

171. Correct answer and rational C
     Autoimmune conditions are inflammation based and steroids treat inflammation.
     Incorrect answers and rationales
     Hormonal and cardiovascular conditions are not specifically treated with steroids.

172. Correct answer and rational A
     Dry mouth is a common side effect of anti-depressant medication.
     Incorrect answers and rationales
     Muscle weakness and joint pain are not common side effects of anti-depressant medication.

173. Correct answer and rational B
     Anticonvulsant medication is used to treat seizures that occur in epilepsy.
     Incorrect answers and rationales
     Antihistamines are a class of drugs commonly used to treat symptoms of allergies. Antineoplastic drugs treat cancer.

174. Correct answer and rational A
     Lying flat can aggravate reflux.
     Incorrect answers and rationales
     The length of the session or pressure depth used would have less affect than the positioning.

175. Correct answer and rational B
     HIV (human immunodeficiency virus) is a virus that attacks the body's immune system.
     Incorrect answers and rationales
     Methicillin-resistant *Staphylococcus aureus* (MRSA) is a cause of staph infection that is difficult to treat because of resistance to some antibiotics. Post-traumatic stress disorder (PTSD) is a mental health condition that's triggered by a terrifying event.

Practice Test 5

Theory and Practice of Massage and Bodywork—175 Questions

1. Correct answer and rational B
   While it is unclear how soft tissue manipulation helps people manage pain most research indicates a shift in the ANS to more parasympathetic dominance.
   Incorrect answers and rationales
   Increased sympathetic arousal would more likely increase pain perception. Localized circulatory changes many or may not occur.

2. Correct answer and rational A
   Mechanisms of action for massage therapy benefit are elusive but consistently research shows ANS affects.
   Incorrect answers and rationales
   Research of blood flow is inconsistent. Massage sensory stimulation is processed through reflex mechanisms.

3. Correct answer and rational C
   It is unclear if and why local blood flow increases in surface tissue when mechanical force is applied but some sort of vasodilation is involved and nitric oxide and histamine are vasodilators.
   Incorrect answers and rationales
   Fibroblast proliferation due to inflammation is a connective tissue function. Interstitial fluid is found around cells.

4. Correct answer and rational C
   Massage may promote sliding in the fascial layers.
   Incorrect answers and rationales
   It is unlikely manual therapy changes the length of collagen fibers or breaks down adhesions.

5. Correct answer and rational A
   Hyperstimulation analgesia refers to the short-term partial or total relief of pain produced by a variety of forms of intense sensory stimulation.
   Incorrect answers and rationales
   Fascial reorganization and increased systemic circulation are not justifiable reasons for short-term pain reduction.

6. Correct answer and rational B
   Regularity responses of the nervous system stimulated by mechanical force application have shown to be valid.
   Incorrect answers and rationales
   Many of the results thought to be related to fluid exchange and posture have not been validated by research.

7. Correct answer and rational A
   Muscle tone pulls on fascial connections and changes in tone may affect the tautness of fascia allowing for ease of movement.
   Incorrect answers and rationales
   Creating inflammation would decrease movement as would creating fibrotic changes in the joint capsule.

8. Correct answer and rational C
   Oxytocin among other actions plays a role in trust between people.
   Incorrect answers and rationales
   Melatonin plays a role in sleep. Leptin decreases appetite and increases metabolism.

9. Correct answer and rational A
   The biopsychosocial model indicates that biological, psychological, and social factors all play a significant role in human functioning in the context of disease or illness and health is best understood in terms of a combination of these factors rather than purely biological.
   Incorrect answers and rationales
   Client outcomes related to massage are flexible not fixed outcomes. General clients would more relate to the biopsychosocial model than population specialization.

10. Correct answer and rational B
    The effects of massage stem from a positive therapeutic relationship and the alliance between practitioner and client.
    Incorrect answers and rationales

Practice setting and practitioner education are important but less responsible.

11. Correct answer and rational A
Kneading presses, twists, and rolls soft tissue
Incorrect answers and rationales
Vibration a rigorous shake/rocking of specific muscles or body segments. Gliding is a method that moves horizontally.

12. Correct answer and rational B
Kneading lifts (which pulls) and rolls tissue.
Incorrect answers and rationales
Oscillation involves rocking and shaking. Hacking is a form of percussion.

13. Correct answer and rational B
Rocking is soothing and can be done over clothing.
Incorrect answers and rationales
Tapotement is more stimulating. Gliding is typically applied to the skin.

14. Correct answer and rational C
Compression can apply pressure to an area without additional movement.
Incorrect answers and rationales
Drag is a method modifier. Friction involves movement.

15. Correct answer and rational A
Compression provides pressure and gliding can elongate tissue using enough drag.
Incorrect answers and rationales
Friction and vibration use focused pressure and contact. While kneading combined with shaking could influence tissue pliability and length, the request for moderate pressure may not be satisfied by kneading as much as gliding.

16. Correct answer and rational C
A lubricant reduces friction on the skin during gliding.
Incorrect answers and rationales
Compression and holding methods do not require lubricant.

17. Correct answer and rational C
Friction is an intervention intended to target local areas.
Incorrect answers and rationales
Joint movement would address a larger area as does gliding.

18. Correct answer and rational A
Twisting is a combined force application resulting in torsion.
Incorrect answers and rationales
Shear stress is created when the mechanical force application causes tissues to slide against other tissues. Compression stress is created by a push/pull force application.

19. Correct answer and rational B
Bending stress is a combination of compression and tensile stress. One side of a structure is exposed to compressive stress as the other side is exposed to tensile stress.
Incorrect answers and rationales

Torsion stress occurs with twisting. Tensile stress occurs with pulling.

20. Correct answer and rational A
Range of motion involves moving the joints.
Incorrect answers and rationales
Traction might produce small separation of joint structures but not ROM assessment. Vibration does not specifically move the joints.

21. Correct answer and rational B
The holding/resting position targets the skin for stimulation of the cutaneous (skin) sensory receptors.
Incorrect answers and rationales
Kneading and shaking are more intense methods than holding.

22. Correct answer and rational A
A relaxation outcome would be smoothly and rhythmically applied.
Incorrect answers and rationales
Frequent pre and post assessments are not performed when relaxation is the targeted outcome. The client positioning prone, supine, or side-lying is not a major factor in achieving the relaxation outcome.

23. Correct answer and rational C
Tissues are addressed from surface layers progressing to deeper layers and then finishing more superficial again.
Incorrect answers and rationales
Supine-prone-seated are ways to position the client. Anterior-lateral-ventral are locations on the body.

24. Correct answer and rational B
Improved mobility outcomes involve more targeted assessment with appropriate intervention.
Incorrect answers and rationales
Outcomes based on relaxation and stress management have fewer focused interventions. A pain management outcome does not mean short frequent sessions are needed.

25. Correct answer and rational B
Thermo relates to temperature.
Incorrect answers and rationales
Force application and psychological responses are not specifically related to temperature-based methods.

26. Correct answer and rational A
All three can be considered complementary approaches but water use indicates hydrotherapy.
Incorrect answers and rationales
Cupping is a vacuum decompression method. Percussion tools apply tapotement type methods.

27. Correct answer and rational C
Cryo means producing cold, especially extreme cold.
Incorrect answers and rationales

28. Correct answer and rational A
Immersion in warm water is the use of both approaches.
Incorrect answers and rationales
Hot stones may be warmed in water but it is not a combined application. Counterirritation ointment

usually containing some sort of menthol will produce cold sensation.

Water can be used at varying temperatures. Sauna thermotherapy is based on heat.

29. Correct answer and rational B

The ability of water to take multiple forms and have a range of temperatures makes it advantageous as a medium for thermotherapy.

Incorrect answers and rationales

Water is a solvent and water application is adaptable but it is the ability of water to vary in temperature that allows for the combined approach.

30. Correct answer and rational A

Ice is not applied directly to the skin.

Incorrect answers and rationales

The pack is typically left on the area for 10 minutes. It would be counterproductive to cover the ice pack with a warm towel.

31. Correct answer and rational B

Contrast therapy alternates temperatures between hot and cold.

Incorrect answers and rationales

Hot water immersion and alternating between a wet and dry sauna are all heat approaches.

32. Correct answer and rational C

Cold applications can act as a counterirritant.

Incorrect answers and rationales

Full body cold exposure could lead to shock but not in a targeted area. Cold only penetrates into surface tissue layers.

33. Correct answer and rational A

Frostbite happens when part of your body freezes, damaging skin cells and tissues.

Incorrect answers and rationales

An ulcer is an open sore on an external or internal surface of the body, caused by a break in the skin or mucous membrane that fails to heal. Anaphylaxis is a serious life-threatening allergic reaction which usually occurs within seconds or minutes of exposure to allergic substances. This involves hives, swelling, and sudden drop in the blood pressure and sometimes shock.

34. Correct answer and rational B

Using heat inappropriately can cause burns.

Incorrect answers and rationales

Bruising is unlikely with thermotherapy. Vasodilation would not be a safety concern.

35. Correct answer and rational C

Vessels constrict in response to cold.

Incorrect answers and rationales

Histamine causes the surrounding blood vessels to dilate. Vasodilation can occur secondary to a cold application but vasoconstriction happens first.

36. Correct answer and rational C

Shiatsu, Japanese massage, and pressure point therapy typically are performed on a mat over clothing.

Incorrect answers and rationales

Swedish and manual lymph drain use gliding on skin.

37. Correct answer and rational A

Myofascial release is an approach to address connective tissue.

Incorrect answers and rationales

Polarity therapy targets proposed energy fields. Lymphatic drainage targets fluid movement.

38. Correct answer and rational B

The massage techniques of Swedish massage are named effleurage, petrissage, tapotement, friction, and vibration. Petrissage refers to kneading motions, effleurage to stroking.

Incorrect answers and rationales

Neuromuscular therapy typically involves locating and treating trigger points. Myofascial release is a hands-on soft tissue technique that facilitates a stretch into the restricted fascia.

39. Correct answer and rational A

Neuromuscular therapy is method of manual therapy applied to the myofascial/soft tissue system which has evolved over the last 65 years.

Incorrect answers and rationales

Classical massage, also called Swedish massage, is seen as the basis of Western massage but not considered modern. Thai massage is an ancient form of bodywork.

40. Correct answer and rational C

Meta-analysis is widely accepted as the preferred method to synthesize research findings in various disciplines.

Incorrect answers and rationales

A medical case report (aka case study) is a detailed description of a clinical encounter with a patient. Clinical trials are medical research studies with volunteers.

41. Correct answer and rational B

Reflexology is a type of bodywork that involves applying different amounts of pressure to the feet, hands, and ears. It's based on a theory that these body parts are connected to certain organs and body systems.

Incorrect answers and rationales

Polarity therapy is a type of "energy medicine" that uses several techniques to alter energy flow and energy balance in the body. Shiatsu (literally meaning "finger pressure") is a Japanese massage modality formalized by Tokujiro Namikoshi during the 1920s.

42. Correct answer and rational B

The client is asking why and how the information is used.

Incorrect answers and rationales

While legislation mandates and requirements are important, the client is asking for a reason related to the session.

43. Correct answer and rational C

Foremost for safety it is necessary to identify possible contraindications before decisions are made regarding treatment planning and referral.

Incorrect answers and rationales

It is necessary to identify possible contraindications before decisions are made related to treatment planning and referral.

44. Correct answer and rational A

Palpation involves physical contact.

Incorrect answers and rationales

Assessing activities of daily living and taking an accurate history involve observation and interviewing.

45. Correct answer and rational B

Movement-related outcomes involve movement-related assessments such as range of motion assessment of joints.

Incorrect answers and rationales

While hot packs and varied positioning may be helpful, ROM assessment is more important regarding mobility outcomes.

46. Correct answer and rational B

First the practitioner needs to determine if the area is contraindicated.

Incorrect answers and rationales

If the condition is determined to be more a caution, methods could be adapted. Avoiding the area may not be necessary.

47. Correct answer and rational C

Joint movement would assess joint range of motion.

Incorrect answers and rationales

Kneading would be used to assess tissue. Percussion is more a method than an assessment.

48. Correct answer and rational A

S stands for "subjective", what the client tells the massage practitioner, such as their chief complaint.

Incorrect answers and rationales

O and P: objective information and plan are based on quantifiable information and ongoing care.

49. Correct answer and rational A

Referral is not indicated but it is important to understand how the condition is being treated to determine contraindications.

Incorrect answers and rationales

Referral is not indicated. Posture and gait assessment are not specifically related to diabetes.

50. Correct answer and rational C

The client is participating in daily living activities, been diagnosed, and has treatment scheduled. Stress management is a logical outcome. The session could be helpful so long as the client is comfortable, the session is general, and the abdominal area is avoided.

Incorrect answers and rationales

The practitioner would not need to postpone the session. The client's doctor does not need to provide specific treatment directions.

51. Correct answer and rational A

The client has been seen multiple times and is of an age where lower leg edema often occurs for multiple reasons. The situation needs to be clarified.

Incorrect answers and rationales

It is unlikely the situation is a medical emergency. Bolstering to promote fluid movement and use of lymphatic drain methods may or may not be indicated.

52. Correct answer and rational B

Head trauma is a medical emergency.

Incorrect answers and rationales

Since the situation is a medical emergency conducting additional assessment and providing the session are incorrect.

53. Correct answer and rational C

Countertransference is a practitioner's reactions and feelings toward a client.

Incorrect answers and rationales

Transference is related to the client's responses. Dual relationships are defined as those when a professional assumes a second role with a client, becoming friend, employer, teacher, business associate, family member, etc.

54. Correct answer and rational B

A dual relationship arises when a client is also a friend, family member, or business associate. These relationships make it difficult to maintain professional boundaries.

Incorrect answers and rationales

Transference is a phenomenon in which one seems to direct feelings or desires related to an important figure in one's life—such as a parent—toward someone who is not that person. Power differential means the basic inequality inherent in the professional relationship.

55. Correct answer and rational A

To avoid or minimize possible harm to the client is the essence of non-maleficence.

Incorrect answers and rationales

Proportionality relates to benefits being more than burden of treatment. Justice means acting in a fair and impartial manner.

56. Correct answer and rational C

Scope of Practice includes everything that the practitioner is trained to do under the specific certificate/license with which they are currently working. Scope of practice for massage excludes diagnosis and prescribing.

Incorrect answers and rationales

A dual relationship can confuse the professional boundaries. Emotional boundaries include transference, countertransference, and the power differential.

57. Correct answer and rational C

The client disclosing that the massage practitioner was complaining during the session about how they were paid is unprofessional and unethical.

Incorrect answers and rationales

The client indicating that the massage practitioner was soliciting them for a cash tip in exchange for sexual acts would be a criminal act more than and ethical violation. The client indicated that the massage practitioner had an unpleasant body odor would not be consider an ethical issue directly.

58. Correct answer and rational A
Self-determination means a person acts with autonomy, makes their own choices, and is free form controlling interference from others.
Incorrect answers and rationales
Ability to pay for services and right to medical insurance are not directly related to autonomy.

59. Correct answer and rational B
Client education on limits of scope of practice is indicated.
Incorrect answers and rationales
Indicating that spinal adjustment naturally occurs and using methods with spinal adjustment potential is unethical.

60. Correct answer and rational A
The most professional action is to schedule a meeting with the chiropractor to discuss the situation.
Incorrect answers and rationales
Ignoring the situation and preparing to leave the business may be a common way to act but is not the most professional. Talking with the other massage practitioner about pay is inappropriate.

61. Correct answer and rational C
Removing draping material to expose the body to the massage practitioner is sexual harassment. Sexual harassment should never be tolerated.
Incorrect answers and rationales
A client being frustrated by the cancellation policy or consistently arriving late for appointments can create conflict leading to client dismissal but not to the level of what is considered "zero tolerance."

62. Correct answer and rational B
All policies are explained during initial contact with the client.
Incorrect answers and rationales
Policies can be posted online and can be reinforced if a violation occurs but explanation should occur prior to the session.

63. Correct answer and rational A
The massage practitioner needs to be aware of their body and avoid contact that can be considered sexual.
Incorrect answers and rationales
Having policies related to clothing and draping is not inappropriate. Talking about irrelevant topics during the massage session is inappropriate. Topics of a sexual nature would be sexually inappropriate.

64. Correct answer and rational B
Sexual harassment is behavior characterized by the making of unwelcome and inappropriate sexual remarks or physical advances in a workplace or other professional or social situation. These should be addressed and not tolerated.
Incorrect answers and rationales

A practitioner explaining sexual boundaries is an important aspect of preventing sexual harassment. A co-worker gossiping about pay scales is unethical but not sexual harassment.

65. Correct answer and rational B
Interest conflicts are caused by competition over perceived incompatible needs. Conflicts of interest result when one or more people believe that to satisfy their needs, the needs and interests of an opponent must be sacrificed. This often occurs during times of scarcity or when it is perceived that there is not enough of something to go around.
Incorrect answers and rationales
Data conflicts occur when people lack information necessary to make wise decisions, are misinformed, disagree on which data are relevant, interpret information differently, or have collected data differently. Relationship conflicts, often called personality conflicts, occur as a result of strong negative emotions, misperceptions or stereotypes, poor communication or miscommunication, or repetitive negative behaviors.

66. Correct answer and rational C
Respect (esteem and regard for clients, other professionals, and oneself).
Incorrect answers and rationales
Client autonomy and self-determination (the freedom to decide and the right to sufficient information to make the decision). Veracity (the right to the objective truth).

67. Correct answer and rational A
Justice is an ethical obligation to treat all people equally, fairly, and impartially. The business owner may be wondering if the conflict between the receptionist and staff member is affecting scheduling fairness.
Incorrect answers and rationales
Beneficence concerns good intentions and outcomes in all our actions. Fidelity is faithfulness to obligations, duties, or observances cultivating trust.

68. Correct answer and rational C
The cord can be a tripping hazard.
Incorrect answers and rationales
Burns would be of a concern for the client. Air quality effects related to this piece of equipment are unlikely.

69. Correct answer and rational A
Essential oils have volatile constituents which evaporate into the air.
Incorrect answers and rationales
If a lotion is hypoallergenic, it is unlikely to contain fragrance. Location in facility may or may not affect air quality.

70. Correct answer and rational B
Lubricant reduces drag on the skin when applying massage methods, especially gliding.
Incorrect answers and rationales
Medicinal or cosmetic use of lubricants is out of the scope of practice for therapeutic massage.

71. Correct answer and rational A

    The portable folding table is constructed with hinges and cables which can become unstable.

    Incorrect answers and rationales

    Hydraulic and stationary tables are not broken down so do not have hinges and cables.

72. Correct answer and rational C

    Disinfectants are primarily applied to non-living surfaces. Do not put disinfectants in or on your body. They can kill you. When using disinfectants, follow the label directions.

    Incorrect answers and rationales

    Antiseptics are applied to living tissues, often to the skin in the form of hand rubs or washes. Air purifiers are devises which clear particles from air.

73. Correct answer and rational B

    An allergic reaction related to either practitioner or client is a safety concern.

    Incorrect answers and rationales

    Cost and manufacturer are not safety issues.

74. Correct answer and rational C

    Nuts and nut products are a common allergen that could produce anaphylaxis.

    Incorrect answers and rationales

    Water and alcohol are not common allergens.

75. Correct answer and rational C

    Expiration date of a product can relate to safe and effective use.

    Incorrect answers and rationales

    Product reviews may or may not be helpful. Concerns regarding discounts on volume include the potential for content expiration before use.

76. Correct answer and rational A

    All are relevant to choosing equipment but a primary concern is ease of cleaning and disinfecting.

    Incorrect answers and rationales

    Storage convenience and manufactures warranty are valuable but safety and sanitation are first priority.

77. Correct answer and rational B

    Pillowcases can be used as coverings for bolsters.

    Incorrect answers and rationales

    While a pillowcase could be used for cleaning and trash, it less appropriate.

78. Correct answer and rational B

    If the practitioner has a contagious illness spread by respiratory droplets, they do not work until the illness is resolved.

    Incorrect answers and rationales

    Contagious illness spread by respiratory droplets can still be transmitted even if face mask and gloves are used. Anyone immune compromised would be more susceptible to becoming ill but only avoiding this group is not sufficient.

79. Correct answer and rational C

    Antiseptics can be used on the skin.

    Incorrect answers and rationales

    Sterilants kill all microorganisms while disinfectants kill only certain microorganisms.

80. Correct answer and rational A

    All fabric which comes in contact with a client needs to be laundered appropriately even if it has antimicrobial properties.

    Incorrect answers and rationales

    All fabric which comes in contact with a client needs to be laundered appropriately even if it has antimicrobial properties. Efficient folding and storage is important but safety and sanitation must be prioritized.

81. Correct answer and rational A

    Isopropyl alcohol is an active ingredient in antiseptics.

    Incorrect answers and rationales

    Sodium hypochlorite and quaternary ammonium are disinfectants.

82. Correct answer and rational C

    Sterilization may be defined as the statistically complete destruction of all microorganisms including the most resistant bacteria and spores.

    Incorrect answers and rationales

    Disinfection is the killing of infectious agents outside the body by direct exposure to chemical or physical agents. Sanitization lowers the number of germs safe levels.

83. Correct answer and rational B

    Keeping the surface wet with a disinfectant for a certain period is the contact time.

    Incorrect answer and rationales

    A variety of dilutions and ingredients can be used but all disinfectants require contact time.

84. Correct answer and rational A

    Disinfecting works by using chemicals to kill germs on surfaces or objects. This process does not necessarily clean dirty surfaces or remove germs, but by killing germs on a surface after cleaning, it can lower the risk of spreading infection.

    Incorrect answers and rationales

    Cleaning works by using soap (or detergent) and water to physically remove germs from surfaces. This process does not necessarily kill germs, but by removing them, it lowers the risk of spreading infection. Sanitizing works by either cleaning or disinfecting surfaces or objects to lower the number of germs to safe levels.

85. Correct answer and rational B

    Soap and water are used for cleaning.

    Incorrect answers and rationales

    Bleach and hydrogen peroxides are disinfectants.

86. Correct answer and rational B

    A risk refers to the likelihood that a hazard will cause specific harm or injury to people or may damage property. The facility should be regularly inspected by staff to identify potential risks.

    Incorrect answers and rationales

An inspection by Occupational Safety and Health Administration (OSHA) is not necessary for performing a risk assessment. Control measures to reduce risks are implemented after the risk assessment.

87. Correct answer and rational C

Products can be dispensed into a single use disposable container to prevent contamination.

Incorrect answers and rationales

Disinfectant should not be used on the skin. Limiting product type does not address contamination.

88. Correct answer and rational A

A risk refers to the likelihood that a hazard will cause specific harm or injury to people or may damage property. Facility-based safety risks involve tripping and fall hazards.

Incorrect answers and rationales

Fans and air filters would be used for ventilation.

89. Correct answer and rational C

Cleaning and sanitizing chemicals are considered hazardous.

Incorrect answers and rationales

Massage lubricants should be safe products. Fire extinguishers are not often encountered.

90. Correct answer and rational B

For safety the parking area needs to have outdoor lighting.

Incorrect answers and rationales

A designated smoking area is not as much a safety concern as lighting. Having multiple trash receptacles may be beneficial but is not specific to safety.

91. Correct answer and rational A

A hard floor can become slippery when wet.

Incorrect answers and rationales

Space size or carpet proximity are not necessarily safety concerns.

92. Correct answer and rational C

Workplace violence can be any act of physical violence, threat of physical violence, harassment, intimidation, or other threatening, disruptive behavior that occurs at the worksite.

Incorrect answers and rationales

A hazard is something, not someone, that may cause harm or injury. Sexual harassment is a specific form of inappropriate behavior.

93. Correct answer and rational A

When a client has any form of behavior that could indicate an underlying condition including using alcohol it is important to communicate with the client by asking questions to understand if massage application or referral is indicated.

Incorrect answers and rationales

Without clarifying the situation it is inappropriate to continue with the session or refuse to provide the session.

94. Correct answer and rational C

Ergonomics focuses on the application of anatomical and physiological science to design equipment and objects, work systems both from management and financial aspects, and their respective environments for human use. Ergonomics also involves the adaptation and optimization involved in matching the job tasks to the worker or use of a product to the user in the interest of ease of use for the overall health and safety of workers.

Incorrect answers and rationales

Biomechanics, or body mechanics, concentrates on the body as a machine and utilizes this perspective to analyze the structures, motions, and muscular forces used to complete tasks. Kinesiology is the study of mechanics and anatomy in relation to human movement.

95. Correct answer and rational B

The duty to report is a professional and ethical responsibility to protect clients and to advocate for safe, competent ethical care.

Incorrect answers and rationales

Discussing this type of information with the client's family or a mentor or supervisor does not eliminate the duty to report.

96. Correct answer and rational A

A major biomechanical concern is improper use of body areas that cannot easily be sustained in a stable position (i.e., the thumb, shoulder, low back, and knee). The saddle joint structure of the thumb is the concern for instability.

Incorrect answers and rationales

A hinge joint is more stable than a saddle joint. Carpal joints are able to withstand some compression.

97. Correct answer and rational B

The structure of the hand consists of many small bones, joints, and intrinsic muscles supporting fine movement instead of gross impact movements involved with massage application.

Incorrect answers and rationales

The hinge joints in the fingers are able to be stabilized. The muscles in the hand are considered intrinsic with all attachments in the hand not at the elbow.

98. Correct answer and rational C

National Institute for Occupational Safety and Health (NIOSH) guidelines indicate the shoulder joint should not exceed 45% of flexion to stay within safe ranges.

Incorrect answers and rationales

Trunk flexion should not exceed 20 degrees and occurs at the hip joint. While supination/pronation action should be limited it is not directly related to excursion/stroke length.

99. Correct answer and rational A

The symmetrical stance should be avoided and long gliding strokes strain the shoulder joint.

Incorrect answers and rationales

Compression using the palm with 15 degrees of trunk flexion at the hip and feet positioned in asymmetrical stance when providing short excursion gliding are accurate recommendations for massage application.

100. Correct answer and rational B
     Kneading involves repeated flexion and extension of the fingers and wrist.
     Incorrect answers and rationales
     Gliding and compression do not involve grasping actions.

101. Correct answer and rational A
     The trunk should be maintained at no more than 20 degrees flexion.
     Incorrect answers and rationales
     The feet position about shoulder width apart and in asymmetrical stance is considered appropriate. Standing on balls of the feet would indicate the table is too high.

102. Correct answer and rational C
     Ergonomics involves effective application of methods related to equipment and workspace.
     Incorrect answers and rationales
     Reception staff and number of rooms are not ergonomic factors.

103. Correct answer and rational B
     Elevated shoulders occurs when the table is too high.
     Incorrect answers and rationales
     Flexed knees are common when the table is too low. Feet should be flat on the floor.

104. Correct answer and rational C
     Shifting center of gravity forward from the feet is a correct strategy for pressure delivery.
     Incorrect answers and rationales
     Symmetrical stance increases protential for using upper body strength. Both should be avoided.

105. Correct answer and rational B
     All options listed are personal protective equipment (PPE), however the situation requires gloves.
     Incorrect answers and rationales
     Face shield and gown would not offer the same protection to the client as gloves.

106. Correct answer and rational A
     A mask limits respiratory disease transmission.
     Incorrect answers and rationales
     Gowns and gloves offer contact protection but do not limit airborne transmission.

107. Correct answer and rational C
     MRSA is contagious.
     Incorrect answers and rationales
     Chronic obstructive pulmonary disease (COPD) and hyperlipidemia are not contagious.

108. Correct answer and rational A
     Gowns and smocks protect clothing.
     Incorrect answers and rationales
     Safety boots, masks, and gloves are not designed to prevent clothing contamination.

109. Correct answer and rational A
     Boundaries supports practitioner self-care.
     Incorrect answers and rationales
     A palliative approach and client intervention are client focused.

110. Correct answer and rational B
     Identifying the balance between professional and personal activities is called work/life balance and is important in self-care.
     Incorrect answers and rationales
     Maximizing income potential may or may not support work/life balance. Professional disclosure relates to information disclosed to the client.

111. Correct answer and rational B
     A mask limits transmission of droplet and aerosol spread pathogen.
     Incorrect answers and rationales
     A face shield does not limit transmission since it is open at the bottom and edges. A smock protects the practitioner's clothing.

112. Correct answer and rational C
     Face shields and goggles help prevent splatter from getting in the eyes, nose, and mouth.
     Incorrect answers and rationales
     Face shields don't protect against droplet or aerosol transmission.

113. Correct answer and rational C
     Feeling over extended often leads to burnout.
     Incorrect answers and rationales
     Motivation involves the biological, emotional, social, and cognitive forces that activate behavior. The resulting stress can be a risk factor for illness but the scenario does not indicate illness.

114. Correct answer and rational B
     The practitioner chose to protect their hands.
     Incorrect answers and rationales
     Application of ergonomics relates more to the environment. Self-care is not a scope of practice issue.

115. Correct answer and rational A
     The practitioner is choosing to respect their need for scheduling flexibility over income. This is self-care.
     Incorrect answers and rationales
     Target marketing and fiscal responsibility are more business related.

116. Correct answer and rational C
     The lift table allows the practitioner to easily adjust table height and lowers potential for repetitive strain injury.
     Incorrect answers and rationales
     Hot towel cabbie and air filter are beneficial but not related to injury prevention.

117. Correct answer and rational A
     The client's body is modestly covered at all times.
     Incorrect answers and rationales
     A blanket many or may not be needed. Other materials such as towels can be used for draping.

118. Correct answer and rational B
     A session can be adapted to work over loose clothing.
     Incorrect answers and rationales
     Disposable material is still draping. Draping would be needed when working on a mat unless the client is wearing loose clothing.

119. Correct answer and rational C

There are many ways to respond and should be guided by conversation and guidance with the client as well as workplace rules and safety and sanitation requirements.

Incorrect answers and rationales

Working with minimal draping or purchasing the linens and detergent used by the client may be alternatives but need to be discussed with the client first.

120. Correct answer and rational C

Draping can be modified such as undraping the feet if a client is hot.

Incorrect answers and rationales

Draping should always occur unless working over clothing. Modifications for client comfort are appropriate as long as safety, sanitation, and modesty are maintained.

121. Correct answer and rational A

Asking the client for guidance is the best response.

Incorrect answers and rationales

Draping is not always secure. A blanket may not address the issue.

122. Correct answer and rational A

A business that is owned and operated by one person only is a sole proprietorship.

Incorrect answers and rationales

A partnership is two or more people. A corporation is a unique business entity.

123. Correct answer and rational B

When an employee it is necessary to follow the established rules and procedures.

Incorrect answers and rationales

I prefer to use my own draping approach and the client guides my draping methods may be appropriate when self-employed but not when employed.

124. Correct answer and rational B

The target market is based on potential clients.

Incorrect answers and rationales

An income projection and business plan may include the target market but are not the actual client base.

125. Correct answer and rational C

Demographics provide information about population segments, especially when used to identify consumer markets.

Incorrect answers and rationales

Business loans and income tax rate are not directly related to fee setting.

126. Correct answer and rational A

National Provider Identification (NPI) number must be entered on all insurance claims.

Incorrect answers and rationales

The Employer Identification Number (EIN), also known as the Federal Employer Identification Number (FEIN) or the Federal Tax Identification Number, is a unique nine-digit number assigned by the Internal Revenue Service (IRS) to business entities operating in the United States for the purposes of identification. When

the number is used for identification rather than employment tax reporting, it is usually referred to as a Taxpayer Identification Number (TIN). A Taxpayer Identification Number (TIN) is an identification number used by the Internal Revenue Service (IRS) in the administration of tax laws.

127. Correct answer and rational A

A budget is an estimate of income and expenditure for a set period of time.

Incorrect answers and rationales

An expense report and income statement are other accounting forms.

128. Correct answer and rational B

Sole proprietor business structure uses the social security number for federal tax purposes.

Incorrect answers and rationales

Partnerships, like corporations, require what is known as an Employer Identification Number (EIN), also called a Federal Tax ID number.

129. Correct answer and rational C

An Employer Identification Number (EIN) is also known as a federal tax identification number and is used to identify a business entity.

Incorrect answers and rationales

Filing for a DBA allows you to conduct business under a name other than your own. Social security number is for personal identification with the IRS in the format 000-00-0000, unique for each individual, used to track Social Security benefits and for other identification purposes.

130. Correct answer and rational B

All health care providers that are considered covered entities under HIPAA, and those who file claims electronically or use a clearinghouse to bill insurance, are required to apply for an NPI. All other health care providers are eligible to receive an NPI if they desire.

Incorrect answers and rationales

The Employer Identification Number (EIN), also known as the Federal Employer Identification Number (FEIN) or the Federal Tax Identification Number, is a unique nine-digit number assigned by the Internal Revenue Service (IRS) to business entities operating in the United States for the purposes of identification. When the number is used for identification rather than employment tax reporting, it is usually referred to as a Taxpayer Identification Number (TIN). A Taxpayer Identification Number (TIN) is an identification number used by the Internal Revenue Service (IRS) in the administration of tax laws.

131. Correct answer and rational C

The Employer Identification Number (EIN), also known as the Federal Employer Identification Number (FEIN) or the Federal Tax Identification Number, is a unique nine-digit number assigned by the Internal Revenue Service (IRS) to business

entities operating in the United States for the purposes of identification.
Incorrect answers and rationales
A retail business may require a state sales tax permit. All health care providers that are considered covered entities under HIPAA, and those who file claims electronically or use a clearinghouse to bill insurance, are required to apply for an NPI. All other health care providers are eligible to receive an NPI if they desire.

132. Correct answer and rational C
A website is a set of related web pages located under a single domain name, typically produced by a single person or organization to be a platform for a social media presence.
Incorrect answers and rationales
Software generally runs on local computer. A blog is an element of social media typically linked to a website.

133. Correct answer and rational A
In business, risk means that a company's or an organization's plans may not turn out as originally planned or that it may not meet its target or achieve its goals.
Incorrect answers and rationales
A tax audit for payroll taxes would be an IRS review. A plan for reducing improper client behavior is part of risk prevention but not a specific process of analyzing business risk.

134. Correct answer and rational B
The social media presence needs to be professional.
Incorrect answers and rationales
Consulting services are provided by a company specializing in development. Social media may or may not contain access to multiple advertising outlets.

135. Correct answer and rational A
Business gross per year needs to be $65,000. The number of sessions per year is 1000.
Incorrect answers and rationales
$50 per session would not meet determined expenses. $90 is more than the minimum fee required.

136. Correct answer and rational C
All would be something to consider but average income is most needed when determining fees.
Incorrect answers and rationales
Distance from location and number of single-family households are considerations but income is most relevant to fee setting.

137. Correct answer and rational B
Payroll burden, also referred to as labor or wage burden costs, is the total cost to the employer to pay an employee. This includes the employee's wages, but it also covers all the payroll taxes and benefits.
Incorrect answers and rationales
A tax burden relates to all tax requirements of the business, not only payroll taxes. A cost benefit ratio

determines whether or not and how much profit will result from an investment.

138. Correct answer and rational C
A strategic business plan is a written document that pairs the objectives of a company with the needs of the market place.
Incorrect answers and rationales
An exit plan is how to leave a business. A facility plan is the physical layout of the location.

139. Correct answer and rational A
All businesses have duties that are not directly income producing or directly related to the service provided. This is office management.
Incorrect answers and rationales
Client records completion is the responsibility of the practitioner. Ergonomics and biomechanics involve how the service is provided.

140. Correct answer and rational B
Maintaining the safety of the practice facility is an example of office management activities.
Incorrect answers and rationales
Fiscal refers to money. Activities of daily living relates to assessment and session goals.

141. Correct answer and rational C
The receptionist is front desk staff.
Incorrect answers and rationales
The spa attendant or massage practitioner are not considered front desk staff.

142. Correct answer and rational A
The franchise structure uses brand recognition as a marketing strategy.
Incorrect answers and rationales
Fees for services are not often adapted. A lead therapist is not always on staff.

143. Correct answer and rational C
Networking is the exchange of information and ideas among people.
Incorrect answers and rationales
Social media is a computer-based technology that facilitates the sharing of ideas, thoughts, and information through the building of virtual networks and communities. Risk management is the continuing process to identify, analyze, evaluate, and monitor to mitigate potentially adverse events.

144. Correct answer and rational B
When working from a home office it is prudent to know the clients prior to scheduling. Word of mouth/referral would be an effective strategy.
Incorrect answers and rationales
The business structure described would not require extensive paid advertising.

145. Correct answer and rational A
Promotion is one of the most important functions of marketing.
Incorrect answers and rationales

Providing an online scheduler and dispensing health-related information are potential website functions but are not part of marketing.

146. Correct answer and rational B

The more information a interviewee has about the business the more prepared they are for a quality interview.

Incorrect answers and rationales

Preparing a market evaluation and organizing accounting records are business management activities.

147. Correct answer and rational B

An interview is a formal consultation to evaluate qualifications for employment.

Incorrect answers and rationales

An application is a process of expressing interest in a position and a job search is the process of looking for potential positions.

148. Correct answer and rational C

A resume is an account of one's professional or work experience and qualifications.

Incorrect answers and rationales

A cover letter is a written document commonly submitted with a job application resume explaining reasons for interest in the position. Form W-4 allows the employer to withhold the correct federal income tax from pay.

149. Correct answer and rational A

A negotiation is a strategic discussion that resolves an issue in a way that both parties find acceptable.

Incorrect answers and rationales

Marketing and budgeting do not relate to negotiation.

150. Correct answer and rational C

The employer needs to have completed payroll tax forms completed before work can commence.

Incorrect answers and rationales

Developing promotional material and organizing the treatment room occur after hiring is completed

151. Correct answer and rational C

A W-2 is a report of employee income and tax withholdings at the end of the year.

Incorrect answers and rationales

W-4 forms serve as a set of instructions for how an employer should withhold taxes from an employee's paycheck. 1099 forms report various types of income to the IRS. 1099-NEC is the form to report nonemployee compensation—sometimes referred to as self-employment income.

152. Correct answer and rational A

Session documentation or charting occurs for every session.

Incorrect answers and rationales

Treatment plans and informed consent are completed at intervals and updated regularly.

153. Correct answer and rational B

The Intake form has information such as name, address, email etc.

Incorrect answers and rationales

Assessment and treatment plan forms may not have address information.

154. Correct answer and rational A

An employee is not responsible for most business records other than reporting work hours.

Incorrect answers and rationales

Supply and rental expenses are the responsibility of the employer.

155. Correct answer and rational B

Form W-4, Employee's Withholding Certificate, is on file for each employee.

Incorrect answers and rationales

Eligibility for workplace benefits is an internal business process. Access to unemployment insurance is available to all employees.

156. Correct answer and rational B

Self-Employment Tax (SE tax) is a social security and Medicare tax primarily for individuals who work for themselves.

Incorrect answers and rationales

Income tax is based on net income. Workers' compensation or workers' comp is a form of insurance providing wage replacement and medical benefits to employees injured in the course of employment in exchange for mandatory relinquishment of the employee's right to sue for negligence.

157. Correct answer and rational A

Only employees are eligible for unemployment compensation.

Incorrect answers and rationales

Self-employed/Independent contractors are not eligible for unemployment.

158. Correct answer and rational C

The employer pays unemployment taxes for employees.

Incorrect answers and rationales

Self-employed/Independent contractors are not eligible for unemployment.

159. Correct answer and rational C

In addition to the payroll tax obligations, small businesses are also required to carry workers' compensation insurance. Workers' compensation insurance is required in most states to cover medical bills, rehabilitation costs, and lost wages for employees who get injured or experience a work-related illness.

Incorrect answers and rationales

Medicare is a federal health insurance plan for people who are age 65 or older. Social security is a federal insurance program that provides benefits to retired people.

160. Correct answer and rational A

A business conducted from a residence may be eligible for some tax deductions if considered a regular, exclusive place of business.

Incorrect answers and rationales

Barrier free access and adjacent restrooms may be required to comply with zoning requirements but are not associated with tax deductions.

161. Correct answer and rational C
Therapeutic touch, or TT, is a noninvasive method of healing that was derived from an ancient laying on of hands technique.
Incorrect answers and rationales
Muscle Energy Techniques (METs) describe a broad class of manual therapy techniques directed at improving musculoskeletal/joint function and pain using various approaches where a client contracts and relaxes targeted muscles. Lymphatic drainage is a manual massage technique that targets the lymphatic system.

162. Correct answer and rational A
Biofields are energy fields generated by and surrounding all living things and while being researched are difficult to explain.
Incorrect answers and rationales
Pain and endocrine function have physical components making research more concrete.

163. Correct answer and rational B
The meridians are directional pathways of energy flow.
Incorrect answers and rationales
A nerve is a physical structure. Self-care involves health maintenance activities.

164. Correct answer and rational A
Quantified outcomes are objectively measurable.
Incorrect answers and rationales
Resuming normal work activities is a subjective qualifiable goal. Reassessment in 12 sessions is part of the treatment plan.

165. Correct answer and rational C
Condition management is a treatment approach focusing on function maintenance.
Incorrect answers and rationales
Assisting in learning to walk or restoring a ROM is a therapeutic change approach.

166. Correct answer and rational B
Head/neck pain and breathing difficulties are related to the cervical plexus.
Incorrect answers and rationales
Shoulder, chest, arm, wrist, and hand pain are related to the brachial plexus. Gluteal, leg, genital, and foot pain are related to the lumbar plexus.

167. Correct answer and rational B
Nerve impingement, known to some as a pinched nerve, occurs where there is too much pressure applied to a nerve by surrounding tissues such as bone, tendon, cartilage, or muscles. Muscle energy techniques and lengthening might increase space around the nerve.
Incorrect answers and rationales
Tapotement, shaking, or deep compression would not be as effective.

168. Correct answer and rational C
Safety and sanitation are the most important factors.
Incorrect answers and rationales
Staying on time is important and having reading material available is helpful but safety and sanitation is essential.

169. Correct answer and rational B
Zoning provides the standards and regulations that apply to land and structure use.
Incorrect answers and rationales
Rental agreements or state occupational licenses do not mandate land use.

170. Correct answer and rational B
A common cause of low back pain in massage therapists is the table being too low. The torso should not be flexed beyond 20 degrees.
Incorrect answers and rationales
Overly flexed knees and forward head positioning would cause additional body strain.

171. Correct answer and rational C
The most stable position of the knees is extension with movement in and out of flexion.
Incorrect answers and rationales
Hard floors would not be as much a cause for knee pain especially if wearing a good work shoe. Positioning would not directly affect the knees.

172. Correct answer and rational B
A professional boundary was breached and the client became uncomfortable.
Incorrect answers and rationales
Feedback might have broken down but this would be secondary to the boundary issue. Gender issues are unlikely in this scenario.

173. Correct answer and rational C
Clients, especially older people, can become dizzy when they have blood pressure issues.
Incorrect answers and rationales
Early stage pregnancy and a diabetes diagnosis are less likely to require assistance or concern.

174. Correct answer and rational A
Gliding on the abdomen can support peristalsis.
Incorrect answers and rationales
Holding is a static application. Tapotement would not be as effective and gliding.

175. Correct answer and rational C
On reflexology charts typically the base of the large toe corresponds with the neck area.
Incorrect answers and rationales
The heel corresponds with the sciatic nerve or gonads. Tips of toes correspond with the sinuses.

INDEX

Note: Page numbers followed by "*f*," "*t*," and "*b*" refer to figures, tables, and boxes, respectively.